T0386136

Evidence-based Education in the Health Professions

PROMOTING BEST PRACTICE IN THE LEARNING AND TEACHING OF STUDENTS

Edited by

TED BROWN
PhD, OT(C), OTR
Associate Professor, Postgraduate Coordinator and Undergraduate Course Convener
Department of Occupational Therapy
School of Primary Health Care, Faculty of Medicine, Nursing and Health Sciences
Monash University – Peninsula Campus, Frankston, Victoria, Australia

BRETT WILLIAMS
PhD, FPA
Associate Professor and Head of Department
Department of Community Emergency Health and Paramedic Practice
School of Primary Health Care, Faculty of Medicine, Nursing and Health Sciences
Monash University – Peninsula Campus, Frankston, Victoria, Australia

Forewords by

PROFESSOR HUGH BARR
MPhil, PhD
Emeritus Professor of Interprofessional Education and Honorary Fellow, University of Westminster, UK
Emeritus Editor, Journal of Interprofessional Care
President, Centre for the Advancement of Interprofessional Education (CAIPE), London, UK

PROFESSOR JOY HIGGS
AM, PhD
Director, The Education for Practice Institute, Division of Student Learning
Strategic Research Professor in Professional Practice
The Research Institute for Professional Practice, Learning & Education (RIPPLE)
Charles Sturt University – Sydney, Silverwater, NSW, Australia

Radcliffe Publishing
London • New York

Radcliffe Publishing Ltd
St Mark's House
Shepherdess Walk
London N1 7BQ
United Kingdom

www.radcliffehealth.com

While every effort has been made to ensure the accuracy of this work, this does not diminish the requirement to exercise clinical judgement and refer to up-to-date evidence when directing care in the clinical setting. Neither the publishers nor the authors can accept any responsibility for the use of information given in this work when used in practice.

British Library Cataloguing in Publication Data

A catalogue record for this book is available from the British Library.

ISBN-13: 978 190936 871 2

The paper used for the text pages of this book is FSC® certified. FSC (The Forest Stewardship Council®) is an international network to promote responsible management of the world's forests.

Typeset by Darkriver Design, Auckland, New Zealand
Manufacturing managed by 21six

Contents

Foreword by Professor Hugh Barr

Few books exemplify better than this the openness that we are coming to enjoy in health professionals' education towards a common understanding within a shared frame of reference. Barriers are coming down. Learning is being liberated following the integration of uni-professional schools into the mainstream of higher education making it easier for students to mix and match their studies as they capitalise on advances in learning technology. Gone are the days when educators in each health profession needed to develop and deliver their courses in isolation. Multiprofessional education is synthesising curricula, optimising the deployment of teaching expertise, widening student choice and winning economies of scale. Interprofessional education is enabling students to learn with, from and about each other in preparation for collaborative practice to deliver better, safer and more cost-effective care.

Assembling evidence to inform health professionals' education was first advocated around the turn of the century,[1] but was slow to gain momentum as Ted Brown and Brett Williams observe in the opening chapter of *Evidence-based Education in the Health Professions: promoting best practice in the learning and teaching of students.* Indeed, the *raison d'être* for their book rests on the need to remedy that omission within and between education systems.

Chapter 2 invokes evidence-based practice (EBP) to inform learning and teaching and to prepare students for their future careers. Much the same evidence may reassure employers regarding workforce needs; professional associations regarding the adoption of standards that they espouse for their members; regulatory bodies regarding adherence to their requirements for validation and review; and policy makers regarding implementation of changes concurrently in education and practice. But EBP is not enough: it must be understood, as Margaret Bearman reminds us, in the context of policy and practice, not only for healthcare but also for higher education, before it can be translated into learning and teaching. Ted Brown explores further the relationship between EBE, education in general, and health professionals' education in particular, helpfully drawing attention to the role of the practitioner turned educator.

Allie Ford, Paula Todd and Ted Brown pick up for EBE where Malcolm Boyle left off for EBP, identifying, describing and applying the range of available research methodologies. They chart five steps in the research process – formulation, planning, collation, analysis and appraisal – which merit critical comparison with the five 'A's – asking, answering, accessing, approving and applying – charted by Karen Saewert and Debra Hagler in the next chapter.

Chapters that follow provide perspectives on health professionals' education. Titles such as student-centred approaches, curriculum development, transformative learning, assessment, pedagogy, e-learning, e-portfolios, simulation, peer assessed learning, interprofessional learning, problem-based learning, case-based learning, team-based learning, service-learning, didactic learning, accreditation and competencies are self-explanatory. Others such as novice to expert, threshold concepts and just-in-time training may intrigue you as much as they did me. If, as Charlotte Rees and Lynn Monrouxe graphically convey, the pieces in nurse education resemble a jigsaw, how much more so the multidimensional puzzle that is health professionals' education?

Lest some readers should fear that their own professions are at risk of being lost in the big picture, the book ends with seven chapters focusing on EBE, profession by profession ranging from nurses to nutritionists and from pharmacists to paramedics.

Such a wealth of material from so many perspectives will surely respond to diverse needs amongst the researchers and educators to whom it is plainly addressed. It prompted me to reflect afresh on the evidence cited in my own field of interprofessional education; a field where evidence is documented in systematic reviews conducted under alternative auspices, adopting different inclusion criteria, resulting in different findings, leading to different conclusions.[2]

Evidence is not self-evident; it is no panacea. It may resolve tension between professions by establishing common ground. Alternatively, it may generate heat rather than light where the relative merits of competing methodologies are in dispute. Health professions towards the scientific end of the spectrum may value findings more highly from experimental research, while those towards the social-behavioural, humanitarian end may be more receptive to findings from descriptive, qualitative and quasi-experimental research. Randomised controlled trials seem set to retain their place at the top of the hierarchy of research paradigms for clinical interventions; not so for educational interventions where their feasibility and desirability is being questioned and other paradigms preferred. Different databases, as Ford, Todd and Brown say, have different hierarchies. For me, their critique is at its most cogent when they cite the research pyramid which may concentrate minds.

Evidence meets muster when it is married from different sources via different academic disciplines and practice professions, respecting each other's perceptions and preferences regarding the means by which it is derived. Only then can it do justice to the complexity of health professionals' education. Ted Brown and Brett Williams, with their 50 contributors from Australia, Canada, the United Kingdom and the United States, make a convincing start on a daunting task. Issues remain but made more intelligible and more manageable with their help.

Professor Hugh Barr, MPhil, PhD
Emeritus Professor of Interprofessional Education
Honorary Fellow, University of Westminster, UK
Emeritus Editor, *Journal of Interprofessional Care*
President, Centre for the Advancement of Interprofessional Education (CAIPE)
London, UK
January 2015

REFERENCES

1. Hargreaves D. *Teaching as a Research-based Profession: possibilities and prospects.* Teacher Training Agency Annual Lecture 1996. London: Teacher Training Agency; 1996.
2. Barr H, Gray R. *Interprofessional Education: learning together in health and social care.* In: K Walsh (ed.) *The Textbook of Medical Education.* Oxford: Oxford University Press; 2013.

Foreword by Professor Joy Higgs

The international world of higher education is demanding good practices in curriculum design and pedagogies. We live in an era of accountability and scrutiny and need to provide supportive rationales for our educational practices. This book *opens the door* to readers and educators who want to enter this world. A strong cast of educators and educational researchers from a variety of locations and roles have come together through this book on evidence-based education (EBE), to inform, challenge and extend this important arena.

Some of the *core topics* examined in this book include:
- The demands on higher education of changing local and international policies and strategies around tertiary education
- The standards agenda and government expectations of high-quality education
- The expectations of professional stakeholders including accreditation authorities
- The demands facing students and educators, for quality performance imposed by educational institutions and workplaces
- The impact of fiscal limitations on educational institutions and how this demands even more of good educational practitioners
- The challenges created by external accreditation alongside internal expectations and procedures, competing with students' marketplace demands
- Patterns of EBE in various disciplines.

A vital aspect of adopting an EBE approach is to remember that we need to understand several key factors relating to *evidence*:
- What is evidence? What counts as good evidence? A lot of emphasis is placed on evidence being the findings of research of various forms. We need to remember that research-generated knowledge and evidence is an insight into the world of practice, and needs to be understood as context and time dependent. What might be sound evidence in one place and time, might not be so in another.
- Evidence is not independent of judgement. Often research is generalised (as in quantitative research) or localised and contextualised (as in many types of qualitative research). The user of evidence cannot simply take evidence and say – this *must* be true for my situation too. Instead, just as we educate our students to be critical appraisers of knowledge and insights arising from research, scholarship and experience, so too, as educators, we need to appraise and judge educational theories and research for their relevance and applicability to our settings and educational programs.

A number of authors in the book reflect on arguments around these issues.

There are many *modes* of teaching, learning, assessment and curriculum design reflecting best practices. Some of these have evolved over long periods of time through review and exploration (including learning in workplaces, role modelling, interprofessional education, problem-based learning), while others are more recently emerged best practices (including cutting-edge approaches to simulated learning). Rich examples are provided throughout this book (from jigsaws to e-portfolios, to peer-assisted learning) to challenge us to identify practices that need refining and those that need exploring before we embrace them in our teaching.

Students – ranging from novice to experienced learners – have a key place in this book. They are the consumers and the future graduates who emerge from the courses. Student-centred learning is a core to many chapters, and many associated educational strategies to deal with the changing student population are presented. Understanding the diversity of students that is linked to changes in student access policies is represented as an important expectation of educators. In many ways, this evolution in the student population is creating escalating demands for a range of good educational practices linked to emerging pedagogies and technologies. Health professional educators need to know not just what graduates will do in practice and what the practice world expects of them, but also who their students are as people, as learners and as members of diverse cultural, age and interest groups. Education is challenged to provide best practices for these numerous groups: 'the student body' is not homogeneous with common needs. Diversity demands diversity and creativity. Student engagement and collaboration is a dominant theme across the book, with many insights provided on how to foster and facilitate this.

Across the book we are introduced to many *terms*. This content is a valuable contribution of the book, even though to the new teacher such a mass of jargon can be bewildering. The authors, however, take the terms (like threshold concepts, peer-assisted learning, Just-in-Time Teaching, service learning, rubrics) and explain them clearly so we can make them part of our working lexicon, and hopefully part of our practice array.

The book provides the reader with a creative opportunity for reflection. The range of *content* asks us to leave behind our 'practised practices' and explore new possibilities. Part I examines the concept and underlying principles of EBE. Part II explores key contextual components of EBE and concepts related to health professional education. Part III introduces a range of teaching and learning approaches linked to EBE. Part IV portrays a landscape of EBE evident across various health professions. The *style* of the book with overviews, reviews, summaries, review questions, reflective questions and a variety of mind-capturing images, encourages readers to keep in touch with the arguments and illustrations presented, as well as holding up a mirror to look at their own educational practices, habits and rationales.

In the end, the book enables reflection, learning and transformation as well as asking us to engage in self-assessment, work collaboratively in communities of practice and envisage the future of good practice for our stakeholders. This is exactly what we want to provide for our students.

Professor Joy Higgs, AM, PhD
Director, The Education for Practice Institute, Division of Student Learning
Strategic Research Professor in Professional Practice
The Research Institute for Professional Practice,
Learning & Education (RIPPLE)
Charles Sturt University – Sydney, Silverwater, NSW, Australia
January 2015

List of contributors

Francis Amara, PhD, Med, BSc, is currently Associate Professor in the Department of Biochemistry and Medical Genetics, Faculty of Medicine at the University of Manitoba in Canada (email: amara@cc.umanitoba.ca). He has served previously as Director of Remediation and Chair of the Committee of Evaluation and is involved in teaching large groups and problem-based learning. He was formerly a Visiting Academic at the Oxford Learning Institute, University of Oxford. His research interests include curriculum development and educational leadership.

Kate Andre, RN, RM, MN, PhD, FRCNA, is Associate Professor of Nursing Education at Edith Cowan University in Perth, Western Australia (email: c.andre@ecu.edu.au). Kate has been involved in the use and teaching of e-Portfolios for many years and is the author of numerous publications about the use of portfolios to support and document learning and professional performance. Most recently, Kate is working with a national team to look at ways to record the clinical performance of students of nursing and midwifery in a secure and reliable format. Kate's interest in e-Portfolio use is driven by a wish to integrate authentic and reliable assessment and professional performance records.

Judith T Barr, MEd, ScD, is an Associate Professor of Pharmacy at the School of Pharmacy, Bouvé College of Health Sciences, Northeastern University, and Director of the National Education and Research Center for Outcomes Assessment in Boston, Massachusetts (email: j.barr@neu.edu).

Margaret Bearman, PhD, BS, BComp, is an Associate Professor and Director of Research at HealthPEER (Health Professions Education and Educational Research) at Monash University in Victoria, Australia, and she convenes the Graduate Certificate in Clinical Simulation (email: margaret.bearman@monash.edu). Margaret began her career within health informatics and she has developed curricula for undergraduate, postgraduate and continuing health professional education programmes. Her recent publications cover a broad range of topics, including simulation; systematic review and research synthesis; underperformance in clinical environments; and transition to clinical practice. She has published on systematic review and evidence synthesis methodologies.

Elizabeth Borycki, RN, MN, PhD, is an Associate Professor in the School of Health Information Science and an Adjunct in Nursing at the University of Victoria in Canada (email: emb@uvic.ca). Elizabeth is a health informatics expert who conducts research in the areas of education in clinical informatics, patient safety, social media in healthcare, quality improvement and organisational behaviour, and education involving health information technology. Elizabeth employs qualitative, quantitative and mixed methods approaches in her study of the effects of health information technology upon patients, caregivers and clinicians (e.g. physicians, nurses). She has represented Canada (as academic representative) and North America (member of the board of directors) to the International Medical Informatics Association and her work is known internationally.

Malcolm Boyle, ADipBus, ADipHSc(Amb Off), MICA Cert, BInfoTech, MClinEpi, PhD, MPA, is a Senior Lecturer in the Department of Community Emergency Health and Paramedic Practice, School of Primary Health Care, Faculty of Medicine, Nursing and Health Sciences, at Monash University – Peninsula Campus, Victoria, Australia, and a Mobile Intensive Care Ambulance Paramedic at Ambulance Victoria (email: malcolm.boyle@monash.edu). Primary research interests include prehospital trauma triage, prehospital trauma management, workplace violence and its effects, and attributes of undergraduate paramedic and allied health students.

Ted Brown, PhD, MSc, MPA, BScOT (Hons), GCHPE, OT(C), OTR, is an Associate Professor, Postgraduate Coordinator and Undergraduate Course Convener in the Department of Occupational Therapy, School of Primary Health Care, Faculty of Medicine, Nursing and Health Sciences, at Monash University – Peninsula Campus, Victoria, Australia (email: ted.brown@monash.edu). Primary research interests include test validation and evaluation, applications of the Rasch Measurement Model, paediatric occupational therapy, assessment of children, education of allied health students and evidence-based practice.

Sharon M Brownie, DBA, M Hlth Serv Mgmt, M Ed Admin, B Ed, RM, RN, GAICD, FCNA (NZ), is a Professor of Workforce and Health Services at the Griffith Health Institute, Griffith University, Queensland, Australia; Griffith University Head of Nursing Capacity Building – United Arab Emirates; and Praxis Research Associate for the Praxis Forum, Green Templeton College, Oxford University (email: s.brownie@ griffith.edu.au). She is an experienced educational and health service leader working in roles with significant workforce development and change management mandates. In 2000 she was awarded an MDC Fellowship for Excellence in the New Zealand Public Service. She is a registered nurse and midwife maintaining active practice, research and publication outputs in health and educational policy settings. In 2011–12, she was the lead author of three major reports relating to competency-based education and training for the Australian health workforce. A major theme in her 2013–14 publications relates to health workforce development and redesign.

Suzanne B Cashman, ScD, has spent the 35 years of her professional career teaching graduate courses in public health, conducting community-based evaluation research and developing partnerships aimed at helping communities improve their health status (email: Suzanne.Cashman@umassmed.edu). Currently, Suzanne is Professor and Director of Community Health in the Department of Family Medicine and Community Health at the University of Massachusetts Medical School, where she co-directs the school's Determinants of Health course, which uses service-learning pedagogy in its required clerkship. She serves as Community Engagement Core Co-Director for the school's Clinical and Translational Research Center and its Center for Health Disparities Intervention Research.

Vanina Dal Bello-Haas, PhD, Med, BSc(PT), is Assistant Dean (Physiotherapy) and Associate Professor at the School of Rehabilitation Science, McMaster University, Canada (email: vdalbel@mcmaster.ca). Vanina's educational research and teaching interests include professional issues, web-based teaching, peer evaluation and strategies to increase capacity of healthcare professionals interested in working with older adults and neurologic populations. Her clinical teaching and research interests and experiences are focused on people with neurodegenerative diseases.

Dale Edwards, BHlthSc(Paramedic), GradCert Ed, MEd, is a Senior Lecturer in Paramedic Practice at the School of Medicine, University of Tasmania, Australia (email: Dale.Edwards@utas.edu.au). Mr Edwards coordinates the Bachelor of Paramedic Practice (conversion pathway) and the Bachelor of Paramedic Practice (Hons). Mr Edwards also teaches into a number of clinical and professional units in these courses. Mr Edwards is chair of the School of Medicine Interprofessional Learning Working Party.

Debbie Faulk, PhD, MSN, RN, CNE, is a Professor of Nursing at Auburn University at Montgomery, Alabama (email: dfaulk@aum.edu). She co-authored a book on transformative learning in nursing with Dr Arlene Morris in 2012. Her presentations and publications focus on transformative learning and learning in the online environment.

Allie Ford, PhD, is a Learning Skills Adviser at Monash University – Peninsula Campus, Victoria, Australia (email: allie.ford@monash.edu). She has worked in higher education for more than 12 years, including as a postdoctoral researcher and an education-focused lecturer in science. She is interested in transition into university and the role of reflective practice in student learning, and she assists with development of critical thinking and academic communication skills in students from a wide range of disciplines.

Jennifer Friberg, EdD, CCC-SLP/L, is an Associate Professor (Speech-Language Pathology) in the Department of Communication Sciences and Disorders at Illinois State University, Normal, Illinois (email: jfribe@illinoisstate.edu). She conducts research in the areas of teaching and learning, and she is particularly interested in methods of increasing student engagement through active learning.

Sarah M Ginsberg, EdD, CCC-SLP, is an Associate Professor in the Department of Special Education at Eastern Michigan University (Ypsilanti), Michigan (email: sarah.ginsberg@emich.edu). She is a qualified speech-language pathologist.

Barbara Gottlieb, MD MPH, has been a primary care physician at a community health centre in Boston, Massachusetts, since 1981 (email: bgottlieb@pchi.partners.org). She is Associate Professor at Harvard Medical School, where she is Co-chair of the Global and Community Health Committee and Chair of the Faculty Committee on Community Service.

Sandra V Graham, PhD, MS, BS, is a member of the Department of Communication Sciences and Disorders at the University of South Florida, Tampa, Florida (email: svgraham@usf.edu). She is a qualified speech-language pathologist with experience as a healthcare provider and as university faculty.

Arthur M Guilford, PhD, is a member of the Department of Communication Sciences and Disorders at the University of South Florida, Tampa, Florida (email: aguilford@sar.usf.edu). He is a qualified speech-language pathologist with experience as a healthcare provider and as university faculty. He has contributed significantly to programme development and assessment of learning outcomes, and he is the current regional chancellor for the University of South Florida Sarasota campus.

Debra Hagler, PhD, RN, ACNS-BC, CNE, CHSE, ANEF, FAAN, is a Clinical Professor at Arizona State University (ASU) College of Nursing and Health Innovation and Coordinator for Teaching Excellence supporting the ASU College of Nursing and Health Innovation and College of Health Solutions (email: debra.hagler@asu.edu). Her experience includes interdisciplinary clinical staff and academic faculty development.

Mowafa Househ, MEng, PhD, is an Assistant Professor and Research Director at the College of Public Health and Health Informatics at King Saud bin Abdulaziz University for Health Sciences, National Guard Health Affairs, Riyadh, Kingdom of Saudi Arabia (email: househmo@ngha.med.sa). Dr Househ is also an adjunct professor at the University of Victoria School of Health Information Science in British Columbia, Canada. He is the Editor-in-Chief of the *Journal of Health Informatics in Developing Countries* and he is a health informatics expert with a specialisation in health and social media in healthcare.

Abbas Hyderi, MD MPH, is the Associate Dean for Curriculum and Associate Professor of Clinical Family Medicine at the University of Illinois at Chicago College of Medicine, Chicago, Illinois (email: ahyder2@uic.edu). He has principal oversight of all 4 years of the curriculum, with a particular emphasis on curricular transformation of the preclinical years. He has championed team-based learning implementation at his home institution and has led faculty development sessions for team-based learning nationally and internationally. He practises full-scope family medicine and is actively engaged in educational research and scholarship, including being the Co-Principal Investigator for the primary care residency expansion grant for the Family Medicine Residency at the University of Illinois at Chicago.

Sharla King, PhD, is an Assistant Professor in the Department of Educational Psychology in the Faculty of Education, and Director of the Health Sciences Education and Research Commons at the University of Alberta in Canada (email: sjk1@ualberta.ca). The Health Sciences Education and Research Commons is an educational research and simulation facility focused on developing and disseminating best practices in interprofessional education and educational technologies for pre-licensure and continuing professionals. Dr King is also Programme Director for the Master of Education in Health Science Education programme. Dr King has worked in the area of interprofessional education and research at the university for the past 12 years. Her research interests relate to interprofessional education and student team interactions, transitions into the workforce, virtual learning communities, blended learning and simulation education.

Andre Kushniruk, PhD, is a Professor at the School of Health Information Science at the University of Victoria in Canada (email: andrek@uvic.ca). Dr Kushniruk conducts research in a number of areas including evaluation of the effects of technology as well as education in health informatics. His work is known internationally and he has published widely in the area of health informatics. Dr Kushniruk has held academic positions at a number of Canadian universities and worked with major hospitals in Canada, the United States and internationally. He holds undergraduate degrees in psychology and biology, as well as a MSc in Computer Science from McMaster University and a PhD in Cognitive Psychology from McGill University.

Tracy Levett-Jones, PhD, RN, MEd & Work, BN, DipAppSc(Nursing), is Professor, Director of the Research Centre for Health Professional Education at the University of Newcastle and Deputy Head of School (Teaching and Learning), School of Nursing and Midwifery, University of Newcastle, New South Wales, Australia (email: Tracy.Levett-jones@newcastle.edu.au). Her research interests include clinical reasoning, interprofessional education and communication, cultural empathy, simulation and patient safety. She has authored eight books, the most recent being *Clinical Reasoning: learning to think like a nurse* and *critical conversations for patient safety*, as well as numerous book chapters and peer-reviewed journal articles. Tracy has conducted a wide range of educational research projects and has been awarded ten teaching awards, including a New South Wales Minister for Education Quality Teaching Award and an Australian Learning and Teaching Council Award for Teaching Excellence.

Deborah MacLellan, PhD, RD, FDC, is a Professor in the Department of Applied Human Sciences, University of Prince Edward Island in Canada (email: maclellan@upei.ca). Her research focuses on the professional socialisation and identity development of dietitians. Dr MacLellan is a past Chair of the Board of Directors of Dietitians of Canada and a Dietitians of Canada Fellow.

Sam Magus, RRT, is a clinical instructor in the Respiratory Therapy Programme, an Interprofessional Faculty Lead and the Preceptor Educator for the School of Health Sciences, Northern Alberta Institute of Technology (NAIT), Alberta, Canada (email: samm@nait.ca). Ms Magus has been teaching at NAIT for 18 years and has been a respiratory therapist for over 30 years. She continues to practise respiratory therapy in a children's community living programme, working closely in interprofessional teams to provide patient- and family-centred care. Ms Magus has been instrumental in the design of the preceptor education programmes at NAIT, and she continues to work closely with all of the health programmes in interprofessional simulation, interprofessional education and collaborative practice.

Stephen Maloney, PhD, MPH, BPT, is currently a Senior Lecturer and Deputy Head in the Department of Physiotherapy at the School of Primary Health Care, Faculty of Medicine, Nursing and Health Sciences, Monash University, Victoria, Australia (email: stephen.maloney@monash.edu). His research interests include curriculum design, the teaching and learning experience, and the measurement of outcomes of cost-effectiveness from the perspective of both the learner and the educational institution.

Trudi Mannix, EdD, RN, RM, NICC, BN(Ed), MN, is a neonatal nurse and academic lecturer based in the School of Nursing and Midwifery at Flinders University, Adelaide, South Australia (email: trudi.mannix@flinders.edu.au). During her studies to gain a doctorate in education, she explored the application of critical thinking to neonatal nursing practice and developed standards for neonatal intensive care nursing education. Her interest in e-Portfolios was sparked in 2010 when Flinders University undertook a 3-year e-Portfolio and personal learning space trial using PebblePad, and Dr Mannix facilitated a pilot to introduce it to the midwifery undergraduate programme.

Sue McAllister, PhD, is an Associate Professor at Flinders University in Adelaide, South Australia (email: sue.mcallister@flinders.edu.au). Sue teaches evidence-based practice and research methods in speech pathology and her research is focused on the nature of health professional competency. This includes researching quality learning and teaching practices at universities and workplaces, development of performance-based assessments, and consultancies with a range of health professions to support quality teaching and assessment of professional competency.

Lisa McKenna, PhD, MEdSt, BESt, RN, RM, is Professor and Head of Clayton Campus in the School of Nursing and Midwifery, Faculty of Medicine, Nursing and Health Sciences at Monash University, Victoria, Australia (email: lisa.mckenna@monash. edu). She has extensive experience in teaching undergraduate and postgraduate nursing, midwifery and other health professional students, and she has led the development of many nursing and midwifery curricula. Lisa has researched and published extensively in education – in particular, in the areas of interprofessional education, simulation, graduate transition to practice, professional attribute development and clinical and nursing education. In 2012, she and a colleague were awarded the Vice-Chancellor's Award for Programmes that Enhance Learning at Monash University for work on peer teaching and learning. Lisa has published five textbooks, the most recent being *Introduction to Teaching and Learning in Health Professions*, which was highly commended at the Australian Educational Publishing Awards in 2013.

Larry K Michaelsen, PhD, BS, is David Ross Boyd Professor Emeritus at the University of Oklahoma, Professor of Management at the University of Central Missouri, a Carnegie Scholar, a three-time Fulbright Senior Scholar and a former editor of the *Journal of Management Education* (email: lmichaelsen@ucmo.edu). Since initially developing team-based learning (TBL) in the late 1970s, he has used TBL with over 1800 teams in his own classes. He has also co-authored four books and numerous journal articles on TBL and conducted TBL workshops in a wide variety of settings. These include workshops at over 250 schools in the United States and in 20 foreign countries and at conferences of more than 20 different professional disciplines.

Anita Witt Mitchell, PhD, MSc, BOT, OTR, joined the Department of Occupational Therapy at the University of Tennessee Health Science Center, Memphis, Tennessee, in 1992 (email: amitche5@uthsc.edu). She has published articles related to occupational therapy education in the *American Journal of Occupational Therapy*, *Occupational Therapy International* and *Occupational Therapy in Health Care*. She has received awards for teaching and research during her tenure at the University of Tennessee Health Science Center.

Lynn V Monrouxe, PhD, CPsychol, FAcadMEd, is a Reader in Medical Education and Director of Medical Education Research at the School of Medicine, Cardiff University, Wales, and she is Fellow of the Academy of Medical Educators (email: MonrouxeLV@ cardiff.ac.uk). With a psychology degree and PhD in cognitive linguistics, Lynn was a Research Fellow and then Lecturer in Clinical Education (Human Sciences) at the Peninsula Medical School, University of Exeter (2003–07) before joining Cardiff. Her current interests focus on identity construction, student-doctor-patient interaction, professionalism in healthcare education and the role of theory in research. She is also Principal and Co-Investigator on a range of healthcare education research projects, is Deputy Editor for *Medical Education* and has published over 50 articles across a range of journals including *Medical Education, Academic Medicine, Social Science & Medicine* and *Qualitative Health Research*.

Arlene H Morris, EdD, MSN, RN, CNE, is a certified nurse educator and Professor of Nursing at Auburn University at Montgomery, Alabama (email: amorris@aum.edu). She is widely published and she authored a book on transformative learning in nursing in 2012. Presentations at national and international levels focus on transformative learning and gerontology.

Curtise KC Ng, BSc(Hons), PhD, is a tenured Senior Lecturer in the Discipline of Medical Imaging in the Department of Imaging and Applied Physics, Curtin University, Perth, Western Australia (email: Curtise.Ng@curtin.edu.au). He is also the Associate Editor of *Journal of Medical Imaging and Radiation Sciences*, and editorial board member or reviewer for 10 international radiography and imaging informatics journals. His research areas include imaging informatics, radiation protection, e-Learning, student-centred learning pedagogies and radiography professional issues.

Gregor Novak, PhD, is Professor of Physics Emeritus at Indiana University–Purdue University Indianapolis, and Distinguished Scholar in Residence at the United States Air Force Academy (email: gnovak@iupui.edu). The culmination of some 50 years of his professional experience is a web-based, classroom-linked strategy termed 'JiTT', or Just-in-Time Teaching. With JiTT now in successful use at Indiana University–Purdue University Indianapolis, the Air Force Academy and many other institutions nationally and internationally, Novak spends some of his time promoting its principles for wider use. He is co-author of *Just-in-Time Teaching: blending active learning with web technology*. His present interests include exploring the possibilities of the flipped-classroom pedagogies and pedagogical applications of mobile technologies.

Lisa O'Brien, PhD, is a Senior Lecturer in the Department of Occupational Therapy at Monash University in Melbourne, Victoria, Australia (email: lisa.o'brien@monash.edu). She has 7 years of experience as both unit coordinator and tutor in problem-based learning units. Lisa also works as Quality Coordinator and Hand Therapist/Researcher at Alfred Health, also in Melbourne, Australia.

Andrys Onsman, PhD, is a Learning and Teaching Advisor in the Centre for the Study of Higher Education at Melbourne University, attached to the Faculty of Architecture, Building and Planning, Melbourne, Victoria, Australia (email: onsman@hotmail.com). His primary interests are in teaching practice in higher education, international higher education and indigenous education.

Dean X Parmelee, MD, FAACAP, FAPA, from the University of Rochester, is the Robert J. Kegerreis Distinguished Professor of Teaching and Associate Dean for Academic Affairs at the Wright State University Boonshoft School of Medicine in Dayton, Ohio (email: dean.parmelee@wright.edu). He has championed team-based learning at his institution, conducted workshops on team-based learning and curriculum design in the United States, Africa, the Middle East, Asia and Europe, and he was the Inaugural President of the Team-Based Learning Collaborative.

Yvonne Parry, RN, BA, MHSM, GradCertEd, PhD, is a Lecturer in the Faculty of Medicine, Nursing and Health Sciences at the School of Nursing and Midwifery at Flinders University, Adelaide, South Australia (email: yvonne.parry@flinders.edu.au). She has research expertise in the areas of mixed methods research, national curriculum evaluations, interprofessional education and student experiences, and vulnerable children's access to health and welfare services. Her primary research focus is the health and welfare needs of vulnerable children and interprofessional child-centred practice. Yvonne has developed industry-certified curricula materials, topics and programmes in pre-service social work, teaching and the health professions (e.g. nursing, paramedics and allied health). She has taught interprofessionally across the health, education and welfare disciplines since 2003.

Charlotte E Rees, PhD, is a social scientist and educationalist by background and is Fellow of the Royal College of Physicians (Edinburgh). Currently, she is Professor of Education Research and Director of the Centre for Medical Education at the Medical Education Institute, School of Medicine, University of Dundee, Scotland (email: c.rees@dundee.ac.uk). She has held previous positions as Associate Professor at the Sydney Medical School, University of Sydney, Australia; Senior Lecturer and Foundation Academic Lead for Human Sciences, Communication Skills and Professionalism at Peninsula Medical School, University of Exeter, UK; and Lecturer at the Nottingham Medical School, University of Nottingham, UK. She is Deputy Editor for the highest-ranked education journal (scientific disciplines) *Medical Education* and has published over 70 articles across a broad range of healthcare, medical education and social sciences journals.

Julie Richardson, PhD, BPhty(Hons), is a Professor in the School of Rehabilitation Sciences at McMaster University, Hamilton, Ontario, Canada (email: jrichard@mcmaster.ca). She teaches community health and community practice in the physiotherapy programme, which includes approaches to the prevention and management of chronic disease. In the Rehabilitation Science Graduate Programme she teaches a course on Research Methods and a course on Rehabilitation and the management of Chronic Disease.

Sylvia Rodger, PhD, BOccThy, MEdSt, is Professor in the Division of Occupational Therapy School of Health and Rehabilitation Sciences at the University of Queensland, Brisbane, Queensland, Australia (email: s.rodger@uq.edu.au). She has 30 years of experience as an occupational therapist, academic and researcher. She led the reform of two interlinked occupational therapy curricula at the University of Queensland during her 12 years as Head of Division (2001–12). She chairs the School of Health and Rehabilitation Sciences Teaching and Learning Committee. She is an Australian Learning and Teaching Fellow who has completed externally funded projects on competency standards, curriculum leadership, capacity building, practice education quality and evaluation.

Karen J Saewert, PhD, RN, CPHQ, CNE, ANEF, is a Clinical Professor at Arizona State University (ASU) College of Nursing and Health Innovation and Senior Director of Educational Support Services and Director of E³: Evaluation and Educational Excellence supporting the ASU College of Nursing and Health Innovation and College of Health Solutions (email: karen.saewert@asu.edu). Her experience includes advancing best practices in academic assessment and evaluation in support of teaching and learning excellence and interprofessional education and collaborative practice.

Jane Scheurele, PhD, is a member of the Department of Communication Sciences and Disorders at the University of South Florida, Tampa, Florida. She is a qualified speech-language pathologist with experience as a healthcare provider and as university faculty.

Michael Sweet, PhD, is Senior Associate Director in the Center for Advancing Teaching and Learning Through Research at Northeastern University in Boston, Massachusetts (email: m.sweet@neu.edu). An educational psychologist by training, his academic and professional work focuses on student learning in small groups at the postsecondary level and he was 2011–12 president of the international Team-Based Learning Collaborative. He has been a college-level faculty developer since 1995 and has published and presented widely on team-based learning, critical thinking and the flipped classroom.

Lynne M Sylvia, PharmD, is a Senior Clinical Pharmacy Specialist in Cardiology in the Department of Pharmacy at Tufts Medical Center, Boston, Massachusetts (email: LSylvia1@tuftsmedicalcenter.org). She also holds the position of Clinical Professor, Northeastern University, School of Pharmacy, Boston, Massachusetts.

Jill E Thistlethwaite, PhD, is a health professional educator and general practitioner who trained in the United Kingdom (email: j.thistlethwaite@uq.edu.au). She has a master's in medical education, and a PhD from the University of Maastricht. Jill is currently an adjunct professor at University Technology Sydney and at the University of Queensland. Her publications include five co-authored books, three edited books and many book chapters and peer-reviewed papers. She is co-editor of the *Clinical Teacher*, deputy editor of the *International Journal of Practice-Based Learning* and associate editor of the *Journal of Interprofessional Care*. Jill has been involved with BEME (Best Evidence Medical Education) since 2009.

Allen Thurston, PhD, is Professor of Education and Director of the Centre for Effective Education, Queen's University Belfast, in Northern Ireland (email: a.thurston@qub.ac.uk). His research interests include peer-assisted learning – in particular, peer tutoring and cooperative learning. He has conducted a significant number of randomised controlled trials in this area. He also researches the socio-emotional effects of visual impairment and the ethics of access to medical information to blind and partially sighted persons.

Dianna Tison, PhD RN, is an Assistant Professor, School of Nursing and Health Professions at the University of the Incarnate Word, San Antonio, Texas, as a nursing educator (email: tison@uiwtx.edu).

Paula Todd, BA GCHE, has worked as a librarian in a variety of higher education libraries (email: paula.todd@monash.edu). She currently holds the position of contact librarian for Medicine, Nursing and Health Sciences at Monash University – Peninsula Campus in Frankston, Victoria, Australia. She has a BA Library and Information Science from Charles Sturt University and a Graduate Certificate in Higher Education from Monash University. She has a keen interest in promoting and developing information literacy and evidence-based practice skills with allied health and medical students.

Colleen F Visconti, PhD, is a Professor in Communication Disorders and Director of the Baldwin Wallace Speech Clinic in the Communication Arts and Sciences Department of Baldwin Wallace University, Berea, Ohio (email: cviscont@bw.edu).

Brett Williams, BAdultVocEd, GradCertIntensiveCareParamed, GradDipEmergHlth, MHlthSc, PhD, FPA, is Associate Professor and Head of Department in the Department of Community Emergency Health and Paramedic Practice, Faculty of Medicine, Nursing and Health Sciences, Monash University, Frankston, Victoria, Australia (email: brett.williams@monash.edu). Brett has an interest in innovative pedagogical approaches, acquisition of non-technical skills, scale development and psychometrics.

Sarah Wojkowski, MSc(PT), PT Reg, is Assistant Professor and Director of Clinical Education at the School of Rehabilitation Science, McMaster University, Hamilton, Ontario, Canada (email: wojkows@mcmaster.ca). Sarah's teaching interests include use of technology to facilitate teaching, professional issues, and integration of population health approaches into clinical practice. Sarah has a special interest in working with youths and adults with chronic conditions. She is pursuing her PhD (Rehabilitation Science) at McMaster University in the areas of health policy and access to rehabilitation services for persons with chronic conditions.

Dedication

Ted Brown

I would like to dedicate the book to the following individuals:

- Sylvia Rodger, friend, mentor, colleague and doctoral supervisor who is an occupational therapy educator, researcher, and advocate extraordinaire;
- David Stevens, life partner and constant source of support and patience for the time my academic pursuits take up;
- Louise Farnworth, friend, colleague, and department supervisor who emphasised the importance of basing a tertiary-level professional curriculum on sound and integrated pedagogical principles and evidence; and
- George and Erma Brown, my parents who instilled in me the importance of education, and pursuing one's life interests and dreams.

Brett Williams

To my family: Angela, Cooper, Parker, Saige and Christian

Acknowledgements

We would like to acknowledge the significant and notable contributions of two individuals who made this edited book possible. Jamie Etherington, Editorial Development Manager, Radcliffe Publishers is thanked for his ongoing advice, insights, encouragement and expertise during all the phases of the publication process of this sizeable edited book. He made the task much less daunting for the two of us as novice editors. We also wish to acknowledge the assistance of Vivianne Douglas of Darkriver Design. Her attention to detail during the copy-editing process, and expertise in typesetting and design of the book, was much appreciated by us. We would also like to thank Professor Hugh Barr from the United Kingdom and Professor Joy Higgs from Australia for each agreeing to write a foreword for this book.

PART I

Evidence-based education in a health professional education context

CHAPTER 1

Introduction

· ·

Ted Brown and Brett Williams

In the healthcare sector, there has been a push for the use of *evidence-based medicine* (EBM) and *evidence-based practice* (EBP). EBM and EBP integrate the best research evidence with clinical expertise and patient values to facilitate clinical decision-making.[1] Clinicians are required to provide the best standard of care to patients and their families that is based on the most current, best-quality research evidence available. Yet, many healthcare academic and clinical educators do not apply the same principle of best practice strategies and pedagogical approaches in the education of healthcare students.[2-5] While EBM and EBP are central to health professionals' clinical practice and the patient care they provide, it appears clear that there is a general lack of consideration given to *evidence-based education* (EBE). This point is illustrated by Boet *et al.*,[6(p160)] who state that

> numerous educational stakeholders have advocated for the movement from opinion-based to evidence-based education whereby educational curricula are based on research findings rather than historical and culturally engrained traditions.

Academic and clinical educators face many challenges in the contemporary landscape of healthcare education. These challenges cross all educational boundaries, from hospital bedsides to lecture theatres at universities, and they come at a time when we are all faced with pressures of improving student learning and satisfaction, while maintaining educational excellence.

Some of these challenges include:
- a growing number of non-traditional and culturally diverse learners
- fluctuating and unpredictable levels of tertiary education funding
- varying models and modes of curricula delivery
- rapid growth in information technology applications and greater levels of sophistication
- increasing competition between tertiary education providers

- sourcing sufficient numbers of clinical fieldwork and practice education placements
- increasing accountability requirements from government agencies (such as Australia's Tertiary Education Quality and Standards Agency, or TEQSA)
- meeting the standards for education programme accreditation by external professional bodies (e.g. the Australian Nursing and Midwifery Accreditation Council, the Australian Physiotherapy Council).[7]

Given these challenges, healthcare educators need to find the best evidence for teaching and learning; we would argue that decisions to change approaches to learning should now be based on empirical evidence, rather than on traditional or time-honoured pedagogical approaches. Examples of mainstream traditional approaches include the delivery of 'sage on the stage' lectures to students in academic settings, and the apprenticeship model of clinical education provision. While educating the next generation(s) of healthcare professions is challenging, it is at the same time very exciting for all of us. While the notion of the scholarship of teaching and learning is not new, we would argue that integration and implementation of this scholarship could be improved through all areas and levels of healthcare education. While we are at a point in time when most educational institutions and healthcare providers are faced with deteriorating financial conditions and other constraints, we have an opportunity to overcome these challenges as educators through transformative teaching and learning that is based on EBE principles.

Moreover, an opportunity exists for raising the standard of learning and teaching by applying the same underlying principles that drive EBM and EBP. To accomplish this, it is essential to begin with a foundation text that outlines the key principles of EBE, building a critical mass of EBE champions, and promoting the scholarship of teaching and learning within the healthcare educator ranks. This edited text aims to provide a starting point. Contributors to the text include authors from Australia, the United States, Canada and the United Kingdom. The text is divided into four sections: Part I covers the underlying principles of EBE; Part II provides some key contextual components and concepts related to health professional education; Part III provides an outline of a number of teaching and learning approaches that have some credible evidence behind them; finally, Part IV provides a landscape overview of the current level of EBE in a number of health professions.

REFERENCES

1. Straus SE, Richardson WS, Glasziou P, *et al. Evidence-Based Medicine: how to practice and teach EBM.* Edinburgh: Churchill Livingstone; 2005.
2. Davies P. Approaches to evidence-based teaching. *Med Teach.* 2000; **22**(1): 14–21.
3. Emerson RJ, Records K. Today's challenge, tomorrow's excellence: the practice of evidence-based education. *J Nurs Educ.* 2008; **47**(8): 359–70.
4. Cannon S, Boswell C. *Evidence-Based Teaching in Nursing: a foundation for educators.* Sudbury, MA: Jones & Bartlett Learning; 2012.
5. Ginsberg SM, Friberg J, Visconti C. *Scholarship of Teaching and Learning in Speech-Language Pathology and Audiology: evidence-based education.* San Diego, CA: Plural Publishing; 2012.

6. Boet S, Sharma S, Goldman J, *et al.* Medical education research: an overview of methods. *Can J Anaesth.* 2012; **59**(2): 159–70.
7. Petersen S. Time for evidence based medical education. *BMJ.* 1999; **318**(7193): 1223–4.

CHAPTER 2

Evidence-based practice in the context of health professional education

....

Malcolm Boyle

OVERVIEW

The evidence-based medicine paradigm came to prominence in the early 1990s with a medical group in Ontario, Canada, using scientific evidence to support history taking, physical assessment and diagnostic tests in the patient management decision process. There are two main approaches to research: (1) quantitative studies, which use numerical analysis of the results, and (2) qualitative studies, which attempt to understand more about the events, situations, cultures and experiences that affect a person. For quantitative studies there is a hierarchical level of scientific evidence, with the systematic review and meta-analysis at the top followed by the randomised controlled trial, cohort study, case-control study, cross-sectional study, case series and case study. For the qualitative studies there are various methods for obtaining the data; these include the phenomenology, ethnography, grounded theory, and case study. There are also studies that use a combination of quantitative and qualitative methods, referred to as mixed methods. The data collection process varies for different studies, from a data collection form to direct observation, one-on-one interviews and focus groups. There are issues within the study that may affect the study outcomes, including bias, confounding and blinding. This chapter provides an overview of evidence-based practice, where the paradigm emanated from, and some of the different study types for both quantitative and qualitative methods. We also discuss how evidence-based practice provides the basis for evidence-based education for the health-related professions.

CHAPTER OBJECTIVES

Upon completion of this chapter, the reader will be able to:

- define evidence-based practice
- describe the key features of quantitative and qualitative research approaches
- outline various methods for obtaining data
- be familiar with issues that affect study outcomes, including bias, confounding and blinding
- reflect on the relationship between evidence-based practice and evidence-based education.

KEY TERMS: evidence-based practice, evidence-based education, levels of evidence, quantitative studies, qualitative studies, mixed methods studies, bias, confounding, blinding, levels of evidence

INTRODUCTION

Evidence-based medicine (EBM) in its early form can be traced back hundreds of years – one example is that of Edward Jenner, who observed that a dairymaid who had cowpox appeared not to develop smallpox when exposed during a smallpox epidemic. Jenner then sought to prove his hypothesis that cowpox protects against smallpox. Jenner vaccinated a young child with cowpox and then exposed him to smallpox, with the result that the child did not present with the clinical features of smallpox.[1] The term 'evidence-based medicine' first came to prominence in 1991, when Gordon Guyatt mentioned it in an article published by the *American College of Physicians Journal Club*.[2] In the early 1990s the Evidence-Based Medicine Working Group, based in Hamilton, Ontario, Canada, outlined a new paradigm for medical student education where the teaching of medical students would encompass clinical experience, the knowledge and understanding of disease processes, and the understanding of evidence and its associated rules. There was a decreased reliance on the 'word' of the authoritarian figure; however, experience was still essential in the areas of history taking, physical assessment and diagnostic processes. The view was that this evidence-based approach to patient management would improve patient outcomes and satisfaction with the information provided to them.

DEFINITION OF EVIDENCE-BASED MEDICINE AND EVIDENCE-BASED PRACTICE

In the late 1990s, Sackett *et al.*[3] sought to clarify what EBM was and what it was not. They defined EBM as 'the conscientious, explicit, and judicious use of current best evidence in making decisions about the care of individual patients.'[3(p71)] and stated that the 'practice of evidence based medicine means integrating individual clinical expertise with the best available external clinical evidence from systematic research.'[3(p71)] Furthermore, they stated that EBM 'is not "cookbook" medicine, it requires a bottom up approach that integrates the best external evidence with individual clinical expertise and patients' choice, it cannot result in slavish, cookbook approaches to individual patient care.'[3(p71)]

Following on from the EBM paradigm is the more generic evidence-based practice (EBP) paradigm, where the practice within a specific discipline or profession is guided by the scientific evidence that supports the day-to-day practice.[4] For the evidence-based education (EBE) paradigm the evidence is used in a variety of ways, including identifying ways in which students learn, methods for teaching and assessment methods.[5]

LEVELS OF EVIDENCE

The information supplied here is by no means exhaustive but aims to give the reader an overview of the different study types and some of the issues associate with them. Owing to the increasing use of a mixed methods approach to education research, the levels of evidence will be divided into *quantitative* and *qualitative*, with a brief description of each study type.

Quantitative

This group of studies refers to a type of study that uses a form of numerical analysis of the study results. The study types are listed in their order of hierarchy, from highest to lowest.

Systematic review

The systematic review study sets about answering a specific research question or focuses on a specific topic. The systematic review normally follows a specific process for identifying relevant articles, determining the quality of the included articles, extracting data from the included articles and synthesis of the extracted data. This process is normally defined in a protocol that is followed precisely.

The Cochrane Collaboration[6] and the Campbell Collaboration[7] are two organisations that promote the conducting of highly rigorous systematic reviews, with these systematic reviews seen as the 'gold standard' of systematic reviews. The Cochrane Collaboration[8] uses predominately randomised controlled trials (RCTs) or controlled clinical trials in the systematic reviews. The Campbell Collaboration uses RCTs, controlled clinical trials and observational studies in the systematic reviews. The systematic reviews that these two organisations publish also incorporate meta-analyses. A meta-analysis is the combining of data extracted from the included articles to produce an overall result for all the included articles – this is represented by a forest plot that includes each study and the overall result. This process is extremely useful for determining an overall outcome from the data of multiple small studies.

Randomised controlled trial

This type of study is the 'gold standard' of study types and normally involves the comparison of two distinct groups of participants – one group is the intervention group and the other group is the control or comparison group. The intervention group participates in a process that is being compared with an existing practice to determine if it provides better outcomes than the existing practice. For example, a comparison between students undertaking a simulation using a high-fidelity manikin and students undertaking the same simulation using a low-fidelity manikin to identify if the type of manikin affects the student performance.

Participants in the study are randomised into one of the two groups. This process can be achieved in a variety of ways: the first method is by a computer-generated randomised number that allocates the participant into one of the groups; the second method is by using a random number table and selecting a specific number sequence as a means of allocating a participant to a group; the third method is not a true randomised allocation but a quasi-randomisation, where the day of the week or month is used to determine the group allocation. Participants are randomised into either of the groups to ensure the characteristics of the study participants are the same in each group. The randomisation process aims to distribute the participants almost evenly into either of the groups.

An RCT can be conducted at one site or multiple sites, a multi-centred study. A multi-centred study is conducted to ensure there are sufficient numbers in the study so if there is a difference between the intervention and control group it will be found. A multi-centred study may also be used to decrease the bias of different student populations or educational systems. The advantages of this study type include an unbiased distribution of study participants into one of the sample groups; the study participants, data analyst or study investigators may be blinded to the group allocation, thereby decreasing the influence upon the study results. The issues with this study are it is an extremely time-consuming process to manage an RCT, it is an expensive study to run, there may be ethical issues with the data collected from the participants, and there is a potential for volunteer bias, meaning the participants may not be a true sample from the general population. Another notable limitation of the RCT approach is that it is not an appropriate methodology for some types of research questions.

Cohort study

This type of study investigates a defined group of students who are then divided into subgroups that are exposed to some process and followed over an explicit time frame to identify specific outcomes of interest. For example, one group of students is exposed to real-time simulation while the other group is exposed to a simulated computer programme, with the outcome of interest being the decision-making ability of the student in an assessment.

A cohort study can be either retrospective, looking backwards in time from a specific point, or prospective, looking forward from a specific point in time. A cohort study can also just involve one group, which is studied either retrospectively or prospectively for the outcome of interest. There are other terms that are commonly used to describe aspects of a cohort study, including (a) a longitudinal study, where students are followed over a period of time to determine changes to specific attributes or characteristics (e.g. attitudes to a person with mental illness) and (b) follow-up studies, where a group or groups of students are followed over time to assess a specific outcome following exposure (e.g. incidence of influenza following community place-ment in students who elect not to be vaccinated against the influenza virus).

The advantages of a cohort study include that it is easier to administer, is less costly and ethically is a lot safer than an RCT; it can determine timing and directionality of the outcomes; and it has the ability to standardise eligibility criteria and outcome assessments. The issues of a cohort study include that it has the ability to 'blind' study participants, data collectors and the data analysis, and the exposure may be associated with a hidden confounder.

Case-control study

This type of study commences with the identification of persons with a specific attribute of interest and a control (comparison or reference) group of persons without the attribute but who are otherwise similar (e.g. similar age range, gender or education level). The two groups are compared to identify factors that may contribute to having the attribute of interest. For example, looking at a specific level of student deafness, the cases (those students with deafness) and the controls (those students not deaf) follow-ing a period of listening to music with headphones or ear buds. The aim of the study is to identify a relationship between listening to music and a specific level of deafness. The advantages of this study type are the low cost and the short period of time in which the study can be undertaken, it requires fewer students than a cross-sectional study does, and it may be the only method for identifying uncommon disorders or problems or those with a long time between exposure and the outcome of interest.

Cross-sectional study

This type of study is essentially a survey or questionnaire that seeks information about a topic or exposure at a specific point in time. For example, the study may seek information about student views or exposure to specific attributes of education over a period of time. The study may use an existing survey document that has been used previously and undergone a validation process. The cross-sectional study is relatively easy to develop and distribute, ethically it is relatively safe, and it is cheap and easy to administer. Some of the issues associated with this study type are that it may be susceptible to recall bias (the tendency for participants to have selective recall of what happened back in time), it may establish an association at most but not causality, its identified confounders may be unequally distributed, and comparison group sizes may be grossly unequal.

Case series study

The case series study is a collation or group of similar individual case reports or stud-ies covering a new or unusual presentation or incident over a short period of time.

The advantages of this study are that it may highlight an issue that requires a more rigorous study to identify if there is a trend or causation to the outcome and it can be undertaken at minimal cost. The issues with this study type are that there is no comparison with a control or unexposed group and it may suggest there is an association with exposure when in fact there is not.

Case report or study

This is a description of a new or unusual presentation or incident that has not previously been described or there have been just a few articles describing the presentation or incident. The case report or study may also be a report of a previously described presentation or incident but within a different context or setting. The advantage of the case report or study is that it may highlight a new or unusual presentation or incident; however, it is prone to author bias and there is no accounting for confounders. A case study format is appropriate for use with rare conditions and diagnoses.

Expert opinion

This is normally an article from an individual who is experienced and is seen as an expert in the field, who has considerable knowledge of the literature in the field, and who may or may not have credibility among his or her peers in the field. There may also be a statement from a professional organisation or college covering their view on a specific topic; this may be in the form of a 'consensus statement' aimed at their membership of practitioners within the field. The expert opinion lacks scientific credibility and is prone to individual or group bias and confounding issues.

Quantitative data collection
DATA COLLECTION FORMS

The data collection is normally undertaken using a specifically designed form on which the data for the study are collected. The data collection form can be either paper-based or electronic. If the data collection is undertaken using a paper-based form, the data are then converted to an electronic format and uploaded into a statistical programme for further analysis.

DIRECT OBSERVATION

The observation process involves the researcher watching the participant undertaking the task of interest. The data are collected by the researcher's written notes of what is observed, a video of what is observed or photographs of what is observed. The researcher may complete a frequency count or rate a participant's performance using a specific set of questions or rating scales.

Issues associated with quantitative studies
BIAS

Although from the late 1970s, the following definition of bias is still referenced by modern-day writers on epidemiology, as it is still relevant: 'a process at any stage of inference tending to produce results that depart systematically from the true value.[9(p117)] There are many forms of bias; however, only a couple will be highlighted here. For a list of biases see the article by Delgado-Rodríguez and Llorca.[10]

Two examples of common bias are *inclusion or selection bias* and *information bias*. Inclusion or selection bias occurs when the sample of participants in the study is not representative of the population the study is aimed at. For example, surveying a group of experienced educators compared with a group of inexperienced ones, when the outcome of the study is aimed at the inexperienced educators. Information bias occurs during the data collection phase when inaccuracies are introduced into the data set. For example, when an interviewer *interprets* the response from the interviewee during the interview process, with the documented response not being a true representation of what was actually stated.

CONFOUNDING

There are several different definitions for confound but the following is one of the more simplistic: 'occurs when two factors are associated (travel together) and the effect of one is confused with or distorted by the effect of the other.'[11(p7)]

BLINDING OR MASKING

This is a process where the participant and researcher associated with the study are blind or masked to aspects of the allocation process and intervention. The blinding or masking process can take place at four different levels: the first level is the researchers who are allocating the patients to the intervention and control group do not know which group the next patient will be allocated to; the second is the patient is not aware of what group he or she has been allocated to; the third is the people working with the participants are not aware which group the participant is allocated to; the fourth is the researchers responsible for analysing the data are not aware which group is the intervention or control group.

Qualitative

This group of studies refers to a type of study that seeks to understand more about the events, situations, cultures and experiences that affect a person. This list is by no means exhaustive but outlines the more common qualitative study types.

Phenomenology

This study type investigates a phenomenon within the natural surroundings; the phenomenon can be an event, a specific situation, experiences of a group of people or different concepts. This study begins by acknowledging there is a gap in the understanding and that clarification or highlighting the issue under investigation will be beneficial. For example, what is it like for the mother of a young child to be studying at university? What problems does it create? Or how does the family cope?

This study type does not provide an absolute explanation of the issue at hand, but increases the insight and awareness.

Ethnography

This study type investigates cultural issues for people from a geographical area, religious group, tribal group, or with shared experiences. The background for this study is from anthropology. For example, this form of study may be used to ascertain the cultural and religious beliefs and needs of foreign students studying at a university, thereby identifying the support services required to assist the students assimilate into university life. Some issues with this study type can be the researchers not understanding the participant's language and social norms, and the researcher as an outsider misinterpreting the information collected. This study type is extremely time-consuming, with multiple sessions of data collection required. The qualitative researcher is expected to be as bias-free as possible and to 'go native' in the surroundings.

Grounded theory

This study type is similar to phenomenology, but it creates a new theoretical base following the data collection process. It extends the phenomenology study by identifying the information that emanated from the study as new knowledge and using this new knowledge to formulate new theories about the phenomena of interest. For example, a researcher using a grounded theory approach may interview a group of 20 first-year occupational therapy students about their professional identifiers and motivations for selecting occupational therapy as a career. After reviewing the results using an in-depth immersive process, the researcher will see if a model of neophyte occupational therapy student identity emerges.

Case study

This type of study ranges from the description of a single event to an analysis of an event over time using the same participants, who may have had exposure to other influences over this time period. The aim of the case study is to define the particular case in detail. The information described is relevant to the population being studied within the situation and system at the time. The results are not meant to be generalisable to the general population; this decision is up to the reader. For example, the response of students to elderly people over the duration of their course and how the interaction changes following increased exposure to elderly people in the clinical setting.

Data collection methods

Interview

The interview can take several different forms, the highly structured interview, the semi-structured or focused interview, or the unstructured interview. The highly structured interview has a set number of questions that are asked the same way to all study participants; it is similar to a questionnaire. The semi-structured interview uses a set of open-ended questions covering specific topic areas. The response to the question allows the interviewer to seek more information about a specific area of the topic. This process also allows the interviewee to seek clarification and further expand on his or her answer. For the unstructured interview the interviewer has an aim of discussing a few topics down to one or two topics. The interviewer starts with a question, with further questions determined by the interviewee responses. The topics are covered in detail, as the lack of structure means the interviewer can seek to clarify each of the interviewee's responses.

Focus groups

Focus groups are commonly used with a small group of participants who have similar attributes, with the interaction between the participants providing useful information. Focus groups can be used when it is impractical to undertake individual interviews.

Observation

The observation may be of a person performing tasks within a work environment, his or her living environment or other areas of interest. The observation process may consist of the researcher's written notes about the participant and his or her actions, a video of the participant and photographs of the participant.

EVIDENCE-BASED PRACTICE PROCESS

There are several ways in which you can identify the scientific evidence to inform educational process change in your setting. The first is to access a data repository where the evidence has already been identified, collated and synthesised. In the medical domain two examples are the Cochrane Collaboration[6] and BestBETs,[12] while in the education, crime and justice, social welfare and international development domain is the Campbell Collaboration.[7] These are large databases where specific research questions have been posed, the appropriate literature identified and synthesised, and an easy-to-understand short summary of the findings is provided for the clinician or educator to review and determine their appropriateness.

The second is a repository where individual articles have been summarised, thereby saving the reader time in not having to read and form a conclusion about the article him- or herself. There are some learned colleges who have their own journal clubs that summarise the scientific literature, such as the American College of Physicians.[13] One or more people review an article and then summarise it into one page, following a specific format, so that busy clinicians or educators can review and determine the appropriateness of the article to their practice.

Finally, it is for you to define a research question, search the specific electronic databases, identify relevant articles and synthesise the data to draw your own conclusion. The research question should be in a structured format – for example, PICO (Problem, Intervention, Comparison and Outcome) or PIO (Problem, Intervention and Outcome). The focused question makes it easier to identify the search terms required in the next step of locating the literature in the electronic databases, and possibly hand searching non-electronic database-listed journals. The identification of relevant articles is based on your inclusion and exclusion criteria. For example, you may exclude articles not written in English as you do not have the time or funds to get them translated. Synthesising data from the identified article means having an understanding of the study design, the statistical analysis and drawing your own conclusion from the published findings. There are software programmes available that allow you to summarise the data presented in multiple studies; these are either incorporated into statistical programmes or are standalone programmes – for example, Review Manager (RevMan) by the Cochrane Collaboration.[14] This can be a time-consuming process; therefore, using an already published review or article summation is preferable.

The decision on whether the findings of the reviews are relevant to your area should be based on the intervention and study population used. For example, there is no point using the results of a review that utilised several US-based studies if the study population, educational system and educational processes are vastly different to those in your setting. You need to find a review or article summary that has the same or very similar systems, student populations and educational processes.

CHALLENGES OF EVIDENCE-BASED PRACTICE

An evidence-based approach to education frees you from a reliance on opinion and tradition, and it allows you to critically evaluate traditional, alternative and emerging processes in a somewhat systematic approach. The evidence-based approach allows you to concentrate on the required outcomes, such as student engagement and interaction using new technologies, in the development of an education programme. The overall challenges are overcoming the barriers or disadvantages to EBP and pursuing the advantages that EBP provides to the development and ongoing improvement of an educational programme, and to a lesser extent keeping in mind the monetary cost of achieving the outcomes of interest.

APPLYING EVIDENCE-BASED PRACTICE PRINCIPLES TO THE EDUCATION OF HEALTH PROFESSIONAL STUDENTS

Applying the principles of EBP to education requires some thought; however, what is presented here is an example of what it can be used for, a starting point for the novice EBP educator. EBP can be used to justify an existing education process, make the transition to a new process based on a significant body of evidence, stop the transition to a different educational process as the evidence does not support the process, and change current practice as it proves to have worse outcomes than that suggested by the evidence. EBP principles can be applied to EBE (*see* Table 2.1).

Undertaking small studies with students can ascertain if what is being taught is preparing the student for the workplace, or if the educational process is making the student work ready. For example, assessing the effectiveness of a student in ventilating a manikin at the required rate and volume during a resuscitation effort as part of a cardiac arrest exercise. Results from this study can then direct curriculum renewal as part of an evaluation of education practices.

Undertaking a study in the first week of first year can determine students' attitudes to specific medical conditions, thereby determining what attitudes and preconceived ideas students bring with them when they start university. The results from this study can guide units/subjects within the curriculum to counteract inappropriate attitudes and ideas students bring with them to the unit/subject, attitudes and ideas that have been developed within their community exposure and home environment. The EBP process may form part of an ongoing staff educational development programme where staff may learn about the EBP process and participate in the evaluation of recently published articles as part of a department journal club. This ensures staff are aware of the EBP process and current evidence to support their educational processes.

TABLE 2.1 Advantages and disadvantages of evidence-based practice (EBP) and evidence-based education (EBE) process

---

Some advantages of EBP include:
- better informed educators
- practice guidelines based on high-level evidence allowing for cross-institutional consistency
- student-centred outcomes
- processes for dissemination of the summarised evidence
- widely available information so all divisions of the education sector are informed
- defined transparent processes, therefore decreasing the possibility of misinterpretation
- identification of what is known about a topic and what further research is required

Some of the disadvantages of EBP include:
- the education and skill development requirement to undertake EBP is time-consuming
- a lack of evidence for the unusual issue or special requirement student subgroup
- a lack of evidence supporting EBP in education
- a lack of support for the lower-level evidence when it is the only available evidence
- potentially decreases educator judgement and/or autonomy

CONCLUSION

EBP is an attitude and a structured process. It has a scientific basis, which some would argue does not fit in an education paradigm; however, it can provide the support to continue or change current practice. As educators we must acknowledge that current practice may be based on tradition or personal views and may lack a scientific basis for what is currently done. EBP is not the panacea for educational change but it does provide a structured approach in which change can be justified based on the evidence, not just the word of an authority in an area of practice, personal beliefs or current fads. While not providing all the answers it does provide some and it highlights areas where further research is required to underpin educational practice. EBP is the way forward for the future and needs to be embraced for the ongoing improvement of educational practice.

SUMMARY POINTS

- EBP is an important part of healthcare and has provided the foundation for EBE.
- There are three approaches to EBP: quantitative, qualitative and mixed methods.
- Quantitative approaches to EBP include systematic review, randomised. controlled trial, cohort, case-control, cross-sectional, case series, case report and expert opinion.
- Three challenges inherent in conducting quantitative research are bias, confounding and blinding or masking.
- Qualitative approaches to EBP include phenomenology, ethnography, grounded theory and case study.
- EBP provides the foundation for EBE to best quality teaching and learning experiences for health professional students.

REVIEW QUESTIONS

- What is the definition of EBP?
- What are two data collection methods for quantitative research?
- Why is bias a potential challenge linked with quantitative research?
- What is the difference between phenomenology and ethnography?
- What are three data collection methods for qualitative research?
- How can EBP assist EBE?

REFLECTIVE QUESTIONS AND ACTIVITIES

- What is the link between EBP and EBE?
- What research approach could be used to evaluate the effectiveness of an online ethics course?
- Given problem-based learning is a commonly used educational approach, what two research approaches could be used to evaluate its effectiveness?
- What could be three challenges linked with conducting education-related research?

REFERENCES

1. Gordis L. *Epidemiology*. 3rd ed. Philadelphia, PA: Elsevier Saunders; 2004.
2. Guyatt G. Evidence-based medicine. *ACP J Club (Ann Intern Med)*. 1991; **114**(Suppl. 2): A-16.
3. Sackett DL, Rosenberg WM, Gray JA, *et al*. Evidence based medicine: what it is and what it isn't. *BMJ*. 1996; **312**(7023): 71–2.
4. Rolfe G. Insufficient evidence: the problems of evidence-based nursing. *Nurse Educ Today*. 1999; **19**(6): 433–42.
5. Bruniges M. *An Evidence-Based Approach to Teaching and Learning: using data to support learning*. Melbourne, VIC: Australian Council for Educational Research; 2005.
6. www.cochrane.org
7. www.campbellcollaboration.org
8. The Cochrane Collaboration. *Cochrane Collaboration Logo*. www.cochrane.org/about-us/history/our-logo (accessed 27 June 2013).
9. Murphy E. *The Logic of Medicine*. Baltimore, MD: The Johns Hopkins University Press; 1978.
10. Delgado-Rodríguez M, Llorca J. Bias. *J Epidemiol Community Health*. 2004; **58**(8): 635–41.
11. Fletcher R, Fletcher S, Fletcher G. *Clinical Epidemiology: the essentials*. 5th ed. Baltimore, MD: Williams & Wilkins; 2012.
12. www.bestbets.org
13. http://acpjc.acponline.org
14. The Cochrane Collaboration. *Review Manager (RevMan)*. www.cochrane.org/editorial-and-publishing-policy-resource/review-manager-revman (accessed 27 June 2013).

CHAPTER 3

Factors affecting health professional education

....

Margaret Bearman

OVERVIEW

The education of health professional students is strongly influenced by policy and practice environments. Any consideration of evidence-based education has to also recognise the particular educational and healthcare implementation contexts. Using Australia as a case example, this chapter discusses how both universities and healthcare services are under a range of pressures that constrain and promote certain types of academic and clinical educator activity, leading to particular trends within the health professional education sector. Higher education sector influences in the Australian context include globalisation, massification, pressures on funding, technological developments and quality assurance mechanisms. Australian healthcare sector influences include pressures on hospitals due to ageing population and rising cost of healthcare, the reform of the primary health sector, increasing complexity of health practice, new forms of standardisation, accreditation and workforce management. Many of these factors are also germane to other countries. Health professional education is strongly influenced by both sectors and five key trends are identified: (1) pressure on clinical placement capacity, (2) simulation-based education, (3) interprofessional learning, (4) accreditation and standardisation frameworks and tools, and (5) the professionalisation of the health professional education educator. Some of these trends are supported by studies while others remain under-researched. It is important that, when reading and interpreting the literature, health professional educators take into account the local, national and international factors before implementing changes within their environments.

CHAPTER OBJECTIVES

Upon completion of this chapter, the reader will be able to:
- describe key international trends in health and higher education sectors that influence health professional education
- debate the links between broad influences on health and higher education and the practice of health professional educators
- reflect on how these trends affect local practice; and how they also affect the application of educational evidence within a particular context

KEY TERMS: health services, higher education, future trends, clinical placements, simulation, interprofessional learning, accreditation, health professional education

---

INTRODUCTION

Health professional education does not take place in isolation. The broader higher education and healthcare contexts have enormous influence over what individual educators and institutions can provide to their students. This chapter discusses at a macro level some of the influences that affect pre-service health professional educators. These context-dependent factors are important to understand when interpreting evidence to enhance educational practice. It is valuable for health professional educators to appreciate some of the system and policy frameworks that enhance or constrain their capacity to deliver the ideal learning experience for prospective students.

This chapter describes the key trends in both higher education and healthcare environments, many of which parallel each other. The example of the Australian context is used to provide a more detailed illustration of how these global issues can play out in a local setting. The nexus of the tertiary education and health service environments is examined, focusing on the implications for the 'on the ground' health professional educator. Five particular developments are discussed: (1) pressure on clinical placements, (2) the role of simulation-based education, (3) the rise of interprofessional learning, (4) the increasing influence of a range of standards and standards frameworks, and (5) the 'professionalisation' of the health professional educator. The reader is encouraged to reflect upon his or her local contexts and how these must necessarily inform the practice of evidence-based education.

TRENDS WITHIN HIGHER EDUCATION ENVIRONMENTS

In the last 2 decades, higher education across the globe has been profoundly affected by a range of significant changes.[1] The 2009 United Nations Educational, Scientific and Cultural Organization (UNESCO) report,[1] which described trends in higher education, detailed some of the phenomena affecting the sector. Issues such as 'globalisation', which can be defined as 'the reality shaped by an increasingly integrated world economy',[1(pii)] strongly influence the tertiary education sector. In particular, the movement of students across national borders is significant, both socially and economically. 'Massification', whereby increasing proportions of the population are seeking professionally oriented qualifications, is also changing the face of higher education. This trend is aligned with the advances in information and communications technology which promote ease-of-access to a more diverse audience. Against this broad backdrop, issues of the world economy, cost, funding and privatisation are seen as being key drivers for change. For example, the 2007 global financial crisis has adversely affected many universities across the globe because of a decrease in public and/or private funding.[2] The rising emphasis on accountability and quality assurance[1] – sometimes critiqued as 'audit culture'[3] – is also seen as significant. Interestingly, the UNESCO report[1] also describes the 'stress' on the academic profession, particularly in response to 'massification'.

These factors affecting higher education practice and experience do not exist in isolation from one another. To illustrate this, consider the recent rise of the massive open online course (MOOC), where there is broad open access for many geographically distributed learners to online learning materials. However, it is important to note that a MOOC not always free, and the number of learners is not always 'massive'.[4] The MOOC is a new technology, and it both illustrates and promotes 'massification' and the tensions of how education is now funded. There is considerable commentary in the popular press that MOOCs will 'disrupt' the current status of higher education through accessing more diverse and larger audiences, with different value placed on more traditional styles of education. However, the completion data on MOOCs suggest that no more than 10% of students who commence, complete.[5] As Breslow *et al.*[5] write:

> it is unlikely that higher educational institutions will not be affected by MOOCs. Those effects will probably not be as dramatic as promoters or detractors would have us believe, but rather will be more nuanced and complex.[(p23)]

The MOOC example illustrates how the influences of technology, massification and funding are substantially interrelated. It also demonstrates how rhetoric with respect to change can overtake the production of evidence.

An individual's experience of the changing higher education sector is strongly influenced by his or her particular nation's policy, as much as by the universities themselves. To illustrate this, it is informative to move from an example of a global cross-nation phenomenon such as the MOOC, to consider a national system. By December 2012, Australia was a nation of 22.9 million people,[6] with 96% of traditional universities owned by the state, against an OECD (Organisation for Economic Co-operation and Development) average of 71%[7] with a strong interest in maintaining or increasing the proportion of population with higher degree qualifications.[8] In 2010, Australia notably had the highest OECD average of international students per capita of total tertiary enrolment, at 19.8%.[7] For many decades this influx of full-fee-paying international students provided diversity to institutions and to the national landscape, as well as fiscal support to the Australian higher education sector.[9] However, there has been a recent reduction in numbers of international students, in part due to the rising Australian dollar, poor publicity based on high-profile assault cases involving international students, increased competition from the rest of the globe and changes to student visa requirements.[10] Simultaneously, the local demand for higher education has also changed, driven by the 2008 Bradley Report into Higher Education,[8] which recommended increasing the proportion of students from disadvantaged backgrounds enrolled at universities while simultaneously deregulating the system so that funding followed the student, not the institution.[8] Additionally, the report recommended a national and more rigorous quality assurance cycle be implemented,[8] which resulted in the formation of the Tertiary Education Quality and Standards Agency, which has the as-yet-unimplemented powers to develop teaching and learning standards.[10] This national snapshot clearly demonstrates the influence of the drivers of globalisation, massification, funding models and quality assurance upon the higher education sector.

What does all this mean at the 'chalkface' level for Australian educators? First, academics are increasingly expected to design courses to be relevant across cultures, both because students come from a wide variety of cultural backgrounds and because graduates should have 'internationally' applicable skills. This process is often referred to as 'internationalising the curriculum'.[11] Second, it can be argued that the real reduction in funding has led to a significant increase in staff-to-student ratios and a rise in casualisation of the academic workforce.[9] Third, technology is often seen as a way of offsetting some of the cost of education as well as attracting 'Generation Tech', also referred to as the 'Click Generation'. Perhaps, less discussed but often encountered by university educators, technology may be responsible for high plagiarism levels, with one 2005 self-report study noting 81% of the cross-university sample (N = 954) admitting to some form of plagiarism.[12] Finally, the quality assurance movement has led to increasing accountability for individuals and departments, such as tracking satisfaction measures with respect to student experience of units and teachers, mapping course objectives against the Australian Quality Framework, and being subject to more stringent course review mechanisms. University educators are now acutely aware that the perceptions of their teaching are important, possibly even privileging this above the actual teaching content itself.[13] In all, these changes represent a significant range of pressures for the average academic. It can be argued that educators must respond to these pressures creatively and collaboratively as they draw from the evidence to improve teaching within their own environments.

TRENDS WITHIN HEALTHCARE ENVIRONMENTS

Healthcare practice is, like higher education, a dynamic and rapidly changing system. The *Harvard Business Review* argues for 'megatrends' in global health systems, which are affecting the practice of healthcare, including the impact of ageing populations; the increasing costs of healthcare; the rise of standardised, evidence-based protocols; and changes in traditional practice roles.[14] Additionally, it is also worth considering the impact of the patient safety movement and its associated increased oversight of healthcare practice, as well as the predicted requirements of the future healthcare workforce.

It is important to understand the impact of these 'megatrends' at a national level, by returning to the case example of Australia. In Australia, the healthcare system is changing to accommodate longer lifespans with more chronic disease.[15] Patients in hospital settings tend to be older and sicker,[16] and while length of stay in hospital is falling relative to a few decades ago, the increasing numbers of sick elderly are putting pressure on hospital admissions[15] and general cost of healthcare is increasing.[17] Of course, healthcare is more than acute level, hospital-based tertiary care. Chronic disease, reducing hospital admissions and length of stay, and uneven provision of primary care services are some of the factors driving reform of primary care systems within Australia.[18]

In Australia, health spending, including government and individual, has increased from 7.9% to 9.4% of spending on all goods and services since the early 2000s[19] and it is predicted to rise further.[17] This rise in spending, which likely reflects the rise in the real cost of healthcare, leads to acute tension when government is trying to rein in overall spending. It is difficult to capture the most recent impact of this tension in the scholarly literature, but there may be some signs from the press. For example, in 2013, media reports that funding issues appear to have led to temporary and permanent bed closure.[20,21] In general, there seems little question that there is fiscal pressure on the Australian state and federal governments, who own and manage many hospitals, and the insurance providers of those who enter private facilities. This subsequently places pressure on the front-line healthcare workers, with a very strong focus on service provision in a tight economic environment. The impact of funding shortages, staff workload, and increased casual workforce on both patient outcome and health worker satisfaction has been reported for a range of environments in a range of countries, including Australia.[22-24] Against this backdrop of fiscal and service pressure, there are new specialised treatments, leading to a need for more a specialised workforce and increasingly fragmented healthcare pathways that require multidisciplinary care.[15]

Alongside the rising complexity of healthcare, and the movement towards care outside acute settings, there has been recognition of the significant impact of medical error. In 1995, the Quality in Australian Health Care Study[17] found that in over 14 000 admissions, 16.6% were associated with adverse events and 8.35% of admissions were associated with highly preventable adverse events. In the 2 decades since this study, the patient safety movement has highlighted this issue from both a systems and individual practice perspectives. A 2013 study has indicated that 43 million adverse events occur globally.[18] Policy is also shaped by high-profile malpractice 'watersheds' such as the Bristol Royal Infirmary case in the United Kingdom, where poor self-regulation led to the deaths of many babies during surgery.[19] Both general patient safety issues plus the high-profile concerns have contributed to an increased oversight of healthcare practitioners' professional performance, underpinned by evidence-based standards. This type of trend is demonstrated in Australia by the creation in 2010 of the Australian Health Practitioner Regulation Agency,[25] where 14 health professions are regulated nationally under the auspices of a single national body (*see* Table 3.1).

TABLE 3.1 Health Professions Regulated by the Australian Health Practitioner Regulation Agency[25]

- Aboriginal and Torres Strait Islander Health Practice Board of Australia
- Chinese Medicine Board of Australia
- Chiropractic Board of Australia
- Dental Board of Australia
- Medical Board of Australia
- Medical Radiation Practice Board of Australia
- Nursing and Midwifery Board of Australia
- Occupational Therapy Board of Australia
- Optometry Board of Australia
- Osteopathy Board of Australia
- Pharmacy Board of Australia
- Physiotherapy Board of Australia
- Podiatry Board of Australia
- Psychology Board of Australia

This standardisation is also required, because the health workforce, like higher education, is now a global industry. Migration has seen many weak economies lose potential healthcare workers to jurisdictions with strong economies; within regions with a strong economy, less desirable areas (such as remote or rural locations) have lost health workforce numbers to more desirable areas. Overall, it is estimated that the current rates of training the Australian health workforce are not sufficient to staff the changing workforce.[26] Because of pressure on the numbers of healthcare personnel available, governments have set up statutory bodies to manage workforce issues. In Australia, for example, this has been Health Workforce Australia (HWA), which reports to all state jurisdictions through the Council of Australian Governments. HWA's stated mandate is 'to address the challenges of providing a skilled, flexible and innovative health workforce that meets the needs of the Australian community'.[27(p2)] Interestingly, HWA views the health workforce as a continuum, one that stretches from pre-service students enrolled in training programmes through to senior specialisations. It also has focused on redesigning practice roles with its 'expanded scope of practice' programme, piloting such initiatives as the 'extended care paramedics', who provide care to patients in the home or expanding the role of nurses in emergency departments.[28]

THE UNIVERSITY–HEALTHCARE NEXUS

The intersection of the broad systems of higher education and healthcare delivery is in health professional education, particularly with respect to teaching and learning that occurs in clinical and practice education environments. The requirements of the healthcare system of the future are placing pressure on the higher education sector, having to educate considerably higher numbers of potential healthcare workers in order to avoid a shortfall of graduates. Moreover, as has been illustrated earlier in this chapter, there are parallels in the trends in both the healthcare and the higher education environments. Both systems are required to be more accountable while seeking to manage rising costs. Health professional educators have to navigate providing clinical education placements for increasing numbers of students and have greater accountability, while at the same time clinical educators must draw from the best available evidence to ensure learning outcomes.

Health professional educators include those who primarily teach in clinical or practice environments, as well as those who mainly teach within academic contexts. Those who work in healthcare systems may be more affected by health developments; those employed by universities may be more influenced by changes within the higher education environment. As such, it is worth discussing five major trends currently occurring within Australia as well as within many other jurisdictions, which flow from the higher-level influences described previously and which affect many health professional educators as well. These are (1) pressure on clinical placements, (2) increasing interest in simulation-based education, (3) the recognition for interprofessional learning at pre-service level, (4) increasingly standardised assessment and accreditation frameworks, and (5) increased requirement for educator professional development and/or formal qualifications. Together, these represent the ways in which the global factors are playing out within the health profession education environment and they represent areas where evidence-based education will be increasingly important.

Pressure on clinical placements

In Australia, there is increasing difficulty in placing undergraduate, graduate-entry master's, and entry-level clinical doctorate health professional students in healthcare environments that are facing a number of pressures simultaneously. This is in part due to the increasing number of students: between 2011 and 2012, the equivalent full-time student load grew by 8%, from 102 456 to 110 816, and hours spent in clinical environments grew by 8.4%, from 31.9 million to 34.6 million hours.[29] This upwards pressure has led to consideration of a wider range of fieldwork placements, with emphasis on various community settings, different models of clinical supervision and the use of simulation-based education.

One interesting development is the increasing emphasis on peer-assisted learning in clinical supervision. A 2008 systematic review[30] notes the rise in peer-assisted learning, describing the move towards models that maximise the availability of practice education opportunities. This review, which included studies from the United Kingdom, Canada, the United States and Australia, pointed to the advantages of peer-assisted learning but concluded that further research was required. Because of the wide diversity of supervision models across professions, there is a wide range of scope to consider how best this should continue. This type and composition of clinical supervision models is an area where evidence will continue to be interrogated as the cost-benefit issues surrounding clinical placements is set to intensify.

The rise of simulation-based education

Simulation-based education is increasingly becoming part of the health professional education landscape both in Australia and internationally. Simulation-based education allows students to replicate the tasks required in real-life clinical practice in university settings, dedicated simulation facilities or in situ within the clinical environment. It lends itself to standardisation by ensuring that students are at identified levels of competence before entering the clinical environment. The use of simulation is also viewed as a way to reduce medical error and improve patient outcomes.[31] There is an increasing range of evidence to support the value of simulation-based education. The first Australian studies in physiotherapy that indicate the capacity of simulation to replace some clinical placements are starting to emerge,[32] and large-scale studies are underway in nursing in California.[33] However, there are strong arguments that simulation should only supplement and support the practice education experience rather than substitute for it in its entirety, as the 'real' health environments and interactions with 'real' patients cannot be replaced in framing the development of health professionals. Additionally, the relative cost benefits of various simulation modalities remain in question, as simulation can be highly expensive (e.g. cost of manikins or paying patient actors). Given the fiscal imperatives of higher education environments, this may require further investigation.

Interprofessional learning

The specialisation and fragmentation of the healthcare system, coupled with the patient safety movement, has triggered another key trend in health professional education: the rise of interprofessional learning. It is increasingly recognised that healthcare takes place in teams, and learners do not have sufficient exposure to learning to work in multidisciplinary teams. The research into interprofessional learning is rapidly increasing; a 2013 updated systematic review into the effectiveness of interprofessional learning concluded that 6 out of 15 studies reported improved patient outcomes, although all 15 studies had limited study design.[34] The requirement for students to learn in interprofessional environments is increasing as accreditation and registration bodies are setting competencies for teamwork.[35] Governments also are supporting further emphasis on interprofessional education. For example, the Japanese government is supporting the Japan Inter Professional Working and Education Network.[36]

Accreditation and standardisation frameworks and tools

Health professional educators may also increasingly find themselves conversant with stringent multiple accreditation frameworks. Many health professional education courses must meet external requirements as well as internal university-based requirements. These are often accreditation standards mandated by professional bodies such as the Dietetics Association of Australia,[37] British Association of Occupational Therapists and College of Occupational Therapists[38] and the Royal College of Physicians and Surgeons in Canada.[39] The universities may have to meet requirements for coursework such as those as outlined by the Bologna Process.[40] Health professional educators must prepare themselves to work across systems and dedicate a significant workload to meet requirements. At best, these privilege learning and encourage teachers towards excellence. At worst, they become a series of time-consuming and meaningless rituals that must necessarily be completed.

There are benefits to increasingly coordinated systems, such as the capacity to match learning across environments. For example, to again draw from the Australian context, an increasing number of health professions are using national coordinated assessment instruments to rate their students. In particular, the Assessment of Physiotherapy Practice assessment tool[41] is being used at both undergraduate and graduate level.[42] The assessment tool may then serve to 'integrate' the learning across the pre-service and service environments. Evidence to underpin these tools is vital to ensure they are optimal. When considering study outcomes, adapting tools to individual environments with respect to implementation and training systems may also be important.

Professionalisation of the educator

Health professional teachers are increasingly receiving professional development in education, with a growing emphasis on formal educational qualifications. This is, in part, due to the previously discussed, more stringent requirements placed upon academic educators and clinical supervisors alike, to deliver high-quality educational experiences for students. Many universities are now mandating that academic staff complete a formal education qualification as one of the eligibility criteria for permanency and tenure (e.g. master's in health professional education, Graduate Certificate in Higher Education). Drawing on a specific Australian example, Nestel *et al.*[43] describe the National Health Educator Training in Simulation programme, which is delivering foundation education in simulation-based education to a target of around 4500 educators across the nation. More broadly, Tekian and Harris[44] write that the numbers of global master's programmes in health professional or medical education has risen from 12 to 76 in 2012. This 'professionalisation' of health professional educators is an exciting development that deserves further research.

CONCLUSION

Reading, interpreting and applying the evidence in local contexts is often made more challenging by factors beyond the control of individual educators. Budgetary and accreditation factors, and difficulties accessing clinical education environments are often a consequence of broader societal trends rather than an individual institution. Evidence-based education is significant, and educators need sound evidence about the contextual factors affecting higher education and practice education to make informed decisions. When considering evidence, educators must make decisions as to how the local environment affects them. It may be worth considering different forms of evidence synthesis, such as realist synthesis, when assessing the health professional education literature.[45]

SUMMARY POINTS

- Educational evidence should be interpreted in light of local, national and international contexts. Alternative forms of evidence synthesis may be helpful.
- Higher education environments are influenced by globalisation, massification, changes in technology, budgetary constraints and increased accountability.
- Healthcare environments are influenced by the changing nature of healthcare, associated rising costs, workforce pressures, budgetary constraints and increased accountability.
- Health professional education sits at the nexus between higher education and healthcare sectors. Key trends are pressure on clinical placements, simulation-based education, interprofessional learning, a shift towards accreditation and standardisation, and the professionalisation of health professional educators.

REVIEW QUESTIONS

- What global factors for change do higher education and healthcare sectors share?
- What are the key trends in health professional education environments?
- What role can a national government play in affecting health professional education?
- What is the impact of rising accountability on health professional education?

REFLECTIVE QUESTIONS AND EXERCISES

- How does your local environment affect how you interpret, apply or synthesise the educational evidence?
- How, in your environment, is the tension between the need for more efficient low-cost education and quality of educational experience resolved?
- What are the ways in which new technologies can assist?
- How might professional development or formal qualifications assist in your environment?

REFERENCES

1. Altbach PG, Reisberg L, Rumbley LE. *Trends in Global Higher Education: tracking an academic revolution; a report prepared for the UNESCO 2009 World Conference on Higher Education.* Paris: United Nations Educational, Scientific and Cultural Organization; 2009.
2. Eggins H, West P. The global impact of the financial crisis: main trends in developed and developing countries. *High Educ Manage Policy.* 2011; **22**(3): 1–16.
3. Shore C. Audit culture and illiberal governance: universities and the politics of accountability. *Anthropol Theory.* 2008; **8**(3): 278–98.

4. Yuan L, Powell S. *MOOCs and Open Education: implications for higher education.* Available at: http://publications.cetis.ac.uk/2013/667 (accessed 30 April 2013).
5. Breslow L, Pritchard DE, DeBoer J, *et al.* Studying learning in the worldwide classroom: research into edX's first MOOC. *Res Pract Assess.* 2013; **8**: 13–25.
6. Australian Bureau of Statistics. *3101.0 – Australian Demographic Statistics, Mar 2013.* www.abs.gov.au/ausstats/abs@.nsf/mf/3101.0 (accessed 29 October 2013).
7. Organisation for Economic Co-operation and Development. *Education at a Glance 2013 – Indicators and Annexes.* www.oecd.org/education/educationataglance2013-indicatorsandannexes.htm (accessed 29 October 2013).
8. Bradley D, Noonan P, Nugent H, *et al. Review of Australian Higher Education: final report.* Canberra, ACT: Department of Education, Employment and Workplace Relations, Commonwealth of Australia; 2008.
9. Welch A. Opportunistic entrepreneurialism and internationalisation of higher education: lessons from the antipodes? *Global Soc Educ.* 2012; **10**(3): 295–315.
10. Norton A. *Mapping Australian Higher Education.* Melbourne, VIC: Gratton Institute; 2012.
11. Sanderson G. Internationalisation and teaching in higher education. *High Educ Res Dev.* 2011; **30**(5): 661–76.
12. Marsden H, Carroll M, Neill JT. Who cheats at university? A self-report study of dishonest academic behaviours in a sample of Australian university students. *Aust J Psychol.* 2005; **57**(1): 1–10.
13. Hardy I. Academic architectures: academic perceptions of teaching conditions in an Australian university. *Stud High Educ.* 2010; **35**(4): 391–404.
14. Dillon K, Prokesch S. Megatrends in global health care. *Harv Bus Rev*; 2010. Available at: http://hbr.org/web/extras/insight-center/health-care/globaltrends/1-slide (accessed 29 October 2013).
15. Duckett SJ. Health workforce design for the 21st century. *Aust Health Rev.* 2005; **29**(2): 201–10.
16. O'Connell TJ, Ben-Tovim DI, McCaughan BC, *et al.* Health services under siege: the case for clinical process redesign. *Med J Aust.* 2008; **188**(6): S9–13.
17. Wilson RM, Runciman WB, Gibberd RW, *et al.* The Quality in Australian Health Care Study. *Med J Aust.* 1995; **163**(9): 458–71.
18. Jha AK, Larizgoitia I, Audera-Lopez C, *et al.* The global burden of unsafe medical care: analytic modelling of observational studies. *BMJ Qual Saf.* 2013; **22**(10): 809–15.
19. Kodate N. Events, politics and patterns of policy-making: impact of major incidents on health sector regulatory reforms in the UK and Japan. *Soc Policy Admin.* 2012; **46**(3): 280–301.
20. Jabour B. Hospital 'quietly' closing beds, says union. *Brisbane Times.* 2013 Jan 10.
21. Medew J. More bed closures alarm nurses. *Age.* 2013 Jul 16.
22. Duffield C, Diers D, O'Brien-Pallas L, *et al.* Nursing staffing, nursing workload, the work environment and patient outcomes. *Appl Nurs Res.* 2011; **24**(4): 244–55.
23. Mann NC, MacKenzie E, Teitelbaum SD, *et al.* Trauma system structure and viability in the current healthcare environment: a state-by-state assessment. *J Trauma Acute Care Surg.* 2005; **58**(1): 136–47.
24. Loan-Clarke J, Arnold J, Coombs C, *et al.* Retention, turnover and return: a longitudinal study of allied health professionals in Britain. *Hum Res Manage J.* 2010; **20**(4): 391–406.
25. Australian Health Practitioner Regulation Agency (AHPRA). *AHPRA Service Charter.* Melbourne, VIC: AHPRA; 2012. Available at: www.ahpra.gov.au/Publications/Corporate-publications.aspx#service (accessed 9 October 2014).
26. Health Workforce Australia. *Health Workforce 2025 – Doctors, Nurses and Midwives.* www.hwa.gov.au/work-programs/information-analysis-and-planning/health-workforce-planning/hw2025-doctors-nurses-and- (accessed 30 October 2013).
27. Health Workforce Australia. *About Us.* www.hwa.gov.au/about-us (accessed 30 October 2013).

28. Health Workforce Australia. *Expanded Scopes of Practice Program.* www.hwa.gov.au/work-programs/workforce-innovation-and-reform/expanded-scopes-of-practice-project (accessed 30 October 2013).

29. Health Workforce Australia (HWA). *Clinical Training 2012: survey results June 2013.* Adelaide, SA: HWA; 2013. Available at: www.hwa.gov.au/sites/uploads/Clinical-Training-2012.pdf (accessed 30 October 2013).

30. Secomb J. A systematic review of peer teaching and learning in clinical education. *J Clin Nurs.* 2008; **17**(6): 703–16.

31. Aggarwal R, Mytton OT, Derbrew M, *et al.* Training and simulation for patient safety. *Qual Saf Health Care.* 2010; **19**(Suppl. 2): i34–43.

32. Watson K, Wright A, Morris N, *et al.* Can simulation replace part of clinical time? Two parallel randomised controlled trials. *Med Educ.* 2012; **46**(7): 657–67.

33. Hayden J, Kardong-Edgren SE, editors. NCSBN National Simulation Study: first results [presentation]. 13th Annual International Meeting on Simulation in Healthcare; Orlando, FL; 2013 January 26–29 (29).

34. Reeves S, Perrier L, Goldman J, *et al.* Interprofessional education: effects on professional practice and healthcare outcomes (update). *Cochrane Database Syst Rev.* 2013; (3): CD002213.

35. Thistlethwaite J. Interprofessional education: a review of context, learning and the research agenda. *Med Educ.* 2012; **46**(1): 58–70.

36. Global Health Workforce Alliance. *Japan Inter Professional Working and Education Network.* www.who.int/workforcealliance/members_partners/member_list/jipwen/en/index.html (accessed 3 February 2014).

37. http://daa.asn.au

38. www.cot.co.uk

39. www.royalcollege.ca

40. European Universities Association. *What is the Bologna Process?* www.eua.be/eua-work-and-policy-area/building-the-european-higher-education-area/bologna-basics.aspx (accessed 3 February 2014).

41. Dalton M, Davidson M, Keating J. The Assessment of Physiotherapy Practice (APP) is a valid measure of professional competence of physiotherapy students: a cross-sectional study with Rasch analysis. *J Physiother.* 2011; **57**(4): 239–46.

42. Physiotherapy Board of Australia. *Supervision Guidelines for Physiotherapy.* Melbourne, VIC: Physiotherapy Board of Australia; 2012. Available at: www.physiotherapyboard.gov.au/documents/default.aspx?record=WD10%2F1394&dbid=AP&chksum=Dv%2F9p8%2BmgiXfLUz7BUd5Uw%3D%3D (accessed 30 October 2013).

43. Nestel D, Watson M, Bearman M, *et al.* Strategic approaches to simulation-based education: a case study from Australia. *J Health Spec.* 2013; **1**(1): 4–12.

44. Tekian A, Harris I. Preparing health professions education leaders worldwide: a description of masters-level programs. *Med Teach.* 2012; **34**(1): 52–8.

45. Bearman M, Dawson P. Qualitative synthesis and systematic review in health professions education. *Med Educ.* 2013; **47**(3): 252–60.

CHAPTER 4

Evidence-based education and health professional education

·····················

Ted Brown

OVERVIEW

It is essential for academics and practice education supervisors to be conversant with evidence-based education (EBE). This chapter reviews factors that affect EBE in the university sector. Two models of EBE are proposed in this chapter: first, the model of EBE for university students is presented; second, the EBE for health professional students is discussed in the context of tertiary-level education.

CHAPTER OBJECTIVES

Upon completion of this chapter, the reader will be able to:
- define the term 'evidence-based education'
- articulate how EBE can be applied in the context of health professional student education
- describe components of the model of EBE for university students
- identify the features of the model of EBE for health professional students

KEY TERMS: education, best practice, research, scholarship of learning and teaching, knowledge

---

INTRODUCTION

This chapter will present an overview of evidence-based education (EBE) and how it can be applied to the education of health professional students. A definition of EBE will be presented, reasons why EBE is significant will be discussed and then sources of EBE will be considered. Then two models of EBE will be introduced: one related to general EBE and a second, more complex, framework that deals with EBE in a health professional education context.

WHAT IS EVIDENCE-BASED EDUCATION?

A number of formal definitions of evidence-based practice, evidence-based medicine (EBM), evidence-based nursing and so on have been proffered in the empirical literature; however, fewer definitions of EBE have been documented.[1-5] Several similar terms have been used to describe EBE, including evidence-based learning, evidence-based teaching, evidence-based instruction and the scholarship of learning and teaching. In this context, EBE will be used as an all-encompassing term. According to the Wing Institute,[6] EBE is

> a paradigm by which education stakeholders use empirical evidence to make informed decisions about education interventions (policies, practices, and programs) [(p1)]

Ginsberg et al.[7] define EBE as

> an educational approach in which current, high-quality scholarship of teaching and learning (SoTL) research evidence is integrated with pedagogical content knowledge ... and teacher-learner interaction in making education decisions in order to maximize student learning outcomes. [(pp28-29)]

Note Ginsberg et al.[7] refer to the scholarship of teaching and learning (SoTL), whereas in the chapter it is referred to as the scholarship of learning and teaching, or SOLT.

The BEME (Best Evidence Medical Education) Collaboration defines EBE as the

> implementation by teachers and educational bodies in their practice, of methods and approaches to education based on the best evidence available.[8,9(p1)]

In the health professions, many educators are clinicians who practised for a number of years before moving into academia and taking on an educator role. That is, health professional educators hold dual roles, those of a health professional with specific *disciplinary content knowledge* and an educator with *general pedagogical knowledge*. When the health professional educator blends these two components, it is referred to as *pedagogical content knowledge*, a concept formulated by Shulman.[10] This definition fits with the three key elements that Ginsberg et al.[7] propose make up EBE: (1) scholarship of learning and teaching, (2) pedagogical content knowledge and (3) teacher–learner interaction. SoTL/SOLT 'is the best available evidence from systematic SoTL research within and across disciplines'.[7(p29)] Pedagogical content knowledge incorporates the health professional educator's content knowledge (e.g. knowledge unique to that specific health profession) together with the 'knowledge about how to teach and how to teach that content'.[7(p29)] Teacher–learner interaction is the best available evidence from the interaction, which is a reciprocal process. The Wing Institute proposes that EBE has four primary components: (1) promoting best practices research and development, (2) facilitating review and evaluation of scientific research, (3) disseminating scientific research and (4) developing and supporting an evidence-based culture.[6]

Sackett *et al.*[11] consider evidence-based practice or EBM to have three parts: (1) patient values and perspectives; (2) clinical knowledge and expertise of the healthcare practitioner; and (3) best empirical evidence available. If this framework is applied to EBE, then it would involve (1) students' values and perceptions; (2) educators' knowledge and expertise; and (3) the body of relevant empirical education and SOLT best evidence available.[12,13] However, in the academic setting, there are other factors that affect the interaction between student and educator, promoting an EBE culture, and the availability and integration of best evidence into day-to-day classroom, laboratory and fieldwork education practices.

WHY IS EVIDENCE-BASED EDUCATION IMPORTANT?

EBE is important for numerous reasons;[14–18] first and foremost, it ensures that students are receiving a contemporary education that is based on teaching and learning best practices and high-quality empirical evidence.

> The concept behind evidence-based approaches is that education interventions should be evaluated to prove whether they work, and the results should be fed back to influence practice.[6(p1)]

It encourages academics to keep abreast and revise their curricula to make it relevant to the higher education market needs. EBE can make an important contribution to the educational empirical body of knowledge. EBE can ensure that value for money is received, particularly for publicly funded educational institutions. In other words, EBE can ensure that the education that university students receive is cost-effective. Another important reason is that it assists to keep education providers current and competitive in the national and international education market. By getting educators to engage in EBE, this will assist them to become informed consumers of education-related research. It also promotes critical reflection about the different educational methodologies that are used. EBE can also facilitate curriculum refreshing, updating, alignment exercises, benchmarking and internationalisation. EBE can inspire academic staff to engage in SOLT activities. Further, all EBE can provide the underpinnings for optimal learning experiences for students.

EBE is crucial for every educator to change and begin to consciously evaluate what is happening within his or her classroom; make conscious decisions about how to meet the learning outcomes for their students; and maximize student learning and retention of information.[7(p36)]

GENERAL MODEL OF EVIDENCE-BASED EDUCATION

Similar to the general EBM model proposed by Sackett *et al.*,[11] there is a general EBE model proposed for students enrolled in arts and science tertiary education programmes (e.g. anthropology, sociology, history, geography, geology, biology, chemistry, physiology). The EBM model proposed by Sackett *et al.*[11] only had three components, while the general EBE model proposed here is made up of five components: (1) academic educator knowledge, expectations and accountability requirements; (2) student values, needs, perceptions and expectations; (3) scholarship of teaching and learning research evidence and empirical knowledge; (4) university policies and procedures, regulations and quality assurance requirements; and (5) federal, state and local government regulations. These components are illustrated in Figure 4.1. Each of these components exerts a different force and has a different set of obligations that need to be met, but the central theme of this EBE model is that it clearly indicates the need for the teaching and learning of activities of educators to be underpinned by strong empirical evidence. These components are broader than the three proposed by Ginsberg *et al.*[7]

MODEL OF EVIDENCE-BASED EDUCATION FOR HEALTH PROFESSIONAL STUDENTS

Students enrolled in health professional programmes at the university (tertiary) level have a number of other factors that affect their education. This is largely due to the unique requirements of educating future healthcare professionals. These include the need to meet professional competency requirements, being a student member of a professional community, the views that the general public and clients have of the professionals, and the need to complete clinical or professional practice education placements or internships as part of their university education. There is a variety of factors and players that affect the education of health professional students (*see* Table 4.1); hence, there are additional factors that involve the EBE of health professional students. While the general model of EBE for university students has five components, the model of EBE for health professional students has 11 factors: (1) scholarship of teaching and learning evidence; (2) academic educator knowledge, expectations and accountability; (3) practice educator provider expectations and accountability; (4) university policies, regulations and quality assurance requirements; (5) professional registration board and regulatory body requirements; (6) federal, state and local government regulations; (7) education programme accreditation board requirements; (8) student values, needs, perceptions, expectations and preferences; (9) employer, industrial and professional community expectations; (10) state, national and international professional association requirements; and (11) clients, consumers and general public expectations.

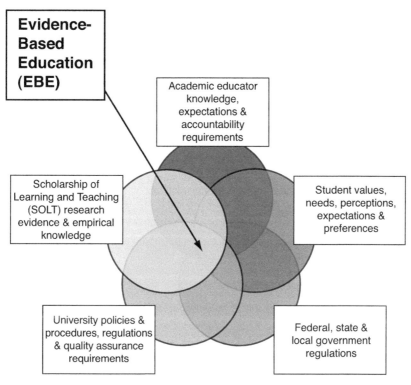

FIGURE 4.1 Model of evidence-based education for university students (© T Brown, 2014)

These components are illustrated in Figure 4.2 and are collectively referred to as the model of EBE for health professional students. For EBE initiatives to be successful, they require 'ongoing, systematic support of scientific research and development of education interventions' and the 'support needs to be financial, institutional, political, and cultural'.[6(p1)] The model of EBE for health professional students includes the many components that are required to be synchronised for EBE initiatives to be successful, relevant, valid and sustainable. Each of these components will now be briefly discussed.

Scholarship of learning and teaching (SOLT) evidence

The SOLT evidence for the health professional student's education can be obtained from several sources, including professional conferences, master's and doctoral dissertations, edited books, peer-reviewed journals and content knowledge experts.[19-23] In order for the SOLT to be successful, a culture of sourcing, critiquing, integrating and then evaluating the use of the evidence in education contexts is needed.

TABLE 4.1 Factors and players affecting evidence-based education (EBE) in the health professions

Factors that affect the EBE process:
- accreditation requirements
- registration board and regulatory body requirements
- research and evidence-based practice traditions within individual healthcare professions
- level of education required to practise (e.g. certificate, diploma, 3- to 4-year undergraduate degree, graduate-entry master's, entry-level clinical doctorate)
- size of profession and number of professionals
- resources of profession: financial, political, personnel
- how well profession is recognised by the general public, funders and other professions
- number of members of profession who have graduate degrees and who are researchers
- body of empirical literature published in education in the profession
- university quality assurance requirements
- government tertiary education regulatory body requirements
- professional education accreditation programme requirements
- professional community, industry and employer requirements
- funding body expectations and requirements

Players who affect the EBE process:
- academic educators
- practice education providers and supervisors
- students: undergraduate and postgraduate; current and past
- funders of education
- journal publishers
- professional associations
- employers and industry
- general public
- professional registration and regulatory bodies
- education programme accreditation bodies
- federal, state and local government
- university policy and procedure requirements

Academic educator knowledge, expectations and accountability

Academic educators who teach in health professional programmes are often members of the specific profession they are teaching about. Often these educators have worked for a period of time in their respective field and then completed additional postgraduate qualifications (often at the master's or doctoral level) when they moved into academia. This group of educators have the opportunity to apply their *pedagogical content knowledge* by combining their previous clinical knowledge and experiences with their current education expertise.[10] Students may view these educators as 'not being current' or as being 'removed from the real life of clinical practice'; however, often these educators are also researchers and active members of their respective professional community (e.g. they may serve as members of a professional association or regulatory body, they may serve on a journal editorial board, they may be on a professional conference organising committee, they may serve as board members in not-for-profit community agencies, they may provide consultation and supervision of students completing practice education placements). Sometimes academic educators also have a cross-appointment with a clinical site where they may work as part-time professionals, consult or supervise students. This helps educators to keep their professional knowledge and skills current and relevant. Academic educators need to be cognisant of and able to apply teaching and learning approaches that are backed up by a body of best research evidence. Often universities will have dedicated centres for teaching and learning (or equivalent) that are able to provide consultations and guidance about where to source the best SOLT evidence.[24,25] This would facilitate the advancement of EBE across the health professional higher education sector.

Practice educator provider expectations and accountability

Another key component of the health professional student EBE model is the role that practice educator providers play in the instruction, orientation and socialisation of student practitioners. In the university classroom environment, students are exposed to theories, models of practice, factual knowledge plus basic practical and professional skills. In the practice education context, students are placed in real-life practice settings where clinicians are working with clients and their families. Students get to put into action what they have studied in the academic environment. Practice education providers are also key socialising agents and role models for students, where they learn what it means to be a professional, to work collaboratively with clients and other service providers, to use the professional terminology and jargon, and to apply their clinical reasoning and problem-solving skills. In many practice-oriented fields, students completing fieldwork education placements often implicitly respond to the professional group cues and quickly learn the nuances of the academic and practice education curriculum expectations.

The methods and strategies used by practice education supervisors need to be underpinned by sound empirical evidence. Often academic educators and practice education providers collaborate on joint research or quality improvement projects. This could be one strategic area where both parties could contribute to the EBE body of knowledge.

University policies, regulations and quality assurance requirements

Universities are the places where student health professionals are accepted into their chosen field of study. This may be at an undergraduate, graduate-entry master's or clinical doctorate level depending on the specific healthcare field. For example, entry-level physiotherapy education in Australia is offered at the undergraduate, master's and clinical doctorate level, whereas occupational therapy is offered at the undergraduate and master's level. Entry-level nursing education in Australia is offered at the diploma, bachelor's and master's level. There has been a move in the United States for many allied health professional entry-level education programmes to move to the clinical doctorate level.[26–28] For example, all physical therapy education programmes in the United States will move to being offered only at the clinical doctorate level (e.g. Doctor of Physical Therapy) by 2018.[28]

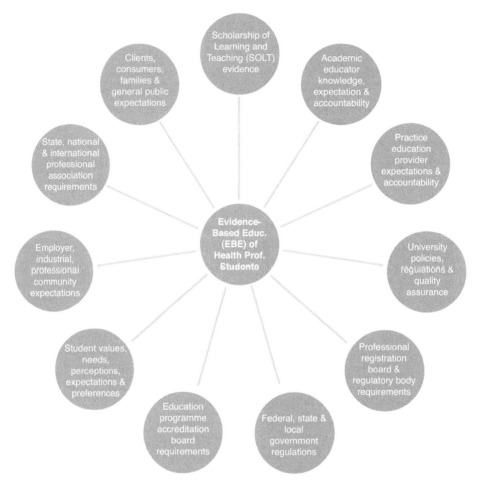

FIGURE 4.2 Model of evidence-based education for health professional students (© T Brown, 2014)

All universities are accountable to a number of internal and external bodies, including the federal and state or provincial governments where they are located. They are answerable to external quality assurance agencies who regulate the higher education sector (e.g. the Tertiary Education Quality and Standards Agency, the Quality Assurance Agency for Higher Education, the Higher Learning Commission of the North Central Association of Colleges and Schools, the Council for Higher Education Accreditation, the United States Department of Education). Also, depending on whether the university is a private or public institution, they are accountable to funders of student education. Universities will also have their own set of internal regulations and quality assurance initiatives that academic programmes have to abide by. For example, if a new academic programme is going to be initiated, a detailed business plan and curriculum outline will need to be submitted to the appropriate department-, school-, faculty- and university-level committees for vetting and approval. Also, most universities have their own round of internal reviews of academic programmes that occur on a cyclical basis (e.g. a programme is reviewed and internally accredited every 5 years by the respective education committee). Another example is that many universities now have statements of graduate attributes that all students who receive a degree from that institution are expected to exhibit (e.g. critical thinking skills, social justice awareness, advanced numeracy and literacy skills). For universities to comply with policy, regulator and quality assurance requirements, they need to operate using best practice EBE principles in the delivery of student education and curricula.

Professional registration board and regulatory body requirements

Professional registration boards (also referred to as regulatory bodies) are established by state or national acts of parliament to protect the public and ensure that profession-als who provide services to the clients and families do so in an ethical manner and that their skills are current. All practising members of a recognised discipline are required to maintain professional registration. For example, all physiotherapists practising in Australia have to maintain membership with the Physiotherapy Board of Australia and all practising occupational therapists in New Zealand have to be members of the Occupational Therapy Board of New Zealand.

Some professions require all new graduates to write a certification examination before they are deemed eligible to practise. In Canada, for example, all occupa-tional therapy graduates are required to write and pass the National Occupational Therapy Certification Examination (NOTCE) that is administered by the Canadian Association of Occupational Therapists. The NOTCE is designed to protect the public by evaluating the application of professional knowledge and professional behaviour of new occupational therapy graduates entering the field in Canada. Passing the NOTCE allows individuals to be eligible for Canadian Association of Occupational Therapists membership and it is a requirement for registration with provincial regulatory bod-ies. Successful completion of certification examinations is often also required for individuals who have completed their professional education in other countries and are seeking employment in other jurisdictions. For example, occupational therapists who are educated outside the United States but are applying to work in US facilities have to sit the Occupational Therapist Registered certification examination that is administered by the National Board for Certification in Occupational Therapy.

Regulatory organisations often will establish codes of ethics and will generate competency statements that members of a profession need to abide by. Professional associations advocate on behalf of the profession, whereas registration boards are designed to represent the best interests of the general public. Education programmes for health professional students need to be aware of professional registration board and regulatory body requirements, and ensure that students are being educated to a standard that meets these requirements. Applying an EBE approach would provide the foundation to ensure that new graduates meet regulatory and registration body requirements.

Federal, state and local government regulations

Federal, state and local governments may establish laws that regulate the scope of practice of healthcare professionals. In addition, governments may pass laws that specify how higher education providers are funded and the rules and regulations that they have to abide by. Higher education may be the domain of federal or state legislation and this varies between countries (e.g. the Australian Department of Education, Employment and Workplace Relations, the United States Department of Education). Acts of parliament often affect how universities are governed, how they are funded, the power of universities to own land and engage in commercial dealings, the authority for universities to award degrees, and how education programmes are delivered to students. Often federal or state governments will pass pieces of legislation to ensure that the curriculum taught to students in the same field, but at different institutions, meets the same baseline requirements. Utilising EBE principles can assist health professional education programmes to stay informed of government regulations that have an impact on them.

Education programme accreditation board requirements

Health professional education programmes are usually accredited by an external accreditation board or agency (e.g. the Commission on Accreditation of Allied Health Education Programmes, the Accreditation Review Commission on Education for Physician Assistants, the Commission on Collegiate Nursing Education). The education programme accreditation agency may be linked with a professional association (e.g. the Accreditation Council for Occupational Therapy Education, which is linked with the American Occupational Therapy Association; the Council on Academic Accreditation in Audiology and Speech-Language Pathology of the American Speech-Language-Hearing Association) or it may be its own independent body (e.g. the Joint Review Committee on Education in Radiologic Technology, the Society for Public Health Education). Universities need to ensure that the education programmes they offer are contemporary, innovative and responsive and that they meet industry standards. Education programme accreditation by a recognised and credible professional body ensures that the curricula taught to health professional students meets the minimum education standards deemed acceptable for that discipline. Education programme accreditation is usually cyclical and is completed every 3–5 years. Documenting EBE activities as part of the accreditation process would provide evidence that health professional education programmes are applying contemporary knowledge and are well informed.

Student values, needs, perceptions, expectations and preferences

Students who select a specific field of study to apply for, and hopefully gain admission into, come to the table with needs, desires, views, opinions, expectations and preferences. This will affect the type of education activities they expect and how they prefer to engage in learning tasks. Students are shaped by the 'generation' they have grown up as part of. Specific labels have been used to identify and characterise various cohorts of students: Boomer Generation, Generation X, Generation Y or Millennial Generation, and Net Generation.[29] This would no doubt have an impact on the expectations, needs and perceptions of students. For example, Generation Y students have some distinct learning preferences and needs that include requiring constant feedback to reinforce their specialness, having high expectations of the relationship with and availability of academic educators, being less comfortable working independently, expecting constant interactions with their peers, and needing clear instructions on what kind of help is acceptable or not in their learning experiences and when performing tasks.[29] Educators need to be aware of the unique traits and needs of the student groups they engage with. Implementing an EBE approach would promote positive outcomes for students by acknowledging their needs and expectations.

Employer, industrial and professional community expectations

There are a number of groups who have direct and indirect effects on an education programme that graduates health professional students. First, there are the employers who hire new graduates from health professional education programmes. They look for specific competencies in new graduates and skills that meet the needs of the agency and the client groups they serve. This can also include the 'professional community' of healthcare professionals that students become a part of once they graduate. The professional community will have certain expectations of behaviour, competency and skills from new graduates. The industrial sector can also affect the student EBE. For example, new graduates may opt to become members of a collective bargaining unit who represents and advocates for specific staff groups. Application of an EBE orientation will assist health professional education programmes to be current and contemporary with regard to employer and professional community expectations.

State, national and international professional association requirements

State, national and international professional associations are established to promote and benefit members of the respective professional group. Each profession will have local, national and international professional associations that education programmes will have direct links with. For example, in the United States there are state-level professional associations of occupational therapy, one national organisation known as the American Occupational Therapy Association, and an international occupational therapy organisation referred to the World Federation of Occupational Therapists. The American Occupational Therapy Association has input into the accreditation of occupational therapy education programmes plus the World Federation of Occupational Therapists specifies that students must complete 1000 hours of practice education fieldwork to qualify and be recognised as an occupational therapist.[30] Often, professional associations encourage students to join as 'student members' and offer them benefits such as discounted conference registration fees or journal subscriptions. Engaging in an EBE approach will promote positive linkages between health professional education programmes and local, national and international professional associations. It will also ensure that education standards are of a level that will facilitate the movement of health professional graduates between countries to practise.

Clients, consumers and general public expectations

The final significant group that affects EBE are the clients (and their families) and consumers of health professional services. Health professional students engage in a long process of education and training so that they can provide expert services to clients and families. The general public has come to expect a certain level of skills, expertise and decorum from healthcare staff and students. Individuals who receive healthcare services from agencies linked with universities often will encounter healthcare students completing practice education placements. Clients and consumers are more informed and assertive in asking questions and requesting information so that they can make informed decisions about the care they receive. Taking on board an EBE approach would promote positive and informed exchanges between health professional students, clients and members of the public.

EBE IN HEALTH PROFESSIONAL EDUCATION

The education of health professional students is unique in several respects. Usually students who are selected into health professional courses are high achieving and have an orientation towards helping people. Students enrolled in a health professional course have also opted into a 'profession' and are socialised into their respective field. Professional courses are unique in that they combine academic education with practice education. Students learn theoretical knowledge and some practical skills, and then they get to apply the knowledge and skills in real-life practice settings with clients and families that students will work with as new graduates. Most students in professional programmes are required to complete a prescribed number of hours in a practice setting. Hence education research completed in the health professional education arena needs to reflect the unique features of the combination of academic education with practice education. There is a large body of research in the area of medical[31-33] and nursing education,[34-36] but smaller bodies of research exist for the other health-related professions.

One source of information is from the BEME Collaboration,[37] an international collaboration between universities and professional organisations devoted to the development of medical and health professional education informed by sound evidence through:

> the dissemination of information which allows teachers and stakeholders in the medical and health professions to make decisions on the basis of the best evidence available; the production of systematic reviews which present the best available evidence and meet the needs of the user; and the creation of a culture of best evidence education amongst individuals, institutions and national bodies.[38(p1)]

Medicine has the largest number of peer-reviewed journals in the area of clinical, academic and professional education. Examples of these include *Medical Education, Medical Teacher, Teaching and Learning in Medicine, British Journal of Medical*

Education, Canadian Medical Education Journal and *Journal of Graduate Medical Education.* Several medical specialties also have their specific education-focused peer-reviewed journals, including *Academic Psychiatry, Academic Radiology* and *Journal of Surgical Education.* Nursing also has a number of refereed journals dedicated to education, and examples of these include *International Journal of Nursing Education Scholarship, Journal of Nursing Education, Journal of Nursing Education and Practice, Nurse Education Today* and *Nurse Education in Practice.* Several centres for nursing education research have been established. For example, the Centre for Research in Nursing and Midwifery Education is located in the School of Health and Social Care, Faculty of Health and Medical Sciences at the University of Surrey in the United Kingdom. Its primary mandate is to support the research strategy around education-focused research. Located at Indiana University in the United States, the mission of the Center for Research in Nursing Education is to develop, evaluate and disseminate new pedagogies for nursing education.

Pharmacy as a profession publishes a number of journals that focus on education, including *Currents in Pharmacy Teaching and Learning, International Journal of Pharmacy Teaching and Practices, International Journal of Pharmacy Education, Journal of the Asian Association of Schools of Pharmacy, Journal of Pharmacy Teaching* and *Pharmacy Education.* Some of the smaller allied health professions have single journals dedicated to education in their field. Examples of these include *Perspectives on Physician Assistant Education, Optometric Education, Journal of Chiropractic Education, Journal of Podiatric Medical Education* and *Journal of Physical Therapy Education.* There are several health professions that have no journals dedicated to the scholarship of learning and teaching in their respective fields, including speech therapy, audiology, respiratory therapy, radiography and medical imaging, and occupational therapy. There are a number of general health professional education journals that publish empirical work that could inform EBE. Some of these publications include *Advances in Health Sciences Education, Evaluation and the Health Professions, Internet Journal of Allied Health Sciences, Journal of Allied Health, Journal of Clinical Problem-Based Learning* and *Journal of Continuing Education in the Health Professions.*

CONCLUSION

The focus on EBE in health professional education is growing, but there is still much groundwork that needs to be done.[39-41] In this chapter, a broad introduction to general EBE and EBE specific to health professional education was provided. A model of general EBE for higher education and a model of EBE for health professional students was presented. Given the importance of EBE, further details of this topic will be provided in later chapters in this book. In summary, 'if our goal as educators is to maximize learning in our students, then we need to use EBE to do so'.[7(p1)]

SUMMARY POINTS

- EBE is the application of best empirical evidence that helps inform in the education of students.
- EBE is significant for a number of reasons but, more importantly, it improves the quality of teaching and instructions that students are exposed to and it encourages educators to become informed, critical consumers of education-related research.
- Two models of EBE have been proposed: (1) the model of EBE for university students and (2) the model of evidence-based education for health professional students.

REVIEW QUESTIONS

- What is EBE?
- Why is EBE important?
- How is EBE similar and how is it different to evidence-based practice?
- What factors contribute to EBE of health professional students?
- Who are some of the primary 'players' that affect the education of health professional students?
- What are the components of the general model of EBE?

REFLECTIVE QUESTIONS AND EXERCISES

- Think of factors that affect EBE in your setting.
- What are some facilitators of EBE where you are employed?
- What are some inhibitors of EBE in your setting?

REFERENCES

1. Buskist W, Groccia JE, editors. *Evidence-Based Teaching: new directions in teaching and learning.* Number 128. San Francisco, CA: Wiley Subscription Services; 2011.
2. Cannon S, Boswell C. *Evidence-Based Teaching in Nursing: a foundation for educators.* Sudbury, MA: Jones & Bartlett Learning; 2012.
3. Davies P. What is evidence-based education? *Br J Educ Stud.* 1999; **47**(2): 108–21.
4. Emerson RJ, Records K. Today's challenge, tomorrow's excellence: the practice of evidence-based education. *J Nurs Educ.* 2008; **47**(8): 359–70.
5. Mennin SP, McGrew MC. Scholarship in teaching and best evidence medical education: synergy for teaching and learning. *Med Teach.* 2000; **22**(5): 468–72.
6. The Wing Institute. *What is Evidence-Based Education?* www.winginstitute.org/Evidence-Based-Education/what-is-evidence-based-education (accessed 25 March 2013).

7. Ginsberg SM, Friberg J, Visconti C. *Scholarship of Teaching and Learning in Speech-Language Pathology and Audiology: evidence-based education.* San Diego, CA: Plural Publishing; 2012.

8. Harden RM, Grant J, Buckley G, *et al.* BEME Guide No. 1: best evidence medical education. *Med Teach.* 1999; **21**(6): 553–62.

9. Harden RM, Lilley PM. Best evidence medical education: the simple truth. *Med Teach.* 2000; **22**(2): 117–19.

10. Shulman LS. Knowledge and teaching: foundations of the new reform. *Harvard Educ Rev.* 1987; **57**(1): 1–22.

11. Sackett DL, Straus SE, Richardson WS, *et al. Evidence-Based Medicine: how to practice and teach EBM.* 2nd ed. London: Churchill Livingstone; 2000.

12. Boet S, Sharma S, Goldman J, *et al.* Medical education research: an overview of methods. *Can J Anaesth.* 2012; **59**(2): 159–70.

13. Greenhalgh T, Toon P, Russell J, *et al.* Transferability of principles of evidence based medicine to improve educational quality: systematic review and case study of an online course in primary health care. *BMJ.* 2003; **326**(7381): 142–5.

14. Beck DE. Pharmacy educators: can an evidence-based approach make your instruction better tomorrow than today? *Am J Pharm Educ.* 2002; **66**(1): 87–8.

15. Ferguson L, Day RA. Evidence-based nursing education: myth or reality? *J Nurs Educ.* 2005; **44**(3): 107–15.

16. Loyola S. Evidence-based teaching guidelines: transforming knowledge into practice for better outcomes in healthcare. *Crit Care Nurs Q.* 2010; **33**(1): 19–23.

17. Petersen S. Time for evidence based medical education. *BMJ.* 1999; **318**(7193): 1223–4.

18. Hammick M. Evidence informed education in the health care sciences professions. *J Vet Med Educ.* 2005; **32**(4): 339–403.

19. Hammer DP, Sauer DA, Fielding DW, *et al.* White Paper on best evidence pharmacy education (BEPE). *Am J Pharm Educ.* 2004; **68**(1): 24.

20. Lilly P, Anderson B, Buckley G, *et al.* Best Evidence Medical Education (BEME): report of meeting – 3–5 December 1999, London, UK. *Med Teach.* 2000; **22**(3): 242–5.

21. Becker WE, Andrews ML. *The Scholarship of Teaching and Learning in Higher Education: contributions of universities.* Indianapolis: Indiana University Press; 2004.

22. Foreman-Peck L, Winch C. *Using Educational Research to Inform Practice: a practical guide to practitioner research in universities and colleges.* New York, NY: Routledge; 2010.

23. Harden RM, Grant J, Buckley G, *et al.* Best evidence medical education. *Adv Health Sci Educ.* 2000; **5**(1): 71–90.

24. Slavin RE. Evidence-based education policies: transforming educational practice and research. *Educ Res.* 2002; **31**(7): 15–21.

25. Vos SJ. Evidence-based education: a fad or the future? *J Evid Based Dent Pract.* 2008; **8**(3): 164–75.

26. Clement DG. Impact of the clinical doctorate from an allied health perspective. *AANA J.* 2005; **73**(1): 24–8.

27. Mundinger M, Starck P, Hathaway D, *et al.* The ABCs of the doctor of nursing practice: assessing resources, building a culture of clinical scholarship, curricular models. *J Prof Nurs.* 2009; **25**(2): 69–74.

28. Royeen CB, Lavin MA. A contextual and logical analysis of the clinical doctorate for health practitioners: dilemma, delusion, or de factor? *J Allied Health.* 2007; **36**(2): 101–6.

29. Ginsburg DB. *Teaching Across the Generations: challenges and opportunities for preceptors.* Austin: College of Pharmacy, The University of Texas at Austin; n.d. Available at: www.pharmacy.utah.edu/pharmacotherapy/adjunct/pdf/Ginsburg_Generation_Preceptor_Presentation_Utah.pdf (accessed 25 March 2013).

30. Hocking C, Ness NE. *WFOT Revised Minimum Standards for the Education of Occupational Therapists.* Sydney, NSW: World Federation of Occupational Therapists; 2002.

31. Salerno-Kennedy R, O'Flynn S. *Medical Education: the state of the art*. Hauppauge, NY: Nova Science Publishers; 2010.

32. Amin Z, Eng HK. *Basics in Medical Education*. London: World Scientific Publishing; 2009.

33. Calman KC. *Medical Education: past, present, and future: handing on learning*. Chatswood, NSW: Churchill Livingstone/Elsevier; 2007.

34. Stevens KR, Cassidy VR. *Evidence-Based Teaching: current research in nursing education*. San Diego, CA: Plural Publishing; 1999.

35. Oermann MH, Gaberson KB. *Evaluation and Testing in Nursing Education*. New York, NY: Springer; 2009.

36. Oermann MH, Heinrich KT. *Annual Review of Nursing Education: strategies for teaching, assessment, and program planning*. Volume 3. New York, NY: Springer; 2005.

37. Thistlethwaite J, Mammick M. The Best Evidence Medical Education (BEME) Collaboration: into the next decade. *Med Teach*. 2010; **32**(11): 880–2.

38. BEME. *The BEME Collaboration*. www.bemecollaboration.org/About+BEME/ (accessed 5 April 2013).

39. Davies P. Approaches to evidence-based teaching. *Med Teach*. 2000; **22**(1): 14–21.

40. McCartney PR, Morin KH. Where is the evidence for teaching methods used in nursing education? *MCN Am J Matern Child Nurs*. 2005; **30**(6): 406–12.

41. Thomas G, Pring R. *Evidence-Based Practice in Education*. Maidenhead, Berkshire: McGraw-Hill Education, Open University Press; 2004.

CHAPTER 5

Finding the evidence for health professional evidence-based education

....

Allie Ford, Paula Todd and Ted Brown

OVERVIEW

This chapter will outline the information research process needed to investigate educational concepts from an evidence-based perspective. The different methods for creating a research question, searching tips and sources of evidence, types of reviews available, and suggestions for critiquing and documenting the evidence will be discussed. Three case studies are provided to illustrate different search purposes and methodologies.

CHAPTER OBJECTIVES

Upon completion of this chapter, the reader will be able to:
- construct an answerable research question using an appropriate mnemonic
- build and document a replicable search strategy
- identify the study type or types most appropriate for the research he or she is undertaking
- appraise evidence that relates to his or her research question.

KEY TERMS: review, search strategy, critical appraisal, research question, information research

INTRODUCTION

Getting started with evidence based education (EBE) can be difficult, especially for researchers or teachers who have not looked at education-focused academic literature before. Sometimes a new vocabulary is needed in order to find and read articles, and databases or journals that target education-focused literature might be different to those a student is more familiar with using. It is important to follow a systematic process, and to make appropriate and smart selections about tools, scopes, terminology and methodology throughout the process. Just like with anything else, you should start small and find your way around the process, developing the necessary skills, before taking on a full-scale systematic review (please refer to the glossary at the end of this chapter for definitions of different review types). EBE involves a number of steps that are outlined in Figure 5.1. Steps 1 through 4 will be covered in detail in this chapter.

STEP 1: FORMULATING THE QUESTION

What is your aim?

The aim is the general intention of the research, and objectives state how the aim is to be accomplished. It is beneficial to outline the aims and objectives before deciding on a research question, as this will help you to define what you are trying to achieve. Try to be specific, as this will refine and focus your search. From a searching perspective it is easier to broaden your search from a narrow focus than to refine from a really broad topic (*see* 'Case study: David (Predictive)' later in this chapter).

Background reading

Find out more about your ideas and possibilities. Particularly, take note of previous research on your topic – has someone done this before? What is the history and what are the future trends? Do you understand all the terminology? Is it useful to provide a definition of your topic as you understand it?

Consider the purpose of your search

- Are you establishing gaps in the scholarly literature for further investigation?
- Are you increasing your understanding of the research area?
- Are you identifying methodologies?
- Is there more than one aspect to your research, as these may require more than one search strategy? (*See* 'Case study: Kerry (Exploration)' later in this chapter)
- Has your background reading of established knowledge identified other search terms?
- What levels of evidence do you need?
- Are you considering what new research has been done (primary sources)?
- Are you establishing an overview of existing research (secondary sources)? (*See* 'Case study: David (Predictive)' later in this chapter)

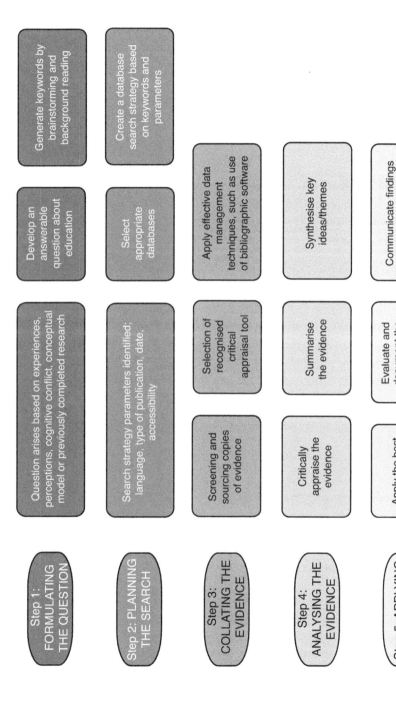

FIGURE 5.1 The evidence-based education process includes five main steps, with several actions necessary at each stage; the process does not always flow linearly, and cycling back to previous stages is often necessary

Construct a research question that is answerable

This is where your aims and objectives will help you develop a research question. This step sounds simple but it is often quite complex. There are a few methods for developing research questions but the principles of drawing concepts out of the research and applying parameters to focus and build a question remain the same. The method may be determined by the type of questions being considered. Eldredge[1] outlines three types of questions.

1. Prediction questions: *will* specific factors affect key outcomes and by how much?
2. Intervention questions: *which* interventions are (most) effective in achieving desired outcomes?
3. Exploration questions: *why/how* do specific factors affect key outcomes?

PICO*[2] is a method commonly used in the health environment to create answerable clinical questions, usually around a treatment or other medical intervention, but it can be applied equally successfully in education. It breaks the research idea into four component parts or concepts:

> **P** = population or problem (what is the issue you are addressing or what group are you focusing on?)
> **I** = intervention or indicator (what is one option you could apply to the problem?)
> **C** = comparison or control (a second possible option as a comparison, or a control group)
> **O** = outcome (what is the measurable result – positive or negative – of applying the intervention?)

If the research question does not fit neatly into a PICO structure, other mnemonics that might be helpful include CLIP or ECLIPSe[3] and SPICE.[4]
CLIP or ECLIPSe:

> **E** = expectation (what is the research going to address?)
> **C** = client group (who are the recipients?)
> **L** = location (the setting being considered?)
> **I** = impact (what is the change expected?)
> **P** = professionals (who is involved?)
> **Se** = service (what part of the organisation will the change impact?).

SPICE:

> **S** = setting (where?)
> **P** = perspective (who is the research intended for?)
> **I** = intervention (what is being considered?)

---

* Sometimes PICO may appear with an additional letter: PICOR (research type), PICOT (time frame) or PICOS (study design). The question would then become 'in (population or problem), does (indicator or intervention) compared with (comparison or control) result in (outcome)?'

C = comparison (what is the alternative to the intervention?)
E = evaluation (the result and its implications).

Regardless of which method is chosen, it is useful to think of your research question as a series of concepts that build into a searchable question. This also serves as a starting point for using two or more concepts for searching.

Concept 1		Concept 2		Concept 3		Concept 4
OR (synonym C1)	AND	OR (synonym C2)	AND	OR (synonym C3)	AND	OR (synonym C4)
OR		OR		OR		OR

STEP 2: PLANNING THE SEARCH
Brainstorm for synonyms or alternative terms for each concept of your search

- It is not necessary to search for all components of a PICO (or other mnemonic) but it is usual to search for at least two.
- Keep the concepts simple and create a table of 'word sets' for each concept (i.e. words rather than whole sentences, nouns rather than verbs).
- Link search terms for the *same* concept with 'OR' to broaden the search.
- Link search terms for *different* concepts with 'AND' to make the search more specific.
- Be prepared to add other terms as you read through initial search results.

Select databases
Select databases according to the focus of your research. For a comprehensive search you should aim for around four to five databases. The search tools selected will also be dependent upon your circumstances and access to information in subscriber databases or whether it is freely available on the Web. A list of key sources in health education, including several open access publications, is provided in Table 5.1.

Background searching
An initial search of a key database can be useful to define the search parameters and identify additional keywords and synonyms. It can indicate the depth and breadth of your topic, which will assist in setting appropriate limits. Searching is not a linear process, it is often a circular procedure, requiring repetition of different steps until you are satisfied that the terms used are the most relevant and effective for finding on-topic results.

Search databases
Search databases separately rather than several at a time, to make the most of database features and thesauri.
- Save your searches. Most databases will allow you to register an account for free.

You can then save your search history and searches to re-run them later, as well as receiving notifications of new articles that meet your search criteria (in some databases).

- Search for each concept separately. Use the database search history to combine your concept searches to allow flexibility when refining your search.
- Use a database's thesaurus if available (such as MeSH for MEDLINE) to determine any appropriate subject headings. These provide a consistent list of headings to label records and enable precise searching, but they are usually database specific.
- Use keyword searching in addition to any thesaurus terms, which will match search terms to most of the text fields in a record. This will provide broader coverage with the following proviso:
  — use subject-heading-only (MeSH) searches where keywords may be common or ambiguous
  — use keyword-only searches if there are no approximate subject terms available.
- Consider advanced search options such as truncation, wildcards, proximity searching (with keyword searches) and phrase searching (NB: the symbols for these options may vary between databases, so check the 'help' functions in each one):
  — truncation replaces the end of a word (e.g. *educat** will retrieve educate, education, educators, educates, educative)
  — wildcards replace letters (e.g. *p#ediatric* will retrieve paediatric, pediatric)
  — proximity searching specifies the distance between search terms (e.g. *health adj(x) education* will find *health* within (x) words of *education*)
  — phrase searching is useful where you wish the words to be located together and in the order that they appear within the quotation marks (e.g. 'evidence-based education').
- Focus your search by applying limits. The exact limits available may be specific to each database, but most include year of publication, age or population groups and publication type. Other limits available in some databases include methodology and levels of evidence.
- Treat your searches as drafts. Refine as you go by looking for additional subject headings or keywords in the abstracts of articles returned. If you are finding irrelevant articles, look at your search terms for any ambiguity. You may need to substitute or remove a term.
- Make note of any additional terms not used in previous database searches. Consider revising earlier searches with these terms.
- Search the grey literature (unpublished material, e.g. technical reports, theses). *See* Table 5.1 for useful resources.
- Use the articles returned from your searches to find other references:
  — use the reference lists at the end of articles.
  — use 'cited reference' searching
  — identify prominent authors in search results and use author searching
  — cross-check key articles in databases to make sure your key terms retrieve these; if not, then look for the search terms you are missing (note, however, that each

database does subscribe to different publishers and journals, so not all articles will be accessible on all platforms).

- Manage your references using bibliographic software to store and annotate your references.
- Create alerts for your saved searches and 'table of contents' alerts for key journals.
- Consider contacting an experienced librarian who can assist you in building a search strategy.

Review search findings

As part of good researching techniques, be prepared to modify your research question and search strategy. Consider further refining your search or question by adding other keywords or concepts or applying more limits if you are retrieving too many results. If you are retrieving too few results, you might need to broaden your question or include additional synonyms. If there are significant gaps in the literature, you might need to include other sources such as grey literature.

Additional sources of evidence

Depending on the information required and the purpose of your search, it is sometimes important to extend the range of sources included into the area of 'grey literature'. This includes recent publications outside journals and books. Patent and technical reports, White Papers, reports from working groups and pre-prints are some examples of such grey literature that might contain useful and relevant information. These can be accessed through the websites of relevant agencies, searches on the open Web, or by contacting relevant authors directly. Conference presentations and presenters can be useful in identifying additional sources of information that might not otherwise be considered or accessible.

Data management

Keep records of your search strategies for each database, as this will allow you to revise searches easily and determine how each result was retrieved. Another useful tip is to print the search screen and put it into a word document, together with any notes about your findings or strategy, or reflections on the process.

Reference management software (such as EndNote[5]) will enable you to sort and manage citations and store full text PDFs. Make sure you keep backups of your work, including citations and other documentation in at least three separate physical and/ or digital locations.

TABLE 5.1 Useful resources for searching and evaluating evidence

Databases (subscriber sources)
- CINAHL (Cumulative Index to Nursing and Allied Health Literature)
- Embase
- ERIC (Education Resources Information Center)
- Informit Education
- MEDLINE
- PsycINFO
- ProQuest Education databases (ProQuest Central)
- Scopus
- Web of Science

Open Web sources, repositories and search engines
- Bandolier (www.medicine.ox.ac.uk/bandolier/)
- BestBETs (http://bestbets.org)
- BioMed Central (www.biomedcentral.com)
- Cochrane Library (www.thecochranelibrary.com/view/0/index.html)
- Directory of Open Access Journals (http://doaj.org)
- ERIC: Institute of Education Sciences (http://eric.ed.gov)
- Free Medical Journals (http://freemedicaljournals.com)
- Health Topics Collection (www.g-i-n.net/library/health-topics-collection)
- HighWire Press (http://highwire.stanford.edu/lists/freeart.dtl)
- MedKnow (www.medknow.com/)
- Mednar (http://mednar.com/mednar) Deep web medical search engine
- National Academies Press (www.nap.edu/content/help/about.html)
- PEDro, Physiotherapy Evidence Database (www.pedro.org.au) Physiotherapy Evidence database
- PLOS (Public Library of Science) (www.plos.org)
- PubMed (www.ncbi.nlm.nih.gov/pubmed)
- Trip (www.tripdatabase.com/index.html)

Theses
- EThOS (UK doctoral theses) (http://ethos.bl.uk)
- ProQuest Dissertations and Theses (worldwide; subscription required) (www.proquest.com/products-services/pqdt.html)
- Trove (Australian theses) (http://trove.nla.gov.au/general/theses)
- Library and Archives Canada (www.collectionscanada.gc.ca/thesescanada/index-e.html)
- The US Library of Congress hosts an annotated bibliography of thesis-access sites from around the world at www.loc.gov/rr/main/alcove9/education/theses.html

Grey literature search
- OpenDOAR (www.opendoar.org)
- OpenSIGLE (www.greynet.org/opensiglerepository.html)
- Grey Literature Report (www.greylit.org)
- Web of Science (conference proceedings)

Status of journal publications
- Ulrichsweb Global Serials Directory (subscriber database, http://ulrichsweb.serialssolutions.com): to check the scientific status or academic merit of a journal publication
- Beall's List of Predatory Publishers (http://scholarlyoa.com), also known as vanity publishers – they produce material that is presented as 'open access' but then charge authors fees to accept and publish in order to generate profit. Many of these publications offer little or no peer review.

Case study: Kerry (Exploration)

Kerry has a PhD in nursing so has a research background but she is new to teaching. She has taken over a unit where the previous assessments do not reflect the key learning objectives and Kerry wishes to look at other forms of assessment that may be more suitable. She feels that preparing her own annotated bibliography on techniques for assessing healthcare students will not only assist her in making informed choices but also form the basis of a good paper to present at an upcoming health conference. Kerry uses the ECLIPSe acronym to clarify her research question.

Research question (Exploration): In a first-year undergraduate nursing unit run as part of a course at EBE University, what types of assessments can be used to improve engagement and performance of clinical tasks during practical labs?

E: Assessment types
C: Undergraduate nursing students
L: Practical nursing unit labs
I: Improved engagement and performance of clinical tasks
P: Nursing lecturers
Se: EBE University nursing course

A preliminary search in CINAHL did not retrieve any relevant results in an academic setting, as the keyword 'assessment' mainly retrieved articles relating to assessment of the patient. ERIC retrieved more relevant results, with combinations of search terms including the following.

Concept 1	Concept 2	Concept 3
assessment	course objectives	nurs*
peer assessment	key learning objectives	
performance based assessment	nursing education	
competency based assessment	practical nursing	
group based assessment		
authentic assessment		
contextually based assessment		
student evaluation		
test construction		
measurement techniques		
educational testing		
simulation		
checklist		

This search retrieved a number of relevant articles to allow Kerry to start her annotated bibliography, and the thesaurus terms and keywords from the citations and abstracts added to her list of concept words. The university she works for uses EndNote,[5] so Kerry creates a library of citations and starts summarising the articles in the bibliographic software by creating groups matching the themes of assessment she begins to identify. Kerry also sets up database alerts to inform her of new articles published that match her searches. She considers other databases to include, such as ProQuest Education and Informit Education (Australasian), to broaden the results and she is keen to see if there are any other search terms she has not found before.

Case study: David (Predictive)

David is an experienced paramedic lecturer with years of on-the-job training combined with several years of teaching in an academic setting. He wants to update his lectures to increase student engagement and has heard the phrase 'blended learning' mentioned in the staff room. He feels that a scoping review of the literature would be beneficial in order to understand the implications of a shift in pedagogy and to share this evidence with his faculty team. David uses the SPICE acronym for setting up his research question.

Research question: Will blended learning be more effective than the traditional lecture model in improving the engagement of part-time postgraduate paramedic students at EBE University?

S: EBE University
P: Part-time postgraduate paramedic students
I: Blended learning
C: Traditional lecture model
E: Student engagement

Some background questions that David considers when formulating his question:
● What is blended learning?
● How is blended learning done?
● How does blended learning differ from lectures?
● Is blended learning linked to student engagement?
● How can we measure effectiveness of teaching strategies?

blended learning	curriculum design	engagement	student
technology mediated instruction	curriculum development	motivation	
web enhanced instruction	classroom management	attitude	
computer mediated activities	classroom instruction	voice	
mixed mode instruction			
flipped classroom			
eLearning			

David starts his search with A+ Education (an Australasian database) and primarily uses 'blended learning' as a search term together with combinations of keywords from the other concepts. His background reading reveals that the concept of blended learning has been around since the turn of the twenty-first century, so he decides to limit to the last 5 years. He is particularly interested in those articles that discuss outcomes of applying the concept of blended learning, rather than discussing specific methods of implementation, so the combination of date limits and keywords enables his search results to be more focused.

Including other databases such as ERIC and ProQuest Education reveals more articles and conference papers on the topic, so he also decides to include some grey literature sources with up-to-date expert opinion from other academics and educational designers. He keeps a table of citations listed under 'advantages' and 'disadvantages' of blended learning, together with his annotations and critiques of the methodologies.

Case study: Maria (Intervention)

Maria is an occupational therapy clinical educator responsible for supervising placement students in a community health centre. She is a keen evidence-based practitioner but wants to extend this into her educational role for her students, as well as sharing knowledge with the other allied health professionals in the clinic. The close working nature of the centre and its interdisciplinary communication culture means that these professionals are open to new ideas such as journal clubs, to help build a better understanding of what each member of the team does and improve referrals for patients with complex needs. Maria takes the initiative to find out more about using journal clubs in student education, with the idea that she will share her findings with the other professionals. Maria uses PICO to format her research question, with C as 'control' (i.e. no intervention).

Question: Do journal clubs improve engagement with research evidence for allied health practitioners?

P: Allied health practitioners
I: Journal clubs
C: N/A
O: engagement with research evidence

Maria's centre does not subscribe to academic databases, so she does most of her research using open access journals and databases. She starts with the Database of Open Access Journals. As the search interface for this database is quite basic, she decides to start with the search 'journal club' AND 'allied health'. Luckily this returns two useful articles that she can use as a starting point.

As she reads the articles she has found, Maria notes where citations point towards other interesting publications on the topic, and she also notes which authors regularly publish in this area so she can search for other works they have written. She then distributes the collection of retrieved articles among members of the clinic, including two placement students, asking everyone to write a brief summary and critique of their article to present and bring together at their first journal club in a few weeks' time.

STEP 3: COLLATING THE EVIDENCE

Evidence sources can be classified as primary, secondary or tertiary, depending on their relation to original research studies. Primary literature comprises original reports about an individual study, written by researchers closely involved with the design, conduct and analysis of the investigation. Journal articles, conference papers, reports and theses form the bulk of primary sources. Secondary sources provide critical commentary on primary sources, with emphasis on synthesising, evaluating or rating primary evidence within a body of evidence. Examples of secondary literature include literature reviews, systematic reviews or scoping reviews. Annotated bibliographies are also secondary studies, although these focus on describing (and sometimes critically analysing) the content of individual articles without significant synthesis. Meta-analyses, where related data from a range of primary studies are collated, statistically aligned and evaluated as a new data set, are at the intersection of primary and secondary literature: authors of these analyses do not collect any original data themselves, but location and collection of the original studies, and processing of the data are both original steps analogous to novel research.

Tertiary information, including textbooks, newspaper articles, encyclopaedias, many websites and some reports, is rarely used as evidence. Fully comprehensive reviews might include information from these sources, however, as might discussions of cultural or social relevance. Tertiary sources can be useful for background reading and idea generation, as well as obtaining unique perspectives, but they do not themselves constitute reliable evidence of efficacy.

In addition to the relation between the authors and the primary content of an article, a number of other factors should be considered when evaluating sources. Various acronyms have been developed to assist with evaluating information (often designed for online information, although the same criteria apply to most sources). These acronyms include:

CARS: Currency, Accuracy, Reasonableness, Support[6,7]
CRITIC: Claim, Role of claimant, Information backing the claim, Testing of the claim, Independent verification, Conclusion[8,9(both adapted from 10)]
RADCAB: Relevance, Appropriateness, Detail, Currency, Authority, Bias.[11]

Peer review

Not all evidence is equal. Material presented in peer-reviewed sources is generally considered to be more reliable than similar information that has not been subject to the peer-review process. Peer-reviewed sources include research articles in peer-reviewed journals, chapters in edited academic books and peer-reviewed proceedings of conferences. The Ulrichsweb Global Serials Directory (*see* Table 5.1) includes an identifier noting whether a particular publication uses peer review. While peer review is not infallible,[12] it does provide a degree of quality control. Theses submitted in fulfilment of the requirements for tertiary qualifications are also considered peer reviewed, as external authorities have evaluated the content. Theses can be accessed through various databases (*see* Table 5.1).

Vanity publishing, predatory publishing and crowdsourced peer review

One important caution relates to an increasing prevalence of 'vanity publishers' who will accept and publish articles with cursory or no peer review, and often with publication titles very similar to reputable journals in the field. Commonly these entities charge authors fees in order to publish. They sometimes extend an option to publish articles not accepted through peer review, offering the authors exposure via an open access platform linked to the journal. Some sites suggest to authors that these platforms allow for crowdsourced peer review, with readers able to rate and discuss articles through 'comments'. While some of these sites are run by reputable publishers (e.g. www.mededworld.org/MedEdWorld-Papers.aspx), the commenters on these systems are not guaranteed to have any knowledge of the specific area or field covered in an article, so such 'reviews' or feedback must also be evaluated carefully. Ulrichsweb and Beall's List of Predatory Publishers (*see* Table 5.1) both provide information on the credibility of various publications.

STEP 4: ANALYSING THE EVIDENCE
Levels of evidence

Numerous systems exist for evaluating the quality of sources included in an analysis. Many studies focus exclusively on either quantitative or qualitative evidence, so different hierarchies of evidence have been established for each data type. Even when considering a specific type of data, it is important to select appraisal tools that match your aims and objectives, as each tool targets slightly different things.

Some examples include a detailed matrix for evaluating evidence, based on the purpose of the review, developed by the Oxford Centre for Evidence-Based Medicine Levels of Evidence.[13] While this tool is largely designed to be used with medical studies, some of the question areas could be adapted for education questions, such as: 'How common is the problem?' 'Does this intervention help?' and 'Is this diagnostic or monitoring test accurate?'

The Centre for Reviews and Dissemination[14] identifies three main quantitative study types, with several subtypes for each.

1. *Highest quality*: randomised control trials, including randomised crossover trials (where randomisation occurs for the *sequence* in which interventions are applied, but all participants are eventually exposed to all interventions), and cluster randomised trials (where *groups* of people, such as different tutorial groups, are randomly allocated to an intervention condition, rather than individuals).

2. *Intermediate*: quasi-experimental studies, where random assignment is not used to allocate participants to intervention groups. This category of studies includes non-randomised control studies, before-and-after studies (where the before and after groups can include the same participants, or different groups) and interrupted time series (multiple observations of participants over time 'interrupted' by the intervention).

3. *Lower quality*: observational studies, where the researchers do not allocate participants to groups or directly intervene. Types of observational studies include cohort studies (different groups are followed over a period of time), case-control studies (groups with and without specific outcomes are compared to identify the role of exposure to an intervention) and case series (descriptive studies presenting outcomes from an intervention where no control group was observed).

The Centre for Reviews and Dissemination[14] wisely cautions that not all studies of a particular type are equal in quality and that every study appraised should be evaluated comprehensively, not solely on the basis of its methodology.

Qualitative evidence can also be evaluated. One set of criteria for this purpose is included in the Rosalind Franklin Qualitative Research Appraisal Instrument.[15] This involves four items, each representing an aspect of trustworthiness as outlined in Guba's model: (1) credibility (internal validity), (2) transferability (external validity), (3) dependability (reliability) and (4) confirmability (objectivity).

It is important to recognise that traditional evidence scales tend to rank quantitative research, especially randomised control trials and meta-analyses more highly than qualitative methodologies or population studies (e.g. Melnyk and Fineout-Overholt[16(p12)]). Often more holistic consideration of the evidence is required (see, for example, Goldsmith *et al.*[17]), especially in an area like education, where outcomes such as self-efficacy are often intangible and subjective rather than concrete. The weight given to rigorous qualitative studies with strong relevance to the topic should be carefully balanced against a more incidental quantitative control trial. One example

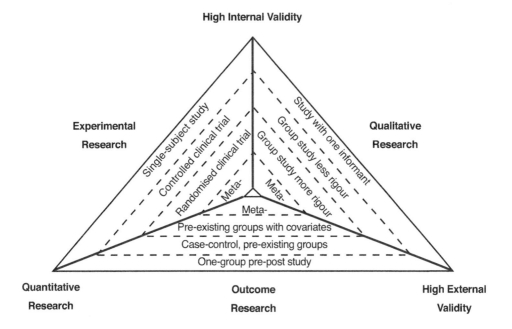

FIGURE 5.2 Research Pyramid model proposed by Tomlin and Borgetto[18] – note, this model aims to encourage consideration of a wide range of research sources and types (reprinted with permission; © Clearance Center ID: 63872982)

Descriptive Research (Base of Pyramid)
1. Systematic reviews of related descriptive studies
2. Association, correlational studies
3. Multiple-case studies (series), normative studies, descriptive surveys
4. Individual case studies

Experimental Research (Side of Pyramid)
1. Meta-analyses of related experimental studies
2. Individual (blinded) randomized controlled trials
3. Controlled clinical trials
4. Single-subject studies

Outcome Research (Side of Pyramid)
1. Meta-analyses of related outcome studies
2. Pre-existing groups comparisons with covariate analysis
3. Case-control studies; pre-existing groups comparisons
4. One-group pre-post studies

Qualitative Research (Side of Pyramid)
1. Meta-syntheses of related qualitative studies
2. Group qualitative studies with more rigor (see a, b, c)
3. Group qualitative studies with less rigor (see a, b, c)
   a. Prolonged engagement with participants
   b. Triangulation of data (multiple sources)
   c. Confirmation of data analysis & interpretation (peer & member checking)
4. Qualitative studies with a single informant

Mega-Syntheses of Descriptive, Experimental, Outcome & Qualitative Research (Top of Pyramid)

that aims to incorporate both quantitative and qualitative research is the *research pyramid* model developed by Tomlin and Borgetto[18] (*see* Figure 5.2). In this model, the faces of the pyramid represent experimental, outcome and qualitative research and are built on a base of descriptive research and support a 'mega-synthesis' keystone. This model aims to encourage consideration of several different types of evidence in an appropriate manner, but the authors themselves identify that there are currently limitations to this approach, especially in identifying the optimal configuration for the qualitative side of the pyramid.

Organising the information

There are numerous ways of recording findings from different studies, in part defined by the ultimate purpose of the investigation. Often tabulating key information can be a useful way of organising and scanning the findings. Such a table can later form the basis of a scoping review (which presents findings from a range of studies, with limited synthesis or analysis, focusing on breadth rather than depth), or a systematic review (where evidence is graded and weighted, synthesised and analysed in depth).

Columns can be adapted for the needs of the research – for example, by breaking down the method (e.g. sample size, focus population, intervention) or results (e.g. different measurable outcomes) further. Columns to record the quality of evidence according to your chosen framework(s) can also be incorporated.

Citation	Aim	Method	Results	Conclusions	Notes

An annotated bibliography is another option for recording information, especially if it is to be shared with others. This consists of a reference list, with each entry followed by a one-paragraph summary and critique of the content of the article. The bibliography does not include synthesis, but it can form the basis of comparisons and thematic synthesis later in the research process. Both scoping reviews and annotated bibliographies can be published, providing useful, collated information for others interested in the topic within academia, practice or governance areas. For example scoping reviews, see Mickan *et al.*[19] and Dryden *et al.*[20] For an example of a published annotated bibliography, see Thomas and Kern.[21]

CONCLUSION

In this chapter we have outlined some methods of structuring an answerable research question utilising a variety of mnemonics and offered practical advice on how to perform a structured search. Reviewing literature, in whichever form you choose, is a continuous process throughout the life of your research project, providing background and context to your research and supplying the evidence for future actions or decisions. It is important, therefore, to develop good practices when searching, critiquing and recording the results. There is no one correct way to work through the process. It is important to select the most appropriate methodology for your situation and context, whether structuring your research question or deciding whether to include grey literature in your review. Review your process often and evaluate your assumptions and progress regularly.

SUMMARY POINTS

- Reviewing literature is an ongoing process throughout the life of the research project.
- Information research is complex set of skills that requires good organisation and regular practice.
- There are different methods for structuring answerable research questions depending on the nature of the enquiry; mnemonics for these include PICO, SPICE and ECLIPSe.
- Numerous methodologies can be used for information research; the most effective option for a particular question will depend on the situation and context.
- All evidence is not equal; each source should be critically evaluated carefully.
- Review your process often and evaluate your assumptions and progress regularly.

REVIEW QUESTIONS

- What are the five main steps in the research process?
- What three types of research questions are there?
- What are the main differences between primary, secondary and tertiary literature?
- How can you find out if a source has been peer-reviewed?

REFLECTIVE QUESTIONS AND EXERCISES

The questions listed here relate to the following scenario:

Kerry, David and Maria (*see* individual case studies) all meet at an EBE conference while sharing their findings. They are interested in forming a collaboration to develop an interprofessional education unit of study for EBE University. In order to get permission for the new unit from the university, they need to prepare a detailed proposal, including a comprehensive review of relevant literature. They must prove the need for, and effectiveness of, interprofessional education for healthcare students at tertiary undergraduate level.

- What research question should they use? Is one of the mnemonics more suitable than others for this question?
- What background information might they review?
- Where could they start their search?
- What keywords could they use?
- How might they need to limit their search? Do they need to include grey literature or other sources of information? If so, what should they look for and why? If not, why not?
- Should they look for qualitative or quantitative literature, or both? Why?
- How can they organise their findings?
- What data management strategies should they use?
- How should they identify the best evidence?

GLOSSARY OF SECONDARY STUDY TYPES (NOT EXHAUSTIVE)

Note that terminology is not consistent; names for different review types are often used loosely (e.g. Harker and Kleijnen[22]).

literature review (traditional review)   Previously the amount of literature on a particular topic, and expert knowledge was needed to locate and bring together the information in a structured way. More recently the opposite problem is true: there is more literature available on given topics than anyone knows what to do with. In this context, the term 'literature review' has now become ambiguous. There are multiple different types of 'literature review', as evidenced in this glossary. Terminology varies depending on purpose, methodology or intended outcome. Literature reviews, in the conventional sense, now form the background of most studies. In this case they are discussions of key articles in a particular field that form the context of a particular study. The term is now more of an umbrella term, describing all the other specific types of review.

mapping review[23] (systematic map)   Used to categorise existing literature and identify gaps.

meta analysis[24]   Combining results of individual quantitative studies using statistical methods to look for patterns that emerge from the new pooled data set.

mini systematic review[25] (mini-review)   Reproducible review with narrow scope and predefined limits, often using easily accessed information rather than all information on the topic. Designed to facilitate more rapid production of reviews on important topics.

narrative review[26]   Three types of narrative reviews are common: commentaries editorials and narrative overviews (or unsystematic narrative reviews). Narrative overviews are the type most associated with narrative review. The author summarises article content in a condensed format but not necessarily critically appraising each article.

rapid review   Similar to a mini systematic review, with a focus on the review being prepared on a short timescale (1–6 months). Petticrew and Roberts[27] have a comprehensive table (Table 2.1) with common approaches to research synthesis including rapid reviews.

scoping review (scoping studies)   No agreed definition; originally conceived by Arksey and O'Malley[28]: 'Aim to map rapidly the key concepts underpinning a research area and the main sources and types of evidence available'. Further developed by Levac et al.,[29] who added clarification of each step and made recommendations to extend the methodology. In Table 1 of their article, Levac et al.[29] summarise definitions and purposes of scoping reviews from a range of sources. Davis et al.[30] maintain that scoping reviews provide the breadth of evidence but not the associated depth.

systematic review (systematic overview/Cochrane review)   'A review of a clearly formulated question that uses systematic and explicit methods to identify, select, and critically appraise relevant research, and to collect and analyse data from the studies that are included in the review. Statistical methods (meta-analysis) may or may not be used to analyse and summarise the results of the included studies.'[31]

REFERENCES

1. Eldredge J. Evidence-based librarianship levels of evidence. *Hypothesis.* 2002; **16**(3): 10–13. Available at: http://research.mlanet.org/hypothesis/hyp_v16n3.pdf (accessed 19 May 2014).
2. Richardson WS, Wilson MC, Nishikawa J, et al. The well-built clinical question: a key to evidence-based decisions. *ACP J Club.* 1995; **123**(3): A12–13.
3. Wildridge V, Bell L. How CLIP became ECLIPSE: a mnemonic to assist in searching for health policy/management information. *Health Info Libr J.* 2002; **19**(2): 113–15.
4. Booth A. Clear and present questions: formulating questions for evidence based practice. *Libr Hi Tech.* 2006; **24**(3): 355–68.
5. http://endnote.com
6. Harris R. *Evaluating Internet Research Sources.* 17 November 1997. Available at: www.niu.edu/facdev/programs/handouts/evaluate.htm (accessed 19 May 2014).
7. Harris R. *Evaluating Internet Research Sources.* 27 December 2013. Available at: www.virtualsalt.com/evalu8it.htm (accessed 19 May 2014).
8. Matthies BS, Helmke J. *Using the CRITIC Acronym to Teach Information Evaluation.* 1 January 2005. Available at: http://digitalcommons.butler.edu/librarian_papers/2/ (accessed 19 May 2014).
9. Matthies BS. The psychologist, the philosopher, and the librarian: the information-literacy version of CRITIC. *Skept Inq.* 2005; **29**(3): 49–52. Available at: http://digitalcommons.butler.edu/librarian_papers/1/ (accessed 19 May 2014).
10. Bartz WR. Teaching skepticism via the CRITIC acronym and the *Skeptical Inquirer. Skept Inq.* 2002; **26**(5): 42–4. Available at: www.siths.org/ourpages/auto/2010/9/20/58992050/1%20Teaching%20Skepticism.pdf (accessed 19 May 2014).
11. www.radcab.com
12. A retrospective of retractions: the striking record in 2011. *Nat Med.* 2011; **17**(12): 1544.
13. Centre for Evidence-Based Medicine. *OCEBM Levels of Evidence.* www.cebm.net/index.aspx?o=5653 (accessed 19 May 2014).
14. Centre for Reviews and Dissemination. *Systematic Reviews: CRD's guidance for undertaking reviews in health care.* York, UK: University of York; 2009. Available at: www.york.ac.uk/inst/crd/pdf/Systematic_Reviews.pdf (accessed 19 May 2014).

15. Henderson R, Rheault W. Appraising and incorporating qualitative research in evidence-based-practice. *J Phys Ther Educ.* 2004; **18**(3): 35–40.

16. Melnyk BM, Fineout-Overholt E. *Evidence-Based Practice in Nursing and Healthcare: a guide to best practice.* 2nd ed. Philadelphia, PA: Wolters Kluwer Health; 2011.

17. Goldsmith MR, Bankhead CR, Austoker J. Synthesising quantitative and qualitative research in evidence-based patient information. *J Epidemiol Community Health.* 2006; **61**(3): 262–70.

18. Tomlin G, Borgetto B. Research pyramid: a new evidence-based practice model for occupational therapy. *Am J Occup Ther.* 2011; **65**(2): 189–96.

19. Mickan S, Tilson JK, *et al.* Evidence of effectiveness of health care professionals using handheld computers: a scoping review of systematic reviews. *J Med Internet Res.* 2013; **15**(10): e212.

20. Dryden R, Williams B, McCowan C, *et al.* What do we know about who does and does not attend general health checks? Findings from a narrative scoping review. *BMC Public Health.* 2012; **12**: 723.

21. Thomas P, Kern D. Internet resources for curriculum development in medical education: an annotated bibliography. *J Gen Intern Med.* 2004; **19**(5): 599–605.

22. Harker J, Kleijnen J. What is a rapid review? A methodological exploration of rapid reviews in health technology assessments. *Int J Evid Based Healthc.* 2012; **10**(4): 397–410.

23. Grant M, Booth A. A typology of reviews: an analysis of 14 review types and associated methodologies. *Health Info Libr J.* 2009; **26**(2): 91–108.

24. Higgins JPT, Green S, editors. 9.4.2 Principles of meta analysis. In: *Cochrane Handbook for Systematic Reviews of Interventions.* Version 5.1.0 [updated March 2011]. The Cochrane Collaboration; 2011. Available at: http://handbook.cochrane.org/

25. Griffiths P. Evidence informing practice: introducing the mini-review. *Br J Community Nurs.* 2002; **7**(1): 38–9.

26. Green BN, Johnson CD, Adams A. Writing narrative literature reviews for peer-reviewed journals: secrets of the trade. *J Chiropr Med.* 2006; **5**(3): 101–17.

27. Petticrew M, Roberts H. *Systematic Reviews in the Social Sciences: a practical guide.* Malden, MA: Blackwell Publishing; 2006.

28. Arksey H, O'Malley L. Scoping studies: towards a methodological framework. *Int J Soc Res Methodol.* 2005; **8**(1): 19–32.

29. Levac D, Colquhoun H, O'Brien KK. Scoping studies: advancing the methodology. *Implement Sci.* 2010; **5**(1): 69–77.

30. Davis K, Drey N, Gould D. What are scoping studies? A review of the nursing literature. *Int J Nurs Stud.* 2009; **46**(10): 1386–400.

31. The Cochrane Collaboration. *Glossary.* www.cochrane.org/glossary (accessed 19 May 2014).

CHAPTER 6

Generating the evidence for health professional education

The five As of the scholarship of learning and teaching – ask, answer, access, appraise and apply

....

Karen J Saewert and Debra Hagler

OVERVIEW

Inquiry in the scholarship of learning and teaching (SOLT) reflects the quality improvement questions asked by educators every day. Opportunities for advancing evidence-based education require attention to the answers arising from questions within and between health education disciplines. When educators share what they have accomplished and publicly report what has worked or not worked, others are advantageously positioned to *access* existing educational evidence to *answer* the SOLT questions they are *asking*. If the purpose of the SOLT is to improve the quality of learning and teaching, determinations need to be made related to outcomes associated with distinct educational interventions. A wide range of research and non-research methodological approaches are available to investigate SOLT questions. Adopting a systematic approach to generating, applying and disseminating educational evidence assists the health professional educator in building a coherent basis for practice. Teachers must critically *appraise* generated evidence to *answer* their SOLT questions and inform *application* to their educational practice. Appraising what is credible and useful in order to make determinations about, apply, or build upon the findings of others is a requisite to evidence-based education practice. When practice recommendations are applied, a determination as to whether the intended or desired outcomes were achieved (e.g. evaluation) is essential to extending the foundation for inquiry. Evaluating outcomes serves to reveal consistent, inconsistent or conflicting findings while producing new evidence, questions and recommendations on which to build. This chapter provides an overview of key concepts relevant to educational evidence and its appraisal by addressing five As: *Asking* and *Answering* SOLT questions and *Accessing*, *Appraising* and *Applying* SOLT evidence.

CHAPTER OBJECTIVES

Upon completion of this chapter, the reader will be able to:
- differentiate the SOLT from other forms of scholarly inquiry
- formulate questions to guide the SOLT inquiry
- identify the broad range of approaches used to generate educational evidence
- distinguish key concepts relevant to appraising educational evidence.

KEY TERMS: scholarship of learning and teaching, evidence-based education, critical appraisal

---

INTRODUCTION

It is not enough to be an expert health professional and an excellent educator. Many such educators work to exhaustion in relative isolation, implementing innovative and effective strategies for their students while the health profession disciplines and other educators remain unaware of and are largely unchanged by the innovations. Health profession educators are increasingly applying evidence in their clinical practices to improve the health outcomes of populations and individuals across healthcare delivery settings; however, applying pertinent evidence to improve their learning and teaching practices is less common. Imagine the outcomes of education if all educators had the benefit of evidence similar to optimal dosing studies and pharmacokinetics for prescribing our educational interventions: might a clinician or teacher deliver a 10% dose of focused clinical care experience followed by alternating doses of discussion with reflection, assessment and feedback until optimal learning was achieved and confirmed by a valid and reliable diagnostic test as an evaluation strategy?

Educators often recreate rather than leverage the prior efforts of others. When educators generously share what they have accomplished and publicly report what has worked or not worked as they had hoped, others are advantageously positioned to *access* existing educational evidence to *answer* the scholarship of learning and teaching (SOLT) questions they are *asking*. To *answer* their SOLT questions, educators must critically *appraise* evidence generated by colleagues to inform *application* to educational practice.

Some educators' efforts are outstanding examples of inquiry, completed on a minimal budget of the educator's unpaid weekend work time, while other projects are lavishly funded and staffed. Some projects are exquisitely designed prospectively while others emerge almost accidentally, requiring an abrupt halt before proceeding in order to obtain relevant institutional review board approvals. Many educational projects have limitations based on the pragmatic considerations in authentic educational settings, such as school holidays and course schedules. Often, consideration for the vulnerability of students and teachers in those authentic educational settings requires using a 'somewhat less-than-experimental' design to respectfully investigate a learning phenomenon.

THE SCHOLARSHIP OF LEARNING AND TEACHING

The SOLT incorporates identifiable characteristics associated with *quality teaching* and *research rigour* but it is not synonymous with either one. As Hutchings and Shulman[1] explained:

> A scholarship of teaching … requires a kind of 'going meta,' in which faculty frame and systematically investigate questions related to student learning – the conditions under which it occurs, what it looks like, how to deepen it, and so forth – and do so with an eye not only to improving their own classroom but to advancing practice beyond it.[p13]

McKinney[2] provided an alternate description that resonates with the work many clinical teaching faculty already perform:

> The *scholarship of learning and teaching* goes beyond scholarly teaching and involves systematic study of teaching and/or learning and the public sharing and review of such work through presentations, performance, or publications.[p8]

The SOLT goes beyond the individual experience of a teacher to the public sharing of the project and its outcomes; teaching innovations are not representative of the SOLT until they are made public and open to review.[3]

But how is the SOLT different from the types of clinical research that health professionals do? Although the SOLT can include traditional research, its range is broader than what is often considered legitimate research in the sciences and allied health fields. The SOLT is also different in how questions are framed, methods are employed, and mechanisms are used for disseminating findings. If the purpose of SOLT is to improve the quality of learning and teaching, how will we know when that improvement has occurred? Educators frequently try new strategies and tweak instructional plans based on anecdotal observations, informal feedback from peers and students, and outcomes associated with prior student cohorts. A more systematic approach to generating, applying and disseminating educational evidence is encouraged to assist the health professional educator in building a coherent art and science of education to guide pedagogical practice. Although evidence does not support a conclusion that conducting research (on topics other than pedagogy) improves individual educators' teaching effectiveness, there are strong reasons to believe that conducting SOLT activities will support the development and delivery of effective teaching strategies and enhance student learning. Weimer[4] articulated seven ways pedagogical scholarship positively affects teaching (*see* Table 6.1).

TABLE 6.1 Seven reasons to do pedagogical scholarship

1. You develop the questions that interest you.
2. You develop instructional awareness.
3. You think more deeply about teaching and learning.
4. You improve for the right reasons.
5. It keeps your teaching fresh over the long haul.
6. It improves your conversations with colleagues.
7. It fosters learning in new ways and from new people.

Note: adapted from Weimer,[4(pp170–4)] © 2006 by Jossey-Bass; this material is reproduced with permission of John Wiley & Sons, Inc.

A requisite to evidence-based education practice is the teacher's ability to appraise what is credible and useful in order to make determinations about, apply, or build upon the findings of others. The purpose of this chapter it to provide an overview of key concepts relevant to educational evidence and its appraisal by addressing five As: *Asking* and *Answering* SOLT questions and *Accessing, Appraising* and *Applying* SOLT evidence (*see* Figure 6.1).

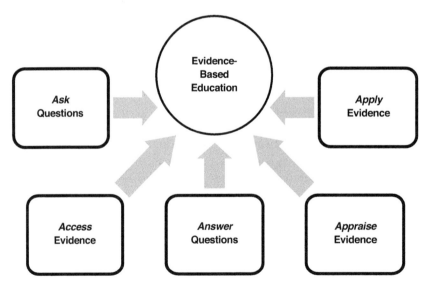

FIGURE 6.1 'The five A's of the scholarship of learning and teaching as a framework for evidence-based education', by KJ Saewert and D Hagler, 2013 (© 2013 by KJ Saewert and D Hagler; used with permission)

ASKING SCHOLARSHIP OF LEARNING AND TEACHING QUESTIONS

> Evidence-based education, like evidence-based health care, is not a pana-
> cea, a quick fix, cookbook practice or the provider of ready-made solutions
> to the demands of modern education. It is a set of principles and practice
> which can alter the way people think about education, the way they go
> about educational policy and practice, and the basis upon which they
> make professional judgements and deploy their expertise.[5(p118)]

What goals do you have for your students' learning? What opportunities exist
to improve students' learning? What challenges are you encountering with your
teaching? How can you reformulate these goals and challenges into searchable and
researchable questions? The SOLT begins with the asking of these and other relevant
questions.[6] Given the different contexts in which learning and teaching occur, the
number of relevant questions approaches infinity.[7]

It is important to recognise that the SOLT in higher education is not divorced from
the content of the discipline being taught.[8] The disciplinary context is powerful in
shaping the way faculty think about, design and conduct their approaches.[9] Specific
features characterising the SOLT include the following.

- Learning and teaching is deeply embedded in a discipline. The questions arise from
the character of the field and what it means to know it deeply.
- The SOLT is an aspect of practice undertaken by faculty looking at their own
practice. It is an element *within* not just *about* teaching.
- The SOLT is characterised by a transformational agenda – that is, scholarship is
undertaken in the name of change; its success measured by its impact on thought
and practice.[9]

Methodological conversations and collaborations *across* fields, as faculty borrow
approaches and perspectives from colleagues in other areas, contribute to the development of a broader repertoire of methods and advance the SOLT as a field.[9,10]

Scholarly and professional fields are defined in part by the questions they ask,
making it useful to examine the taxonomy of questions that characterise the SOLT.

- *What is?* These questions examine a current learning and teaching situation in an
attempt to describe it fully.
- *What works?* These questions seek evidence about the relative effectiveness of a
particular learning and teaching method or approach.
- *What could be?* These questions provide a vision of what is possible related to goals
for learning and teaching.
- *Theory building.* These questions are designed to build theoretical frameworks to
shape thought about practice.[9]

Hubball and Clarke[11] proposed a model for investigating potential SOLT questions that embraces exploratory learning, discovery, and/or problem-solving and

self-educating techniques (e.g. evaluation of feedback) contextualised across diverse higher education settings.

- *Context questions*: these questions focus on the critical structures that shape educational initiatives.
- *Process questions*: these questions focus *formatively* on issues of importance that arise over the course of an educational initiative.
- *Impact questions*: these questions focus *summatively* on issues of importance that arise as a result of an educational initiative.
- *Follow-up questions*: these questions focus on issues of importance that arise as a result of longer-term impacts of educational initiatives.

Foundation for inquiry

Inquiry in the SOLT reflects quality improvement questions asked by teachers every day, such as whether a new strategy adopted by a school or programme is really changing the learning outcomes, or what methods best support the motivation of a particular group of learners. Table 6.2 provides examples of common teaching activities that lend themselves to reflection and inquiry.

ACCESSING EVIDENCE TO ANSWER SCHOLARSHIP OF LEARNING AND TEACHING QUESTIONS

'Teaching and learning are complex processes, and no single source or type of evidence can provide a sufficient window into the questions we most want to explore.'[9(p6)] The best opportunities for advancing health professions education require attention to findings from colleagues both within and beyond our own disciplines. Gathering the best available evidence that currently exists on the subject of interest from a variety of credible sources is an essential to engaging in the SOLT,[6] and will be demonstrated for a number of specific topics and disciplines in later chapters of this book.

An important aspect of scholarly teaching is formulating the types of good questions that arise from intentional reflection on learning and teaching. Applicable evidence accessed in response to a well-articulated question may provide relatively more or less satisfactory 'answers'. What work have others done that relates to your inquiry questions? When the best available evidence in an area of inquiry does not adequately address the questions of interest, conducting an original inquiry to generate new evidence may be appropriate. Enhancing clinical judgement and building confidence in clinical practice guidelines requires striving for 'better evidence' as urgently as using the 'best available' evidence.[12] This requirement holds true for education practice as well; however, inquiries about learning and teaching lend themselves to a broader range of approaches than what may be considered legitimate for research in some disciplines.

TABLE 6.2 Examples of teaching and learning inquiry amenable to the scholarship of learning and teaching

Category of inquiry	Related areas	Activities for reflection and possible inquiry
Instructional knowledge from reflection and inquiry on *content*	Course design Instructional materials Teaching methods	Writing learning objectives Constructing tests Developing teaching materials Preparing a lecture or learning activity Facilitating discussion Using a variety of instructional methods Organising or sequencing instruction
Pedagogical knowledge from reflection and inquiry on *process*	Learning style Cognitive processes Group dynamics Teaching content within a discipline Assisting student in understanding concepts Facilitating critical thinking and self-directed learning beyond the discipline	Motivating students with different learning styles Selecting various teaching materials Delivering an interesting lecture Facilitating collaboration among students Helping students overcome learning difficulties Encouraging students to think critically Using specific techniques for fostering learning Providing meaningful feedback Judging the quality of specific techniques
Curricular knowledge from reflection and inquiry of *premise*	Merit and functional relevance of teaching Critical reflection on practice Goals and rationale for course, programme, sequence or system of higher education	Judging the quality of course goals Explaining how a course fits into the existing programme Describing contributions that a course may make to the student's existing knowledge Articulating how a course or programme may affect students' learning outcomes

Note: adapted from Kreber C, Cranton PA. Exploring the scholarship of teaching. *J High Educ.* 2000; **71**(4): 479–81. © 2000 by The Ohio State University; adapted with permission.

Diverse methodological approaches for the scholarship of learning and teaching

There is a wide range of methodological approaches to investigate SOLT questions in diverse higher education settings; each approach is rooted in particular disciplinary assumptions, as well as embodied in ethical considerations for the processes and outcomes of research. Selecting an appropriate methodology for a SOLT inquiry will largely depend on situational practicalities as well as the appropriate alignment of clearly articulated SOLT questions that one wants to ask in order to gain the sorts of insights to enhance institutional, curricula or classroom practices. These determinations also enable the development of a clear sense of who and how many people are likely to be involved, the sort of data that will need to be collected, over what time period and under what conditions.[11]

The range of SOLT inquiry options are described as research or non-research inquiries and are summarised in Tables 6.3, 6.4 and 6.5. Research methods for SOLT inquiries include traditional types of designs common to clinical studies in the health professions. However, research in pursuit of objectivity based on precise control of variables is not always ethically acceptable or practically feasible in authentic educational settings. Non-research methods include personal accounts of change and reports of recommended practices or content.[4] A major critique of such methods is the lack of critical assessment of the processes and outcomes, although the current evidence-based practice movement strives to promote rigour in reports of innovative practices. The International Committee of Medical Journal Editors has been very influential in elevating the reporting standards for all types of inquiry through requirements for more complete and transparent reporting that facilitates readers' critical appraisal and interpretation. Table 6.6 presents guidelines and related sources for the reporting on various types of SOLT inquiry.

TABLE 6.3 Scholarship of learning and teaching inquiry: research

Type	Characteristics	Examples
Experimental	Randomised assignment to an intervention or control group	Randomised controlled trial
Quasi-experimental	May have a control group Participants are not randomly assigned	Repeated measures Participants as self-controls 'Pre- then post-test' evaluation
Non-experimental	No random assignment, control group or manipulation of variables	Descriptive study Case study
Qualitative	No random assignment, control group or manipulation of variables	Ethnography Grounded theory Narrative analysis Phenomenology

TABLE 6.4 Scholarship of learning and teaching inquiry: summative research

Type	Characteristics	Examples
Systematic review	Compilation of evidence from multiple studies of the same (or similar) question	Clearly defined search strategy and appraisal process
Meta-analysis	Synthesis and analysis of quantitative evidence	Statistically pooled data from several studies Summarised findings based on a larger pooled sample and estimate of effect size
Meta-synthesis	Synthesis and analysis of qualitative evidence	Identification of concepts across several qualitative studies for translation into theory

Note: adapted from Poe and Costa.[13(pp86–7)] Adapted with permission. © 2012 by the Johns Hopkins Health System Corporation. All rights reserved. No part of this work may be modified, redistributed, or reproduced in any form or by any means, electronic or mechanical, including photocopying, recording, or by any information storage and retrieval system without the written permission of Johns Hopkins. This work is intended for use to assist hospital and healthcare audiences, however, Hopkins makes no representations or warranties concerning the content or clinical efficiency of this work, its accuracy or completeness, and Hopkins is not responsible for any errors or omissions or for any loss, liability, or damage resulting for the use of this work. This work is not intended to be a substitute for professional medical advice, diagnosis, treatment, or individual root cause analysis.

TABLE 6.5 Scholarship of learning and teaching inquiry: non-research[14(pp125–44)]

Type	Characteristics	Examples
Opinion	Individual insights drawn from experience	Personal narratives Personal accounts of change Recommended practices Recommended content Case reports
Organisations' documents	Reports produced for internal workflow and process review May be published as benchmarks	Quality improvement data Programme evaluation data Financial data
Evidence summaries	Recommendations based on research and/or experience Variable rigour in level of evidence appraisal	Clinical practice guidelines Consensus statements Position statements Integrative or narrative literature review

TABLE 6.6 Scholarship of learning and teaching inquiry: reporting guidelines

Reporting guidelines		Type
CONSORT	Consolidated Standards of Reporting Trials www.consort-statement.org/consort-statement/	Randomised controlled trials
COREQ	Consolidated Criteria for Reporting Qualitative Research www.equator-network.org/resource-centre/library-of-health-research-reporting/reporting-guidelines/qualitative-research/	Qualitative methods
ENTREQ	Enhancing Transparency in Reporting the Synthesis of Qualitative Research www.equator-network.org/reporting-guidelines/entreq/	Systematic reviews of qualitative research
GLISC	Grey Literature International Steering Committee www.glisc.info/	Scientific and technical reports
PRISMA	Preferred Reporting Items for Systematic Review and Meta-Analyses www.prisma-statement.org/	Systematic reviews, educational interventions
SQUIRE	Standards for Quality Improvement Reporting Excellence http://squire-statement.org/	Quality improvement projects in healthcare
REPOSE	REPOrting of primary empirical research Studies in Education http://eppi.ioe.ac.uk/cms/Default.aspx?tabid=759	Educational research methods (varied)

APPRAISING SCHOLARSHIP OF LEARNING AND TEACHING EVIDENCE

At the core of evidence appraisal is skilled critical thinking needed to evaluate the robustness and scientific rigour of evidence.[12] Entire books, book chapters and other literature sources address the process of conducting critical appraisal, offer tools for appraising non-research and research evidence, and provide a variety of hierarchies for use in rating evidence quality and strength. Drawing upon available resources and experts to guide the process of judging the use of statistics and their interpretation is encouraged to strengthen knowledge, skill and confidence in applying these concepts, practices and principles.

Level of evidence

Level of evidence is determined by the type of study design;[13] subsequently, levels of evidence hierarchies will vary by the types of questions being asked.[15] Evidence hierarchies or rating scales, while providing a structure should encourage the application of the educator's knowledge, skills, experience and critical thinking abilities.

Quality of evidence: critical appraisal

A large number of checklists and rating instruments with explicit criteria and varying degrees of specificity are available for grading the *quality of evidence* determined by *critical appraisal* of study design (*level of evidence*); methodological strengths, limitations and execution (*study quality*); and the extent to which subjects, interventions and outcome measures are similar to those of interest (*directness*).[13] The process of *critical appraisal* is organised around three key questions:

1. Are the results of the study valid?
2. Are the results of the study reliable?
3. Are the results applicable to my situation?

Answers to these and other questions relevant to *critical appraisal* guide determinations related to the relevance and transferability of the evidence and the effectiveness of a specific intervention for a population of interest.

A basic understanding of *validity* (extent to which a study measures what it is intended to measure and how well the findings will approximate the truthfulness of the subject of interest), *reliability* (the consistency or repeatability of measurement), *precision* (statistical measures of significance) and *practical significance* (application importance) are needed to consider information presented in reports of research evidence.[13] Application of the more advanced concepts of *internal validity* (causal inference) and *external validity* (generalisability) supports critical decision-making for knowledge transfer. Although statistically significant (e.g. unlikely to have occurred by chance) results are more likely to have clinical significance (or educational significance in the case of evidence-based education), this is not always the case. Findings that are not statistically significant for a variety of reasons, including small sample size, can still have clinical or educational significance. Conversely, results that are statistically significant may lack important practical application.

As discussed earlier in this chapter, when research evidence does not exist or where it is insufficient to answer the questions of interest, non-research evidence may be useful. Strategies for appraising non-research evidence vary according to types. While non-research evidence does not have the rigour of research evidence, it provides important information to inform practice decisions.[14]

Strength of evidence

Finally, the *strength of evidence* is determined though synthesis of the *level* and *quality* of evidence leading to a practice recommendation.[13] It is important to consider the body of evidence for its consistency across sources of evidence.

APPLYING SCHOLARSHIP OF LEARNING AND TEACHING EVIDENCE

Implementing practice recommendations is the essence of the evidence-based practice process and the cornerstone of best practice.[16] However, the inquiry process does not end with application. Once implemented, evaluation of findings to determine whether the intended or desired practical outcomes were achieved extends the foundation for inquiry. Evaluating outcomes serves to reveal the level of consistency with previous findings and produce new evidence, questions and recommendations on which to further build evidence-based education.

Knowledge does not flow only from science to practice; it also results from direct experiential learning and inquiry.[12] The educator must contextualise (e.g. to learner audience and educational setting) the practice of evidence-based education to allow for informed development of relevant educational guidelines and facilitate scholarly dialogue regarding best educational practice options. The values, concerns, preferences and expertise of stakeholders affected by the educational enterprise should be central to these discussions.

The chapters that follow provide examples of a variety of educational interventions and contexts, including examples of the generation of evidence for application. As you read these chapters, consider and apply the key concepts presented in this chapter relevant to educational evidence and its appraisal for translation to practice. Are the five As *Asking* and *Answering* SOLT questions and *Accessing*, *Appraising* and *Applying* SOLT *evidence*?

CONCLUSIONS

Evaluation of whether and how educational interventions within and across educational settings result in improved health outcomes of populations and individuals across healthcare settings is the gold standard for inquiry in health professions education. Despite the valuable scholarly work that has been done, we are far from reaching this gold standard. For health professions evidence-based education to move forward, knowledgeable and skilful educators must intentionally and conscientiously make use of the best available evidence, or, in its absence, generate new knowledge. Accountability and adherence to standards for the design, relevance and reporting of SOLT inquiries across health professional education has the potential to support ongoing collaborative progress, strengthen health professions education and ultimately contribute to improved health outcomes.

SUMMARY POINTS

- There are variety of sources of evidence that educators can access to answer pedagogical questions they might have.
- A wide range of research and non-research methodological approaches are available to investigate SOLT questions.
- Utilising a systematic approach to generating, applying and disseminating educational evidence assists health professional educators in building a viable body of knowledge for evidence-based education.
- Educators must critically *appraise* generated evidence to *answer* their SOLT questions and inform *application* to their educational practice.

REVIEW QUESTIONS

- How is the SOLT different from other forms of scholarly inquiry?
- What experiences and questions from your own roles in education would you like to explore through the SOLT?
- What are the most common research methods and non-research methods used to generate educational evidence?
- How are the concepts of validity and reliability and the use of level of evidence hierarchies relevant to appraising educational evidence?

REFLECTIVE QUESTIONS AND EXERCISES

- *Asking* SOLT questions: What challenges are you encountering with your teaching? How can you reformulate these challenges into searchable and researchable questions?
- *Accessing* evidence to *Answer* SOLT questions: What work have others done that relates to your inquiry questions? How can you access evidence from your workplace?
- *Appraising* SOLT evidence: What considerations are important when critically appraising the quality and strength of evidence?
- *Applying* SOLT evidence: How can you thoughtfully incorporate current evidence with your clinical and pedagogical knowledge to improve practice?

REFERENCES

1. Hutchings P, Shulman LS. The scholarship of teaching: new elaborations, new developments. *Change.* 1999; **31**(5): 10–15.
2. McKinney K. The scholarship of teaching and learning: past lessons, current challenges, and future visions. In: Wehlburg C, Chadwick-Blossey S, editors. *To Improve the Academy: resources for faculty, instructional, and organizational development.* Volume 22. Bolton, MA: Anker; 2004. pp. 3–19.
3. Goto ST. Who is the 'public' when you make teaching public? Conceptions of audience in the scholarship of teaching and learning. *J Scholarship Teach Learn.* 2009; **9**(3): 1–14.
4. Weimer M. *Enhancing Scholarly Work on Teaching and Learning: professional literature that makes a difference.* San Francisco, CA: Jossey-Bass; 2006.
5. Davies P. What is evidence-based education? *Br J Educ Stud.* 1999; **47**(2): 108–21.
6. MacMillan M, Mitchell M. Opening the door to SoTL: Teaching evaluations as part of the inquiry cycle. Available at: www.kpu.ca/sites/default/files/Teaching%20and%20Learning/TD.5.2.1.Macmillan_etal_Teaching_Evaluastions.pdf (accessed on 9 October 2014).
7. Buskist W, Groccia JE. Evidence-based teaching: now and in the future. *New Dir Teach Learn.* 2011; **2011**(128): 105–11.
8. Healy M. Developing the scholarship of teaching in higher education: a discipline-based approach. *High Educ Res Dev.* 2000; **19**(2): 169–89.

9. Hutchings P. Approaching the scholarship of teaching and learning. In: Park CA, editor. *Opening Lines: approaches to the scholarship of teaching and learning.* Menlo Park, CA: Carnegie Foundation for the Advancement of Teaching; 2000. pp. 1–10.

10. Dewar JM. An apology for the scholarship of teaching and learning. *Insight.* 2008; **3**: 17–22.

11. Hubball H, Clarke A. Diverse methodological approaches and considerations for SoTL in higher education. *Can J Scholarsh Teach Learn.* 2010; **1**(1): Article 2.

12. Benner PE, Leonard VW. Patient concerns, choices, and clinical judgment in evidence-based practice. In: Melnyk BM, Fineout-Overholt E, editors. *Evidence-Based Practice in Nursing and Healthcare: a guide to best practice.* 2nd ed. Philadelphia, PA: Wolters Kluwer Health/Lippincott Williams & Wilkins; 2011. pp. 167–85.

13. Poe S, Costa L. Evidence appraisal: research. In: Dearholt SL, Dang D, editors. *Johns Hopkins Nursing Evidence-Based Practice: model and guidelines.* 2nd ed. Indianapolis, IN: Sigma Theta Tau International; 2012. pp. 83–124.

14. Shaefer SJ, Mark HD. Evidence appraisal: non-research. In: Dearholt SL, Dang D, editors. *Johns Hopkins Nursing Evidence-Based Practice: model and guidelines.* 2nd ed. Indianapolis, IN: Sigma Theta Tau International; 2012. pp. 125–44.

15. Melnyk BM, Fineout-Overholt E, editors. *Evidence-Based Practice in Nursing and Healthcare: a guide to best practice.* 2nd ed. Philadelphia, PA: Wolters Kluwer Health/Lippincott Williams & Wilkins; 2011.

16. Newhouse RP, White K. Translation. In: Dearholt SL, Dang D, editors. *Johns Hopkins Nursing Evidence-Based Practice: model and guidelines.* 2nd ed. Indianapolis, IN: Sigma Theta Tau International; 2012. pp. 145–60.

PART II

Concepts that underpin health professional evidence-based education

CHAPTER 7

Applying student-centred approaches to learning in health professional education

. . . .

Yvonne Parry

OVERVIEW

This chapter provides an overview of student-centred approaches to education for undergraduate health professionals. It discusses the contextual issues related to health professional student education that include the importance of the learning environment, teacher education and institutional factors. These topics are presented in three separate sections of this chapter.

CHAPTER OBJECTIVES

Upon completion of this chapter, the reader will be able to:
- describe student-centred learning and its impact on student learning
- explain the principles of reflective practice and its importance in health professional practice
- discuss the relationships between the various aspects of context and student learning.

KEY TERMS: student-centred education, health professionals, reflective practice, teaching impacts on student learning, context of learning

INTRODUCTION

This chapter endeavours to explore some of the influences that affect the student's experience of university education. Teachers' knowledge of student learning – namely, how students learn and the learning environment – can be limited by individual contextual variations (such as the social, cultural, discipline and institutional constraints in meeting students' and teachers' needs); however, some understanding of the student cohort is important. Any development of learning materials needs to take into account the learning environment. This chapter explores some of the issues that are crucial to students in the health professions. These include the students as potential health professionals, teachers supporting the students, and university environment including the institutional infrastructure.[1-3] According to Benson and Samarawickrema,[4] in education

> Context is a complex, multifaceted, perspective-dependent concept which may include a range of factors … specific to the learning and teaching environment, to disciplinary, institutional … social influences and personal issues affecting students' lives.[(p61)]

Students and their environments are thus inextricably interconnected in their learning experience. For health professional students, their own learning needs and the learning environment can influence their future career pathway and the requisite need for reflective practice.

STUDENT-CENTRED LEARNING

Learning is a process rather than an end product.[5] The process involves a long-term and permanent change in a student's knowledge, beliefs and attitudes that is initiated by the student's participation in his or her own process of learning.[5,6] Furthermore, learning that explicitly demonstrates the values of social justice, where high student attainment is expected and where student and teacher self-reflection is used will be beneficial for student.[6]

Student-centred learning (SCL) is explained as learning that places the student at the centre of the learning process.[7] This instructional approach has an impact on the provision of materials, activities, content and pace of learning provided to the students.[8] It has implications for teaching and service provision in universities, as an SCL curriculum requires flexible design, content sharing and interactivity between the teachers, materials, activities and the student.[7,8] SCL seeks to identify and provide learning that is inclusive of the range of instructional methods that reflects the vast array of learning styles students require to augment their learning needs and styles. Universities are expected to address SCL throughout their curricula.[1-3,7,8]

HEALTH PROFESSIONAL STUDENTS

The uniqueness of first-year health professional students

The ultimate role for health professional students is the provision of care for others. This focus is an important point of distinction between health profession students and students studying generalist courses, such as Bachelor of Arts. The first-year experience for health professional students involves more than learning about university and university study: it also requires understanding of how to be a health professional and take on the responsibility of caring for others. University study requires students to develop an awareness of complex information and to integrate this into their existing knowledge, and to also engage in higher-order thinking, self-awareness, self-monitoring and time management practices.[3,9–11]

Reflective practice

Health professional students need to develop the complex skills of reflective practice[12,13] to enable them to engage in professional reflective practice. This means developing the ability to think critically to be able to identify their own learning needs and to understand their own personal beliefs, attitudes and values that may affect the delivery of care to others.[13,14] Developing reflective skills is essential for professional competence in the health sector.[13] The ability for reflection in professional practice is an important attribute for health practitioners, allowing them to determine the appropriate action when faced with an unfamiliar problem through logically deducing the possible consequences of their action, and predicting alternative possible outcomes.[13,14] This process explores evidence-based practice and applies it to the provision of care in busy emergency environments.[12] Educators need to productively engage with students to ensure learning opportunities incorporate aspects of reflective learning and enhance developmental reflective practices. Explicitly linking the theoretical components to clinical practice assists students in understanding the possible applications of their new knowledge.

Engaging with students

Students' background, their economic status, educator modes of relating to students, institutional supports for teaching staff ('teaching staff' here refers to the instructor, teacher or tutor providing direct teaching in the tutorial, laboratory or classroom) and students all have an impact on student motivation and the engagement of students in higher education.[4,15] Environments where students are provided with learning experiences that are supportive and enhance their sense of community promote deeper learning.[4,15] Curricula based on SCL assist in promoting engagement.[8] Successful engagement enriches the students' experience, encourages them to be a part of institutional culture and promotes the development of lifelong learning habits. For example, university cultures that welcome and accommodate students from diverse backgrounds (e.g. cultural backgrounds, socio-economic status, geographical location) and which invest in and promote education through staff education and student support services sustain student engagement, support the students sense of belonging and promote student inclusiveness.[4,15] SCL and teaching practices, combined with university culture, need to be inclusive of diversity in order to enhance the student outcomes and the experience of tertiary education.

Student diversity is an important issue for educators and tertiary institutions within Australia and internationally. Currently in Australia over 54% of the student populations are of mature age (over 24 years).[1,3,16] Therefore, it cannot be assumed that students have the same learning issues, computer skills and technology knowledge,[1-3,17] nor that these skills are present in all student populations. Thus programmes need to accommodate a variety of life experiences, learning styles and modes of delivery within education materials to enhance SCL and to cater for such diversity.[3] Teaching and learning that incorporate learning tasks, learning resources and learning supports that are informed by the diversity of the student cohort provide learning experiences that support students.[4,12] In addition, for some of the student population, such as the secondary school leavers, their university experience will be the first time they have encountered a learning environment that includes learners from across the age spectrum. Learning environments therefore need to accommodate not only the school leaver but also mature age students. Tertiary institutions also need to accommodate students who have completed previous community college or certificate- or diploma level studies and wish to pursue university-level studies.

Student diversity encompasses a complexity of student issues such as backgrounds; for example, non-traditional tertiary education participants may have an impact on retention rates. Students from lower socio-economic backgrounds have traditionally withdrawn from university studies after the first year.[18] It is important that teaching staff are able to relate to students regardless of their background[18,19] and socio-economic status, to ensure that health professionals complete programmes of study and are thus able to promote workplace and societal diversity.

The levels of student maturity and learning approaches that are student centred can significantly enhance the learning environment. Preparing health professional students for their future practice entails developing materials that promote reflective learning, critical thinking and professional identity. Health professional students' enhanced development is facilitated by the accommodation of students' varied learning styles and the incorporation of evolving student expectations.[2,3,20] Conversely, approaches to teaching and learning that are teacher centred are less flexible and unable to contribute to high-quality student outcomes.[3,20]

Student-centred institutions provide students with the information and support they need to evolve. Educational research has established a set of principles that enrich SCL and that includes timely and appropriate feedback,[3,19,21] scaffolding of programmes and topics across the degree,[2,20-22] adequate time on tasks,[20] incorporation and respect for diversity of learning and students,[2,19] increasing student and staff interaction,[3] and high expectations of students and staff.[3,20] In addition, the institutional practices, teacher education and training[3] further enhance student support programmes and also provide areas where students' learning spaces can promote student-centred practices.[2,20]

CONNECTING EDUCATORS WITH STUDENTS' NEEDS
Potential disconnections with educators

The extent to which educators can connect with students to enhance learning opportunities is an important aspect of the university teaching environment. The provision of teaching that enhances students' experience of university is often dependent on learning and teaching quality. Poor teaching quality, poor academic processes, poor course fit, financial strain, resource constraints, poorly maintained physical facilities (such as computer labs, audiovisual equipment and classrooms), and limited student–staff interaction all impact negatively on student outcomes. These factors are both student and institutionally based issues that create disconnects for the students and limit the quality of the student outcomes.[1-3,20]

Actively addressing teaching quality through educator training, academic processes through timely student and faculty feedback, course fit through the scaffolding of assessments and tasks across the programme of study, and increasing opportunities for student–staff interaction can all improve student outcomes. The financial strain endured by some students and institutions is a multifaceted issue that often incorporates societal and political intervention and may include increased student subsidies and low-cost student accommodation. These issues also add to the strain placed on the provision of quality teaching and learning by tertiary institutions and can create a potential disconnect between students and teaching staff. One major factor limiting educator–student interaction time is the trend in academic institutions of hiring sessional staff who are only salaried for direct teaching time. The issue of the casualisation of education staff within the higher education sector is an ongoing and, unfortunately, increasingly frequent issue for employees and students alike. It is challenging for education staff to be student focused when they are only funded for the face-to-face provision of lectures and tutorials.

By addressing the areas of disconnection between students and educators the 'transactional distance' between the student and teacher can be limited.[4] The transactional distance refers to the psychological space between the student and educator and is important for facilitating the incorporation, comprehension and application of the subject or unit materials.[3,4] Taking into account the transaction distance is more important than the mode of study (e.g. example internal or external) and plays a significant role in the development and delivery of effective learning materials.[4] Therefore, institutions that minimise the transactional distance between the student, educational materials and teaching are able to enhance the students' outcomes and their experience of university. This is important when considering that the role of health professions in society requires them to be highly educated professionals. However, in many instances the economic and budgetary constraints faced by individual departments and schools cause the transactional distance to be increased between the two parties.

The transactional distance is a factor when students enter generic courses in order to transfer into their destination course at a future time. Students' knowledge on entering a pathway course (such as a broader-based Bachelor of Health Sciences programme) before transferring to their destination course could create disconnects with the materials and educators conducting the pathway courses, as students may not believe the material to be as important as that of their destination courses. For example, many health professional courses have moved up to the graduate-entry master's level or entry-level clinical doctorate. In order for students to gain entry to these courses, they must complete a related feeder undergraduate degree programme. Students enrolled in the broader-based pathway course may perceive an increased transactional distance.

Student pathways

One key issue facing university students today is the modern phenomenon of tertiary transfer. This complex issue results when students feel pressure to enter a programme with a career endpoint rather than a generalist programme, such as a Bachelor of Arts or Bachelor of Health Sciences. Students want to enter programmes that provide clear pathways to a defined profession and employment. Combined with this is the highly competitive nature of tertiary entrance criteria that can result in the more popular career-based programmes being more difficult to enter in the first instance. For example, medicine and physiotherapy courses traditionally receive many more applicants than places available and are hence much more competitive.

Tertiary transfer students: the experience of two transitions

The impact of increasing tertiary entrance scores requirements and competition for niche programmes results in undergraduate students looking for alternative pathways to their preferred health profession course of study. For example, universities offer programmes that provide pathways into health-based career programmes, resulting in an increase in students using the first-year general health studies programmes, such as the Bachelor of Health Science, as a pathway programme to the paramedic, nutrition and dietetics, radiography, occupational therapy and speech pathology majors. Research undertaken in the United States with students moving from vocational or community colleges to 4-year degree programmes describes a 'transfer shock' experience.[23] This can be countered by supporting students with academic support and programmes such as peer mentoring that can enhance student learning programmes.[17,24,25] In the United States, it is common for students to transfer several times in young adulthood from high school to college and then to university.[26]

Both the causes and consequences of these transfers require further research in the Australian context.[27,28] In Australia, however, the phenomenon for transferring within a university course is relatively new and thus as tertiary transfers are increasing the transfer experience requires further understanding. The recommendations from a review by Bradley et al.[29] suggested uncapped student numbers into programmes, yet this will have consequences in the increased pressure on entry into generic open access courses, such as Bachelor of Health Science, placing greater demand on limited places in preferred programmes and increasing the number of students entering tertiary transfer pathways. Despite Bradley et al.'s[29] premise of broadening participation in higher education, this practice will increase the numbers of students transferring to alternative courses after the completion of their first year. Australian students often enter an open access course in order to improve their grade average to achieve entry into a higher-rated or more prestigious professional stream. Currently, some universities offer guarantees for first-year students attaining distinction average grades to enter the course of their choice – for example, a Bachelor of Health Science student who obtains a distinction average grade may be guaranteed entry into a paramedic science degree.

The role of the education staff in tertiary transfer

Part of the role of education staff is to support students wishing to succeed and gain entry into highly sought-after tertiary courses.[30] Research has noted that the type of input, social acceptance and student support improve the overall student experience and their grade outcomes.[15,19,30,31] Furthermore, students' high self-efficacy and belief in their ability to learn is increased with tutor support.[19,31] Education staff also offer those students with lower university entrance score a means to improve their grade in their first year and to transfer into their final course of choice by providing extra support where feasible.[32,33] In programmes where the student is required to transition from a broader generic course to their course of choice, there is pressure for them to maintain a high tertiary score or grade point average in order for them to successfully transfer. This heightens the importance of educator feedback and academic support to enable a successful transfer for the student. Feedback and support can take many different forms, including large group feedback, peer-to-peer feedback, formal written comments and the use of well-designed, comprehensive marking rubrics.

In research undertaken to understand the pressures on students, several studies have documented the student experience as they transition from generic programmes (such as the Bachelor of Health Science) into their preferred course of study.[30,31,33,34] Research by Parry and Reynolds[33] captured key aspects of the student experience. Issues such as student support, curriculum development and the connection between assessment and learning were highlighted by the students as important in assisting them to attain their desired objective of a successful tertiary transfer. The successful building of relationships between students, academics and student learning support services is also important for students wishing to achieve a tertiary transfer.[34] Universities with tertiary transfer programmes need to invest in student support services and tutor training specific to the transfer experience in order for these programmes to succeed, not only in attracting students but also in retaining them. Again, for many higher education providers, this has become challenging, with exponential increases in number of students accepted into universities (resulting in larger classes sizes) without the concurrent increase in the number of education staff employed to manage the larger student cohort numbers.

UNIVERSITY SECTOR IMPACTS ON STUDENT OUTCOMES

The experience of university students in a changing university environment has impacted on their outcomes. The uncapping of programmes has led to an overall increase in the numbers of university students, as already mentioned. One such increase is in university students from non-traditional backgrounds.[29,35] Another factor is a global trend in the employment sector that requires workers to complete higher levels of education, thereby leading to a proliferation in courses. These major trends have seen an increase in the overall growth in the tertiary education sector.[3,36]

The role of the teaching staff is crucial in providing quality education; uniting educators and learners in the common goals of preparing students for professional practice is a critical aspect in modern university education.[3,4] One of the major outcomes of quality staff and student interactions is the students' increased sense of belonging within the university or institution,[3] thereby improving student outcomes. Despite the importance of high-quality experienced educators for student outcomes, the majority of teaching is invariably performed by sessional, casual and junior teaching staff.[3] Increasing student numbers, the casualisation of the university sector workforce and decreasing provision of teacher education all have the potential to increase the pressure on the university sector and negatively impact on student outcomes.[3]

EDUCATOR IMPACT ON THE LEARNING EXPERIENCE

The constructivist view of learning explores the impact of the teaching and peer-learning experience on student experiences.[31] Differences in teaching staff and teaching staff effectiveness may have an impact on student motivation, grades and learning;[15,31,37] therefore teaching can be one of the most effective educational interventions. Bloom[38] found that students supported by teaching staff (e.g. tutored) perform, on average, one to two standard deviations above those not supported (e.g. not tutored). Ideally, every student needs to receive expert teaching from education staff; however, the pressure to provide a plethora of courses in order to meet the increasing demand has led to some open online courses providing little direct educational support (see King[35]).

Researchers found that educator aptitude has an impact on student learning, with caring support responses from educators eliciting more help-seeking behaviour from students.[3,15,38,39] Additionally, educators with attitudes and behaviours that engage and encourage students assist undergraduates to develop independent, productive, autonomous and self-determining behaviours that enhance their learning experiences in the higher education context.[3,15] Given the increasing numbers of students in classes, a future tertiary educational sector with uncapped undergraduate numbers, and the increasing use of casual tutors, the transactional distance* between learner and teaching staff will more than likely expand, which is not optimal for either party on either side of the teaching–learning equation.

---

* Transactional distance: the psychological space between the student and educator important for facilitating the incorporation, comprehension and application of the subject materials.

DISCUSSION

The role of the educator in assisting the student through his or her degree is of crucial importance for successful high-quality student outcomes. Given the importance of the health professional's role in the care of others, is it important that programmes developing future health professionals engage their students, not just with the course materials but chiefly with reflective practice. The support afforded students by the teaching staff clearly assists students in this process. This may be achieved by encouraging students through motivation and compassionate understanding of the pressures on the students. As discussed previously, the input of education staff on students' experiences of the university sector can assist the students not only in aspects such as the transfer journey but also in their sense of belonging, academic achievement and adjustment to their professional career. Furthermore, it remains important, especially in a competitive university environment, that educators are supported in providing quality learning and teaching opportunities and this needs to remain an important component of future health professional workforce planning and student outcomes.

For tertiary transfer pathway students, the development of clear choices and pathway journey is paramount to the success of their transition. Given the increasing numbers of students in generic entry programmes in universities, their career path via tertiary transfer processes are increasing and there needs to be clearly outlined process available to both students and academics to ensure students are aware of their commitments, such as clear explanations of their course pathways.

IMPLICATIONS FOR HIGHER EDUCATION

Educators make a difference on the overall student experience, yet feedback and the perception of providing feedback remains an issue. Parry and Reynolds[33] explored the differences in providing and receiving assessment-related feedback. While educators are perceived by students as good at providing feedback, the use of that feedback seemingly does not correlate to students improving their grades. Clearer processes for feedback and student understanding of the application of feedback for academic improvement and professional development are important to this outcome and need to be explicit.

The understanding of the student experience provides important insights for course administrators, academics and student support services and can then assist in enhancing a successful first-year experience of students. The flow-on effect of ensuring that students are retained and attrition rates are minimised is invaluable to maintaining the viability and productiveness of tertiary courses. While tertiary transfer students and health professional students have demonstrated several aptitudes[12] that ensure their academic and future health profession success[40] the support and encouragement of education staff should not be underestimated in this process. Academic staff and the tertiary sector need to harness this unique health profession student aptitude in order to enhance the university experience of future health professionals.

CONCLUSION

Student-centred teaching and teaching staff remain the most effective educational interventions, allowing students and teaching staff to accommodate various teaching and learning needs. Despite cost limitation pressures constraining teaching hours, every student needs to receive expert teaching. The tertiary transfer experience is increasingly occurring in highly competitive courses and the supportive role of the educators and teaching are integral to student success. Students require the teaching environment to include support to assist their transition journey.

The use of curricula material that assists in the development of reflective practice is important for first-year health professional students. It is important that educators understand the role of reflection in the development of future health professionals and provide activities that promote its use in tutorials.

SUMMARY POINTS

- Student-centred approaches to learning and teaching of health professional students are essential to ensure optimal student outcomes.
- There are many students from non-traditional backgrounds who are seeking admission to health professional courses via alternate pathways; this group of students has unique learning needs.
- Consideration of the transactional distance between educators and students is a significant factor related to students' experience and learning success in the tertiary sector.
- Ongoing research into student-centred approaches to the learning and teaching of health professional students is essential and this will contribute to the evidence-based education body of knowledge.

REVIEW QUESTIONS

The topics presented as follows are possible future research questions:
- What is the impact of tertiary transfer programmes on Australian students?
- What academic support programmes do tertiary transfer students need?
- What is the role of teaching staff in supporting students to achieve their goals?
- How does this differ between tertiary transfer and non-tertiary transfer students?
- What is the role of academic support programmes for first-year university students and how do these programmes affect student outcomes?
- What is the impact of university structures on student diversity and tertiary transfer experiences?
- What is the impact of increasing student numbers on teaching staff?
- Outline the factors involved in high-quality student outcomes.
- Discuss the impact of increasing student numbers on teaching.
- How do societal pressures (e.g. requiring more people to have degrees) affect the university sector?

REFLECTIVE QUESTIONS AND EXERCISES

- James is a first-year university student from rural Australia. He wants to be a paramedic and return to his country town to provide health services for his community. He feels a great pressure on him to succeed and he misses his family. He does not feel as though he is 'fitting in' at university.
  - As a student, what could you do to assist James with 'fitting in'?
  - What could the teaching staff do to assist James?
  - What programmes could the university put in place that would assist James with fitting in?
- James wishes to become a paramedic; you may also wish to become a health professional. If so, what qualifications do you need to fulfil the entry requirements into your future profession? What is your profession's code of ethics and conduct? Describe how you would meet these professional standards. Where would you find this information?

REFERENCES

1. Coates H. *Australasian Survey of Student Engagement (AUSSE). Working on a dream: educational returns from off-campus paid work. Research briefing paper.* Camberwell, VIC: Australian Council for Education Research; 2011.
2. Coates H, Ransom L. *Australasian Survey of Student Engagement (AUSSE). Dropout DNA, and the genetics of effective support. Research briefing paper.* Camberwell, VIC: Australian Council for Education Research; 2011.
3. Richardson S. *Australasian Survey of Student Engagement (AUSSE). Uniting teachers and learners: critical insights into the importance of staff-student interactions in Australian university education. Research briefing paper.* Camberwell, VIC: Australian Council for Education Research; 2011.
4. Benson R, Samarawickrema G. Teaching in context: some implications for e-Learning design. *ICT: Providing choices for learners and learning. Proceedings ascilite Singapore 2007.* 2007: 61–70. Available at: www.ascilite.org.au/conferences/singapore07/procs/benson.pdf (accessed 9 October 2014).
5. Ambrose S, Bridges M, DiPietro M, *et al. How Learning Works: 7 research-based principles for smart teaching.* San Francisco, CA: Jossey-Bass & Wiley Publishers; 2010.
6. Korach S. You are the curriculum: participant identification of experience and practice with impact. *Plan Changing.* 2012; **43**(1–2): 149–60.
7. Di Napoli R. *What is Student-Centred Learning?* London: Educational Initiative Centre, University of Westminster; 2004.
8. Attard A, Di Ioio E, Geven K, *et al. Student Centred Learning: an insight into theory and practice.* Bucharest: EU Educational International; 2010.
9. Bandura A. *Social Foundations of Thought and Action: a social cognitive theory.* Englewood Cliffs, NJ: Prentice-Hall; 1986.
10. Erikson EH. *Identity and the Life Cycle.* New York, NY: Norton; 1980.
11. Van der Meer J, Jansen E, Torenbeek M. It's almost a mindset that teachers need to change: first-year students' need to be inducted into time management. *Stud High Educ.* 2013; **35**(7): 777–91.
12. Ash JK, Walters LK, Prideaux DJ, *et al.* The context of clinical teaching and learning in Australia. *Med J Aust.* 2012; **196**(7): 475.

13. Mann K, Gordon J, MacLeod A. Reflection and reflective practice in health professions education: a systematic review. *Adv Health Sci Educ Theory Pract.* 2009; **14**(4): 595–621.

14. Steketee C, Bate F. Using educational design research to inform teaching and learning in health professions. *Issues Educ Res.* 2013; **23**(2): 269–82.

15. Zepke N, Leach L. Improving student engagement: ten proposals for action. *Active Learn High Educ.* 2010; **11**(3): 167–78.

16. Australian Bureau of Statistics. *Education and Training: participation in education.* 1301.0 – Year Book Australia, 2012. Belconnen, ACT: Australian Bureau of Statistics; 2012. Available at: www.abs.gov.au/ausstats/abs@.nsf/Lookup/by%20Subject/1301.0~2012~Main%20 Features~Participation%20in%20education~108 (accessed 24 May 2012).

17. Strahn-Koller BL. *Academic Transfer Shock and Social Integration: a comparison of outcomes for traditional and nontraditional students transferring from 2-year to 4-year institutions* [PhD thesis]. Iowa City: University of Iowa; 2012. Available at: http://ir.uiowa.edu/etd/2992 (accessed 24 May 2012).

18. O'Shea H, Onsman A, McKay J. *Students from Low Socioeconomic Status Backgrounds in Higher Education: an annotated bibliography 2000–2011.* Higher Education Research Group. Sydney: Australian Learning and Teaching Council; 2011. Available at: www.lowses.edu.au/assets/LSES-Annotated-Bibliography.pdf (accessed 15 January 2014).

19. Mullin C. *The Road Ahead: a look at trends in the educational attainment of community college students. American Association of Community Colleges – Policy Brief 2011–04PBL2011.* Washington, DC: American Association of Community Colleges; 2011.

20. Matthews PH. Factors influencing self-efficacy judgments of university students in foreign language tutoring. *Mod Lang J.* 2010; **94**(4): 618–35.

21. Boud D, and associates. *Assessment 2020: seven propositions for assessment reform in higher education.* Sydney: Australian Learning and Teaching Council; 2010. Available at: www.uts.edu. au/sites/default/files/Assessment-2020_propositions_final.pdf (accessed 15 January 2014).

22. Vygotsky L. *Mind in Society: the development of higher psychological process.* London: Harvard University Press; 1978.

23. Laanan FS. Transfer students: trends and issues. In: Cohen AM, Brawer B, Zeszotarski P, editors. *New Directions for Community Colleges. Number 114.* San Francisco, CA: Jossey-Bass Adult Education Series; 2001. pp. 5–13.

24. Berger JB, Malaney GD. Assessing the transition of transfer students from community college to a university. *NASPA J.* 2003; **20**(4): 1–23.

25. Eggleston LE, Laanan FS. Making the transition to the senior institution. In: Cohen AM, Brawer B, Zeszotarski P, editors. *New Directions for Community Colleges. Number 114.* San Francisco, CA: Jossey-Bass Adult Education Series; 2001. pp. 87–97.

26. Hagedorn LS, Lester J. Hispanic community college students and the transfer game: strikes, misses, and grand experiences. *Community Coll J Res Pract.* 2006; **30**(10): 827–53.

27. Townsend BK. Feeling like a freshman again: the transfer student transition. *New Dir High Educ.* 2008; **2008**(144): 69–77.

28. Kozeracki C. Studying transfer students: designs and methodological challenges. In: Cohen AM, Brawer B, Zeszotarski P, editors. *New Directions for Community Colleges. Number 114.* San Francisco, CA: Jossey-Bass Adult Education Series; 2001. pp. 61–75.

29. Bradley D, Noonan P, Nugent H, *et al. Review of Australian Higher Education: Final Report.* Canberra City, ACT: Department of Education, Employment and Workplace Relations, Commonwealth of Australia; 2008.

30. Malik S. Students, tutors and relationships: the ingredients of a successful student support scheme. *Med Educ.* 2000; **34**: 635–41.

31. Chi MTH, Roy M, Hausmann RGM. Observing tutorial dialogues collaboratively: insights about human tutoring effectiveness from vicarious learning. *Cogn Sci.* 2008; **32**(2): 301–41.

32. VanLehn K, Graesser AC, Jackson GT, *et al.* When are tutorial dialogues more effective than reading? *Cogn Sci.* 2006; **31**(1): 3–62.
33. Parry Y, Reynolds L. Scaffolding key academic skills in a Bachelor of Health Science program [presentation]. 13th Pacific Rim First Year in Higher Education Conference; Adelaide, SA; 2010 June 27–30. Available at: http://fyhe.com.au/past_papers/papers10/content/pdf/6A.pdf (accessed 9 October 2014).
34. Reynolds L, Kutileh S. Academic support for first year students transferring to other programs [oral presentation]. 13th Pacific Rim First Year in Higher Education Conference; Adelaide, SA; 2010 June 27–30. Available at: www.fyhe.com.au
35. King S. MOOCs will mean the death of universities? Not likely. *The Conversation.* 28 August 2012. Available at: http://theconversation.edu.au/moocs-will-mean-the-death-of-universities-not-likely-8830 (accessed 15 January 2014).
36. Carnevale AP, Strohl J, Smith N. Help wanted: postsecondary education and training required. *New Dir Commun Coll.* 2009; **2009**(146): 21–31.
37. Roscoe RD, Chi MTH. Tutor learning: the role of explaining and responding to questions. *Instr Sci.* 2008; **36**: 321–50.
38. Bloom BS. The 2 sigma problem: the search for methods of group instruction effective as one-to-one tutoring. *Educ Res.* 1984; **13**(6): 4–6.
39. Stephenson PM. Aspects of the nurse tutor-student nurse relationship. *J Adv Nurs.* 2006; **9**(3): 283–90.
40. Wilson K, Lizzio A. *First Year Tutor Training.* Mt Gravatt, QLD: Griffith University; 2007.

CHAPTER 8

Professionalism education as a jigsaw

Putting it together for nursing students

....

Charlotte E Rees and Lynn V Monrouxe

OVERVIEW

Nursing students learn professionalism and how to *become* professionals through the formal, informal and hidden curriculum. While nursing students are taught professionalism through codes of practice, and teaching in ethics, law and humanities, it is known that they often witness and participate in events that flout that teaching, such as breaches of patient safety and dignity – illustrated starkly in the recent Mid Staffordshire NHS Foundation Trust Public Inquiry report. This chapter begins by discussing professionalism education using the metaphor of a *jigsaw*, with interlinking pieces: the formal, informal and hidden curriculum. The formal, informal and hidden curriculum for professionalism education is first discussed and then an example of evidence-based education related to professionalism is presented in order to demonstrate how these puzzle pieces do not always neatly fit together. In this chapter, we present and interpret three written narratives from British nursing students to illustrate their lived experiences of professionalism lapses involving nurses, healthcare assistants and doctors. Through the discussion of these narratives, how nursing students make sense of their developing professional identities and professionalism is illustrated against a constantly shifting backdrop of interprofessional hierarchies, roles and conflicts. The chapter concludes by outlining the implications of evidence-based education research and further research. The chapter also includes discussion questions and reflective exercises for nursing and other healthcare students in order to prepare them better for future workplace professionalism dilemmas.

CHAPTER OBJECTIVES

Upon completion of this chapter, the reader will be able to:
- discuss how nursing professionalism is learned through the formal, informal and hidden curriculum
- present an illustrative example of evidence-based education related to nursing students' professionalism development
- facilitate nursing and other healthcare students' critical reflections on their lived experiences of professionalism dilemmas in order to better prepare them for future dilemmas.

KEY TERMS: professionalism, professionalism dilemmas, professionalism lapses, formal curriculum, informal curriculum, hidden curriculum, narratives, identities, evidence-based education, nursing students

---

INTRODUCTION

> A toxic culture can pollute good people ... through constant change, chronic under-staffing and unrelenting pressure, staff have kindness and compassion eroded from them.[1(p3)]

Professionalism education for healthcare students is of paramount importance.[2] Although there is no single overarching definition of healthcare professionalism and understandings vary by person, place and time,[3-5] regulatory bodies in the United Kingdom such as the Nursing and Midwifery Council have articulated clearly their understandings of and expectations for professional values:

> All nurses must act first and foremost to care for and safeguard the public. They must practise autonomously and be responsible and accountable for safe, compassionate, person-centred, evidence-based nursing that respects and maintains dignity and human rights.[6(p13)]

Professionalism education can be conceptualised as a *jigsaw*, with smaller pieces meant to fit together to make a whole: these pieces can be thought of as the formal, informal and hidden curriculum.[7] However, these pieces do not always fit together easily or neatly and this is often the case for professionalism education, with students receiving mixed messages about the way things *should be* done as part of the formal curriculum versus the way things *are* done as part of the informal and hidden curriculum. Professionalism dilemmas created by this lack of fit can cause students distress and can also have a negative impact on their further professionalism development.[8] This chapter will discuss each piece of the jigsaw and will provide an example of evidence-based education related to professionalism in order to demonstrate how these jigsaw pieces sometimes do not fit together. This chapter will assist students to reflect critically on their lived experiences of professionalism dilemmas and facilitates discussion among students and educators about professionalism education.

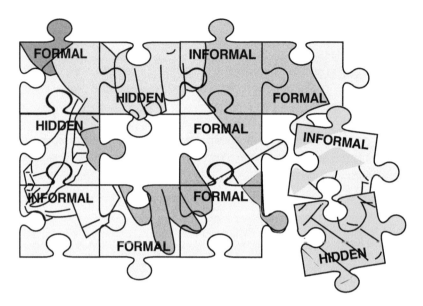

FIGURE 8.1 The jigsaw of professionalism education

THE FORMAL CURRICULUM: TEACHING PROFESSIONALISM IN NURSING EDUCATION

The formal curriculum is the specified and avowed curriculum.[7] In the United Kingdom, nursing students participate in a minimum of 4600 hours of training, less than half of which could be described as the formal curriculum taking place in the classroom.[6] Included in the formal curriculum is essential content such as professionalism codes of practice, ethics, law and humanities.[6] The starting point for much teaching of professionalism in health professions education is the codes of practice. The UK Nursing and Midwifery Council includes four core principles in their code: (1) prioritising patient care and treating patients as individuals and respecting their dignity; (2) working with others to promote the health and well-being of patients, carers, family members and the community; (3) providing high standards of care consistently; and (4) being open and honest and acting with integrity to uphold the profession.[2] Although codes have been criticised for being unrealistic and too theoretical to guide practice, they are thought to be central to professional identity formation.[9] Various instructional methods have been reported in the literature for teaching professionalism codes, ranging from interactive, student-centred methods that integrate theory with clinical practice (e.g. case-based discussion, problem-based learning, written reflection, simulation and role-play) to individually oriented, educator-centred methods that separate theory and practice (e.g. lectures and seminars).[10–12] Although educators typically state their preference for interactive, student-centred methods that bridge the theory–practice gap, students complain that individually oriented and educator-centred methods that fail to integrate practice with theory are all too common.[10] Therefore, the formal nursing professionalism curriculum is not always evidence-based.

THE INFORMAL CURRICULUM: LEARNING PROFESSIONALISM IN THE HEALTHCARE WORKPLACE

The informal curriculum can be described as serendipitous teaching and learning that occurs between students and teachers.[7] Nursing students in the UK spend over 50% of their time learning across a range of placement experiences and those placement experiences should be supervised, either by their mentor, practice teacher or another suitably qualified healthcare professional.[1,6,13] Mentors are registered nurses who have successfully completed approved programmes to supervise and assess students in the clinical workplace.[14] Nursing students are advised to work with their mentors to maintain patient safety, to seek advice from their mentors if they are in doubt about how to act within the workplace, and to inform their mentors if they perceive themselves or anyone else to be putting patients at risk.[15] Mentors and other clinical teachers have complex educational roles within the workplace: they are instrumental in role-modelling professionalism; they help students develop their professional knowledge, skills, values and identities; they facilitate students' reflective practice about professionalism; and they help them navigate the routines and norms of the clinical environment and develop a sense of belonging as they are socialised into the profession.[14,16] However, both grey and academic literature suggests that nursing students are too often inadequately supervised while on placement and witness the poor practice of their role models – poor practice that contradicts the codes that students are taught as part of their formal curriculum.[1,8,14] As we can see, the informal and formal curricula do not always fit neatly together (*see* Figure 8.1).

THE HIDDEN CURRICULUM: LEARNING PROFESSIONALISM THROUGH THE INTERPROFESSIONAL HEALTHCARE CULTURE

The hidden curriculum is about institutional structures and cultures that communicate to students what *is* and what is *not* valued by an institution, so: 'the norms, values and belief systems … imparted to students through daily routines, curricular content, and social relationships'.[17(p6)] Traditionally, nursing was understood as a semi- or quasi-profession because it lacked its own knowledge base and professional autonomy and nurses were consequently seen and treated as the subordinate 'handmaidens' to other professionals such as doctors.[14,18–20] However, nurse education has shifted away from that of a vocational occupation based on a diploma to a professional degree programme in the United Kingdom in order to produce flexible, responsive and highly skilled practitioners capable of meeting the complex care needs of today's patients.[14,19,20] Through this professionalisation of nursing, there has been changes in the division of healthcare labour. Nurses are increasingly taking on some of the physician's roles and simultaneously trying to protect their own roles, like that of personal care, from lower-skilled and lower-paid workers such as nursing auxiliaries and healthcare assistants.[14,18,20,21] Some scholars have discussed the subjugation of relational care within this new professionalism discourse with some nurses being branded as *too posh to wash*.[22,23] Others continue to problematise the professionalisation of nursing, arguing that nurses still lack autonomy in the healthcare workplace: their ability to make decisions is still thought to be limited through traditional medical dominance but also increasingly through increased managerial control and bureaucracy.[20,21] Ultimately, it is through this interprofessional culture of the healthcare workplace and this constantly shifting backdrop of interprofessional hierarchies, roles and conflicts that students learn what it means to be a nurse, and how they should act and interact with other healthcare professionals.

THE PROFESSIONALISM PUZZLE: EXAMPLE OF EVIDENCE-BASED PROFESSIONALISM EDUCATION

Research on healthcare professionalism education has mushroomed over the last decade or so, with questions focusing on four areas related to the formal, informal and/or hidden curriculum: (1) What is professionalism? (2) How should it be taught? (3) How is it learned? (4) How should it be assessed? While various methods have been used to answer questions in these four domains, it is common for research exploring professionalism teaching and assessment (the formal curriculum) to use quantitative methods (e.g. psychometric analyses of assessment instruments), while research investigating what professionalism is and how it is learned (informal and hidden curriculum) typically employs qualitative methods (e.g. discourse analyses of academic and grey literature, and students' talk). In order to explore how the jigsaw pieces of the formal, informal and hidden curriculum fit together in terms of our own research, we explored healthcare students' narratives of professionalism dilemmas. Encompassing four related studies across the United Kingdom (England, Northern Ireland, Scotland and Wales) and Australia, and with 4065 participants (from 41 group and 25 individual interviews and two questionnaires), over 2000 written and oral professionalism dilemma narratives from nursing, physiotherapy, pharmacy, dentistry and medical students have been collected.

Narratives of events are not the events themselves. We choose what to include and what to omit depending on to whom we are telling our story. In that sense, narratives are constructions of events. Thus they are sense-making activities both for the self and the other. Narratives can be described as reports of sequences of events that have 'entered into the biography of the speaker'.[24] Narratives can include multiple elements such as the gist of the story (abstract); details about protagonists, setting, and timing (orientation); the sequence of what happens in terms of actions, problems and turning points (complicating action); one event that has the greatest impact on the narrator (most reportable event); what happens after the most reportable event (resolution); the narrator's commentary on the event (evaluation); and a return from the story to the present (coda).[24,25] Narratives therefore help individuals make sense of their experiences, actions and identities, and through the act of storytelling narrators tend to engage in identity work, sometimes trying to portray themselves in a positive light.[26-28] Thus by attending to the content of these narratives, alongside the ways in which individuals narrated the events, research has demonstrated that key aspects of a person's identity can be revealed.[8,29-31] These aspects include professional and moral identities as constructed through talk.[32]

The preliminary thematic framework analysis of these narratives shows more similarities than differences between the five healthcare student groups. Common themes across all student groups include dilemmas involving patient safety and dignity breaches (by qualified healthcare professionals and students), consent, student identity and student abuse.[8,27,31] In this chapter, three narratives from the most recent study employing an online questionnaire with nursing, physiotherapy, pharmacy and dentistry students to collect their 'most memorable' professionalism dilemmas prompted by the Labovian structure outlined here are presented. Through this questionnaire, we collected 456 written narratives amounting to 59 800 words (narratives ranged from 15 to 537 words, with an average of 131 words). The majority of narratives in this study came from nursing students (N = 294, 65%), so nursing narratives are focused on in this chapter. Narratives from other healthcare students can be found elsewhere.[8,27,31,32] Three narratives are presented – the first being intraprofessional and the second and third being interprofessional – to illustrate various points already identified in this chapter.

Jilly's narrative

The narrative on the following page is a fairly typical 'regret' narrative, from a white, female nursing student aged 36–40 years and in the second year of her training.[32] The experience recounted in the narrative occurred over a year previously, so it took place near the start of her first year. In this narrative, the student describes a common type of professionalism dilemma narrated across our research programme (the breach of patient safety and dignity) and a common response on the part of students (doing nothing and therefore going along with the professionalism lapse).

In this narrative, the student stated that she and her nurse mentor left a male patient on a neurological ward soiled in his own excrement and in extreme pain for several hours, action that flouts the professional code.[2] She explained that the reason she did nothing and participated in this action was because she was following her mentor's behaviour and she lacked the confidence to advocate for the patient. So, her narrative illustrated the important influences of role-modelling and hierarchies in terms of her own professionalism.[14,16] It also emphasised the mismatch between the formal and informal curriculum pieces of the professionalism education jigsaw: what she was taught by her mentor contradicted what she was taught by the professional code.

What was particularly interesting in this narrative was how the student constructed the patient as victim, her mentor as the villain, and herself as both villain (towards the patient) and victim (of her mentor). Her mentor was constructed as

---

BOX 8.1 'I was following my mentor'

What is the gist of your dilemma? I left a patient in his own faeces and in terrible pain for hours because I was following my mentor and this is what she did. We even had a cup of tea and a biscuit.

Where were you and who was present? On a neuro. ward. I was present with the patient and my mentor behind closed curtains.

What happened? A patient was left in terrible pain and discomfort for several hours.

What did you do? Nothing.

Why did you do that? I didn't have the confidence to speak up for the patient.

How do you feel about it now? Terrible guilt and pain for the patient.

Any other comments about this? I would never do it again.

---

unprofessional, dispassionate and uncaring (e.g. the neglectful carer) through being the person primarily responsible for ignoring (and thereby failing to attend to) the patient's discomfort and pain.[32] The narrator constructed herself as a villain (also the neglectful carer) right at the start of her narrative (for example, her use of 'I' in the first sentence demonstrates that she takes personal responsibility for leaving the patient in his own faeces and in pain) but then shortly thereafter she constructed herself as the victim (also slave) of her mentor ('because I was following my mentor', 'I didn't have the confidence to speak up').[32] The second time she stated that the patient was left in pain she shifted from an active voice, including the pronoun 'I', to the passive voice, excluding 'I' ('a patient was left in terrible pain'), illustrating that she abrogated personal responsibility for the professionalism lapse, thereby laying the blame squarely on the shoulders of her mentor. She further constructed herself as victim as she stated that she also felt 'terrible guilt and pain'.

Throughout her narrative it was clear that she knew how she should have acted with care and compassion in accordance with the code but that she failed to enact this for the patient. She concluded her narrative by saying that she would never again behave in this way, suggesting that she has recommitted to the professionalism code.[2]

Clair's narrative

The second narrative is from a white, female nursing student aged 17–25 years and in the second year of training. The experience recounted in the narrative occurred 6–12 months previously, so it took place at the end of her first year. Similar to the previous narrative, the student describes a common type of dilemma across our research, a breach of patient dignity, but this time a communication violation by a healthcare worker to patients. Unlike the previous narrative, this student does something about this professionalism lapse.

**BOX 8.2 'The HCA [healthcare assistant] entered the end
of the ward shouting'**

What is the gist of your dilemma? A young, very confident, HCA on my placement ward walked down the entire length of the 30 bedded ward shouting 'no
one's getting a wash, unless you've wet your … bed!'

Where were you and who was present? I was finishing my assistance with a
patient during a wash, as the HCA entered the end of the ward shouting.

What happened? There was a RN [registered nurse] present who simply raised
her eyebrows and looked at me, not saying anything to the HCA.

What did you do? I walked over to the young HCA, and said to the HCA that
she can't say those things, and although we were extremely short staffed, the
morning washes would still be performed for everyone, and it would just take a
bit longer than usual.

Why did you do that? Because I felt outraged that she exclaimed that to the
patients. And, the fact that she wasn't prepared to assist with washing more
patients than normal, due to the lack of staff. I felt disgusted with her remarks to
the patients and embarrassed at her lack of care, or empathy for them …

How do you feel about it now? I am annoyed that the RN said very little to her
on the matter, because she was young and she had had previous warnings for
behaviour, that she didn't want to get her into more trouble.

Any other comments about this? I reported it to my mentor on the next shift,
who promptly told the sister in charge and the HCA was disciplined accordingly
due to her unacceptable behaviour. Thankfully.

In this narrative, the student states that a healthcare assistant (HCA) shouted at the
patients on a large 30-bedded ward that none of them were getting washed unless
they had soiled themselves, behaviour that is inconsistent with the professional code.[2]
The narrator explains that she verbally challenged this HCA and reported the incident to her mentor, actions that are consistent with the professional code.[2] So, while
a mismatch between what she is taught as part of the formal curriculum is viewed
and what she sees as part of the informal and hidden curriculum, it is also seen that
this student was fitting together these pieces of the jigsaw by challenging this HCA.

She positioned herself as hero in this story: she constructed her identity as assertive,
moral, hard-working and caring, and this professionalism was repeatedly emphasised
by her negative emotional talk ('outraged', 'disgusted', 'embarrassed', 'annoyed') when
talking about the HCA's professionalism lapse and the inaction of the registered nurse
(RN) in the face of that lapse. Conversely, she positioned the HCA as the villain of the
story: she was constructed as uncaring, dispassionate and lazy (also neglectful carer),
and her lack of professionalism was further emphasised by the narrator's revelation
that the HCA had received previous warnings about her 'unacceptable behaviour'.[32]

The narrator therefore blames the HCA for her own behaviour rather than the fraught context of having to wash many patients while being extremely understaffed. The narrator referred to the HCA as 'very confident' and 'young', implying that her behaviour might have been attributable to her personality and the naivety of youth. That she repeatedly referred to this HCA as 'young' was interesting, given that she was only 17–25 years old herself (this possibly implied that she was older than the HCA). The RN was simultaneously constructed as passive bystander (she failed to challenge the HCA) and diplomat (her inaction was to try to avoid the HCA getting into trouble).[32]

What was most interesting about this narrative was that although the student nurse raised her concerns about the HCA's behaviour, she failed to raise concerns about the RN's inaction, which also flouted the code.[2] This narrative raises important issues about professional roles and hierarchies: the student nurse may have challenged the HCA because the HCA was younger and a nursing assistant and therefore subordinate to her, and/or because it was ultimately the HCA's role to conduct the lower-skilled task of personal care.[22,23] By contrast, the student nurse may have failed to challenge the RN because she was older and superordinate to herself. So, while this student seems to fit together pieces of the professionalism jigsaw in terms of her action towards and about the HCA, she failed to do this in terms of the RN (her clinical teacher).

Lisa's narrative

The final narrative was from a white, female nursing student aged 17–25 years and in the second year of her training. The experience recounted occurred 2–3 months previously, so it took place at the start of her second year. In this narrative the student described two common types of professionalism dilemmas narrated across this research: a lack of patient consent and a breach of patient physical dignity. Similar to the previous narrative, this student nurse acted in the face of this professionalism lapse.

In this narrative, the student stated that an anaesthetist tried to insert a cannula into a teenager's arm without her valid consent, by grabbing her arm in the induction room prior to surgery and then thrusting a mask into her face, behaviour inconsistent with the code.[2] She explained her own behaviours, all of which are consistent with the code: she verbally challenged the anaesthetist by calling for everything to stop, she acted to show concern for the patient by explaining the anaesthetic induction to her and involving the teenager's mother, and she took the teenager back to the ward once it was determined that she did not want her operation. Although a mismatch was seen between what she was taught as part of the formal curriculum and what she saw as part of the informal and hidden curriculum, this student can be seen fitting together the jigsaw pieces by challenging the anaesthetist.

As a narrator, she positioned the anaesthetist as the villain: he is constructed as clinically and communicatively incompetent, unprofessional and physically aggressive. By contrast, she positioned herself as the heroic patient advocate: she constructed herself as assertive, clinically and communicatively competent and caring.[32] What was interesting in this narrative was that she repeatedly excluded pronominal talk during her explanations of what happened, making it sometimes difficult to work out *who*

BOX 8.3 'Feel the anaesthetist was inappropriate and threatening'

What is the gist of your dilemma? An anaesthetist coercing an anxious 13-year-old girl to have cannulation, no consent, no explanation, bullish.

Where were you and who was present? In the induction room, 2 ODPs [operating department practitioners], student nurse, mum and anaesthetist.

What happened? Very nervous patient, calmed and reassured by student nurse, on entering induction room, little introduction, no explanation, anaesthetist physically grabbed patients arm to cannulate. Patient struggled and withdrew arm. Inappropriate communication, bullish and semi aggressive. Move to gas induction, again no explanation mask thrust into patient's face.

What did you do? Called for everything to stop. Gained patient's trust again, explained gas induction fully, pros and cons, got mum involved said she could hold the mask, got her agreement. After poor attempt by anaesthetist patient withdrew again, asked patient if she wanted operation, she replied no. So I took her back to the ward.

Why did you do that? No consent, 13 years old, competent, understood. Acted as advocate for the child.

How do you feel about it now? Feel the anaesthetist was inappropriate and threatening. Hope the girl hasn't suffered emotional effects of experience. Feel I acted in the best way I could although I wish I could have said more.

---

did *what*. Such pronominal ellipsis seems consistent throughout the narrative and probably reflected her succinct writing style. However, there were two sentences that did include the pronoun 'I': 'So *I* took her back to the ward' and '*I* acted in the best way *I* could although *I* wish *I* could have said more'. Her use of 'I' here demonstrated her taking ownership and responsibility for her positive actions and thoughts. She clearly regretted that she could have said more although the reader was left wondering at the end of her narrative to whom she should have said more: the anaesthetist, the patient or both?

This narrative raises important issues about interprofessional roles and hierarchies: that the student nurse challenged this anaesthetist despite his superordinate position (he is both qualified and a doctor) probably reflects their different 'curing' and 'caring' roles within this encounter.[33] The anaesthetist was clearly focused on the technical task of anaesthetising this teenager so that she can be operated on. The student nurse, on the other hand, was focused on the patient's psychological and emotional well-being. It was perhaps by donning the cloak of patient advocacy that this student felt sufficiently empowered to challenge this anaesthetist who was higher in the healthcare hierarchy.

Conclusions: completing the picture

Nursing students learn professionalism in the classroom and the workplace. As part of the formal curriculum they are taught how to act with teaching methods that are often not evidence-based (e.g. individually oriented, educator centred and fail to bridge the theory–practice gap).[10] As part of the informal curriculum they learn how professionals act within the workplace: through their interactions with mentors and other clinical role models (both intra- and interprofessional) students commonly witness, and can be socialised into, suboptimal professional practice.[16] As part of the hidden curriculum they see how professionals interact with each other; they learn the roles and responsibilities of different professionals and how those groups inter-relate in terms of the healthcare hierarchy.[19] Importantly, they learn their own roles and responsibilities and their place within the pecking order. However, these pieces of the professionalism education jigsaw do not always fit together effortlessly, since students often receive mixed messages about how they should act and this can be dis-tressing. As illustrated by the three narratives in this chapter, nursing students witness healthcare professionals flouting the codes they learn in school: they fail to care for and safeguard patients; they fail to provide safe, compassionate and person-centred care; and they breach patient dignity and human rights [2]

How students act in the face of such professionalism lapses varies from one student to the next. Some students fail to challenge professionalism lapses and in doing so go along with them (such as Jilly did); others challenge some protagonists yet fail to challenge others (for example, as Clair did); and others still seem to do everything they can to right the wrongs of their healthcare colleagues (like Lisa attempted to do). Whether students challenge or not appears to depend on a complex interplay between intra- and interprofessional roles and hierarchies. Through the narratives we can see how three nursing students make sense of their professionalism dilemmas and their own actions as they attempt to fit together the pieces of the professionalism education jigsaw. We also see how they make sense of themselves and others through their nar-ratives. There are some patterns of identity construction across these three narratives, with patients constructed as victims, healthcare professionals exhibiting professional-ism lapses constructed as villains, and the narrators constructing themselves as heroes when they challenge professionalism lapses, and villain or victim when they do not.

It is recommended that students be given the opportunity to reflect on their pro-fessionalism dilemmas through narrative as part of the formal curriculum. It is also suggested that students share their dilemmas with their peers through small group interprofessional learning sessions in order to gain support and formulate strategies for dealing with future dilemmas in the healthcare workplace. Such formal curricula should give students the interactive and student-centred methods that integrate theory and practice that both students and teachers desire. Through small group learning, students should have a safe forum to discuss the different pieces of the jigsaw: the formal, informal and hidden curriculum, and how and why these pieces sometimes do not fit together.

CONCLUSION

The narratives discussed in this chapter are rich with emotional talk, revealing the personal meanings these events hold for students. Analysing students' professionalism dilemmas through narrative has helped us understand the different pieces of the professionalism education jigsaw, particularly the informal and hidden curriculum from the student perspective. While quantitative and qualitative methods abound in the healthcare education literature to explore various aspects of the formal, informal and hidden professionalism curriculum, few studies employ observational methods.[34] Drawing on the authors' video observation research of bedside teaching encounters,[35] it is recommended that further video observation of the formal, informal and hidden aspects of the professionalism education curriculum be completed to assist in making these other components more visible and overt. Such video observation allows for video reflexivity, whereby edited video could be played back to students and clinical teachers to help them better understand the different facets and how they fit together.[36,37] Video reflexivity could provide students and clinical teachers with the opportunity to see a more complete picture, rather like looking at the whole picture of a jigsaw on the box it came in. Video reflexivity might therefore allow students and teachers to work together to better integrate the pieces and complete the jigsaw that is professionalism education.

SUMMARY POINTS

- Nursing students learn professionalism through interlinked pieces of the curriculum jigsaw: the formal, informal and hidden curriculum.
- Sometimes these curriculum jigsaw pieces do not fit easily or neatly together: what students are taught is not necessarily what they learn.
- Students faced with professionalism lapses act in various ways, ranging from going along with lapses to doing something about them (e.g. challenging).
- Students often construct the patient as victim, the perpetrators of professionalism lapses as villains, and themselves as heroes in their narratives.
- In terms of evidence-based education, students should share their dilemmas as part of the formal curriculum in order to integrate theory and practice.
- In terms of the development of educational evidence, more observational methods are needed to help make the formal, informal and hidden aspects of the curriculum of professionalism education more visible.

REVIEW QUESTIONS

- How would you define professionalism within your own healthcare profession?
- How is professionalism taught in your own setting?
- How is professionalism learned in your own setting?
- How is professionalism assessed in your own setting?
- What elements of culture within the interprofessional healthcare workplace do you think are most important in shaping your professionalism?

REFLECTIVE QUESTIONS AND EXERCISES

- Reflect critically on the three narratives provided in this book chapter. Put yourself in the shoes of the student nurse in each narrative. You may have already experienced a similar situation on placement and/or you might experience similar situations in the future. Thinking about your professional code, write down all the things that each student could or should have done.
- Thinking about your answers to the previous point, write down what you think are the barriers to taking such actions and how you might overcome these barriers in practice.
- You have already read three narratives by nursing students. You may have experienced something similar or something quite different that you would also consider a professionalism dilemma. Write down your own dilemma, answering the following questions: What is the gist of your dilemma? Where were you, who was present and when did it occur? What happened? What did you do and why did you do that? How do you feel about it now?
- Once you have written down your dilemma, reread it and reflect critically on your action. Think about what you could or should do differently if this similar situation happened again.
- Reflect critically on the way that you have constructed yourself and others within your narrative. What does this say about your professional identity now and who you want to be in the future?

REFERENCES

1. Royal College of Nursing (RCN). *Mid Staffordshire NHS Foundation Trust Public Inquiry Report: response of the Royal College of Nursing.* London: RCN; 2013.
2. Nursing and Midwifery Council (NMC). *The Code: standards of conduct, performance and ethics for nurses and midwives.* London: NMC; 2008.
3. Hafferty FW. Definitions of professionalism: a search for meaning and identity. *Clin Orthop Relat Res.* 2006; **449**: 193–204.
4. Hutchings H, Rapport F, Wright S, *et al.* Obtaining consensus about patient-centred professionalism in community nursing: nominal group work activity with professionals and the public. *J Adv Nurs.* 2011; **68**(11): 2429–42.

5. Monrouxe LV, Rees CE, Hu W. Differences in medical students' explicit discourses of medical professionalism: acting, representing, becoming. *Med Educ.* 2011; **45**(6): 585–602.
6. Nursing and Midwifery Council (NMC). *Standards for Pre-registration Nursing Education.* London: NMC; 2010.
7. Hafferty FW. Beyond curriculum reform: confronting medicine's hidden curriculum. *Acad Med.* 1998; **73**(4): 403–7.
8. Monrouxe LV, Rees CE, Endacott R, *et al.* 'Even now it makes me angry': health care students' professionalism dilemma narratives. *Med Educ.* 2014; **48**(5): 502–17.
9. Numminen O, van der Arend A, Leino-Kilpi H. Nurse educators' and nursing students' perspectives on teaching codes of ethics. *Nurs Ethics.* 2009; **16**(1): 69–82.
10. Numminen O, Leino-Kilpi H, van der Arend A, *et al.* Comparison of nurse educators' and nursing students' descriptions of teaching codes of ethics. *Nurs Ethics.* 2011; **18**(5): 710–24.
11. Lin C-F, Lu M-S, Chung C-C, *et al.* A comparison of problem-based learning and conventional teaching in nursing ethics. *Nurs Ethics.* 2010; **17**(3): 373–82.
12. Smith KV, Witt J, Klaassen J, *et al.* High-fidelity simulation and legal/ethical concepts: a transformational learning experience. *Nurs Ethics.* 2012; **19**(3): 390–8.
13. Nursing and Midwifery Council (NMC). *NMC Response to the Francis Report.* London: NMC; 2013.
14. Willis Commission. *Quality with Compassion: the future of nursing education.* London: Royal College of Nursing; 2012.
15. Nursing and Midwifery Council (NMC). *Guidance on Professional Conduct for Nursing and Midwifery Students.* London: NMC; 2011.
16. Brown J, Stevens J, Kermode S. Supporting student nurse professionalisation: the role of the clinical teacher. *Nurs Educ Today.* 2012; **32**(5): 606–10.
17. Margolis E, Soldatenko M, Ackers S, *et al.* Peekaboo: hiding and outing the curriculum. In: Margolis E, editor. *The Hidden Curriculum in Higher Education.* New York, NY: Routledge; 2001. pp. 1–19.
18. Manninen E. Changes in nursing students' perceptions of nursing as they progress through their education. *J Adv Nurs.* 1998; **27**(2): 390–8.
19. Rutty JE. The nature of philosophy of science, theory and knowledge relating to nursing and professionalism. *J Adv Nurs.* 1998; **28**(2): 243–50.
20. Wall S. 'We inform the experience of health': perspectives on professionalism in nursing self-employment. *Qual Health Res.* 2013; **23**(7): 976–88.
21. Daiski I, Richards E. Professionals on the sidelines: the working lives of bedside nurses and elementary core French teachers. *Gender Work Organ.* 2007; **14**(3): 210–31.
22. Scott SD. 'New professionalism': shifting relationships between nursing education and nursing practice. *Nurs Educ Today.* 2008; **28**(2): 240–5.
23. Young L. Too posh to wash? *Prim Health Care.* 2004; **14**(5): 12–13.
24. Labov W. Some further steps in narrative analysis. *J Narrat Life Hist.* 1997; **7**: 395–415.
25. Labov W, Waletzky J. Narrative analysis: oral versions of personal experience. In: Helm J, editor. *Essays on the Verbal and Visual Arts.* Seattle, WA: American Ethnological Society, University of Washington Press; 1967. pp. 12–44.
26. Smith B, Sparkes AC. Contrasting perspectives on narrating selves and identities: an invitation to dialogue. *Qual Res.* 2008; **8**(1): 5–35.
27. Rees CE, Monrouxe LV, McDonald LA. Narrative, emotion and action: analysing 'most memorable' professionalism dilemmas. *Med Educ.* 2013; **47**(1): 80–96.
28. Riessman CK. *Narrative Methods for the Human Sciences.* Thousand Oaks, CA: Sage Publications; 2008.
29. Monrouxe LV. Negotiating professional identities: dominant and contesting narratives in medical students' longitudinal audio diaries. *Curr Narrat.* 2009; **1**: 41–59.

30. Monrouxe LV. Solicited audio diaries in longitudinal narrative research: a view from inside. *Qual Res.* 2009; **9**(1): 81–103.

31. Monrouxe LV, Rees CE. 'It's just a clash of cultures': emotional talk within medical students' narratives of professionalism dilemmas. *Adv Health Sci Educ Theory Pract.* 2012; **17**(5): 671–701.

32. Monrouxe LV, Rees CE. Hero, voyeur, judge: understanding medical students' moral identities through professionalism dilemma narratives. In: Mavor K, Platow M, Bizumic B, editors. *The Self, Social Identity and Education*. Hove, UK: Psychology Press; in press.

33. Hanson S. Teaching health care ethics: why we should teach nursing and medical students together. *Nurs Ethics.* 2005; **12**(2): 167–76.

34. Stern DT. In search of the informal curriculum: when and where professional values are taught. *Acad Med.* 1998; **73**(10 Suppl.): S28–30.

35. Rees CE, Ajjawi R, Monrouxe LV. The construction of power in family medicine bedside teaching encounters: a video-observation study. *Med Educ.* 2013; **47**(2): 154–65.

36. Iedema R, Long D, Forsyth R, *et al.* Visibilising clinical work: video ethnography in the contemporary hospital. *Health Sociol Rev.* 2006; **15**(2): 156–68.

37. Iedema R, Merrick ET, Rajbhandari D, *et al.* Viewing the taken-for-granted from under a different aspect: a video-based method in pursuit of patient safety. *Int J Multiple Res Approach.* 2009; **3**(3): 290–301.

CHAPTER 9

Curriculum development, implementation and maintenance in the health professional education context

Andrys Onsman

OVERVIEW

This chapter discusses issues related to curriculum development and implementation in health professional student education. It argues that the creation of a successful, purposeful curriculum depends a great deal on a sound conceptual basis, and that each aspect of every part of the course curriculum needs to be aligned to ensure that the students move through it in a coherent and cohesive manner, with each step clearly organised and each assessment task transparent. Moreover, systemic maintenance and ongoing quality control need to be a structural part of its implementation. To that end, this chapter is organised in the following structure: first, it will present a brief overview of current theory, with an emphasis on curriculum alignment; second, it will discuss the principles of curriculum implementation; third, it will outline the issues to be addressed in terms of curriculum maintenance; fourth, it will put forward some points for consideration and reflection.

CHAPTER OBJECTIVES

Upon completion of this chapter, the reader will be able to:
- summarise the features of 'curriculum development theory'
- describe components of curriculum alignment
- outline principles of curriculum implementation
- describe the features of curriculum maintenance.

KEY TERMS: curriculum development and implementation; constructive alignment; health profession education

---

INTRODUCTION

It is relatively easy to list the defining characteristics of an effective curriculum. Although there will be contestation about the relative importance of each element, it is generally agreed that curricula ought to be constructively aligned, informed by research, learning centred, future focused, discipline specific, communicatively clear, personally transformative, professionally and vocationally preparatory, intellectually engaging and stimulating – and preferably cost neutral to deliver. Curricula are obliged to ensure that students who complete the programme can demonstrate that they have the qualities that the institution advertises as graduate attributes: that specifically they are ready to enter the vocation or profession that their degree qualifies them for and generally that they are better human beings for having completed the course of study. All of this rests Atlas-like on the shoulders of the curriculum.

The development and delivery of sound curricula requires first and foremost an understanding of the conceptual framework on which any curriculum is built. On the other hand, the structure of a curriculum needs to facilitate the student's progress through it in a purposeful manner, and its structural coherence depends on research rather than tradition. Although this chapter is very much concerned with conceptual issues, much of the commentary will be based on research evidence from health professional student education and cognate disciplines, because while curriculum development and implementation is context specific to health sciences education, its conceptual underpinnings borrow from disparate fields including organisational behaviour, social psychology and constructivist pedagogy.

CURRICULUM DEVELOPMENT THEORY

Slattery,[1] in his internationally influential analysis of the current state of curriculum development, argues that the contemporary curriculum lags behind the contemporary world. Traditional approaches to curriculum design and implementation rely on notions of sanctity and imperturbability, whereas the real world demands accountability and relevance. Slattery[1] promotes an approach to curriculum development based on postmodernist discourse, delving deeply into the apparently irreconcilable differences between humanist ambition for personal growth and neo-liberal demand for utilitarian reward. Slattery[1] argues that the two approaches to functionality affect curriculum development. However, in health professional education, it is crucial that the two approaches are reconciled, and much of curriculum development theory in this area is concerned with achieving a practical amalgam. To some extent at least, this can be achieved through evidence-based education.

Although some individual commentators[2] had long sought to accommodate both the formal and the informal content and processes that lead to new knowledge, understanding, skills, attitudes, appreciations and values, much of what is now generally referred to as 'curriculum development theory' originated in the early 1970s, when the work of curriculum theorists such as Elliot Eisner[3] and Daniel and Laurel Tanner[4] took curriculum definitively away from being a summary of what was to be taught and emphasised a learning-centred base. While still retaining the intention of guiding learning according to some institutional norm, there was increased acknowledgement that learning ought to have agency beyond the physical and temporal constraints of the immediate teaching and learning environment. Tanner and Tanner[4] as an example defined a curriculum as the

> planned and guided learning experiences and intended outcomes, formulated through the systematic reconstruction of knowledge and experience, under the auspices of the school, for the learner's continuous and willful growth in person-social competence.[p13]

Fundamentally, the curriculum became a road map of study that led to the acquisition of capabilities that acknowledged the changing nature of both the learner and the world where graduates would be expected to operate. Essentially the curriculum was underpinned by neo-liberal ideas and focused on preparing learners to be able to meet the demands and challenges that they would face in their futures, primarily in terms of employment. What students were to learn would still be based on the collected knowledge of the past but it ought to prepare them for the (vocational) future.

Most contemporary health professional curricula retain a predominantly neo-liberal basis and focus on vocational capacity – that is, health professionals are still trained. However, over the last 2 decades two further, complementary aspects of curriculum development have influenced health professional students' education. First, the narrow focus of vocational training that neo-liberalism creates is being increasingly contested. Second, the notion of a curriculum being confined to a predetermined intention is also being challenged.

Vocational prerequisites have broadened beyond what strict neo-liberal utilitarianism generally focuses on and the acquisition of disparate competencies is no longer seen as preparing learners to operate effectively as practitioners upon graduation. For example, Hojat et al.[5] argue compellingly that successful practice in the health professions relies upon the ability to interact effectively with patients as much as it does on clinical knowledge and skill, and that empathy is one of the core skills of the health professional. Hojat et al.[5] define empathy as a cognitive attribute, contrasting it with the affective attribute of sympathy, an overabundance of which can be detrimental to patient care. Training in empathetic practitioner–patient interaction has superseded the acquisition, often through some assumed, nebulous form of pedagogic osmosis, of a 'good bedside manner.' Empathy is more often seen as a human capacity that requires development through experience and/or teaching. Since healthcare workers' professional developmental needs evolve and refine over the course of their (often prolonged) training and continue to evolve and refine during their practice, qualities such as empathy should be taught iteratively and with increased sophistication throughout their career.[6]

Another example of where specific curricular changes are designed to influence particular issues in professional practice is in the area of practitioner–patient collaboration, especially in terms of devising treatment programmes that afford patients greater autonomy. Because practitioners generally show a reluctance to work in meaningful partnerships with patients,[7] the inclusion in the curriculum of the theoretical principles underlying patient empowerment can result in a framework of understanding and behaviour that will inform future practice.

This trend in curriculum development to actualise all aspects of practice reflects the growing concern with humanising the extant neo-liberal approach that retains a great deal of traction and agency in current curriculum development. Other functional skills demanded of the contemporary health practitioner include collaboration, team building and cross-cultural communication and negotiation skills that are most effectively learned during varying phases of training, indicating that a spiral curriculum, wherein they are revisited throughout the programme at appropriate times and with differing emphasis, may be the most effective structure.

The second area where research is having a discernible impact on development questions the assumption that a curriculum necessarily involves a perimeter defined solely by the accrediting institution, often in consultation with or at the behest of the relevant professional body that will accredit the graduate as a professional practitioner. There are three distinct but related issues that have the attention of academics currently. First, there is general consensus that a health professional curriculum requires input from industry. Second, and less generally accepted, is input from students. Finally, there is an increasing emphasis on including consumers (e.g. patients who health professionals provide services to) in the curriculum consultation process.

Although the negotiated curriculum in higher education generally is a controversial notion, accommodating input from the students from the beginning is seen as meaningfully incorporating critical thinking skills into the learning process. In health professional education, the idea of allowing students to have input about what is to be learned is a pill still particularly difficult to swallow for most educators and administrators. The counterargument generally revolves around the notion that graduates are rightfully expected to have a defined skill set, specialised knowledge and preferred attitudes and values. More specifically, there is an argument that without these the graduate will not be admitted into the various health professions anyway.

There is a good measure of truth in the argument. However, the notion of negotiation in the health professional education curricula must be considered within the framework of a constructive alignment. Given that the intended learning objectives are clearly stated, that the teaching and learning events are planned to support their acquisition and that the assessment tasks are structured as opportunities for students to demonstrate their mastery or acquisition, negotiation assumes a different purpose. Negotiation then becomes learners assuming an active role in decision-making about how they can best achieve the required learning targets. Decisions made in the process can have serious repercussions and are not to made lightly or to be uninformed.

One of the main benefits of empowering learners to have a meaningful say in curriculum development is to facilitate the development of critical thinking skills.[8] Most Western universities cite critical thinking as a graduate attribute. In the health professions, along with attributes such as good communication skills, appropriate ethical values and lifelong learning, critical thinking has assumed near-universal importance as a desirable practitioner attribute. However, the actual teaching of such attributes is often vague and left undefined.[9] Leicester[10] characterises critical thinking as consisting of four broad components: (1) recognising dubious assumptions and generalisations; (2) taking account of context; (3) imagining alternatives; and (4) developing reflective scepticism. In the first instance, these components are particularly appropriate to the health professional student in training. Further, they will also serve the graduate well in practice.

DEVELOPING CURRICULA TO FOSTER COMMUNITIES OF LEARNING IN HEALTH PROFESSIONAL EDUCATION

As has been outlined already in this chapter, there are a number of factors that have a direct impact on the creation and implementation of a curriculum that is relevant to the learner, to the institution that is providing the qualification, and to the industry that the graduates are expected to be prepared to enter. The next section of this chapter considers how they and others directly affect curriculum development. Although there is contestation about the exact proportions, the notion that 70% of learning is experiential, 20% of learning is expository and only 10% is formally educational is increasingly widely accepted as likely.[11] Particularly in the health professions, such a distinction among the learning environments has important ramifications for curriculum development, not least of which is the increasing focus on evidence-based education.

The cognitive or affective accommodation of new knowledge is ultimately an individual activity. However, learning in terms of accessing, formulating, verifying and acquiring knowledge can also be a social process. Learning occurs informally through everyday experiences, either individually or socially when someone learns from others.[12] When social learning is intended or planned it refers to a curriculum based on a 'community of learning' approach.[13] A community of learning curriculum deliberately blurs the distinction between formal and informal education by creating meaningful bonds between all the people involved in the process: students, staff and industry professionals.

An essential component of a community of learning style curriculum is that it also allows an individual's learning objectives and personal needs, skills and preferences to be personalised.[14] Within the socio-educative setting, learning is increasingly self-directed, with the aim of scaffolding it for lifelong professional learning. Learning that is personalised to the individual challenges any standardisation of learning experiences.[13] More purposeful exploitation of learning analytics provides increasingly more detailed data about the learner's activity and achievement, creating a steady stream of information that shapes future learning and allows learners to respond individually.

Furthermore, the increased utility and affordability of mobile technology has resulted in ubiquitous learning and the development of curricula that foster lifelong learning.[15] Communities of learning are no longer encased by traditional classroom boundaries but exist as and within new modes of communication.[16] The combination of the physical and virtual aspects of the learning environments allows students to respond to individually specific feedback in a variety of modes and times – such freedom is at the heart of contemporary curriculum design.

One direction in which this has been taken is by major universities allowing open access to course materials. Open practices promote innovative pedagogical models that support learners to become lifelong learners, particularly those previously excluded from formal learning.[17] Although internationally uneven, there is a steady increase among higher education institutions towards not only providing their accredited courses online but also to provide free access to courses and materials – MOOCs, or massive open online courses. The availability of MOOCs can act as a catalyst for innovation and change by encouraging open collaboration and sharing,[18] which in turn can have a positive effect on the creation of broad communities of learning. Open resource courses do not distinguish pedagogically between participants who are studying for recognised qualifications and those simply interested[19] and thereby demand and achieve innovative pedagogical models that encourage lifelong learning and engagement. Further, the line between accredited and non-accredited students is being blurred by a number of initiatives underway to create formal credentialing of studies undertaken using open education resources, which will result in recognised qualifications from higher education providers other than those offering the course materials. Health professional education is still grappling with how best to embrace this particular development.

How these and other trends will eventually affect health professional education courses remains to be seen but any curriculum that is seeking to prepare learners for a professional future will emphasise skills over facts and it will embrace individual learners' values and motivations, recognising that the skills that the twenty-first-century health professional will be expected to have mastery of include critical thinking, innovation and creativity, self-direction and collaborative practice, and information literacy. In order to attain these goals, health sciences education is increasingly moving towards curricula that foster meaningful, functional and normalised communities of learning that will 'naturally' graduate into community of practice.

CONSTRUCTIVELY ALIGNED CURRICULA

As well as socially constructed it will be constructively aligned, in that learning objectives will align to teaching and assessment tasks. Devised by Biggs and Tang,[20] constructive alignment aims to create curricula that have transparent and clearly stated intended learning objectives articulated at the commencement of a course of learning. Learning objectives for each learning event are articulated with the learning objectives of the unit of study, which in turn are articulated with the course learning objectives, which are in turn articulated with the degree programme learning objectives, which are in turn articulated with the institutional graduate attributes. Within this dendritic structure, each learning objective links to targeted assessment tasks with clearly articulated assessment rubrics. Students will know what they are expected to be able to demonstrate in terms of learning, including what kind of (quantitative or qualitative) response will be assessed according to characteristics. The challenge to the educator is to ensure that learning guidance maximises the likelihood of success. Hence, the setting of the intended learning outcomes assumes a critically important role in curriculum design and delivery.

When health professional learning objectives reflect the twin emphases on being both personally transformational and preparatory in terms of employment, a curriculum that is constructively aligned allows all the agents in the learning environment to be actively involved in the learning process. The teacher assumes a responsibility to guide the learner as to how the learning objectives can be best acquired, in terms of both method and information. The learners assume a concomitant responsibility to be proactive in their learning, both individually and collectively. Teaching assumes guiding, expository and modelling as its primary tactics, and learning assumes the setting and achieving of targets in the way of project management as core strategies.

CURRICULUM IMPLEMENTATION

There are a number of factors that have a direct impact on the implementation and particularly on the delivery of a curriculum that is relevant to the learner, to the institution that is providing the qualification, and to the industry that the graduates are expected to be prepared to enter. The distinction between lectures, tutorials and practical sessions is becoming increasingly less rigid in health professional courses, moving away from didactic lectures followed (often after some delay) by dialectic tutorials and discovery practical sessions and being replaced by more integrated seminar-style delivery, wherein information can be transmitted in shorter bursts, followed by immediate dialogue and hands-on experience. The decisions as to when and for how long the teaching should be didactic or dialectic is left to the judgement of the teacher and the individual requirements of the learner.[21] It is important therefore that the learner is aware that his or her learning environment extends far beyond the immediate teaching environment. The curriculum needs to accommodate the entire learning environment rather than be confined to those parts that are educator led. In other words the old notion that learning objectives are to be articulated only for those learning and teaching events that are led by teachers needs to be disregarded.

Informal learning is an important part of the negotiated, aligned curriculum that forms the bedrock of evidence-based education.

In their seminal book on curriculum, Ornstein and Hunkins[22] point out that curriculum implementation in higher education often involves a great deal of change management; however, as a general strategy, Lewin's[23] deconstruction of organisational change as a three-step process (destabilise the extant, implement the change, normalise the new) retains currency today. For example, John Kotter applied the strategy in higher educational settings, and expanded the process to eight steps to include the buy-in from all active agents. Table 9.1 outlines the steps in Kotter's[24] sequence in thumbnail terms.

TABLE 9.1 Kotter's[24] curriculum implementation steps

Step 1
1. Establish the necessity for the change
2. Allocate leadership of the change
Step 2
3. Formulate and articulate a vision and strategy
4. Communicate vision to all agents
5. Empower all agents to act by removing perceived barriers
6. Recognise incremental changes to demonstrate progress
Step 3
7. Consolidate gains using credibility to encourage more change
8. Integrate into culture by normalising the change

Extrapolating from a number of studies where Kotter's[24] guide has been used and evaluated as a strategy for curriculum change and implementation, it seems that the amount of rigour with which these steps are to be applied depends on the degree of change that is proposed.[25] Whereas change in industry is characteristically a long-term process, the advantage of implementing organisational change in health sciences education curricula is that each year presents new cohorts. However, it should also be acknowledged that the majority of health science education curricula in Australia already incorporate elements of negotiation. Many health science education curricula successfully utilise simulations or scenario-based learning to inculcate general problem-solving skills.[26] Within these contexts it is relatively easy to create a focus on, for example, critical thinking, given that the defining characteristics of critical thinking have been formulated and clearly articulated.

Before ending this section on curriculum implementation, a note of caution must be added. While there is compelling evidence that curriculum implementation is most effectively and efficiently achieved when it refers to a conceptual, theoretical framework, there remain a number of concerns about the extent to which the structures of such frameworks limit the implementation process. Trowler *et al.*[27] argue that institutional change is creative, unpredictable in its specifics and not simply the implementation of an executive blueprint. They demonstrate that the approach chosen affects not only the change but also how the change is managed. In short, as well as subscribing to the value of the curriculum to be implemented, stakeholders also need to agree on the manner of implementation, particularly in health sciences education.[28] Ultimately, successful curriculum implementation depends on all agents taking personal responsibility for process by proactively adapting to the new learning environment.[29]

CURRICULUM MAINTENANCE

Maintaining the relevance, effectiveness and the quality of a health sciences education curriculum is a central aspect of curriculum development and implementation and demands a systemic approach. Rather than leave quality assurance processes to be add-ons that are employed only when demanded by external agencies, maintenance should be seen as an essential part of creation and delivery.

At the heart of it, quality assurance of curriculum seeks an answer to one question: does the curriculum do what it says it will do? Hence the importance and centrality of constructive alignment to curriculum development, for it is in the learning objectives as much as in the course content that the department, faculty or university says what it will provide for and to the learner.

Before setting a system for curriculum maintenance in place, it is (again) profitable to consider the underlying concepts. We should ask not only what is expected of quality assurance of the curriculum but also how quality assurance can be systematically optimised in terms of curriculum enhancement. Rather than seeing it as a box to be ticked, we need to ask how it can be used as a mechanism for improvement. In their study looking at the compatibility of quality assurance and quality enhancement as part of reviewing a nursing curriculum, van de Mortel *et al.*[30] conclude that the two key elements are clear communication and closing the feedback loop. Educators are more likely to sustain their commitment to successful implementation of curriculum development if they are clear as to what is to be changed and why. They will also maintain commitment to ensuring the development is successfully implemented if they are informed of progress. These findings echo the strategies proposed in the sections on curriculum development and implementation earlier in this chapter.

Referring to the principles espoused in constructive alignment, any quality assurance process needs to confirm that the course curriculum contributes to the realisation of the institutional mission. As well as practical outcomes, quality assurance needs to reflect the institutional beliefs and aims: the key indicators of its (either intended or observed) culture. Excellence in terms of both student learning and teaching environment is a consequence of an academic culture that has normalised the implementation of an architecture of quality principles.[31] For that to happen requires more than seductive rhetoric: all agents need to accept and respond proactively to clearly articulated and understood achievement targets. When that occurs, quality assurance becomes a force for transformative change.[32]

For curriculum quality assurance to be effective as a transformative change agent, it needs to be cyclical and iterative as a matter of course, not only to check on what has been done but also to stimulate what can be done. Formal quality assurance is still often considered an unwarranted imposition, an institutional mistrust of teacher competence and commitment, a threat to professional autonomy and authority. That attitude needs to be discarded by all those involved in curriculum development and implementation and replaced by a commitment to effectiveness.

REFLECTION, REVIEW AND CONCLUSION

Creating and implementing new curricula in health professional education is an exciting business: matching vocational requirements with personal development. But how do we balance the pedagogical and the personal with institutional accountability, equitable and fair assessment and formal accreditation? How do we get the personal into a set and defined curriculum? The increasing utility and availability of mobile technologies seem tailor-made for enthusiastic educators but universities are more cautious about investing extensively in mobile technologies, pointing to the speed with which new models emerge, as well as the speed with which devices become obsolete. Web-based courses are increasingly commonplace, even as we accept that Internet access is far from universally even.

This chapter has argued that the trend to empowering students in order to create interactive learning communities, wherein they take responsibility for their own learning under the guidance of teachers and according to a well-constructed curriculum, forms the key to health sciences education curriculum development. We generally want critical thinking to lead to empathetic and skilful practice. Preparing a student for post-study professional life involves much more than simply walking him or her through a collection of information and skills. The health professions often include activities wherein you can't make mistakes without seriously affecting the well-being of others. As well as best practice knowledge and skills, graduates should also have best practice attitudes and values.

SUMMARY POINTS

- The curriculum of a health professional education programme can be thought of as an academic programme's road map that is constantly changing and evolving.
- Curriculum alignment is a crucial aspect of an academic programme.
- Curriculum implementation and curriculum maintenance are also two important features of a dynamic, evolving and contemporary health professional education programme.

REVIEW QUESTIONS

- What are the features of an academic programme's curriculum?
- What are some strategies to ensure that the curriculum of an academic programme remains dynamic, informed and contemporary?
- What are the features of curriculum alignment?
- What are the similarities and differences of curriculum implementation and curriculum maintenance?

REFLECTIVE QUESTIONS AND EXERCISES

- Two of the most fundamental questions that should guide educators when they reflect critically upon the curricula they are intending to present to health professional students are as follows: (1) Is what the curriculum is presenting to the students the *best* preparation for their professional life? (2) Will the students be actively engaged in acquiring everything that the curriculum covers?
- One interesting exercise all of us can (and many should) do regularly is to list what in past curricula or informal learning environments have had the greatest impact on us – both at the time or later, after graduation. It is often startling to realise that so much of what we have acquired that has proven useful to us in our professional lives has come from unexpected sources and at unpredictable times. Modern health professional curricula understand and accommodate that.

REFERENCES

1. Slattery P. *Curriculum Development in the Postmodern Era: teaching and learning in an age of accountability*. New York, NY: Routledge; 2012.
2. Hammick M. Evidence shaped health professional education: can we talk about a new paradigm? *Med Teach*. 2012; **34**(6): 435–8.
3. Eisner EW. Creative curriculum development and practice. *J Curriculum Super*. 1990; **6**(1): 62–73.
4. Tanner D, Tanner LN. *Curriculum Development: theory into practice*. New York, NY: Macmillan; 1975.
5. Hojat M, Louis DZ, Maio V, *et al.* Empathy and healthcare quality. *Am J Med Qual*. 2013; **28**(1): 6–7.
6. Stoller JK, Taylor CA, Farver CF. Emotional intelligence competencies provide a developmental curriculum for medical training. *Med Teach*. 2013; **35**(3): 243–7.
7. Cooper HC, Booth K, Gill G. Patients' perspectives on diabetes health care education. *Health Educ Res*. 2003; **18**(2): 191–206.
8. McKie A, Naysmith S. Promoting critical perspectives in mental health nursing education. *J Psychiatric Mental Health Nurs*. 2013; **21**(2): 128–37.
9. Rudinow J, Barry VE. *Invitation to Critical Thinking*. Belmont, CA: Wadsworth Cengage Learning; 2007.

10. Leicester M. *Teaching Critical Thinking Skills*. London: Continuum International Publishing Group; 2010.
11. Jennings C, Wargnier J. Experiential learning: a way to develop agile minds in the knowledge economy? *Dev Learn Organ*. 2010; **24**(3): 14–16.
12. Reed M, Evely AC, Cundill G, *et al*. What is social learning? *Ecol Soc*. 2010; **15**(4): r1.
13. Keamy RL, Nicholas HR, Mahar S, *et al*. *Personalising Education: from research to policy and practice*. Paper No. 11. Melbourne, VIC: Department of Education and Early Childhood Development, State Government Victoria; 2007.
14. Deakin CR. Pedagogical challenges for personalisation: integrating the personal with the public through context-driven enquiry. *Curriculum J*. 2009; **20**(3): 185–9.
15. Beddall-Hill NL, Raper J. Mobile devices as 'boundary objects' on field trips. *J Res Center Educ Technol*. 2010; **6**(1): 28–46.
16. Schauble L, Glaser R. *Innovations in Learning: new environments for education*. Mahwah, NJ: Lawrence Erlbaum Associates; 2013.
17. Mackintosh W. Opening education in New Zealand: a snapshot of a rapidly evolving OER ecosystem. In: Glennie J, Harley K, Butcher N, *et al*., editors. *Open Educational Resources and Change in Higher Education: reflections from practice*. Vancouver, BC: Commonwealth of Learning; 2012. pp. 263–79.
18. Geser G. Open educational practices and resources: the OLCOS roadmap 2012. *Revista de Universidad y Sociedad del Conocimiento (RUSC)*. 2007; **4**(1); 1–150,
19. De Boer J, Ho AD, Stump GS, *et al*. Changing 'course': reconceptualizing educational variables for massive open online courses. *Educ Res*. 2014; **43**(2): 74–84.
20. Biggs J, Tang C. *Teaching for Quality Learning at University*. Maidenhead, UK: Open University Press; 2007.
21. Ashley KD, Desai R, Levine JM. Teaching case-based argumentation concepts using dialectic arguments vs. didactic explanations. In: Cerri SA, Gouardères G, Paraguaçu F, editors. *Proceedings of the Sixth International Conference on Intelligent Tutoring Systems*. Berlin: Springer; 2002. pp. 585–95.
22. Ornstein AC, Hunkins FP. *Curriculum*. Boston, MA: Pearson; 2013.
23. Lewin K. *Resolving Social Conflicts: selected papers on group dynamics*. New York, NY: Harper & Row; 1948.
24. Kotter JP. Leading change: why transformation efforts fail. *Harv Bus Rev*. 1995; **73**(2): 59–67.
25. Bates T. Changing cultures in higher education: moving ahead to future learning. *Dist Educ*. 2011; **32**(1): 143–8.
26. Baroffio A, Vu NV, Gerbase MW. Evolutionary trends of problem-based learning practices throughout a two-year preclinical program: a comparison of students' and teachers' perceptions. *Adv Health Sci Educ Theory Prac*. 2012; **18**(4): 673–85.
27. Trowler P, Hopkinson P, Comerford Boyes L. Institutional change towards a sustainability agenda: how far can theory assist? *Tert Educ Manage*. 2013; **19**(3): 267–79.
28. Cleverly D. *Implementing Inquiry-Based Learning in Nursing*. London: Routledge; 2003.
29. Ghitulescu BE. Making change happen: the impact of work context on adaptive and proactive behaviors. *J Applied Beh Sci*. 2013; **49**(2): 206–45.
30. Van De Mortel T, Bird JL, Holt JI, *et al*. Quality assurance and quality enhancement of the nursing curriculum: happy marriage or recipe for divorce? *J Nurs Educ Pract*. 2012; **2**(3): 110–18.
31. Freed JE. *A Culture for Academic Excellence: implementing the quality principles in higher education*. ASHE-ERIC Higher Education Report, Vol. 25, No. 1. Washington, DC: The George Washington University, Graduate School of Education and Human Development; 1997.
32. Harvey L, Knight PT. *Transforming Higher Education*. Bristol, PA: Open University Press, Taylor & Francis; 1996.

CHAPTER 10

Programme accreditation and professional competencies in health professional education

....

Sharon M Brownie

OVERVIEW

Health professions are defined by a range of significant responsibilities including the responsibility of being bound by accountability and trust to society. Inherent in this accountability is the responsibility for health professionals to engage in lifelong processes of fostering and enhancing competence and continual improvement in an open, transparent and verifiable manner.[1] Congruent with this mandate, processes of programme accreditation and professional competencies are now unequivocally embedded in the contemporary health professional education models of developed nations and in the context of increasing globalisation are now central to preparing health professionals for the twenty-first century.[2]

The focus of this chapter is to discuss issues related to programme accreditation, professional standards, fitness to practise and professional competencies in health professional education. Research evidence about evidence-based best practices in programme accreditation and professional competencies in health professional student education is included in the discussion. The chapter concludes with recommendations related to best practice in education, teaching and learning, along with areas for further research and reflective exercises for readers.

CHAPTER OBJECTIVES

Upon completion of this chapter, the reader will be able to:

- discuss the topic of competencies in the context of health professional education
- describe three different interprofessional competency frameworks
- outline how the six-step Gibbs Reflective Practice Cycle can be used to assist with health education programme accreditation
- articulate the key points related to the design, delivery and accreditation of competency-based health professional education.

KEY TERMS: accreditation, competency, health professionals, health professional education, competency-based education, health workforce

---

INTRODUCTION

Contemporary health professional education is designed, delivered, reviewed and evaluated within a complex system of standard setting, licensing and accreditation. Today's health professional educator requires an in-depth understanding of the graduate outcomes and competency expectations of employers, professional bodies, accrediting authorities, regulators and others from which to deploy evidence-based educational practice strategies. The health professional educator also requires an understanding of the higher education, medico-legal, health service and professional systems in which their programme is taught and quality affirmed. The challenge for health professional educators is in ensuring the delivery of evidence-based learning and teaching practices within this context.

DEFINITIONS AND CONTEXT

A shared understanding of definitions is an important beginning in establishing the context for the discussions in this chapter. However, this is a complex task, as review of literature to source an agreed set of definitions indicates significant debate and lack of consensus in the field.[3-5] An example highlighting definitional difficulties is the definition of competence, where the only consistency or commonality of findings is that no common definition exists.[6-10]

The lack of understanding and consensus of concepts such as competence, competency-based education and accreditation is increasingly apparent in the writings of educators and researchers working in the field. For example, those resulting from the International Consensus Conference on Competency-Based Medical Education,[11] the recent reports about competency-based education and training commissioned by Health Workforce Australia,[4,5,12] and publications associated with the L-TIPP (Aus) project (Learning and Teaching for Interprofessional Practice in Australia).[13] Inherent within each of these examples are recommendations and calls for national leadership involving a range of leadership strategies and consensus forums to identify and agree more commonly accepted definitions. Despite these difficulties, it is important for the discussions in this chapter to be bounded by a series of evidence-based understandings that can serve as a guide to the reader. The following definitions have been sourced and included on this basis, with two definitions of competency included in acknowledgement of the breadth of this concept.

- **Accreditation**: a process by which a statutory authority evaluates and recognises an educational institution and/or its programmes with respect to meeting approved criteria.[1]
- **Competence**: a dynamic combination of knowledge, understanding, skills and abilities. Fostering competence is the objective of educational programmes. Competences will be formed in various course units and assessed at different stages.[14]
- **Competency (1)**: a component part of competence. It refers to specific capabilities in applying particular knowledge, skills, decision-making attributes and values to perform tasks safely and effectively in a specific health workforce role.[15,16]
- **Competency (2)**: the consistent application of knowledge and skills to the standard of performance required in the workplace (doing). It embodies the ability to transfer and apply skills and knowledge to new situations and environments.[17]
- **Fitness to practise**: a comprehensive concept including clinical competence, professional conduct and compliance with regulatory standards assessed during supervised practice.[3]
- **Policy**: the process of making organisational or systems decisions by considering a number of options and their potential effects.[18]
- **Professional standards**: measurable performance outcomes to which an individual is expected to work in a given occupation.[19]

HEALTH PROFESSIONAL EDUCATION IN THE TWENTY-FIRST CENTURY

A multitude of forces are currently driving an unprecedented growth and interest in global health and health professional education. Long-standing professional boundaries, geographic disparities, differences in regulation and licensing standards and incongruities in educational programmes are highlighted as compromising the ability of nations to meet the health demands of the twenty-first century.[20] The forces of globalisation have heightened public visibility and expectation of health services. Combined with factors such as escalating burdens of non-communicable disease and increased mobility of the health workforce, these factors contribute to calls for major reform in the education and training of healthcare professionals to ensure they are better prepared for the twenty-first century.[20]

In 2010, calls for reform were heightened by a commission of academic and professional leaders whose formal report entitled *Health Professionals for a New Century: Transforming Education for Health Systems in an Interdependent World* was published in the *Lancet*, thus increasing the opportunity for global discussion.[2] Review of this report and related literature highlights that clear and consistent global competencies are essential to the successful achievement of global health goals and that a high level of accountability should exist in respect to minimising variability of competence internal to and between nations.[2,20–23] Translated, this means that an increased expectation exists for health professional educators to ensure that their programmes include well-defined competency expectations and graduate outcomes and that these are consistent across providers nationally and internationally.

COMPETENCIES IN HEALTH PROFESSIONAL EDUCATION

In the early parts of the twentieth century, the assessment of health professionals was primarily undertaken by written and/or oral examination of factual knowledge. Over the past 20 years a growing consensus has developed that mastery of knowledge alone is an insufficient indicator of clinical competence.[24] Few educators today would argue with the fundamentals of the Miller pyramid, which defines 'knowing' not as the final destination but simply as a beginning step on a much longer pathway to 'doing'.[25] Subsequently, higher-order 'doing' skills are now known as 'competencies'. Congruent with these concepts, actual performance is recognised as the gold standard for the demonstration of competency, and observation of competency as the gold standard of competency assessment.

Despite the relative ease with which these competency concepts can be articulated and understood, they have proved devilishly complex to develop and implement. After more than 2 decades of work, consensus has not yet been reached regarding how to define or assess the competencies across and between the various health professions, and there is no global agreement on how this could be achieved.[20,25,26] Extensive discussion continues on how best to craft well-designed competencies and learning outcomes, and how to gain consensus of these within and between professions both nationally and globally.[4,5,27] It is harder than many think. Widespread variance persists within and between professions and components of the health sector. The higher education literature reveals a continuing concern that the competency approach may be reductionist in nature.[4] Specifically, much of the concern has revolved around the fear that narrowly defined task orientated competencies may compromise the ability of educators to develop higher-order competencies such as the reflection and clinical reasoning skills required within expert practice – concepts recently described as 'tacit knowledge'.[28] The challenge for health professional educators is how best to teach the 'complex ensemble of analytic thinking, skilful practice, and wise judgement upon which each profession rests'.[29(p195)]

Despite the difficulties, the competency movement is now well established and all health professionals have, to varying extents, developed a range of competencies and/or standards to define the expected areas and levels of competence.[11,14] Equally, expectations regarding competency-based programmes are now strongly embedded within educational programmes for health professionals in both vocational and higher education settings.

PROFESSION- AND ORGANISATION-SPECIFIC COMPETENCIES

The health workforce comprises an extensive and broad range of highly skilled and competent health professionals educated in more than four million universities and many more non-university settings across the globe. On the basis of numbers, medicine, nursing and midwifery form the majority groupings within the health workforce. The health workforce is further strengthened by the essential expertise and contributions of a growing range of allied health specialties, with as many as 35 distinct specialties now recognised by organisations such as the Association of Schools of Allied Health Professions.[30]

TABLE 10.1 Standards and competency requirements necessary for accreditation of a nursing programme

Practice area	Standards and competency requirements	Source
Nursing practice	National Standards for Registration and Licensure	Nursing and Midwifery Board of Australia: www.nursingmidwiferyboard.gov.au
	Australian National Competency Standards for the Registered Nurse	Working in partnership with the Australian Health Practitioner Regulation Agency: www.ahpra.gov.au
	Code of Ethics and Code of Conduct	
Educational practice	Nurse Educator Competencies	National League for Nursing: www.nln.org/facultyprograms/Competencies/educator_core_competencies.htm
Nursing programme accreditation	ANMAC Quality Accreditation Standards	Australian Nursing and Midwifery Accreditation Council: www.anmac.org.au/accreditation-standards
	National framework for the accreditation of nursing and midwifery courses	Nursing and Midwifery Board of Australia: www.nursingmidwiferyboard.gov.au/Accreditation.aspx
Higher education regulatory standards	Higher Education Standards	Higher Education Standards Framework: www.teqsa.gov.au/higher-education-standards-framework
		Australian Government Tertiary Education Quality Standards Agency: www.teqsa.gov.au

In most instances, a simple external Internet search combined with an internal organisational or intranet search will enable health professionals and professional educators to identify and locate competency standards related to their particular profession, programme of study, employing institution and/or governing accrediting entity. A key issue is that these are not yet standardised within and across professions and nations. Thus, each health professional and professional educator needs to ensure he or she is familiar with the specific competency requirements within his or her particular profession and practice settings and know how to source these locally, nationally and globally. Table 10.1 sets out an outline of the minimum required knowledge for a nurse educator wanting to get a programme accredited in Australia. This is an example of the range of standards and competency requirements that an educator must address in order to meet mandated programme quality and accreditation standards.

In summary, health professionals and educators involved in programme delivery accreditation need to be cognisant of, and meet the standards and competencies required for, their particular profession. Increasingly, a range of interprofessional standards and competencies are also of relevance. Professional educators must also meet standards related to other regulatory and legislated requirements such as those mandated by various tertiary or higher education entities.

PROFESSIONAL STANDARDS

Because of the personal and confidential nature of most professional services and the expert and specialist skills required to ensure client safety, professions are bound by strict codes of conduct and rigorous moral and ethical obligations. A range of literature is available detailing 'best practices' in health professional regulation and licensure – most of which is embedded within the legislation of the particular host nation. Models are often profession specific and may be contained within state-based boundaries, as per the American and Canadian contexts, where standards, regulation and licensure commonly fall within the jurisdiction of the particular state, province or territory.[31,32] Further, professional standards are usually linked to formally legislated health professional regulation and licensing systems, as per the example of the International Council of Nurses principles regarding the regulation of nursing.[33] In the Australian context, professional standards are formally overseen and implemented by the Australian Health Practitioner Regulation Agency, which represents all professional groups. Meanwhile, the UK-based Health and Care Professions Council has recently established a database that aims to assist in the identification of global organisations that set standards, regulate or control the practise of healthcare workers (www.hpc-uk.org/aboutregistration/regulators/worldwide/).[34]

Professional standards underpin the complex intertwining of requirements for providers of health professional education to develop learning outcomes for competency-based educational programmes and achieve accreditation of these programmes. Professional standards also underpin the certification and licensure requirements of individual practitioners – a process often referred to as credentialing.

INTERPROFESSIONAL COMPETENCY FRAMEWORKS

Best practices in health professional education involve a strong partnership between the health industry and education sector. Today's health sector is challenged by increasing levels of chronic disease, co-morbidity and healthcare complexity that demand significant levels of health service reform and redesign, including an increased focus on interprofessional collaboration and teamwork. This in turn creates parallel demands on the education sector to develop health professionals capable of working effectively alongside and collaboratively with others rather than within the bounds of their own professional paradigm.[35]

A number of well-resourced and well-researched global initiatives are available to health professional educators for use in the process of ensuring that their courses keep pace with the evidence base of developments in the field of interprofessional practice. Of particular note are the Canadian National Interprofessional Competency Development,[36] a major globally recognised development, and the UK National Interprofessional Competency Framework, from which interprofessional education has been extended into the workplace.[37] Each of these frameworks is aligned to significant workforce developments and health service reform initiatives in their respective nations. Development of shared competencies has emerged in tandem with the emphases on improved coordination of health service teams and interprofessional models of collaborative care. The Canadian National Interprofessional Competency Framework groups common competencies under six key domains, specifically:

1. interprofessional communication
2. patient-, client-, family-, community-centred care
3. role clarification
4. team functioning
5. collaborative leadership
6. interprofessional conflict resolution.[36]

A further example of large-scale cross-professional competency projects is the work recently completed by the International Union for Health Promotion and Education in developing competencies and professional standards for health promotion capacity building in Europe (CompHP).[38] A parallel example is the developments of the UK-based Council on Linkages between Academia and Public Health Practice. This groups the expected core competencies into eight domains or topic-based areas of knowledge and skill:

1. analytic and assessment skills
2. policy development and programme planning skills
3. communication skills
4. cultural competency skills
5. community dimensions of practice skills
6. public health sciences skills
7. financial planning and management skills
8. leadership and systems thinking skills.[39]

In contrast, the European CompHP competency framework outlines a required expectation that all health professionals working in public health roles will possess the following nine competencies.

1. *Enable change*: enable individuals, groups, communities and organisations to build capacity for health promotion action to improve health and reduce health inequities.

2. *Advocate for health*: advocate with, and on behalf of, individuals, communities and organisations to improve health and well-being and build capacity for health promotion action.
3. *Mediate through partnership*: work collaboratively across disciplines, sectors and partners to enhance the impact and sustainability of health promotion action.
4. *Communicate effectively*: communicate health promotion action effectively, using appropriate techniques and technologies for diverse audiences.
5. *Demonstrate leadership*: contribute to the development of a shared vision and strategic direction for health promotion action.
6. *Undertake assessments*: conduct assessment of needs and assets in partnership with stakeholders, in the context of the political, economic, social, cultural, environmental, behavioural and biological determinants that promote or compromise health.
7. *Plan effectively*: develop measurable health promotion goals and objectives based on assessment of needs and assets in partnership with stakeholders.
8. *Implement*: implement effective and efficient, culturally sensitive, and ethical health promotion action in partnership with stakeholders.
9. *Evaluate and research*: use appropriate evaluation and research methods, in partnership with stakeholders, to determine the reach, impact and effectiveness of health promotion action.[40]

These projects arose on the basis that, globally, nations are challenged by an escalating burden of non-communicable disease – much of which is chronic in nature – with significant impact upon health service demand and utilisation.[41,42] An increasing evidence base exists that improvement against these trends is dependent upon large-scale behaviour and social change, which cannot be achieved by medical practitioners alone. Thus the rationale for the development of public health competencies across all health professions and inclusion in all education programmes for the preparation of the current and emerging health workforce.[43]

Recently, two major Australian-wide projects have been established with the aim of significantly increasing the capacity of the Australian higher education sector to produce future health professionals with well-developed interprofessional practice capabilities. The projects are funded by the Australian Learning and Teaching Council, with each project being freely available via open web access, specifically:

- the Curriculum Renewal for Interprofessional Education in Health project (www. ipehealth.edu.au/portal/)
- the L-TIPP (Aus) project (Learning and Teaching for Interprofessional Practice in Australia) (www.aippen.net/docs/LTIPP_proposal_apr09.pdf).

The open access reflects the recognition that successful implementation of competency frameworks with shared competencies across all professions is dependent upon wide stakeholder engagement and culture change across both health and education sectors.

FITNESS TO PRACTISE

It has long been accepted that health professionals should be both professional and competent in their practice. Over the decades, society has trusted individual practitioners to discharge this responsibility. Society has also trusted professional regulatory bodies to protect health service users from unethical and incompetent practitioners.[3] However, high-profile cases, such as that of Dr Death in Bundaberg in Australia,[44] the Shipman case in the United Kingdom,[45] and the most recent case of the New South Wales nursing home murderer Roger Dean,[46] have called to question the rigour and processes associated with the regulation and licensure of health professionals.

Against this backdrop, reported analysis of the literature highlights the fact that the concept of professionalism is as difficult to define as the concept of competency and that professionalism has been defined in many different ways by many different authors, institutions and organisations.[3,47-50] Subsequently, a new and broader concept of 'fitness to practise' has emerged that includes notions of both professionalism and competence and which carries with it higher levels of personal accountability, regulation and reporting.[49] A useful model that draws together the tenets of this discussion is the 'Star of Practice' model.

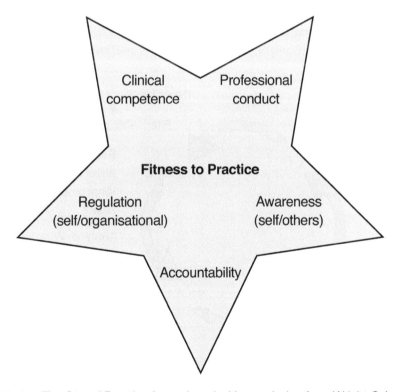

FIGURE 10.1 The Star of Practice (reproduced with permission from Wright C A, Jolly B, Schneider-Kolsky M E, Baird M A. Defining fitness to practise in Australian radiation therapy: A focus group study. *Radiography*. 2011; **17**: 6–13).

The Star of Practice model usefully illustrates the complexity and multi-component nature of fitness to practise, highlighting that it is a comprehensive concept that includes clinical competence, professional conduct and compliance with regulatory standards assessed during supervised practice.[3] Regulatory bodies have a major role in the assessment of fitness to practise. Guidelines established by the International Council of Nurses highlight the overriding purpose of statutory regulation as that of 'service to and protection of the public' along with the obligation of statutory regulators to 'satisfy this intent in a comprehensive manner'.[33]

PROGRAMME ACCREDITATION

Accreditation is noted as a process by which 'a statutory authority evaluates and recognises an educational institution and/or its programmes with respect to meeting approved criteria'.[1] Within the context of contemporary health professional education, the accreditation process is now widely viewed as an essential quality improvement and social accountability responsibility, whereby programmes are measured against transparent, internationally and professionally recognised standards[1,28,51,52] and where professional competencies are aligned with accreditation standards.[53]

Accreditation is a process whereby state-mandated statutory authorities monitor and assure the maintenance of education and professional standards. The process of accreditation intrinsically offers the potential for organisations and individual health

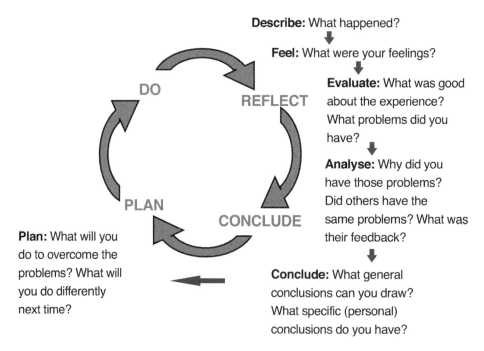

FIGURE 10.2 Gibbs Reflective Cycle (reproduced with permission of EAP Foundation: www.eapfoundation.com/studyskills/learningcycle/)

professional educators to reflect upon practice and engage in ongoing evidence-based educational improvements of teaching and learning delivery, including the assessment of professional competencies.

Embedded within this notion are the concepts of reflective practice and the use of a reflective practice cycle. The Gibbs Reflective Cycle is a useful and well-published reflective practice framework[54] that health professional educators can use to underpin reflections on experience through an accreditation process and as a basis for planning subsequent programme improvements.

The literature contains a range of models of reflective practice, several of which can be used for post-accreditation reflections. The Gibbs model is particularly useful for post-event analysis, as it builds upon Kolb's[55] earlier 'experiential learning cycle' by use of structured debriefing via a structured six-step process: (1) description, (2) feelings, (3) evaluation, (4) analysis, (5) conclusions and (6) action plan, as shown in Figure 10.2.

Throughout and following an accreditation process, health professional educators can use the six-step Gibbs Reflective Cycle to assist reflections and quality improvement strategies as follows.

1. *Description*: What happened during the accreditation preparation stages and visit processes? Were we sufficiently prepared? Was I personally prepared? What were the accreditors' views and comments?
2. *Feelings*: What are our/my reactions and feelings?
3. *Evaluation*: What was good and/or not so good about the situation? What value judgements can we/I make?
4. *Analysis*: What sense can we/I make of all of this? How can our collective experience be portrayed? Were our individual experiences different or similar in any important ways?
5. *Conclusions*: What are our collective experiences? What are our individual experiences? How will these contribute to the best practice evidence base that will guide our ongoing learning and teaching strategies?
6. *Action plan*: What are we/I going to do differently from now on? What steps will we/I take on the basis of what we/I have learned?

Thus, accreditation can be viewed as more than a just an audit or monitoring process. It can be viewed as an organisational and individual learning tool: 'the hope of accreditation is to support the further learning and accomplishment of individuals as they reach higher levels of experience and wisdom.'[51(p323)]

POLICY AND IMPLEMENTATION CONSIDERATIONS

The implementation of professional competencies within educational programmes and accreditation systems involves major policy and infrastructural considerations.[4,56] Successful implementation requires careful attention to, and coordination of, a wide range of factors across the system in which health professionals are prepared and practise, as summarised in Table 10.2.

TABLE 10.2 Implications in the introduction of professional competences in health professional education and accreditation

Core principles of competency-based education	Implementation requirements
Flexibility and learner-centeredness	Flexibility in planning in clinical placement rotations
Focus on outcomes from programme design, through delivery, evaluation and accreditation	Ongoing development on valid and reliable competency standards
	More work needed to define competencies with consistent links between programme and accreditation
New roles for teachers and students	Greater involvement from faculty
	Faculty development required
	Students required to demonstrate actual competence rather than knowledge only
New methods of assessment	Development of new clinical assessment and examination tools
New definitions of competence and fitness to practise	Ongoing work in respect to challenges of competency concepts including. • balance between individual competences and overall competence • avoiding reductionism through over focus on individual competences

Note: adapted from Taber *et al.*[56]

Implementation can only be successful if adequate commitment, resourcing and support are provided to faculty and students. Equally, ongoing work needs to occur in developing standards and competencies via a research oriented and evidence-based approach.

CONCLUDING REMARKS: PUTTING IT ALL TOGETHER

As highlighted, the design, delivery and accreditation of competency-based health professional education occurs within a system from which it should not be isolated. As Figure 10.3 shows, excellence in competency-based education and accreditation requires a process of ongoing development and review. Development of a credible evidence base requires ongoing consultation with all key stakeholders and a close working partnership between education and practice.

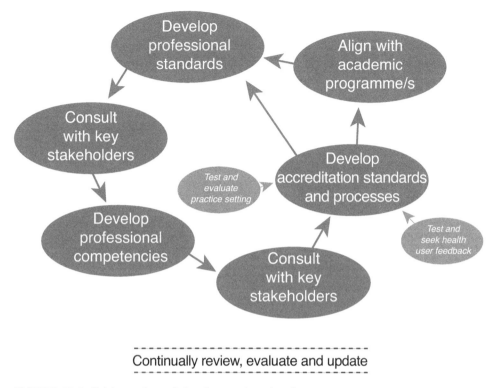

FIGURE 10.3 Evidence-based development and review

AREAS FOR FUTURE RESEARCH

While the competency approach is now well embedded in contemporary health professional education, there is still a great deal of work to be undertaken and things to be understood. As highlighted, the competency movement has now gained a high level of momentum. Review of the literature yields an extensive arrange of health professional competency frameworks and competency standards. In contrast, little research relates to the effectiveness or evaluation or competency standards and competency-related teaching and learning methods.

Major areas for further research relate to the need to:
● increase consensus in respect to definitions and concepts related to professional competence, fitness to practise and professional accreditation
● enhance understanding of how best to craft well-designed competencies and learning outcomes and how to gain consensus of these within and between professions (nationally and globally), and, within the overall system of health professional educators, providers, regulators and accreditors
● increase evaluative studies related to competency-based teaching and learning effectiveness.

SUMMARY POINTS

- Health professional programme accreditation and professional competencies are key components in the education of new healthcare graduates.
- Because of changes in the healthcare sector and increasing complexity of the level of care required for patients, there has been an increased focus on interprofessional collaboration and teamwork; this has generated parallel requirements in the education of new healthcare professionals who need to be capable of working effectively alongside and collaboratively with others rather than within the bounds of their own professional paradigm.
- Fitness to practise as a concept has emerged, which includes notions of both professionalism and competence and carries with it higher levels of personal accountability, regulation and reporting.
- The accreditation of health professional education programmes has become more rigorous and closely monitored in parallel with the importance of professional competencies.

REVIEW QUESTIONS

- Define what professional competency is in the context of health professional education.
- What are six key interprofessional competencies?
- What are the steps in the Gibbs Reflective Practice Cycle?
- Explain the relationship between professional competencies and the accreditation of health professional education programmes. What are the implications in the introduction of professional competences in health professional education and accreditation?

REFLECTIVE QUESTIONS AND EXERCISES

- Competency-based education provides professional entities, educators and accreditors with a framework for a significant rethink of assessment processes, with a much stronger focus on learning outcomes and competencies. How are the competencies and learning outcomes defined and reviewed in the programme with which you are associated? What process do you adopt to align learning outcomes and competencies with the standards set by the multivariate agencies and professional bodies of relevance to your programme?
- LeBlanc[27] asserts that professional educators are very good at defining how long students need to sit at desks and participate in a course but are very poor at confirming how much they have learned or if they even learned at all during a session. He further asserts that 'competency-based education flips the relationship – let time be variable and make learning well defined, fixed and non-negotiable.'[27(p2)] Reflect upon the implications of this statement on your programme. Do you think that students need to 'do the time' to become safe practitioners or can this be judged by competency-assessment alone?

REFERENCES

1. Lindgren S, Karle H. Social accountability of medical education: aspects on global accreditation. *Med Teach*. 2011; **33**(8): 667–72.
2. Frenk J, Chen L, Bhutta Z, *et al*. Health professionals for a new century: transforming education to strengthen health systems in an interdependent world. *Lancet*. 2010; **376**(9756): 1923–58.
3. Wright C, Jolly B, Schnieder-Kolsky M, *et al*. Defining fitness to practise in Australian radiation therapy: a focus group study. *Clin Oncol*. 2011; **23**(3): S57–8.
4. Brownie S, Bahnisch M, Thomas J. *Competency-Based Education Training and Competency-Based Career Frameworks: informing Australian health workforce development*. Brisbane, QLD: University of Queensland Node of the Australian Health Workforce Institute in partnership with Health Workforce Australia; 2012.
5. Brownie S, Bahnisch M, Thomas J. *Exploring the Literature: competency-based education and raining and competency-based career frameworks*. Brisbane, QLD: University of Queensland Node of the Australian Health Workforce Institute in partnership with Health Workforce Australia; 2012.
6. Boon J, van der Klink M. *Scanning the Concept of Competencies: how major vagueness can be highly functional*. Proceedings of the 2nd Conference on HRD Research and Practice across Europe; University of Twente, Enschede; 2001.
7. Whiddett S, Hollyforde S. *A Practical Guide to Competencies: how to enhance individual and organisational performance*. London: CIPD; 2003.
8. LeDeist F, Winterton J. What is competence? *Hum Res Dev Int*. 2005; **8**(1): 27–46.
9. Lans T, Mulder M. Competence, empirical insights from a small-business perspective. *Development of Competencies in the World of Work and Education: conference proceedings*. Ljubljana, Slovenia, 24–26 September, 2009. pp. 265–70.
10. Winterton J. Competence across Europe: highest common factor or lowest common denominator? *J Eur Ind Train*. 2009; **33**(8–9): 681–700.

11. Frank JR, Snell LS, Cate OT, *et al.* Competency-based medical education: theory to practice. *Med Teach.* 2010; **32**(8): 638–45.

12. Brownie S, Bahnisch M, Thomas J. *Listening to our Stakeholders: analysis of interviews regarding competency-based education and training and competency-based career frameworks.* Brisbane, QLD: University of Queensland Node of the Australian Health Workforce Institute in partnership with Health Workforce Australia; 2012.

13. Nisbet G, Lee A, Kumar K, *et al. Health Education: a literature review overview of international and Australian developments in interprofessional health education (IPE).* Sydney, NSW: University of Sydney; 2011.

14. www.unideusto.org

15. Scott Tilley DD. Competency in nursing: a concept analysis. *J Contin Educ Nurs.* 2008; **39**(2): 58–64.

16. Verma S, Broers T, Paterson M, *et al.* Core competencies: the next generation comparison of a common framework for multiple professions. *J Allied Health.* 2009; **38**(1): 47–53.

17. National Quality Council. Melbourne, VIC: National Quality Council; 2009.

18. Torjman S. *What is Policy?* Ottawa, ON: Caledon Institute of Social Policy; 2005. Available at: www.caledoninst.org/publications/pdf/544eng.pdf (accessed 2 March 2011).

19. Torterat J. The International Standard Classification of Occupations (ISCO) in the European Union. *Courrier des Statistiques.* 2009; English series No. 15: 22–26. Available at: www.insee.fr/en/ffc/docs_ffc/cse15d.pdf (accessed 2 March 2011).

20. Calhoun JG, Spencer HC, Buekens P. Competencies for global health graduate education. *Infect Dis Clin North Am.* 2011; **25**(3): 575–92.

21. Bruno A, Bates I, Brock T, *et al.* Towards a global competency framework. *Am J Pharm Educ.* 2010; **74**(3): 56.

22. Becker C, Rager RC, Wright FE. Update on validity of required competencies for worksite health professionals. *Am J Health Educ.* 2013; **44**(2): 67.

23. Shilton T. Health promotion competencies: providing a road map for health promotion to assume a prominent role in global health. *Glob Health Promot.* 2009; **16**(2): 42–6.

24. Lurie SJ. History and practice of competency-based assessment. *Med Educ.* 2012; **46**(1): 49–57.

25. Miller GE. The assessment of clinical skills/competence/performance. *Acad Med.* 1990; **65**(9): 63–7.

26. Kuhlmann E, G. Competency-based social work education: a thirty-year retrospective on the behavioural competency movement. *J North Am Assoc Christian Soc Work.* 2009; **36**(1): 70–6.

27. LeBlanc P. Competency-based education and regional accreditation. *Inside Higher Ed.* 2013: 1–4. Available at: www.insidehighered.com (accessed 2 March 2014).

28. Australian Medical Council (AMC). *Competence-Based Medical Education: AMC consultation paper.* Kingston, ACT: AMC; 2010.

29. Sullivan WM. *Work and Integrity: the crisis and promise of professionalism in North America.* San Franciso, CA: Jossey-Bass; 2005.

30. www.asahp.org

31. Canadian Psychological Association. *Provincial and Territorial Regulatory Bodies.* www.cpa.ca/public/whatisapsychologist/regulatorybodies/ (accessed 2 March 2014).

32. Tennessee Department of Health. *About Health Professional Boards.* https://health.state.tn.us/boards/ (accessed 2 March 2014).

33. APRN Consensus Work Group & the National Council of State Boards of Nursing APRN Advisory Committee. *Consensus Model for APRN Regulation: licensure, accreditation, certification and education.* 2008. Available at: http://nursingworld.org/DocumentVault/APRN-Resource-Section/ConsensusModelforAPRNRegulation.pdf (accessed 9 October 2014).

34. Health and Care Professions Council. *Health Regulation Worldwide.* www.hpc-uk.org/about registration/regulators/worldwide/ (accessed 2 March 2014).

35. Kuipers P, Ehrlich C, Brownie S. Responding to health care complexity: suggestions for integrated and interprofessional workplace learning. *J Interprof Care.* 2014; **28**(3): 246–8.

36. Canadian Interprofessional Health Collaborative. *A National Interprofessional Competency Framework.* Vancouver, BC: Canadian Interprofessional Health Collaborative; 2010. Available at: www.cihc.ca/files/CIHC_IPCompetencies_Feb1210.pdf

37. Hughes L. *Creating an Interprofessional Workforce: an education and training framework for health and social care in England.* Fareham, UK: Centre for the Advancement of Interprofessional Education; 2007.

38. Dempsey C, Battel-Kirk B, Barry MM. *Developing Competencies and Professional Standards for Health Promotion Capacity Building in Europe (CompHP).* Paris: International Union of Health Promotion and Education; 2011. Available at: www.nuigalway.ie/health-promotion/documents/Annual_Report/comphp_2012.pdf (accessed 2 March 2014).

39. Public Health Foundation. *About the Core Competencies for Public Health Professionals.* www.phf.org/programs/corecompetencies (accessed 2 March 2014).

40. Barry MM, Battel-Kirk B, Dempsey C. The CompHP core competencies framework for health promotion in Europe. *Health Educ Behav.* 2012; **39**(6): 648–62.

41. Beaglehole R, Bonita R, Horton R, *et al.* Priority actions for the non-communicable disease crisis. *Lancet.* 2011; **377**(9775): 1438–47.

42. Wagner K-H, Brath H. A global view on the development of non communicable diseases. *Prev Med.* 2012; **54**(Suppl.): S38–41.

43. Ezzati M, Riboli E. Behavioral and dietary risk factors for noncommunicable diseases. *N Engl J Med.* 2013; **369**(10): 954–64.

44. Sandall R. Doctor Death in Bundaberg. *Quadrant.* 2005; **49**(12): 11–20.

45. Pounder DJ. The Case of Dr. Shipman. *Am J Forensic Med Pathol.* 2003; **24**(3): 219–26.

46. Ralston N. Killer nurse joins ranks of inmates never to be released. *Sydney Morning Herald.* 3 August 2013.

47. Epstein RM, Hundert EM. Defining and assessing professional competence. *JAMA.* 2002; **287**(2): 226–35.

48. Kearney RA. Defining professionalism in anaesthesiology. *Med Educ.* 2005; **39**(8): 769–76.

49. Holmes B, Mann K, Hennen K. Defining fitness and aptitude to practice medicine. *Med Teach.* 1990; **12**(2): 181–8.

50. Morrow G, Burford B, Rothwell C, *et al. Professionalism in Healthcare Professionals.* London: Health and Care Professions Council; 2011. Available at: www.hpc-uk.org/assets/documents/10003771Professionalisminhealthcareprofessionals.pdf (accessed 2 March 2014).

51. Wood BP. Competency-based training: accreditation as a pathway to wisdom. *Radiol.* 2009; **252**(2): 322–3.

52. Moskowitz EJ, Nash DB. Accreditation Council for Graduate Medical Education competencies: practice-based learning and systems-based practice. *Am J Med Qual.* 2007; **22**(5): 351–82.

53. Allison M, Dickerson P. Assessing competency: a new accreditation resource. *J Contin Educ Nurs.* 2008; **39**(6): 244–5.

54. Gibbs G. *Learning by Doing: a guide to teaching and learning methods.* London: Oxford Centre for Staff and Learning Development, Oxford Polytechnic; 1988.

55. Kolb DA. *Experiential Learning: experience as the source of learning and development.* Englewood Cliffs, NJ: Prentice Hall; 1984.

56. Taber S, Frank J, Harris K, *et al.* Identifying the policy implications of competency-based education. *Med Teach.* 2010; **32**(8): 687–91.

CHAPTER 11

Applying threshold concepts in a health professional education context

Sylvia Rodger

OVERVIEW

This chapter provides an overview of threshold concepts developed by Meyer and Land.[1,2] Specifically, it will (a) define and describe threshold concepts, (b) outline the characteristics that must be met for concepts to be called threshold concepts and (c) discuss student learning journeys and the liminal space through which students must traverse in order to master learning of such concepts.[3] Threshold concepts are a relevant concept to consider in the domain of evidence-based education. In addition, assessment of these concepts will be explored. The focus of this chapter will be on the use of threshold concepts within higher education and tertiary curriculum design. This will be followed by a few examples of use of threshold concepts in health professional education, with a focus on allied health. The chapter will conclude with a summary of their potential use and application to enhance teaching and learning as well as student engagement with learning activities within the health professions.

CHAPTER OBJECTIVES

Upon completion of this chapter, the reader will be able to:

- define what threshold concepts are
- outline the five characteristics that must be met in order for something to be considered a threshold concept
- describe what ritual knowledge, inert knowledge, alien knowledge and tacit knowledge are
- explain the concepts of liminality and liminal spaces in the context of student learning
- outline how threshold concepts can be used to inform curriculum design
- discuss how assessment is understood within a threshold concept framework.

KEY TERMS: curriculum, threshold concepts, student learning, assessment, professional education

---

INTRODUCTION

The scholarship of teaching and learning in higher education has recently become an important focus for academics. Over the past decade there has been an increasing emphasis on quality teaching and learning environments and the enhancement of student learning experiences within Australian higher education. This has in part been influenced by quality management systems utilised within higher education institutions and in part by government funding drivers whereby key performance indicators are externally evaluated with financial rewards provided as an incentive for improved institutional teaching and learning outcomes.[4]

Congruent with this, there has also been a focus on the identification of learning outcomes for particular courses (referred to as separate units of study or subjects) and programmes (learning within a whole sequence of study, such as a degree). The concept of constructive alignment is also germane to this discussion.[5] Constructive alignment is a principle conceived by Biggs[5] used for devising teaching and learning activities as well as assessment tasks that directly address intended learning outcomes. Consistent with social constructivist views of learning, Biggs[5] proposed that students construct meaning for themselves through undertaking relevant well-designed learning activities. The instructor provides the alignment by setting up a learning environment and activities that will lead to the desired outcomes. Biggs[5] proposed four major steps in setting up an aligned teaching and learning system: first, intended learning outcomes are defined; second, teaching learning activities likely to lead to the intended learning outcomes are selected; third, students' actual learning outcomes are assessed as per the match with the intended learning outcomes; and fourth, a final grade is derived.

At the same time that Biggs[5] was proposing that academics needed to carefully examine how they designed course learning objectives, learning activities and assessment tasks, Meyer and Land[1] introduced the notion of a threshold concept as a way of differentiating between core learning outcomes that require students to see things differently or in a new way, and those that do not. They hypothesised that these concepts may represent 'troublesome knowledge', a term introduced by Perkins[6] to describe knowledge that is conceptually difficult and appears not to make sense initially, counterintuitive and at times 'alien'.

WHAT ARE THRESHOLD CONCEPTS?

Originating from the discipline of economics and the work of Meyer and Land,[1,2] threshold concepts have been proposed as specific concepts that meet defining characteristics. These concepts require complex understanding by students and are regarded as 'thresholds' that students must cross in order for them to master their selected academic discipline or profession. The use and application of threshold concepts in education contexts has been documented in a wide range of fields, including literature,[7] economics,[8] engineering,[9] biology,[10] dentistry[11] and statistics.[12] There is an emerging body of evidence in relation to threshold concepts.

Meyer and Land[1] described these concepts as being 'akin to a portal, opening up a new and previously inaccessible way of thinking about something'.[(p1)] Threshold concepts are central to the discipline, in that without this understanding or new perspective, the learner is unable to move forwards. They are frequently difficult to grasp, hence this knowledge has been referred to as being 'troublesome'.[6] Once the learner grapples with this knowledge, his or her view of the subject matter or indeed his or her identity changes or evolves in some way. This transformation may be sudden or extended over a period of time, with the transition to a new understanding being troublesome and at times uncomfortable.[1] This transformed view may represent how people 'think' within a given discipline. For example, within the health professions, the way that practitioners think, problem-solve and process information has been referred to as clinical reasoning.

Threshold concepts are different to 'core' concepts, which are viewed as 'conceptual building blocks that progress understanding of the subject; it has to be understood but it does not necessarily lead to a qualitatively different view of subject matter'.[1(p1)] The latter transformed view of the subject matter is unique to threshold concepts. They are considered to be 'conceptual gateways' or 'portals' that lead to a new way of thinking about something.[2] Hence, in order for something to be considered a threshold concept, Meyer and Land[1] proposed that five characteristics must be met. These characteristics have been found to be consistent across a range of subject areas and disciplines.

Threshold concepts are:

1. *transformative*, in that they change the learners' way of knowing or understanding such that once understood there is no going back; this often involves an affective component or a shift in values, feelings or attitudes
2. *irreversible*, in that once understood they are unlikely to be forgotten or unlearned
3. *troublesome*, hence they tend to be difficult to grasp or problematic for the learner,

as the knowledge is sometimes counterintuitive or different to a common-sense view, requiring unlearning of earlier perspectives

4. *bounded* within disciplines (although not always), hence the meaning of the concept may well be understood in a nuanced way within a particular discipline
5. *integrative*, in that understanding of one threshold concept may well unlock understanding of other related disciplinary concepts.[1,2,6]

HOW IS KNOWLEDGE TROUBLESOME?

Perkins[6] proposed that knowledge might be troublesome for different reasons. These reasons will be illustrated here using examples from the occupational therapy field. First, *ritual knowledge* has a routine or 'meaningless' character. This type of knowledge often features where students are required to learn foundational concepts with limited practical experience and understanding of their application or relevance. An example might be anatomical, physiological, psychological or profession-specific theoretical concepts that must be learned but may be decontextualised from real-life clinical practice. Instead, students may approach such knowledge in a ritualised way until they encounter actual clients in professional practice settings.

Second, *inert knowledge* refers to concepts that are understood but not actively used. In many occupational therapy programmes, students undertake courses in sociology but its application and relevance to their clients' lives is not immediately clear, thus they frequently struggle to make connections between sociological concepts and societal participation. For example, sociology makes overt the structures of society that contribute to unequal access to health and rehabilitation services, but students frequently struggle to see this.[13]

Third, *alien knowledge* refers to information that conflicts with one's own perspectives and may not be recognised as foreign. For example, students often share the normative view predominant in Western, First World society that health equals the absence of disease. However, they need to learn that occupational therapy's view of quality of life is broader than just eliminating physical, psychosocial and developmental deficits, and that it focuses as much on facilitating clients' exploration of alternative and meaningful ways of living their daily lives, regardless of their disabilities and impairments.[13]

Fourth, *tacit knowledge* is often implicit. One dominant yet implicit assumption is an individualistic understanding of health. This has been critiqued by authors such as Iwama[14] who emphasised that this is a Western view and that in collectivist societies, health and well-being are based on the assumption that individuals are inseparable from their environment. The centrality of independence has not until recently been contested or recognised as tacit knowledge.[13] Challenging such tacit perspectives is an important role of health professional educators.

Finally, one example of *alien language* is use of the term 'occupation'. Lay understandings usually relate to employment or the field of paid work one pursues. However, occupational therapists understand the term to refer to all of the daily activities people engage in, including paid work, play and leisure, rest, sleep, social participation and self-care. It is important that students transition from a lay to a profession-specific understanding early in their education and training.[13]

LIMINALITY AND LIMINAL SPACES

Cousins[3] focused on the emotional states experienced by students when traversing difficult spaces frequently encountered in mastering troublesome concepts. These difficult spaces have been referred to as *liminal spaces* or *states of liminality*.[2] The threshold is viewed as the entrance into the transformational state of *liminality*. When students occupy this space they challenge 'old' conceptualisations and frequently struggle to take on new meanings and incorporate new understandings within their world view. Once this state is entered into there is no capacity to fully return to the *pre-liminal state*, although regression may be temporarily experienced. From an educational perspective, students in these *liminal spaces* may engage in a form of ritualised learning or mimicry, which involves an attempt to understand but may also involve misunderstanding or limited discernment. These liminal spaces are also referred to as 'stuck places' where epistemological obstacles are experienced.[2]

Cousins[3] highlighted that this learning is both cognitive and affective and that it may require a shift in a student's identity. Educators need to tolerate learner confusion and potential irritation within this space and to create learning experiences that require them to tackle these concepts. In addition, educators must assist students to traverse these liminal spaces by providing appropriate structure and scaffolding of their learning to enable conceptual mastery. They also need to enable students to articulate their confusion when in this space, to prevent isolation.[3] From a pedagogical perspective, while constructive alignment[15] can assist students in stuck places through alignment of objectives and learning activities, it is not sufficient in and of itself. In addition, educators need to consider redesigning activities and instructional sequences, using scaffolding, recursive approaches, provision of support materials and technologies, mentoring and peer collaboration to assist students to move forwards.[2]

Appropriate design of and supported engagement with assessment activities and tasks are critical to facilitate students bridging these thresholds. Meyer and Land[2] advocated that if teachers are to be student centred they need to understand why some students traverse this space easily and why others become stuck. To some extent this requires an understanding of variations in student learning and engagement. Hence designing learning and assessment tasks and ensuring that they require high levels of student engagement becomes an essential pedagogical task.

HOW CAN THRESHOLD CONCEPTS INFORM CURRICULUM DESIGN?

Given that these concepts are central to disciplines, they become important in planning sequences of learning and the development of curriculum, and their troublesome nature becomes pedagogically significant.[1] It is from this premise that threshold concepts may be used to inform curriculum design. In addition, they may be useful in avoiding the traps inherent in an 'overstuffed curriculum',[3] as they provide a view about where the curriculum needs to focus so that students can master concepts central to that body of professional knowledge.

Threshold concepts can be used to inform curriculum design, as they are 'jewels in the curriculum',[16] allowing a focus on concepts that require mastery. Cousins[3] proposed that one approach to curriculum design was to first enquire about the concepts that students have difficulty mastering. This was the approach described by Rodger and Turpin[13] who used *troublesome knowledge* as a springboard to the synthesis of five threshold concepts that underpinned the occupational therapy curriculum reform at the University of Queensland, Brisbane, Australia. This approach evolved from the standpoint that threshold concepts are fundamental to ways of thinking and practising in a particular profession[16] and hence might enable students to 'think like an occupational therapist.'[13] With a threshold concept framework in mind, teaching and learning programmes can be designed and evaluated in relation to:
- sequence of content
- processes or learning opportunities developed to help students encounter threshold concepts
- assessment for the attainment of threshold concepts.[16]

Land *et al.*[16] identified a number of considerations in the design of curricula in the higher education environment. First, if viewed as 'jewels in the curricula', threshold concepts can be used to design transformative experiences for students at pertinent points within an education programme.

Second, they highlighted the need for active student engagement with the requisite conceptual material – explaining it, representing it in new ways, integrating it into their schemas, applying it and relating it to their own life contexts. From a course design perspective, they recommend designing a framework for engagement that leads to ways of thinking and practising that are expected of practitioners within given professions. The work of Wenger[17] related to authentic learning within real communities of practice is also relevant in this context.

Third, Land *et al.*[16] recommended 'listening for understanding' to help educators 'listen for' what students know and where they might be stuck. This is particularly critical as educators are usually content experts within the field, who have traversed these professional knowledge thresholds and whose thinking is forever transformed. Therefore, it is difficult to recognise where and what students' learning obstacles might be.

Fourth, they contend that curriculum designers need to attend to the discomforts of troublesome knowledge (recognising its troublesome nature) and how students reconstruct who they are as a result of encountering and interacting with this knowledge. They need to create a 'supportive liminal environment'.

Fifth, educators and instructors need to tolerate learner uncertainty and be comfortable in making students aware of the nature of the transition they are likely to encounter. Students are more likely to manage liminal states if they are prepared for the difficulty and discomfort that they are likely to experience.

Sixth, learning tasks will require a recursive approach with learners attempting different 'takes' on the conceptual material. This requires recognition by both students and educator that the learning process and curriculum design are not linear, but that the learning journey is likely to be an excursion with unexpected and unintended outcomes.

Seventh, *pre-liminal variation* needs to be recognised – namely, the prior knowledge, learning styles, and approaches of students who commence a programme or course in which thresholds need to be traversed.

Next, generic good pedagogy which requires simplifying or breaking down concepts to make them accessible may be counterproductive, leading to 'false proxies' and ritualised learning or mimicry.

Finally, Land *et al.*[16] recommended consideration of whether there is 'an underlying game' or threshold conception that might be required in order to understand the difference between authorised understanding (within the professional community) versus alternative understanding (everyday common sense) of concepts.[16] One example of the latter might be that of client-centred practice in the occupational therapy field whereby the student has to 'let go' of the concept of therapist as expert (intuitive or lay understanding) who tells the client what to do and how to do it, and embrace the concept of the client as an expert in his or her own life, coming together with therapist in a partnership to share the client's expertise about his or her life, his or her personal narratives, together with the therapist's knowledge of health conditions, prognosis, treatment and skills to promote a match between person, occupation and environment to optimise his or her occupational performance and societal participation.

HOW IS ASSESSMENT UNDERSTOOD WITHIN A THRESHOLD CONCEPT FRAMEWORK?

When using threshold concepts in curriculum design, a dynamic approach to assessment is recommended,[18] which takes into account the fact that what is being assessed is likely to lie outside of students' prior knowledge and experiences and where there may be no precise or correct answer. Importantly, Meyer and Land[18] proposed that educators need to understand the variation in learning that is experienced by learners in pre-liminal space (how the portal comes into view and is perceived and the cognitive and ontological mindset it is viewed from). This is known as *pre-liminal variation*. When students approach the portal, how it is experienced, negotiated and made sense of is referred to as *liminal variation*. Finally, the exit point creates *post-liminal variation* or a view of the trajectory of future learning. This recognises that not all students reach the same conceptual understanding at the exit point from a course, and that some indeed pass with residual difficulties and misconceptions or partial understandings. Finally, there is a need to understand students' awareness and understanding of the underlying game or 'episteme' (ways of knowing) within the field. These modes of variation provide a conceptual basis for developing new and creative methods of assessment.[18]

When using threshold concepts as a pedagogical framework, assessment needs to uncover what each student knows, how this knowledge is organised, the interrelationships with other knowledge, and causal links between a student's ideas and thinking. Additionally, Meyer and Land[18] promoted the need to develop more nuanced terminology to discuss the assessment of threshold concepts and for understanding students' learning journeys rather than simply looking at 'snapshots' of learning. Activities such as portfolios, logs and sequential conceptual maps are assessment protocols that may be useful to provide evidence of this. Techniques such as using 'talk aloud' and 'write aloud' protocols such as blogs that promote reflection also elucidate the learning journey and can make students' thinking more explicit. These techniques may help to elicit the change in students' identities or the ontological shifts that are an important part of mastering threshold concepts. Educators need to signal what lies ahead – namely, the uncertainty and unfamiliarity of the liminal space encountered in the assessment task; students need to be prepared for and deal with intellectual uncertainty.[18] For example, when the assessment task lies beyond the students' experience or zone of proximal development,[19] it is difficult for them to know what it means to think like a clinical practitioner. Hence the challenge for the educator is to ensure that students have access to the materials, resources, technologies, supports and discussions they might need to engage with the learning tasks, as part of the required scaffolding to enable them to deal with the uncertainty of learning.

This requires a lot more than clear objectives, criterion and constructive alignment as proposed by Biggs.[1] A rich feedback environment is also required so that students can be assisted to work through points of conceptual difficulty and be aware of their learning in relation to threshold concepts. Assessment of threshold concepts has been explored to some extent in medical education[20] and more recently in occupational therapy.[21] Meyer and Land[18] in referring to threshold concepts as the 'jewels in the curriculum' argued that this could assist in the development of a simplified model of assessment at a programme level, as they can identify crucial points of engagement that teachers can construct to enable students to gain important conceptual understandings. They also provide insights into students' learning journeys regarding key transformations that educators wish to bring about. There are not likely to be too many such transformations in a single programme and 'in the assessment of threshold concepts less is probably more in this regard.'[18(p15)]

BEST EVIDENCE OF USE OF THRESHOLD CONCEPTS IN HEALTH PROFESSION EDUCATION

This section provides several examples of the use of threshold concepts within health profession education. There is a growing body of empirical evidence in the use and application of threshold concepts. Clouder[22] studied British occupational therapy and physiotherapy students regarding their transformation in self-identity with regard to the threshold concept of 'caring'. She argued that students grapple with 'caring' particularly on clinical placements, as it is not explicitly addressed in most educational programmes. Intuitive views of caring are different to those experienced by professionals treating patients in medical contexts. The latter requires questioning of fundamental beliefs and grappling with 'detachment and responsibility, with altruism and selflessness.'[22(p506)] Through traversing this troublesome space, students develop identities as healthcare professionals. Given that learning to care as a professional is bounded with emotions, she argued that assisting students to learn the limits of their capacity to care is critical to their professional survival. Moderated online discussion forums may be useful in connecting students to enable discussion about such concepts when they are geographically dispersed during fieldwork placements.[22]

Within occupational therapy, threshold concepts have been explored as a theoretical framework that can underpin curriculum redesign,[13,23] in terms of those that exist in practice education,[24] and with respect to students' learning journeys during their undergraduate years.[25] Tanner[24] interviewed practice educators who supervised students on clinical placements and identified three threshold concepts that led to transformations in students' understanding. These were (1) client-centred practice and the use of self, (2) developing a professional self-identity and (3) practising in real world settings. She highlighted the importance of these concepts with regard to ensuring that preclinical curriculum better prepares students for clinical work and in terms of preparing practice educators who will support students traversing this liminal space during placements.

Rodger and Turpin[13] described how they used an action research process to redesign two preregistration occupational therapy curricula (bachelor's and master's levels) and how they identified a set of unifying threshold concepts. After systematically identifying troublesome knowledge (through review processes based on student feedback, assessment results, staff reflection and peer review), thematic clustering enabled threshold concepts to emerge. Subsequently, specific emergent concepts were interrogated to ensure that they met the characteristics specified by Meyer and Land.[1] Five threshold concepts evolved that were then used to underpin curriculum redesign at the University of Queensland – namely, (1) purposeful and meaningful occupation, (2) client-centred practice, (3) the inseparable nature of theory and practice, (4) integrated reasoning (thinking critically, reflecting) and (4) professional identity.[13] These concepts have been integrated within each occupational therapy course and are explained to students by way of information guides, course outlines and are revisited by coordinators within each course undertaken. It is noteworthy that both Tanner[24] and Rodger and Turpin[13] identified client-centred practice and professional identity as being threshold concepts for occupational therapy students, suggesting they may be relevant beyond specific programmes and institutions.

In a more recent study, Rodger *et al.*[23] explored the perceptions of academic staff at the University of Queensland about the usefulness of threshold concepts when designing and revising curriculum. Many benefits were identified, including staff cohesion, a shared language and ownership of the curriculum, horizontal and vertical integration, clearer expectations and language for students through a consistent approach, and making troublesome knowledge explicit. Rodger *et al.*[23] also described transformations in student identity across the programme as recognised by academic staff. The development of professional identity may well be a fundamental threshold for students in occupational therapy, but this also applies in other healthcare professions.

RECOMMENDATIONS FOR FUTURE RESEARCH

There are several means of increasing the evidence base related to threshold concepts. While threshold concepts have been embraced in many areas of higher education, they are still contested territory. There is much that needs researching in order to determine whether they are useful within curriculum development in health profession education. Lucas and Mladenovic[26] argued that rather than being a research field on its own, threshold concepts provide a framework with potential to draw together a number of fields of research into a 'productive educative framework.'[(p237)] They contended that the threshold concepts framework provided a different lens for educators to view their current curriculum concerns by focusing attention on the social construction of disciplines and disciplinary knowledge and the nature of students' understanding of this knowledge.[26]

Some examples of research questions that still need to be addressed include the following: Are there threshold concepts that are germane to many health professions or are these truly bounded within particular fields? For healthcare educators who are already using threshold concepts to drive curriculum development, questions include the following: What do staff and students perceive to be the specific benefits? For those using threshold concepts to underpin assessment tasks, how is this being done? What do students need to scaffold their learning? What do students and staff members perceive to be the benefits of assessment tasks that measure students' understanding of a threshold concept or concepts, and what are the associated ontological shifts experienced? What are the emotional and cognitive barriers to students' engagement with threshold concepts? What student preconceptions might be problematic in conceptual mastery? What are the best ways to document ontological shifts – for example, what are the benefits of written formats such as blogs versus talk-aloud methods that might be incorporated into vivas/oral examinations?

CONCLUSION

This chapter has provided an overview of threshold concepts and their characteristics. It has provided some examples of how threshold concepts have been used within health professional education, such as in occupational therapy. Specific terminology linked with threshold concepts has been described and the implications for understanding these pre-liminal, liminal and post-liminal spaces as part of students' learning journeys. There is some preliminary evidence that threshold concepts hold potential for reforming curricula and improving students' learning experiences, but much still needs to be done to advance this agenda and provide conclusive evidence regarding threshold concepts as a framework for unpacking professional curricula within the health professions. Threshold concepts can be a key component in the arena of evidence-based education of health professional students.

SUMMARY POINTS

- Meyer and Land[1] describe threshold concepts as the 'concepts that bind a subject together, and that are fundamental to ways of thinking and practicing in that discipline'.[p1]
- Meyer and Land[1] propose threshold concepts have five characteristics: transformative, irreversible, troublesome, bounded and integrative.
- Perkins[6] proposed that knowledge might be troublesome for different reasons. He identified four types of knowledge: ritual, inert, alien and tacit.
- When students are mastering key threshold concepts, they often encounter difficult emotional spaces and these difficult spaces have been referred to as liminal spaces or states of liminality.
- Threshold concepts can be used to inform curriculum design, as they are key conceptual components in a curriculum allowing a focus on concepts that require mastery.
- Threshold concepts can be used to inform curriculum design and how student knowledge is assessed.

REVIEW QUESTIONS

- What is the definition of threshold concepts?
- What are the key features for something to be considered a threshold concept?
- Why is new knowledge considered troublesome?
- Define the four types of knowledge proposed by Perkins.
- Explain the concepts of liminality and liminal spaces in the context of student learning.
- How can threshold concepts be used to provide a framework for curriculum design?

REFLECTIVE QUESTIONS AND EXERCISES

- Think about how threshold concepts might fit within a health professional education curriculum.
- List four key threshold concepts that you think are relevant to your healthcare profession.
- Take the five characteristics that Meyer and Land[1] proposed true threshold concepts must have, apply them to key concepts (e.g. transformative, irreversible, troublesome, bounded and integrative) in your own healthcare profession and see if the concepts stand up.
- Recall a situation when you were teaching students a new concept, method or idea and how they reacted in that context. Were there any signs of students finding the new knowledge troublesome?
- Think about how threshold concepts might be able to inform any new developments in your health professional curriculum.

REFERENCES

1. Meyer JHF, Land R. Threshold concepts and troublesome knowledge: linkages to ways of thinking and practising. In: Rust C, editor. *Improving Student Learning: Theory and Practice Ten Years On.* Oxford, UK: Oxford Centre for Staff and Learning Development; 2003. pp. 1–15.
2. Meyer JHF, Land R. Threshold concepts and troublesome knowledge (2): epistemological considerations and a conceptual framework for teaching and learning. *High Educ.* 2005; **49**(3): 373–88.
3. Cousin G. An introduction to threshold concepts. *Planet.* 2006; **17**: 4–5.
4. Tertiary Education Quality and Standards Agency (TEQSA). *Higher Education Standards Framework (Threshold Standards) 2011.* Canberra, ACT: TEQSA; 2011. Available at: www.comlaw.gov.au/Details/F2012L00003/Download (accessed 29 January 2013).
5. Biggs JB. *Teaching for Quality Learning at University.* 2nd ed. Buckingham: Open University Press for Research into Higher Education; 2003.
6. Perkins D. The many faces of constructivism. *Educ Leadership.* 1999; **57**(3): 11.
7. Wisker G, Robinson G. Encouraging postgraduate students of literature and art to cross conceptual thresholds. *Innov Educ Teach Int.* 2009; **46**(3): 317–30.
8. Davies P, Mangan J. Threshold concepts and the integration of understanding in economics. *Stud High Educ.* 2007; **32**(6): 711–26.
9. Quinlan K, Baillie C, Male S, *et al.* A developing methodology to locate curricula thresholds in first year engineering. *Abstract Proceedings of the 4th Biennial Threshold Concepts Conference* (p.19). 28–29 June 2012. Dublin, Ireland; 2012.
10. Taylor C, Tzioumis V, Meyer JHF, *et al.* Using a mixed methods approach to understanding of hypotheses in biology. *Abstract Proceedings of the 4th Biennial Threshold Concepts Conference* (p. 19). 28–29 June 2012. Dublin, Ireland; 2012.
11. Kinchin IM, Cabot LB, Kobus M, *et al.* Threshold concepts in dental education. *Eur J Dent Educ.* 2011; **15**(4): 210–15.
12. Bulmer M, O'Brien M, Price S. Troublesome concepts in statistics: a student perspective on what they are and how to learn. In: Johnston I, Peat M, editors. UniServe Science National Conference – *Symposium Proceedings Science Teaching and Learning Research including Threshold Concepts* (pp. 9–15). 28–29 September 2007. Uniserve Science, University of Sydney; 2007.

13. Rodger S, Turpin M. Using threshold concepts to transform entry level curricula. In: Krause K, Buckridge M, Grimmer G, *et al.*, editors. *Research and Development in Higher Education: Reshaping Higher Education*, 34. Gold Coast, Australia, 4–7 July 2011. pp. 263–74.

14. Iwama MK. *The Kawa Model: culturally relevant occupational therapy.* Edinburgh: Churchill Livingstone-Elsevier; 2006.

15. Biggs J. *Aligning Teaching for Constructing Learning.* York: The Higher Education Academy; 2003. Available at: www.bangor.ac.uk/adu/the_scheme/documents/Biggs.pdf (accessed 12 October 2014).

16. Land R, Cousin G, Meyer JHF, *et al.* Threshold concepts and troublesome knowledge (3): implications for course design and evaluation. In: Rust C, editor. *Improving Student Learning: equality and diversity.* Oxford: Oxford Centre for Staff and Learning Development; 2005. pp. 53–64.

17. Wenger E. *Communities of Practice: learning, meaning, and identity.* London: Cambridge University Press; 1998.

18. Meyer JHF, Land R. *Threshold Concepts and Troublesome Knowledge: dynamics of assessment.* 2nd International Conference on Threshold Concepts, Threshold Concepts from Theory to Practice. 25–27 June 2008; Kingston, Ontario, Canada; 2008.

19. Vygotsky LS. Thinking and speech. In: Reiber RW, Carton AS, editors. *The Collected Works of L S Vygotsky.* (Vol. 1. Problems of generaly psychology.) New York, NY: Plenum Press; 1987.

20. Meyer JH, Cleary EG. An exploratory student learning model of clinical diagnosis. *Med Educ.* 1998; **32**(6): 574–81.

21. Springfield L. *Using assessment activities to engage students with threshold concepts.* Abstract Proceedings of the 4th Biennial Threshold Concepts Conference (p.105). 28–29 June 2012. Dublin, Ireland; 2012.

22. Clouder L. Caring as a threshold concept: transforming students in higher education into health(care) professionals. *Teach in Higher Educ.* 2005; **10**(4): 505–17.

23. Rodger S, Turpin M, O'Brien M. Experiences of academic staff in using threshold concepts within a reformed curriculum. *Stud Higher Educ.* Epub 2013 Sept 25.

24. Tanner B. Threshold concepts in practice education: perceptions of practice educators. *Br J Occup Ther.* 2011; **74**(9): 427–34.

25. Fortune T, Ennals P, Kennedy-Jones M. *Understanding troublesome moments and transitional states along the journey from learner to graduate among occupational therapy students.* Abstract Proceedings of the 4th Biennial Threshold Concepts Conference (p. 61). 2012 June 28–29. Dublin, Ireland; 2012.

26. Lucas U, Mladenovic R. The potential of threshold concepts: an emerging framework for educational research and practice. *Lond Rev Educ.* 2007; **5**(3): 237–48.

CHAPTER 12

Transformative learning for health professional education

Arlene H Morris and Debbie Faulk

OVERVIEW

In the context of adult education, transformative learning involves cognitive and non-cognitive processes whereby adults examine thoughts, beliefs, feelings and underlying assumptions through critical reflection, critical self-reflection and critical dialogue. The outcome of transformative learning is development of new perspectives for personal and/or professional change. A synthesis of literature related to use of transformative learning as a planned process for teaching and learning in health professional education provides evidence to inform teaching and learning practices, with the caveat that educators, researchers and students should not rely solely upon the evidence without further questioning of conclusions. Transformative learning is often embedded in learning activities such as case studies, problem-based learning, reflective journaling, service-learning, simulation and storytelling in education of health professionals. Best teaching practices for evidence-based education include the need for teacher authenticity, willingness to invest time in transformative learning, willingness to take risks, understanding that transformative learning is voluntary, role-modelling, and sharing power with students for collaboration and engagement. The student role in transformative learning mirrors those of teacher, but it also includes accepting personal responsibility for transformative learning and commitment to improvement. Transformative learning research involves theoretical underpinnings, the influence of relationships, context and settings for transformative learning and studies to test transformative learning as an outcome. Recommendations for future research to foster scholarship of teaching and learning across health professional education include testing the processes of transformative learning, measurement of transformative learning outcomes, identification of learning

activities that stimulate critical reflection, critical self-reflection and critical dialogue, and comparison of transformative learning in online, hybrid and traditional
educational settings.

CHAPTER OBJECTIVES

Upon completion of this chapter, the reader will be able to:
- explain transformative learning within the context of adult education
- define transformative learning terms as used in original adult education
  research
- discuss findings from evidence regarding transformative learning in health
  professional education
- consider application of transformative learning processes within the reader's
  health professional education setting.

KEY TERMS: transformative learning, critical reflection, critical self-reflection, critical dialogue, evidence-based education, health professional education

INTRODUCTION

The focus of this chapter is a synthesis of literature related to use of transformative
learning as a planned process for teaching and learning in health professional education. Evidence is presented to inform teaching practices across a variety of health
professions. The authors have grounded their teaching of nurses in transformative
learning for the past 15 years and believe transformative learning 'enables learners to
become engaged to imagine alternatives to prior assumptions and their own role in
nursing and healthcare delivery systems.'[1(p4)] Within the context of adult education,
transformative learning involves cognitive and non-cognitive processes whereby
adults examine thoughts, beliefs, feelings and underlying assumptions through critical
reflection, critical self-reflection and critical dialogue. The outcome of transformative
learning is development of new perspectives for personal and/or professional change.

SEARCH METHODS

Google Scholar, ProQuest and CINAHL (Cumulative Index to Nursing and Allied
Health Literature) using combinations of terms 'healthcare professions education',
'health professional students' AND 'Mezirow's Transformative Learning Theory', or
'transformative learning' were used in the search for evidence. Search limits included
scholarly articles written in English and published between the years 2007 and 2013.
Titles and abstracts were initially scanned to determine relevance to the questions:
'Is transformative learning used in education of healthcare professional students?'
and 'What evidence supports use of transformative learning in education of health

professionals?' Because of a lack of consistency in terms, articles related to transformative education rather than transformative learning were eliminated. For example, a number of authors used the term transformative or transformation to describe curricular revisions rather than actual intentional use of transformative learning.

TRANSFORMATIVE LEARNING THEORY

Transformative learning is an adult education theory developed by Jack Mezirow in 1974 after his seminal work with females returning to college. Mezirow's definition of transformative learning, frequently cited in adult education literature, is the

> process by which we transform our taken-for-granted frames of reference (meaning perspectives, habits of mind, mindsets) to make them more inclusive, discriminating, open, emotionally capable of change, and reflective so that they may generate beliefs and opinions that will prove more true or justified to guide action.[2(p73)]

Two well-noted researchers of transformative learning postulate that Mezirow's theory is one of the most closely scrutinised education theories.[3] Disciplines outside of education have become interested in transformative learning as an educational approach that subsumes some practices that are inherent in good education of adults.

At the heart of transformative learning is the premise that adults learn and relearn leading to transformation of perspectives and resultant changes in actions or behaviours. Adult learners come to learning situations with unique backgrounds that include life experiences, prior learning and assumptions that contribute to frames of reference and habits of mind. Experiences recalled from a person's history have an associated emotion that is essential for opinions and world view.[4] Adults move from one frame of reference to another and reject ideas that do not fit comfortably within current ways of thinking and behaving. When adults are exposed to planned educational or happenstance situations and are asked to voluntarily participate in critical reflection, critical self-reflection and critical dialogue, prior thinking may be reconsidered, leading to new thinking, revision or recommitment to current thinking that can be transformative, resulting in changes in behaviours or actions.

Adult learners may progress through stages to develop new attitudes and actions. These stages begin with triggering events, causing disorienting dilemmas, and may result in recommitment to a prior perspective or internalisation of a new perspective. The process repeats in cycles and may involve clarification of existing relationships or negotiation of new relationships.[5] For example, consider an adult learner returning to school to obtain a baccalaureate degree in nursing who experienced a sudden triggering event, causing a disorienting dilemma while taking an algebra test. The learner began crying during the test and realised that there had to be some deep-seated reasons for the distress. After turning in the test, the learner began a critical self-examination of assumptions related to prior experiences regarding ability to learn mathematics.

One of the outcomes of the learner's reflection was the realisation that there was no self-confidence in learning mathematics. The learner began to question personal intelligence and learning abilities, actually admitting the belief that everyone else was smarter. The learner began to consider and question if other females had experienced the same point of view or may have gone through this same experience. Over time the learner began to explore prior thinking about past roles, relationships and actions related to learning algebra and learning in general, including past teachers who did not challenge the learner. Through continuing critical self-reflection, the learner slowly began to form a different way of thinking by developing and implementing a plan of action. The plan was to seek tutoring and to have discussion with the tutor to further explore prior thinking about learning abilities. It was through this dialogue that the learner came to understand that past methods for learning, particularly memorisation of facts, was not an effective learning strategy. The learner realised that learning must include application of information. In the end, the learner gained new knowledge, not only about algebra but also about self as a learner. Algebra skills were conquered, but the broader understanding led to implementing new plans for learning. New learning skills were tried out in other learning situations. With each new learning experience, the learner gained competence and self-confidence. This new point of view about personal learning abilities was re-evaluated and integrated into a new point of view, which had lifelong implications.

Transformative learning involves deeper analysis using the process of reflection. Reflection can be substantive, in that new concepts are pondered (*critical reflection*), or it can involve consideration of how the concept relates to self and past mindsets (*critical self-reflection*). Interaction and discussion with others (*critical dialogue*) helps promote awareness of differences in thinking and alternative possibilities, furthering critical reflection and critical self-reflection.[6] These three approaches are basic to the process of transformative learning and can be used to develop a multitude of teaching and learning strategies across all healthcare professions.

Consider a class about principles of movement in which a student of occupational therapy ponders amazing new concepts (*critical reflection*). If the learner then decides to further consider how this information regarding movement could increase independent functioning of individuals who have experienced a stroke, he or she becomes engaged. *Critical self-reflection* occurs when the learner further considers, 'Is this relevant or important to me?' and 'Do I want to include this concept in how I view the world and will I use it in my anticipated role?' The learner considers how movement principles relate to past personal experiences and assumptions based on a family member who experienced a stroke. Discussion with patients, peers or faculty in face-to-face or online discussions (*critical dialogue*) can lead to revision of past thinking based on the choice to integrate the new concept into a new or revised personal view, or to recommit to past or current thinking and behaviours.

Transformative learning research within the context of adult education in traditional and non-traditional settings has spanned a period of 30 years. It is beyond the scope of this chapter to present an analysis of this research. However, in a synthesis of research for years 2006–10, two well-recognised adult education researchers note that while studies continue to consider theoretical foundations, influence of relationships, and context and setting, fostering transformative learning is still the primary focus of the published research findings. Evidence specific to fostering transformative learning provides new considerations related to context for transformative learning, meaning of holistic learning, and use of pleasure and humour to stimulate transformative learning. Of note is Taylor and Synder's[3] assertion that

> basic assumptions for fostering transformative learning have been accepted
> .... there is a lack of a clear understanding of what it looks like in practice.
> This lack of clarity further complicates the task of assessing transformative
> learning.[(p53)]

Their recommendations for future research include the need to be consistent with historical use of transformative learning terms within various research contexts and more studies that measure the outcome or outcomes of transformative learning.

HEALTH PROFESSIONAL EDUCATION

Common challenges in teaching inform the use of transformative learning in health professional education. In 2005 the World Health Organization[7] in collaboration with JHPIEGO (an affiliate of the Johns Hopkins Hospital in the United States) developed a reference manual for effective teaching in health professional education. This document identified common challenges in curricular design and selection of teaching methodologies and strategies across disciplines. Challenges included, for example, how to accommodate teaching large numbers of students, the growing problem of finding relevant practice experiences, and the vast amount of ever-changing information. Additionally, awareness regarding use of most current national and state policies, guidelines and standards is required for healthcare providers to be able to address the needs and problems of specific populations.

Each healthcare profession has core or essential competencies for performance within their specific scopes of practice. These core and essential competencies are used to determine content, teaching methodologies, strategies and evaluation processes. Although pedagogical decisions are founded on evidence or expertise, research in education practices has revealed ubiquitous concepts and principles that are best addressed through application of learning in real life situations. This evidence is especially important to health professional educators.

Commonalities are also seen in teaching strategies. Across a variety of discipline-specific health professional education, educators are using problem-based learning, journaling, case studies, portfolios, service-learning, simulation and storytelling.[8-11] Interestingly, transformative learning is inherent in many of these strategies. For example, *critical reflection* is used to ponder information presented through case studies, simulations and in problem-based learning, while *critical self-reflection* is used in journaling, in portfolios and in decision-making related to identification of assumptions and the power assumptions have on actions. Within planned activities such as service-learning or use of stories, *critical dialogue* helps learners develop an appreciation for how others think and provides further reflection for possible alternative ways of thinking about a concept or issue. Use of these prevalent teaching strategies which promote transformative learning situates learning as relevant for future healthcare providers.

TRANSFORMATIVE LEARNING IN HEALTH PROFESSIONAL EDUCATION

The question, 'Why is transformative learning needed in health professional education?' is relevant to a scholarship of teaching and learning. As stated previously in this chapter, transformative learning is an adult learning theory for how adults learn and relearn. Health professional students are adult learners who come to educational programmes with preconceived ideas, values, beliefs and assumptions (habits of mind) regarding health, healthcare, health delivery systems, health consumers, patient populations, diseases, and so forth. Preconceived thinking may manifest as negative attitudes that influence actions and behaviours of learners.

For example, evidence indicates that nursing students may have negative attitudes towards elderly patients.[12] Valuing youth, a focus on productivity, or past experience of taking care of older grandparents or parents may affect beliefs and values related to this population. Negative perceptions may have a profound effect on ability to recruit nurses to work in long-term care or other gerontology settings. Negative perceptions can also affect the care of individuals with certain diseases. Findings from a qualitative study demonstrated that despite gender, profession or clinical experience, healthcare professionals continue to exhibit negative attitudes related to cancer.[13] A fear of developing cancer or a past personal experience with the disease may influence communication and teaching behaviours.

Development of professional role identity is imperative in all health professions. Professional development prepares the learner for effective practice. Negative habits of mind may create a barrier to professional development. For example, students who are cynical regarding politics may not embrace the importance of political advocacy for leading change for healthcare delivery and for the profession as a whole. Using evidence-based education for transformative learning, educators can help students examine negative habits of mind with a goal of producing healthcare professionals who make sound, rational, caring, unbiased clinical judgements based on evidence and valuing of human beings.

TRANSFORMATIVE LEARNING FOR EVIDENCE-BASED EDUCATION

Evidence demonstrates that transformative learning is being used in the education of occupational therapists, physicians, nurses, dentists and physician assistants (*see* Table 12.1). Specific examples of teaching and learning activities to promote critical reflection, critical self-reflection or critical dialogue included service-learning, problem-based learning, portfolios, case studies, videos, reflection activities and storytelling. It is pertinent to note that measurement of transformative learning was not the focus of the evidence reported in the studies. However, attainment of transformative learning was inferred from authors' reports of findings and opinions. The predominant outcome identified was desire to cultivate socialisation of learners across healthcare professions for role identity. Health professional educators used this goal as a guide for developing transformative learning activities. Lack of studies with the purpose of measuring transformative learning supports the need for future research.

Evidence to inform teaching practices is presented in Table 12.2. Intentional use of transformative learning involves taking risks and is time-consuming. The first step is to explain transformative learning to elicit student engagement. Teachers must be authentic and create safe and trusting learning environments that engage learners. Sharing power with students, an intimidating proposition for some educators, is critical to enhancing learner collaboration. Educators should model transformative learning by sharing transformation of perspectives related to the teacher role.

Teaching practices should also include awareness that critical self-reflection and dialogue can be anxiety producing. For example, students in health professions will encounter individuals, families and communities that differ from personal backgrounds. When asked to reflect on assumptions regarding these encounters, students can experience cognitive dissonance that is painful or uncomfortable. Educators should inform learners about the potential for experiencing disorienting dilemmas and ways to help students effectively deal with conflicts related to prior beliefs and values. Educators should anticipate potential discomfort and encourage students to allow time to process and potentially grow from these experiences. Planning for transformative learning should include awareness that changes in learner behaviours may occur quickly or may be revealed after the learner begins professional practice.

Educators using transformative learning must understand the role of learner in the learning process (*see* Table 12.3). Students must make the decision to participate in transformative learning. The decision is voluntary and cannot be forced on the student. Students must be willing to take risks and accept personal responsibility for personal and/or professional transformation in perspectives and resultant changes in behaviours. Voluntary participation, risk-taking and acceptance of personal responsibility and commitment to improvement allow the learner to become engaged with the content.

TABLE 12.1 Overview of relevant evidence

Author (year), journal, location	Purpose	Relevant findings
Bagatell *et al.* (2013),[14] *Occupational Therapy in Mental Health*, the United States	Understand occupational therapy students' transformative learning during clinical experiences	Use of transformative learning theory as a framework for clinical experiences in mental health settings resulted in greater understanding of needs of clients and professional role development

(continued)

Author (year), journal, location	Purpose	Relevant findings
Branch (2010),[15] *Patient Education and Counseling*, the United States	Determine if use of reflection activities in physician education programmes increased communication competencies and development of physicians committed to professional values	Longitudinal educational programmes that use critical reflection in combination with clinical experiences enhance development of humanistic values and may result in transformation of perspectives of physicians
		Reflective learning approaches can effectively influence learners' skills, values, attitudes and behaviours
Faulk *et al.* (2010),[16] *International Journal of Nursing Education Scholarship*, the United States	Evaluate graduate nursing students' progression through Mezirow's phases of transformative learning	Increased awareness of self-concept and nursing role fulfilment
		Graduate education experiences paralleled Mezirow's transformative learning phases
Hanson (2013),[17] *Nurse Education Practice*, Australia	Presentation of a value-based learning activity grounded in transformative learning	Critical reflection promoted development of professional role identity in nursing students
Horton-Deutsch and Sherwood (2008),[18] *Journal of Nursing Management*, the United States	Report use and outcomes from teaching/learning activities that focus on reflection	Learning activities that prompt deeper reflection of issues in clinical settings link nursing education, research and practice
Langley and Brown (2010),[19] *Nursing Education Perspectives*, the United States	Examination of graduate nursing students and faculty perceptions related to use of reflection	Students and faculty report enhanced development of professional self-identity and empowerment through reflective journaling
Mann *et al.* (2009),[20] *Advanced Health Science Education Theory and Practice*, Canada	Identify variables in health professions educational processes, evidence gaps, and explore implications of using reflection as a teaching and learning approach	Reflection as a teaching approach was reported in 14 medicine, 11 nursing, 2 health sciences, 1 dentistry, and 1 physiotherapy education programme/s
		Reflective practice is difficult to measure; call for studies with rigorous designs and consistent term use to evaluate effectiveness of reflection as a strategy to promote professional development

Author (year), journal, location	Purpose	Relevant findings
McAllister *et al.* (2013),[21] *Educational Action Research*, Australia	Test use of the *Sensitise Take Action and Reflection (STAR)* framework that incorporates transformative learning approaches to evaluate development of nursing, nutrition, public health, occupational therapy, paramedic students' competencies related to understanding and planning care for health inequity situations	STAR was easy to understand and relevant for health professional education STAR holds promise for achieving stated purpose STAR may be an effective tool for interprofessional collaboration across disciplines
Morris and Faulk (2007),[6] *Journal of Nursing Education*, the United States	Determination of professional role changes following completion of baccalaureate education Identification of specific learning activities in returning Registered Nurse (RN) to Bachelor of Science in Nursing (BSN) nursing education that resulted in perspective transformation	Use of transformative learning theory as framework for planning teaching and learning activities affects resocialisation Planned learning activities using transformative learning processes (critical reflection, critical self-reflection, critical dialogue) result in perspective transformation
O'Connell (2010),[22] *Journal of Physician Assistant Education*, the United States	Recommend use of transformative learning theory as a framework in development of learning activities to enhance physician assistant (PA) students' professional development	Transformative learning theory provides a framework for educators planning learning activities for PA students Transformative learning processes can challenge PA students to examine values, beliefs and frames of reference through reflection on new and challenging experiences encountered during education Educators must anticipate and plan for cognitive dissonance that can occur in PA education experiences PA students may experience the phases of transformative learning

(continued)

Author (year), journal, location	Purpose	Relevant findings
Sandars (2009),[23] *AMEE Guide No. 44*, Scotland	Report ways to incorporate reflection in secondary and tertiary medical education	Development of therapeutic relationships and professional expertise can be enhanced through reflection using reflective journals, critical incident reports, digital media and storytelling
Wittich *et al.* (2010),[24] *Academic Medicine*, the United States	Report results of incorporating transformative learning using critical reflection to conceptually link and teach practice-based learning improvement and systems-based practice to medical residents	Transformative learning using critical reflection helps residents and faculty understand and make connections between improvement competencies
		Residents' reflection of personal experience in difficult patient care situations can lead to identification of personal and/or system limitations
		Critical reflection for quality improvement efforts may lead to healthcare system improvements
		Residents' reflection regarding personal limitations can improve individual practice

TABLE 12.2 Evidence-based teaching practices

Teaching practices	Examples of application
Create a safe, trusting and inclusive learning environment	• Provide an introductory overview for students about transformative learning including concepts and definitions • Set ground rules • Use a case study to introduce potential stereotypes and prejudices
Take risks	• Recognise that transformative learning is time-consuming • Plan learning activities to stimulate critical reflection, critical self-reflection and critical dialogue • Recognise and capitalise on happenstance learning situations • Willingness to examine self as educator • Recognise that transformative learning may not occur suddenly
Consider content and context	• Provide pre-session questions to evaluate students' points of view regarding issue(s) and current emotional and stress levels • Use digital storytelling • Consider factors influencing quality healthcare outcomes • Discuss specific topics through questioning in traditional and online classrooms

Teaching practices	Examples of application
Focus on individual learner needs	• Aggregate information related to individual learner styles and personalities in planning teaching approaches • Recognise that students cannot be forced to participate in transformative learning • Recognise that transformative learning may produce anxiety in students • Prepare opportunities for learners to cope with cognitive dissonance
Set the stage through modelling	• Exhibit transparency in use of reflection and openness to new learning • Incorporate personal stories as applicable
Share power	• Collaborate with learners regarding structure, outcomes and evaluation of learning • Share experiences, including service-learning opportunities • Incorporate creative, non-traditional sources of information • Allow student choices regarding learning activities
Strike a balance between support and challenge	• Accept alternate learning activities • Accept potential for delayed or lack of perspective transformation • Encourage learners to use deeper analysis for critical self-reflection
Allow time for transformative learning	• Plan sequential or extended time for learning activities • Anticipate unplanned opportunities for critical reflection, critical self-reflection and critical dialogue

TABLE 12.3 Student role in transformative learning

Student role	Examples of application
Willingness to take risks	• Interact with previously unknown or diverse situations (e.g. inner-city outreach experience of needle exchange programme) • Reflective journaling • Dialogue in face-to-face or online environments
Accept personal responsibility for creating a transformative learning environment	• Be open to consider alternate ways of thinking (personal and in relation to peers) • Engage in learning activities (e.g. narratives, case studies or simulation) to explore biases, prejudices, alternative points of view • Reflect on additional application of new concepts in personal and professional roles
Engage in content with other learners	• Critically reflect and self-reflect regarding constructs and content in relation to prior habits of mind and future applications • Actively engage in collaborative activities • Dialogue in face-to-face or online environments
Willingness to critically examine thinking, values, belief systems, assumptions, habits of mind and recognise impact on behaviours	• Values clarification activities • Interaction in diverse situations • Community advocacy programmes • Work with underserved populations • Clinical experiences

(*continued*)

Student role	Examples of application
Willingness to critically reflect on personal strengths and areas of needed improvement	• Identify personal habits of mind and areas of needed development • Focus on cognitive and non-cognitive skills to determine strengths and areas for improvement
Commitment to improvement	• Identify areas for quality improvement in healthcare systems • Continuous quality improvement in personal practices • Lifelong learning

RECOMMENDATIONS FOR FUTURE RESEARCH

The need for further evidence related to use of transformative learning as a planned process for health professional education includes:

- explaining processes of transformative learning
- use of learning activities that stimulate critical reflection and dialogue
- outcomes of transformative learning
- outcomes linked to specific teaching strategies
- comparison of transformative learning outcomes in online, hybrid and traditional educational settings
- comparison of outcomes across and within all healthcare professions
- longitudinal research of learners who engaged in transformative learning to determine learner behaviours and commitment to safe practice and quality outcomes
- identification of structures required in higher education settings that promote effective use of transformative learning, including educator competencies and educator-to-student ratios.
- identification of cross-cultural implications for use of transformative learning and challenges inherent within some cultures
- identification of challenges related to generational characteristics among teachers and learners.

Educators who desire to conduct research related to transformative learning within an adult education context should consider using a variety of research methodologies and data collection tools. Research must be grounded in the terms and results from primary resources rather than depending on critiques of prior studies. Collaboration among researchers can enable planned, intentional designs of studies that can reveal a more in-depth analysis of transformative learning use in health professional education. This would lead to teaching practices based on evidence and further develop a scholarship of teaching and learning for health professional education.

CONCLUSION

The primary purpose of this synthesis of literature was to provide educators with evidence to inform use of transformative learning as a teaching/learning approach in health professional education. Findings should serve as a starting point and should not be solely relied upon without further questioning and analysis. As nurse educators, we believe the transformative learning process is powerful for both teachers and learners, as we have seen changes in ourselves as educators and in student behaviours indicative of a commitment to providing quality healthcare and lifelong learning. Evidence reveals that a number of health professional programmes are using learning activities that promote transformative learning. Both nursing and medicine are using transformative learning processes as instructional tools and in a few instances in design of individual courses or curricula. Further research to clarify specific questions, processes, settings and context, and outcomes of application of transformative learning can advance the scholarship of teaching and learning in health professional education.

SUMMARY POINTS

- Transformative learning involves cognitive and non-cognitive processes whereby adults examine thoughts, beliefs, feelings and underlying assumptions through critical reflection, critical self-reflection and critical dialogue.
- The outcome of transformative learning is development of new perspectives for personal and/or professional change.
- Transformative learning is often embedded in learning activities such as case studies, problem-based learning, reflective journaling, service-learning, simulation and storytelling in education of health professionals.
- Best teaching practices for evidence-based education include need for teacher authenticity, willingness to invest time in transformative learning, willingness to take risks, understanding that transformative learning is voluntary, role-modelling, and sharing power with students for collaboration and engagement.
- The student role in transformative learning mirrors those of the teacher, but also includes accepting personal responsibility for transformative learning and commitment to improvement.
- Individual learner commitment to quality and safe healthcare practices may begin in learning activities planned to promote transformative learning.
- Collaboration among researchers can enable planned, intentional designs of studies that can reveal a more in-depth analysis of transformative learning use in health professional education, leading to teaching practices based on evidence that would further develop a scholarship of teaching and learning for health professional education.

REVIEW QUESTIONS

- Explain transformative learning within the context of adult education.
- What are the three core processes within transformative learning?
- How can transformative learning be used as a foundation for decisions about teaching approaches within courses and curricula?
- What teacher practices are based in best evidence for transformative learning?
- What is required for learners who voluntarily participate in transformative learning?
- What are the recommendations for future research regarding transformative learning within health professional education?

REFLECTIVE QUESTIONS AND EXERCISES

- Critically self-reflect on personal strengths, beliefs, values and biases, and recognise potential influence on teaching.
- Reflect on ways educators could improve the perception of authenticity, safety and trust in all types of classroom settings.
- Develop teaching/learning activities that promote transformative learning.
- Identify specific learner outcomes that reflect transformative learning within a selected course.
- Propose a purpose statement for a research study that would measure outcomes of transformative learning within or across one or more specific health professional discipline(s).

REFERENCES

1. Morris AH, Faulk D, editors. *Transformative Learning in Nursing: a guide for nurse educators.* New York, NY: Springer Publishing; 2012.
2. Mezirow J. Learning to think like an adult: core concepts of transformation theory. In: Taylor EW, Cranton P, editors. *The Handbook of Transformative Learning: theory, research, and practice.* San Francisco, CA: Jossey-Bass; 2012. pp. 73–95.
3. Taylor EW, Synder MJ. A critical review of research on transformative learning theory, 2006–2010. In: Taylor EW, Cranton P, editors. *The Handbook of Transformative Learning: theory, research, and practice.* San Francisco, CA: Jossey-Bass; 2012. pp. 37–55.
4. Mezirow J, Associates. *Learning as Transformation: critical perspectives on a theory in progress.* San Francisco, CA: Jossey Bass; 2000.
5. Mezirow J. *Transformative Dimensions of Adult Learning.* San Francisco, CA: Jossey-Bass; 1991.
6. Morris AH, Faulk D. Perspective transformation: enhancing the development of professionalism in RN to BSN students. *J Nurs Educ.* 2007; **46**(10): 445–51.
7. World Health Organization (WHO); JHPIEGO. *Effective Teaching: a guide for educating health-care providers.* Geneva: WHO; 2005. Available at: www.jhpiego.org/files/EffTeach_man.pdf (accessed 12 October 2014).

8. Polverini PA. A curriculum for the new dental practitioner for a prospective oral health care environment. *Am J Public Health.* 2012; **102**(2): 1–3.
9. Buckley S, Coleman J, Davison I, *et al.* The educational effects of portfolios on undergraduate student learning: a Best Evidence Medical Education (BEME) systematic review. *Med Teach.* 2009; **31**(4): 340–55.
10. Brendel W. A framework of narrative-driven transformative learning in medicine. *J Transformative Educ.* 2009; **7**(1): 26–43.
11. Christiansen A. Storytelling and professional learning: a phenomenographic study of students' experience of patient digital stories in nurse education. *Nurse Educ Today.* 2010; **31**(3): 289–93.
12. Lovell M. Caring for the elderly: changing perceptions and attitudes. *J Vasc Nurs.* 2006; **24**(1): 22–6.
13. Kearney N, Miller M, Paul K, *et al.* Oncology health care professionals' attitudes to cancer: a professional concern. *Ann Oncol.* 2003; **14**(1): 57–61.
14. Bagatell N, Lawrence J, Schwartz M, *et al.* Occupational therapy student experiences and transformations during field work in mental health settings. *Occup Ther Mental Health.* 2013; **29**(2): 118–96.
15. Branch WT Jr. The road to professionalism: reflective practice and reflective learning. *Patient Educ Couns.* 2010; **80**(3): 327–32.
16. Faulk D, Parker F, Morris AH. Reforming perspectives: MSN graduates' knowledge, attitudes, and awareness of self-transformation. *Int J Nurs Educ Scholarsh.* 2010; **7**(1): Article 24.
17. Hanson J. From me to we: transforming values and building professional community through narratives. *Nurse Educ Pract.* 2013; **13**(2): 142–6.
18. Horton-Deutsch S, Sherwood G. Reflection: an educational strategy to develop emotionally-competent nurse leaders. *J Nurs Manag.* 2008; **16**(8): 946–54.
19. Langley ME, Brown ST. Perceptions of the use of reflective learning journals in online graduate nursing education. *Nurs Educ Perspect.* 2010; **31**(1): 12–17.
20. Mann K, Gordon J, MacLeod A. Reflection and reflective practice in health professions education: a systematic review. *Adv Health Sci Educ Theory Pract.* 2009; **14**(4): 595–621.
21. McAllister M, Oprescu F, Downer T, *et al.* Evaluating STAR – a transformative learning framework: interdisciplinary action research in health training. *Educ Action Res.* 2013; **21**(1): 90–106.
22. O'Connell CB. Enhancing transformative learning in physician assistant education. *J Physician Assist Educ.* 2010; **21**(1): 18–22.
23. Sandars J. The use of reflection in medical education: AMEE Guide No. 44. *Med Teach.* 2009; **31**(8): 685–95.
24. Wittich CM, Reed DA, McDonald FS, *et al.* Transformative learning: a framework using critical reflection to link the improvement competencies in graduate medical education. *Acad Med.* 2010; **85**(11): 1790–3.

CHAPTER 13

Best practice assessment in health professional education

....

Sue McAllister

OVERVIEW

Evidence for best practice assessment is sparse, particularly with regard to allied health students and, where it exists, may be poor quality or not derived from expert opinion. This chapter provides an overview of current issues in educational assessment design in the health sciences as a foundation to a scholarly approach to assessment. A strategy is described and illustrated that will assist readers to engage in scholarly research and practice with regard to educational assessment. The principles of evidence-based educational assessment (EBEA) practice are applied to identifying types of evidence, developing inquiry directed to the desired assessment outcomes, locating a range of evidence and using this to guide decision-making and related research and scholarship.

CHAPTER OBJECTIVES

Upon completion of this chapter, the reader will be able to:
- define the term 'evidence-based educational assessment'
- explain the components of the EBEA cycle for assessment design
- articulate how validity and reliability are important components of the EBEA process
- outline the concept of objectivity in relation to EBEA
- describe the EBEA process using the elements of SESACO (Student or Student group; Environment; Stakeholder; Assessment; Comparison or Control; Outcome).

KEY TERMS: evidence-based educational assessment, evidence-based education, allied health

---

INTRODUCTION

Assessing students is a key activity in health professional education programmes. It is tempting to simplify the process of assessment – we just want to know if our students have learned what we have taught them. How hard can that be? We give them a test. However, there are so many assessments to choose from, so many issues to consider when choosing and very little high-quality research evidence available to guide us. Where evidence is available, it often evaluates the qualities of a specific type of assessment but not whether it is the best choice for a particular assessment situation or desired outcome. Furthermore, much of the current evidence rests on expert opinion. However, as assessment is an important and required part of our curriculum, we need to evaluate the best available evidence and use it to make decisions about current practice and future research.

Davies[1] identifies that evidence-based education (EBE) should inform two courses of action: (1) using evidence to inform educational decisions and (2) generating high-quality evidence through research. This chapter aims to support best practice in evidence-based decision-making in assessment by providing a process for selecting and evaluating assessment tools and approaches. The same process can also be used to design research questions that are well grounded in current evidence regarding assessment and which use rigorous methodology most likely to address the assessment outcomes of interest. The process is based on elaborations of clinical evidence-based practice (EBP) for allied health developed by Dollaghan[2] and Schlosser and Raghavendra.[3] Figure 13.1 illustrates this EBP cycle as applied to evidence-based educational assessment (EBEA), and the sections that follow in this chapter will step through each stage. Throughout this process the primary question is: What is the desired outcome for the assessment? Ginsburg *et al.*[4] state that evidence maximising student learning outcomes should be the focus of EBE. This is clearly a priority, but are there other relevant outcomes specific to assessment within the educational process or EBEA? Are there outcomes specific to educating and assessing allied health students? An understanding of the current issues in assessment is useful for deciding on a desired outcome(s), assessment tools or approaches that may support the outcome(s), and the kind of evidence that should be sought to design or evaluate an assessment approach.

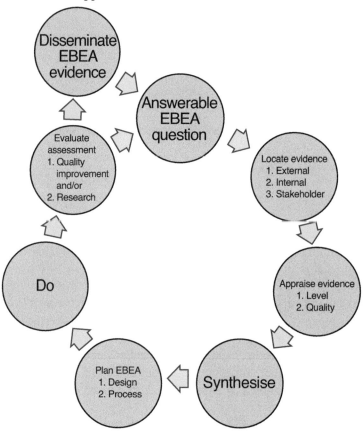

FIGURE 13.1 Evidence-based educational assessment (EBEA) cycle for assessment design

CURRENT ISSUES AND THEORIES IN ASSESSMENT
Assessment outcomes

If student learning outcomes are the focus of EBEA, what kind of outcomes does assessment serve? As educators, we generally consider assessment to have two primary outcomes: (1) learning and (2) measurement or certification of learning.[5] Assessment focused on facilitating learning is usually referred to as formative assessment, or assessment for learning. For example, providing feedback on assignment drafts, or cycles of feedback and discussion between clinical educator and student on placement. However, it has long been accepted and demonstrated that all assessment has the potential to influence learning.[5,6] Measurement of learning or summative assessment intends to collect definitive evidence about how much students know or can do. In both these assessment outcomes, the student is the object of assessment and is being encouraged to internalise the assessor's learning targets and develop goals in relation to these. Boud and Falchikov[7] suggest that this may result in professionals who are not prepared for lifelong learning. They propose that assessment should facilitate the development of the ability of students to assess their own performance rather than rely on how they are judged by others.[7] Therefore, students should be engaged as agents or participants in assessment so that they are able to make judgements in the future about their own work, their learning needs and appropriate strategies to meet them.

Assessment processes can also have negative or positive backwash into curriculum (e.g. they influence what and how knowledge, skills, and practices are taught).[8,9] Therefore, aspects of process and meaning in EBEA should be considered as well as learning outcomes.[1] The influence of assessment on curriculum may be intentional or unintentional. Educational philosophies such as constructive alignment[10] intentionally aim for assessment to influence how students are taught, by considering assessment as one element of an interconnected, or constructively aligned, curriculum. Assessment, therefore, is not considered separately from the curriculum but, rather, as one element of a learning outcome-focused curriculum where learning objectives, learning activities, assessment tasks and grading are congruent.

Other assessment stakeholders have three desired assessment outcomes that are more focused on what learning has occurred: (1) fitness for practice, (2) fitness for award and (3) fitness for purpose.[11] All three are focused on measuring the learning that has occurred and identifying the level that has been achieved. *Fitness for practice* assessments measure students' performance against standards for acceptable practice of the profession. This reflects an accreditation perspective where the boundaries of professional practice need to be defined and status or reputation protected.[11] *Fitness for award* assures the university and the students that the assessments have provided enough evidence to grant the final qualification. Assessment of *fitness for purpose* ensures that graduates are properly prepared for the professional practice, an important outcome for the graduate, his or her employer, health service users and the whole profession.

Thus assessment processes can have multiple and sometimes competing desired outcomes and may be addressed by different kinds of assessment strategies. Furthermore, assessment may be directed at various stages of the educational process. For example, it may focus on sub-elements such as the demonstration of specific knowledge, skills and practices or on how these might be integrated and applied to create competent professional performances.[12] Regardless of whether the primary focus is learning or measurement, ultimately educators and stakeholders want assessment to be fair and accurate. As such, gathering evidence on these aspects of assessment falls under the umbrella of assessment validity and reliability.

Validity and reliability

This aspect of assessment relates to psychometrics – a large and complex discipline with its own contested theories and practices. However, we need to be informed consumers if we are to review, understand and appropriately apply evidence-based approaches to assessment that draw upon psychometric theories and measurement practices. Most academics teaching in health professional programmes have a working knowledge of validity and reliability concepts, particularly if their first degree is within a health discipline. It is readily known that validity relates to whether an assessment really samples the knowledge, skills or outcomes of interest, which will depend on its purpose, while reliability describes how reproducible an assessment's results are for individuals or groups. This concept speaks to concepts of fairness, a key concern for educators and their students.[8]

It is commonly assumed that validity is a property of an assessment itself. However, the recommended approach to evaluating assessment validity for over 20 years has been to focus on the validity of interpretations and actions based on the measures or results from an assessment.[13] Other outdated conceptual approaches to validity continue to be employed, such as evaluating evidence against traditional and separate concepts of face, content, criterion and construct validity. Modern approaches to validation require an integrated judgement that considers multiple aspects of validity. The validation process should provide evidence that supports the conclusion that the assessment measures can be validly used for a particular purpose.[14] Therefore, when evaluating whether the results of an assessment can be validly used to make decisions with regard to students' learning, a range of information should be sought. This includes the purpose of the assessment; the theoretical framework underlying the validation process and how it has guided choices for content development; assessment and scoring procedures; and recommendations for interpretation and actions based on the resulting measures.

Therefore, a range of evidence should be collected and integrated. Some evidence is qualitative and relates to the rigour of the processes used to develop aspects such as assessment content. Other evidence is statistical and examines the properties of items, relationships between them and the purpose of the assessment. There is a tendency to employ customary statistical strategies such as Cronbach's alpha, factor analysis and correlations without connection to a validity framework resulting in diminished validity.[15] Modern test theory now requires statistical evaluation of items, measures and relevant relationships against models of well-functioning assessments, tests and scales.[16]

Reliability should not be considered separately from validity, as validity can be easily sacrificed for reliability.[17] Aiming for high reliability may require undesirable compromises to content or processes and therefore validity (e.g. reducing complex aspects of professional practice into simpler components to ensure highly similar judgements by assessors). These efforts to control error and randomness in assessment may result in reliable assessments where the relationship between the skills, pratices, or knowledge assessed to the context in which it will be used must be assumed. For example, research evidence now informs the content and processes of objective structured clinical examinations (OSCEs) so that the measures inform reliable and valid assessment judgements but the students' ability to reproduce these performances in the real, complex world of workplace action must be inferred.

Objectivity

The assumption that assessment should and can be completely objective contributes to this tension between objectivity and reliability. In reality, all assessment can be considered an exercise in judgement based on evidence that will fall somewhere along a continuum of objectivity.[18,19] This is more obvious when assessing products such as reports, essays and reflective portfolios. However, even apparently highly objective validated assessment processes involve a series of judgements during development and application: experts make judgements about content to include; developers decide on evidence to collect; assessors decide if a response meets criteria; and so on and so forth. This valuing of objectivity is closely linked to what Hager[20] describes as the 'folk theory' of learning, where learning is the accumulation of definable and unchanging products provided by educators who then measure the amount the student has acquired.

Assessment can be more usefully considered as a process of gathering and evaluating a range of evidence to make an ethical and attentive judgement about achievement.[21] This process is similar to clinical reasoning in that EBEA also requires us to evaluate and combine evidence that varies along the continuum of objectivity. Thus, subjectivity is always present to a greater or lesser degree along with a mandate to critically evaluate our assessment choices against appropriate criteria and continually seek evidence to inform these choices. The need to gather and evaluate a range of evidence to inform our assessment judgements also suggests that a programmatic approach to assessment should be considered for high stakes and/or crucial decision points.[19,22]

LEVELS OF LEARNING OUTCOMES

A programmatic level approach to assessment design requires all stakeholders for the health professional education programme to consider learning outcomes and related levels or standards for the whole programme. The aim is to manage the problem of subjectivity with sufficient sampling and variety of evidence across the programme to make a fair judgement as to whether graduates from the programme have achieved the learning outcomes to an adequate level.[19,22] Therefore, within a programme, assessment may focus on samples of evidence against learning outcomes for the whole programme or each year or logical stage of a health professional education programme to decide if students are fit for progression to the next stage. Assessment is also, of course, directed to learning outcomes for specific subcomponents of a programme. Finally, in some circumstances, specific learning outcomes may need to be addressed for a particular student.

Even where an agreed-upon programmatic assessment framework is not in place, every academic can determine learning outcomes and assessment approaches for his or her curriculum component in relation to the overall programme outcomes. The academic can consider where his or her component and assessment fits within the overall developmental trajectory of the programme and how it will contribute to preparing the students for professional practice. Identifying what students have learned previously and what they will learn next will help decide if the assessment should assess mastery of specific areas of knowledge and skills or their integration and application, and to what level of complexity. For example, will you be locating evidence to inform your design of an assessment where the students demonstrate mastery of specific sets of knowledge (such as multiple choice) versus integrating aspects of knowledge and skills in a highly controlled environment (such as an OSCE)? Or evidence of the students' ability to integrate and apply knowledge, skills, and practices in complex unpredictable workplace environments (such as a work performance rating assessment)?

ENACTING EVIDENCE-BASED EDUCATION IN ASSESSMENT DESIGN

Moving from the wide range of issues outlined so far in this chapter regarding assessment practice and its link to learning outcomes to locating and appraising evidence to inform our educational practice is challenging. Particularly when some of these issues have been identified via research processes and some are articulated in educational theory or philosophy that draws upon different types of evidence. However, we know that sourcing quality evidence for assessment practices starts with a well-designed or 'answerable' question (*see* Figure 13.1).

Defining an answerable question

Designing an answerable EBE question ensures that we clearly articulate what we want to know and why, and this in turn supports effective searching for and appraisal of relevant evidence. Usual EBP question design considers four question elements, or PICO, to structure the question.
1. **P**: Patient, Population or Problem
2. **I**: Intervention, Indicator or Index text
3. **C**: Comparison or Control group
4. **O**: Outcome[2]

Emerson and Records[23] suggested that answerable questions in EBE should be structured as follows:

> **S**: Student/Problem
> **T**: Teaching strategy
> **C**: Comparison
> **O**: Outcome.

However, neither of these approaches sufficiently addresses the challenges of EBEA where, as already outlined, current issues and theories acknowledge the important role of stakeholders and contexts. Consideration of stakeholders is important to ensure quality assessment practices and to prevent lack of engagement with assessments perceived as irrelevant or unwieldy.[24] Furthermore, factoring in the perspective of stakeholders will support decision-making about relevant evidence and effective communication of findings, which may be critical for managing pressures exerted upon our EBEA decisions by stakeholders, such as university strategic plans, professional accreditation and societal demands.[23] Assessments also occur in multiple contexts or environments and in multiple ways in universities (e.g. paper based, OSCEs, viva voce, virtual reality) as well as workplaces.

Schlosser and Raghavendra[3] have elaborated the standard PICO design framework for application to the multidisciplinary disability field to include consideration of 'environment' and 'stakeholders', creating a PESICO framework to guide question design. The process outlined here adapts the PESICO framework for EBEA in the form of **SESACO**.

> **S**: Student or Student group – *Who is the question about?*
> **E**: Environment – *Where can or should the assessment be conducted?*
> **S**: Stakeholder – *For whom is the outcome most relevant?*
> **A**: Assessment – *What aspect of assessment is in focus?*
> **C**: Comparison or Control – *Are we comparing this aspect of assessment with an alternative one?*
> **O**: Outcome – *What is the outcome of interest?*

Table 13.1 identifies how the issues to consider during assessment design that were elaborated on earlier in this chapter relate to this adapted format. Adapting this EBP process for EBEA accrues similar benefits – for example, supporting development of a well-targeted search strategy and providing a point of reference against which to appraise the relevance of evidence. It will also guide the synthesis of the evidence and inform the development of planning, implementation and evaluation of the assessment approach. Box 13.1 shows some examples of how to use these SESACO elements to construct a question.

Locating evidence

Well-structured and answerable questions provide a strong framework for developing search terms for an effective search strategy and subsequent appraisal. Generally EBP in healthcare includes two sources of evidence – research and practice – which are then integrated with patient preferences. Davies[1] maps this approach on to EBE by highlighting that educators should also consider evidence developed through professional judgement and experience. Dollaghan,[2] however, makes the case that EBP in allied health should weight the patient's preferences as an equally important third source of evidence. Adapting this approach to EBEA ensures that evidence from the multiple stakeholders identified in Table 13.1 receives equal consideration.

Therefore, the three sources of evidence for EBEA are as follows. The first source is external evidence, from systematic research that builds theory and evaluates assessment approaches. The most relevant external evidence or empirical evidence from qualitative and/or quantitative research will depend on the question being asked. For example, questions about what students perceive as being the fairest assessment of

TABLE 13.1 Question elements for consideration when designing an answerable question to inform evidence-based educational assessment design

S: Student or Student group	*Who is the question about?*
	For example:
	• a particular student's learning outcomes (e.g. adapting performance assessment to evaluate strategies used by a student who has a physical disability)
	• a specific subgroup within the programme (e.g. first-year students, international students)
	• all students by the end of a programme
E: Environment	*Where can or should the assessment be conducted?*
	For example, in a specific kind of university learning space, or in a workplace or virtually
S: Stakeholders	*For whom is the outcome most relevant?*
	For example:
	• students
	• clients or patients
	• academics
	• educational institution (if so, at what level? – professional programme, faculty or university, e.g. strategic plan)
	• professional bodies
	• employers
	• society
A: Assessment	*What aspect of assessment is in focus?*
	For example:
	• the assessment strategy – OSCE, workplace observation, and so forth
	• the assessors – self or peer assessment, clients/patients, practitioners, lecturers, employers
C: Comparison	*Are we comparing this aspect of assessment with an alternative one?*
O: Outcome	*What is the outcome of interest?*
	For example:
	• type of learning outcome
	— specific aspects of knowledge, skills or practices (KSPs)
	— integration and application of KSPs
	— fitness for practice, award or purpose
	• level of learning outcome – topic, year/stage or programme
	• validity and reliability of an assessment approach
	• process
	• meaning

Note: adapted from Schlosser and Raghavendra[3]

BOX 13.1 Designing answerable questions

EXAMPLE 1

Scenario

You coordinate a problem-based learning curriculum, and a colleague has observed a similar programme where each week the students generate a group concept map after each problem-based learning case. She is excited by what she has observed and believes that it will promote students' integration and application of knowledge, skills, and practices to cases. The first issue you decide to investigate is whether there is evidence that concept mapping assessments are effective for this purpose.

Question elements

S = Students
E = Any type of university-based assessment
S = Students
A = Concept mapping assessments
C = Any other assessments
O = Clinical reasoning

Question statement

Do concept mapping assessments improve students' clinical reasoning performance on subsequent university-based assessments more than other kinds of assessments?

EXAMPLE 2

Scenario

Your university assessment policy requires that all topics must include a formative as well as a summative assessment component, so that you can identify students' learning needs and develop strategies to meet them. You would like to know more about the relationship between formative assessment and student achievement, as you are not convinced that this policy has sufficient merit to justify the time involved.

Question elements

S = All students
E = All assessment environments
S = Academics and university
A = Formative and summative assessment
C = Summative assessment only
O = Improved student achievement

Question statement

Does formative followed by summative assessment improve student achievement compared with summative assessment only?

their performance in the workplace would be answered with a qualitative research method. A question regarding how to design multiple-choice questions that effectively sample students' ability to apply theoretical knowledge to practice would be answered with a quantitative method. Many assessment design questions have considerations of validity at their heart, and therefore require both qualitative and quantitative methods.

The second source is internal evidence, which includes knowledge developed through rigorous evaluation of our own assessment practices, expert opinion and the opinion of our peers.

The third source is stakeholder evidence or preferences, which should be factored into assessment design to ensure that their practical constraints and expectations are appropriately addressed, increasing the likelihood of successful outcomes. This may include students and requirements that have to be addressed such as university strategic plans, policy and procedure, professional bodies (accreditation), employers and last, but not least, clients or patients who will access services provided by our graduates. Once the best-quality evidence from each of these sources is located, standard EBP practices should be applied (e.g. the evidence should be critically evaluated and synthesised into a decision and action, which is subsequently evaluated (*see* Figure 13.1).

Appraising evidence

External evidence regarding the best assessment can be appraised in the same two-step process as any research evidence. Begin by identifying the highest level of evidence available and therefore how likely it is to generalise to your context. Then, appraise the quality of the evidence found with regard to rigour in design, execution, analysis and interpretation. Even evidence at the level of expert opinion can be appraised in this way. Harden *et al.*[25] provide useful guidance for adapting the appraisal process to EBE under the acronym of QUEST (Quality, Utility, Extent, Setting, Target).

Internal evidence for assessment practice is derived from reflection on our experience and that of our colleagues. This evidence is important, as it is highly relevant and specific to the context in which we are going to apply the assessment approach and it is grounded in our knowledge of our profession and our students. However, we must be critical in our reflection on our assessment practice, as evidence derived from personal experience is prone to error because of our cognitive tendencies to bias. These include being more likely to notice information that confirms our expectations; requiring substantial amounts of information to change our position; remembering information that co-occurs with strong emotions; being primed to seek patterns and causations even where they do not exist; our tendency to resist new ideas or change our opinions; and our general need for certainty, control and simplicity.[26]

Sources for stakeholder evidence will vary widely. They may include feedback from students and service recipients, policy documents from accrediting bodies or government, or university strategic plans – to name just a few. This evidence can be evaluated with regard to its relevance and the rigour of the processes of collection and interpretation.

Synthesising, planning, doing and evaluating

Once the best evidence available from each of the three sources has been identified, we need to go through a process of weighing it up and integrating it into a decision to answer our original question and meet our desired assessment outcomes. Every assessment situation is unique, so it is highly unlikely that we will find evidence for an assessment approach that can be directly applied.[25] Therefore, we will need to consider how to prioritise the evidence, how well it can be translated or adapted to the outcome(s) we are seeking to address, and how feasible it is, given the resources, barriers and enablers in our setting. The focus should be on 'what can be done' rather than 'what can't be'. A thoughtful approach that is clear about the desired outcome(s) of the assessment and which then gathers, appraises and combines evidence from all relevant sources will equip us to make well-informed and reasoned decisions about key priorities for change. It will also identify what can and should be adapted or applied to the assessment approach we are developing. Furthermore, awareness of the strengths and weaknesses of our decision lays a strong foundation for planning an evaluation process to collect evidence regarding how well the assessment meets our intended outcomes.

Dissemination

Emerson and Records[23] highlight that EBE is a subset of a scholarship of learning and teaching approach to educational practice. They identify that a scholarship of learning and teaching approach has a moral dimension, as does a knowledge translation approach in EBP, that includes the imperative to disseminate findings and contribute to cultural changes and paradigm shifts in educational practice. This approach is supported by organisations such as the Australian Office for Learning and Teaching[27] that provide practical guidance and resources for disseminating findings of EBE projects beyond the usual research publication channels to foster rapid translation of EBE into educational practice and promote the active uptake of educational research evidence.

APPLYING EVIDENCE-BASED EDUCATION TO ASSESSMENT DESIGN AND/OR SELECTION

It is beyond the scope of this chapter to undertake an evidence-based review of the large and somewhat overwhelming array of assessment approaches available for consideration. For example, Brown[28] identifies 23 assessment approaches suitable for inquiry-based learning approaches alone. No doubt there are more approaches than this, particularly given the recent rise of e-assessments. Therefore, a strategy to build answerable questions focused on learning outcomes that are situated in current theory has been outlined. Good-quality questions provide direction for locating, appraising and applying evidence to make an informed decision. There are many questions to be asked, all of which will contribute to the quality of our academic practice and outcomes for students. For example, we may be concerned with improving an assessment we currently use and will therefore be focused on questions regarding validity and reliability. We may wish to identify the most effective assessment strategy to meet a particular outcome, which could be as specific as particular knowledge and skill acquisition, or broader, such as integration and application of knowledge and skills to practise, or development of skills to support ongoing professional development. We may want to evaluate a specific assessment strategy for our students, programme or desired learning outcomes or, indeed, develop and evaluate a new assessment. Table 13.2 provides a briefly worked example of the latter two.

TABLE 13.2 Evidence-based education assessment selection example

A course review of your allied health programme has suggested introducing a portfolio to support development of students' professional skills across the programme. You are aware that portfolios include students collecting and reflecting on evidence of achievement and that they can be done in hard copy or electronically. You would like to know what the evidence is regarding learning outcomes before investing more time and resources.

1. *Answerable question:*
   S = all students by the end of your undergraduate programme
   E = university assessed
   S = students
   A – reflective portfolio across the programme
   C = none
   O = development of professional skills (integration and application of KSPs).

Does a university-assessed reflective portfolio promote undergraduate students' integration and application of professional KSPs across a programme?

2. *Locate evidence:*
   a) *internal* – you haven't used portfolios so you consult with colleagues within your programme, your discipline and other allied health programmes
   b) *stakeholders* –
      • course review committee, included stakeholders and recommended using portfolios
      • university, no specific guidance regarding portfolios but a commitment to quality assessment strategies and demonstrating that students have achieved graduate outcomes
      • consultation with student year representatives
   c) *external (databases)* – you consult with your university librarian to develop a search of databases; two systematic reviews [29,30] reviewed material up to 2008; you limit your search to journal articles in English and from 2008 to the present; see the following list of key words used and databases that were searched; you review the abstract and then the article for relevance to the question; total articles relevant to question = two systematic reviews and five subsequent studies

Database	Search terms	Numbers
Scopus	((TITLE-ABS-KEY(**portfolio*** OR **e-Portfolio*** OR **'e-portfolio*'**) AND TITLE-ABS-KEY(**student*** AND **education***) AND TITLE-ABS-KEY(**health*** OR **audiology** OR **speech** OR **'physical therapy'** OR **physiotherapy** OR **'occupational therapy'** OR **nutrition** OR **dietetics**))) AND (**evaluat*** OR **valid*** OR **reliability** OR **outcome*** OR **measure***)	97

Database	Search terms	Numbers
ERIC (Educational Resources Information Center)	(exp Allied Health Occupations/ or exp Allied Health Occupations Education/ or allied health.mp.) AND (exp Portfolio Assessment/ or portfolio.mp.)	0
CINAHL (Cumulative Index to Nursing and Allied Health Literature)	(Portfolio MESH OR portfolio e-Portfolio OR portfolio assessment) AND (MM Education Health Sciences+) yielded most results (296), when filtered by year, abstract available and 2008+	65
MEDLINE	(Students, Premedical/ or Students, Dental/ or Students, Nursing/ or Students/ or Students, Medical/ or Students, Public Health/ or Students, Health Occupations/ or Students, Pharmacy/) AND (portfolio*.mp.) AND (reflect*.mp.)	43

 d) *external (sources of expert opinion)* – Office of Learning and Teaching project reports, UK Academy Higher Education, university websites and links.

3. *Appraise evidence:* you only have time for rapid appraisal and you identify that the highest levels of external evidence available have been found, all sources are of good quality and strong consensus exists between your colleagues' opinion and expert opinion, but student opinion is mixed.

4. *Synthesise:* a university-assessed portfolio has the potential to promote students' integration and application of professional KSPs but this will depend on careful design and implementation.

5. *Plan assessment:*
 a. *design* – collaborate with stakeholders to adapt elements from relevant models and design a progressive portfolio. Design will also be guided by reference to the SESACO elements to identify key decisions and with evidence sources
 b. *process* – develop quality improvement plan including own ongoing seeking and evaluation of evidence; investigate feasibility of research to evaluate the portfolio outcomes.

6. *Do:* trial the portfolio.

7. *Evaluate:* implement quality improvement plan and research plan if feasible.

TABLE 13.3 Evidence-based education assessment design example

The speech pathology discipline recognised that their assessment of students' performance on practicum lacked evidence and rigour. An evidence-based approach to assessment design was undertaken over a 3-year period.[31,32] A critical review of the assessment evidence at that time (2001) found that there were no evidence-based Australian tools and only one tool overseas that had minimal validation some time prior. The design and evaluation process can be characterised using the EBE assessment design cycle elements (*see* Figure 13.1) and was activated as follows.

1. *Answerable question:* Can a validated competency-based assessment be designed that will validly and reliably measure speech pathology students' development of professional practice and readiness for entry to the profession?

2. *Locate evidence:*
 a. *external evidence* – existing research evidence and expert opinion regarding performance assessment

(continued)

2. *Locate evidence:* (*cont.*)
    b. *internal evidence* – current practice in health professional education
    c. *stakeholder evidence* – opinions and preferences of students, clinical educators, university educators and the professional body.

3. *Appraise:* the quality of relevance of evidence was evaluated.

4. *Synthesise:* evidence regarding key issues was combined to inform assessment design, including reliability and validity of performance assessment; assessment as judgement; nature of speech pathology competence and practice; development of expertise; impact of assessment on learning; content and processes that support quality assessment practices and fairness; and feasibility.

5. *Plan:* an assessment tool and a process were designed for trialling and collecting evidence to answer the question.

6. *Do:* a national field trial was conducted.

7. *Evaluate:* a research evaluation was conducted through combining qualitative evaluation by students and clinical educators and quantitative statistical evaluation.

8. *Disseminate:* the assessment tool COMPASS®[33] was developed and provided to universities[34] and an active dissemination process was undertaken.[35]

9. Further EBE cycles have been undertaken to collect evidence and data to answer subsequent questions regarding the utility of the assessment design and maintenance of validity and reliability.

MOVING FORWARD: ENGAGING IN DEVELOPMENT OF EVIDENCE-BASED EDUCATION ASSESSMENT

The systematic reviews located for the example in Table 13.2 identified that the quality of research evidence related to portfolio assessments was generally poor, although improvements were noted in the more recent literature appraised. Buckley *et al.*[29] also suggested that only low-level learning outcomes were being addressed (e.g. level one or two on the Kirkpatrick framework, where the highest level – improving patient outcomes – is the one we all aspire to as educators). Furthermore, while some literature was located from disciplines other than medicine, this was sparse. This poses difficulties for allied health academics as they are educating their students to enter cultures and contexts of practice that may be very different to that of medicine. More pragmatically, the allied health academic professions may not have sufficient funding to translate the strategies developed in medical education and apply them within their teaching contexts.

The example given regarding portfolio assessments is only atypical in that the evidence located regarding portfolios included systematic reviews. While external and research evidence regarding assessment practices is growing, much of the evidence available to guide our assessment practices will be sourced internally and from stakeholders. This is not new territory for the allied health professions. They prepare their graduates to engage in evidence-based professional practice where high-quality external (research) evidence is often not available. Educators in the health professions need to accept the same challenge: to be open to changing their practice; to go beyond their 'gut feeling' and engage in developing clarity about their questions and desired outcomes; to critically evaluate and integrate all three sources of evidence; developing research-based evidence through their practice; and to take responsibility for disseminating this evidence.

Applying EBE steps, even when there is only time for rapid appraisal, will support a scholarly approach to assessment as an integral part of quality teaching and learning processes. It will also provide a strong foundation for developing research questions, establishing effective communities of practice and collaborating with stakeholders. As so much unexplored territory exists, there are many opportunities for health professional academics to contribute to evidence-based changes to their assessments that will have a positive impact on the outcomes for their students, their future clients or patients, and their families, as well as their communities and workplaces.

SUMMARY POINTS

- EBEA is an important component of EBE.
- It is recommended that education researchers follow the EBEA cycle for assessment design.
- Validity and reliability are important components of the EBEA process.
- Using the SESACO (Student or Student group, Environment, Stakeholder, Assessment, Comparison or Control, Outcome) format to generate research questions is recommended.

REVIEW QUESTIONS

- What are the current issues in assessment?
- What are the six key steps for evidence-based education assessment practice?
- Design an answerable question with reference to the SESACO elements.
- What sources of evidence should be considered?
- What issues should be considered when appraising external, internal and stakeholder evidence?
- What should be considered when implementing and evaluating this inquiry?

REFLECTIVE QUESTIONS AND EXERCISES

- What assumptions currently govern my assessment practices?
- Which ones would I like to evaluate?
- What skills, knowledge, and pratices do I need to develop to support my ability to use an evidence-based approach to assessment of my students?
- What resources currently exist to support me to develop my skills, knowledge, and practices?

REFERENCES

1. Davies P. What is evidence-based education? *Br J Educ Stud.* 2009; **47**(2): 108–21.
2. Dollaghan CA. *The Handbook for Evidence-Based Practice in Communication Disorders.* Baltimore, MD: Paul H Brookes; 2007.
3. Schlosser R, Raghavendra P. Evidence-based practice in augmentative and alternative communication. *Augment Altern Commun.* 2004; **20**(1): 1–21.
4. Ginsburg S, Friberg J, Visconti CF. *Scholarship of Teaching and Learning in Speech-Language Pathology and Audiology: evidence-based education.* San Diego, CA: Plural Publishing; 2012.
5. Boud D. Sustainable assessment: rethinking assessment for the learning society. *Stud Cont Educ.* 2000; **22**(2): 151–67.
6. Wass V, van der Vleuten C, Shatzer J, *et al.* Assessment of clinical competence. *Lancet.* 2001; **357**(9260): 945–9.
7. Boud D, Falchikov N. Aligning assessment with long-term learning. *Assess Eval High Educ.* 2006; **31**(4): 399–413.
8. McAllister S, Lincoln M, Ferguson A, *et al.* Dilemmas in assessing performance in fieldwork education. In: McAllister L, Paterson M, Higgs J, *et al.*, editors. *Innovations in Allied Health Fieldwork Education: practice, education, work and society.* Vol. 4. Rotterdam: Sense Publishers; 2010. pp. 247–60.
9. Wall D. Impact and washback in language testing. In: Clapham C, Corson D, editors. *Encyclopedia of Language and Education: language testing and assessment.* Vol. 7. Dordrecht: Kluwer; 1997. pp. 291–302.
10. Biggs J. What the student does: teaching for enhanced learning. *High Educ Res Dev.* 1999; **18**(1): 57–75.
11. Eraut M. *Developing Professional Knowledge and Competence.* London: Falmer Press; 1994.
12. McAllister S, Lincoln M, Ferguson A, *et al.* Issues in developing valid assessments of speech pathology students' performance in the workplace. *Int J Lang Commun Disord.* 2010; **45**(1): 1–14.
13. Messick S. Validity. In: Linn RL, editor. *Educational Measurement.* 3rd ed. New York, NY: Macmillan Publishing; 1989. pp. 13–103.
14. Brualdi A. *Traditional and Modern Concepts of Validity.* Washington, DC : ERIC Clearinghouse on Assessment and Evaluation; 1999. Available at: www.ericdigests.org/2000-3/validity.htm (accessed 13 February 2002).
15. Schuwirth LW, van der Vleuten CP. A plea for new psychometric models in educational assessment. *Med Educ.* 2006; **40**(4): 296–300.
16. Embretson SE. The new rules of measurement. *Psychol Assess.* 1996; **8**(4): 341–9.
17. Van der Vleuten C, Norman G, de Graaff E. Pitfalls in the pursuit of objectivity: issues of reliability. *Med Educ.* 1991; **25**(2): 110–18.
18. Leach L, Neutze G, Zepke N. Assessment and empowerment: some critical questions. *Assess Eval High Educ.* 2001; **26**(4): 293–305.
19. Schuwirth LW, Van der Vleuten CP. Programmatic assessment: from assessment of learning to assessment for learning. *Med Teach.* 2011; **33**(6): 478–85.
20. Hager P. Lifelong learning in the workplace? Challenges and issues. *J Workplace Learning.* 2004; **16**(1–2): 22–32.
21. Jones A. It's a judgement call … and consistency isn't all it's cracked up to be. *Australian Vocational Education and Training Research Association Conference*; 28–30 March 2001; Adelaide, SA, Australia.
22. Van der Vleuten CP, Schuwirth LW. Assessing professional competence: from methods to programmes. *Med Educ.* 2005; **39**(3): 309–17.
23. Emerson RJ, Records K. Today's challenge, tomorrow's excellence: the practice of evidence-based education. *J Nurs Educ.* 2008; **47**(8): 359–70.

24. Cross V, Hicks C, Barwell, F. Exploring the gap between evidence and judgement: using video vignettes for practice-based assessment of physiotherapy undergraduates. *Assess Eval High Educ.* 2001; **26**(3): 189–212.

25. Harden R M, Grant J, Buckley G, *et al.* BEME Guide No. 1: best evidence medical education. *Med Teach.* 1999; **21**(6): 553–62.

26. Shermer M. *Why People Believe Weird Things: pseudoscience, superstition, and other confusions of our time.* New York, NY: AWH Freeman/Owl Book; 2002.

27. www.olt.gov.au

28. Brown G. *Assessment: a guide for lecturers.* York, UK: Learning and Teaching Support Network; 2001.

29. Buckley S, Coleman J, Davison I, *et al.* The educational effects of portfolios on undergraduate student learning: a Best Evidence Medical Education (BEME) systematic review. BEME Guide No. 11. *Med Teach.* 2009; **31**(4): 282–98.

30. Driessen E, van Tartwijk J, van der Vleuten C, *et al.* Portfolios in medical education: why do they meet with mixed success? A systematic review. *Med Educ.* 2007; **41**(12): 1224–33.

31. McAllister S, Lincoln M, Ferguson A, *et al.* A systematic program of research regarding the assessment of speech-language pathology competencies. *Int J Speech Lang Pathol.* 2011; **13**(6): 469–79.

32. McAllister S, Lincoln M, Ferguson A, *et al.* Validating workplace performance assessments in health sciences students: a case study from speech pathology. *J Appl Meas.* 2013; **14**(4): 356–74.

33. McAllister S, Lincoln M, Ferguson A, *et al. COMPASS*®: *competency assessment in speech pathology.* 2nd ed. Melbourne, VIC: Speech Pathology Australia; 2013.

34. Speech Pathology Australia. *COMPASS*®. www.speechpathologyaustralia.org.au/resources/compassr (accessed 15 January 2014).

35. Ferguson A, Lincoln M, McAllister L, *et al. COMPASS*™ *Directions: leading the integration of a competency based assessment tool in speech pathology learning and teaching.* Canberra, ACT: Carrick Institute for Learning and Teaching in Higher Education; 2008.

CHAPTER 14

Modes of pedagogy delivery in health professional education

Brett Williams and Stephen Maloney

OVERVIEW

The tertiary education sector, typically in conjunction with the health services, strives to facilitate optimum performance of our present and future clinicians through effective teaching and learning techniques. The wealth of literature within the field of health professional education is growing daily, even though the scholarship of educators monitoring, reviewing and improving their educational techniques to enhance student learning commonly occurs without report. Whether effective teaching is a science or an art, few would argue that it cannot be influenced by the careful design and consideration of the approach or mode taken. This chapter will explore modes of pedagogy for health professional education. The difficulty from the point of view of leading a comprehensive discussion is that there are no real limits on the number of approaches available. How does one choose the appropriate mode for a particular activity?

CHAPTER OBJECTIVES

At the conclusion of this chapter the reader should be able to:

- compare and contrast traditional and alternative modes of pedagogical delivery
- appraise the positives and negatives of near-peer teaching and learning
- summarise the effect of modes of delivery and their impact on student feedback
- examine the evaluation methods for alternative modes of delivery
- differentiate between face-to-face and web conference case-based learning modes of delivery
- relate the capacity and long-term impact of MOOCs (massive open online courses) for health professional education.

KEY TERMS: case-based learning, feedback, MOOCs, near-peer teaching, web conference

INTRODUCTION

This chapter will touch upon a range of pedagogies, including evidence for those in the mainstream such as case-based learning (CBL), small group learning, blending learning, simulation and reflective practice. It will then focus on alternative pedagogies such as near-peer teaching, along with emerging techniques afforded by developing technologies such as student self-video of performance and MOOCs (massive open online courses) and small group learning via web conferences. It will conclude by discussing insights into future directions for modes of pedagogy in health professional education and trends in research methods and evaluation; particularly the use of head-to-head comparisons and economic evaluations. This chapter looks to raise the profile and importance of choosing the mode of pedagogy for an activity in the consciousness of the critical and creative academic.

'MAINSTREAM' TECHNIQUES

It is an exciting time to be examining the scholarship of teaching and learning and evidence-based education of health professionals. Today, in many universities and other teaching institutions around the country, there are passionate, engaging and innovative teachers who are 'pushing the envelope' when it comes to the type of mode of their pedagogical delivery. This is almost second nature for some teachers, many of whom are instinctively curious and critical – these are the lecture theatres or classrooms that are filled with almost palpable energy and engagement in the room. However, what of those teachers who do not possess such skills or innate abilities? Are these lecture theatres or classrooms still echoing mainstream or traditional modes of pedagogy? Are the same types of small group activities or hybrids of CBL being used? If so, what are the levels of engagement or actual student numbers attending classes?

What employability skills or competitive edge are we providing learners with? Are students provided with flexibility and accessibility 24 hours a day? Or are these not the types of questions that are important if quality learning outcomes and competencies are being measured or appropriately aligned?

These types of questions are central to the very point of evidence-based education for many of us who teach into health professional education programmes, and why this book will provide many teachers with important pragmatic and contemporary points of reference in their teaching journeys.

ALTERNATIVE MODES OF DELIVERY
Near-peer teaching

The teaching of peers and others is a professional requirement for all health professionals in Australia. In clinical settings, health professions regularly teach students from their respective profession and often other health professions, peers, patients and their families. However, few, if any, academic programmes formally prepare health professionals for this dimension of their future roles as teachers or educators. Near-peer teaching is a term that unites a number of similar cooperative learning approaches from the same professional discipline.[1] These include peer teaching and learning, peer learning, and peer mentoring. The basic premise is that senior peers teach (often in laboratories, tutorials or practical demonstrations) peers from the same or more junior levels of their programme. Regardless of the precise strategy, both peer teachers and peer learners are actively involved in a 'fluid' knowledge exchange.[2]

The evidence-based education of near-peer teaching is growing and overall is very positive. Numerous papers and scholars have shown or argued that both 'learning' as a peer and 'teaching' as a peer has been largely very positive.[1,3-6] Benefits for peer teachers include improved academic and clinical performance, better understanding of the content and syllabus acquisition of communication, improved interpersonal performance and confidence at public speaking, and dealing with conflict or difficult learners.[7-9] Benefits for peer learners include better understanding of the hidden curriculum through having more comfortable conversations with peer teachers than with academic staff, feeling less anxious or isolated and perceptions of feeling more confident in their own abilities.[3,7-9] These positives are also balanced with negatives for both peer teachers and peer learners, centring on perceptions of cost-saving measures by the institution, underprepared peer teachers, peer teachers not having adequate knowledge, and propensity for surface learning to occur.

While the current evidence suggests that any form of peer-based teaching is good for the teacher and the learner, the challenge for health professional education is the construction and alignment of where to include this type and mode of pedagogy. Not many health professions or programmes of study can embed an actual unit of study on near-peer teaching; however, many opportunities do exist for programmes to integrate near-peer teaching as an extracurricular activity for students. This is where leaders or designers should consider the first step as being.

Incorporating student self-video of performance

The clinician–patient interaction is the interface between health professional education and patient care. It is within these interactions that experienced and developing clinicians participate in the management of health service delivery and further develop their skills, combining their health knowledge with competent handling and communication in order to affect their client's well-being. Practical skills are commonly taught in the campus-based preclinical environment using face-to-face methods such as lectures, small group learning and live demonstration tutorials.[10,11] Tutor feedback is given during the session as students practise the skill with their peers following the tutor's 'live' demonstration of the skills mastery. The traditional approach to practical skills creates a number of limitations. Physical limitations are created by the time constraints associated with creating and adhering to room booking schedules. Limitations in access and equity of tutor feedback are created from student competition for tutor time and attention to provide feedback.[12]

Likewise, the delivery medium of live face-to-face interaction does not allow the learner the ability to view his or her performance from the perspective of an observer, as would occur if the student were to view a video playback of his or her performance. Considering your performance from another's perspective can be a valuable learning opportunity for focusing on potential deficits, particularly in nuances of a performance such as the verbal and non-verbal communication.[13,14] Emerging technologies such as Web 2.0, and devices equipped with digital multimedia capability, along with increased social drive and accessibility to these technologies, is allowing exploration of innovative teaching methods with potential to overcome some of the limitations of the traditional approaches.[15]

Oblinger[16] argued that the university education of Generation Y should include instructional modes with which students are familiar. Generation Y are typically familiar with mobile web-enabled devices, which can assist practical skill learning in tertiary education.[17–20] Web-based delivery of educational content provides flexibility of access and promotes a student-centred approach to learning, with the timing of learning occurring when the student is in a frame of mind for interacting with the resources.[21] Increased student familiarity and access to multimedia and web-based technologies creates opportunities overcoming the limitations of on-campus learning, particularly for decentralising teacher observation and feedback on student skill performance, as well as new avenues for facilitating student reflection on performance.[14]

The ability to reflect on performance is a cornerstone of effective lifelong learning and a vital attribute of professional behaviours.[22] However, the link between reflection and demonstrable enhancement of clinical performance remains less certain.[23] One reason for persistent performance deficits during psychomotor skill acquisition is inaccurate learner perception of performance.[24] A key limitation for student reflection on performance is the overestimation of competence by underperformers.[25] Accuracy of a student's self-assessment may be improved by increasing the learner's awareness of the required benchmark of competency.[26] This increased learner awareness can be afforded through the use of video and other multimedia. Schwan and Riempp[27] and Mayer[28] found deeper learning outcomes from the use of a multimedia format such as video in conjunction with regular tutor instruction. For example, Emmen *et al.*[13] used video playback to help sportspeople improve their performance, such as a tennis players improving their serve. However, results in the sporting arena are arguably not generalisable to learning interplay between complex 'hands on' clinical skills and physical assessment, strong communication skills and high levels of professionalism.

Aspegren[29] argued that instructional teaching is less valuable than a student experiencing the activity itself, and that instructional elements need to be ongoing and integrated over time. Requiring students to submit self-video of performance tasks forces experiential learning. Students require well-choreographed communication and manual handling skills, body language and thought processes when they interact with simulated patients. A video self-modelling task fosters the development of skills in self-evaluation as well as providing the ability for students to repeatedly view their own performance, facilitating self-evaluation.[30] An example of how video self-modelling of performance can be utilised within a clinical skills programme is illustrated in Figure 14.1. This example has been taken from a physiotherapy training programme. Key elements within the activity design include opportunities for briefing students, remote tutor feedback, and feeding forward of observed skill deficits into the next class.

This method has been evaluated within two published randomised controlled trials (RCTs). The first RCT compared student self-video as an additional resource with 'face-to-face' teaching and found a statistically significant increase in skill performance using blinded outcome assessment within an observed structured clinical examination.[31] The RCT study compared student self-video with traditional teaching methods in a direct head-to-head comparison, finding that neither method was superior. These results indicate that student self-video of performance is likely to be a viable alternative to traditional pedagogy, rather than only being used as an additional resource.[32]

Web-conferenced case-based learning

There are a number of advantages and disadvantages to moving to 'new' versions of existing pedagogies in a web-based environment. An example of this would be moving the 'traditional' face-to-face CBL, using small group 'constructivist' learning, into a web conference. Unpublished data examining the student's first attempt at a web-conferenced CBL, compared with traditional 'face-to-face' CBL, found no significant difference in learning outcomes. The outcomes were measured under RCT conditions, consisting of a brief multiple-choice examination on the content covered at the completion of the CBL. However, the web-conferenced CBL group did experience difficulties with obtaining an effective stable Internet connection, due to the load placed on the bandwidth to complete the activity. The students also reported a perception that the activity discussions were not covered in as much depth.

This finding aligns with 'willingness to pay' data collected from another educational RCT investigating web-based versus online education, where students rated their willingness to pay for online education at a lesser value than the face-to-face mode of delivery.[33] This was in spite of the course delivery methods producing comparable learning outcomes and levels of learner satisfaction. Another argument for the decreased 'value' of the education is that students may perceive the education as being cheaper to deliver and therefore expect it to be discounted accordingly. The weaknesses in the web-conferenced CBL delivery were counteracted by the flexibility in learning, with the student being able to engage in the learning activity from a remote environment (as indicated in Figure 14.2), and decreased burden on faculty space requirements.

Engaging in web-conferenced CBL obviously contains both risks and rewards. This method should be chosen after careful consideration of the education institution's information technology capabilities, accessibility for students and the training available to students.

Massive open online courses

World-leading universities are beginning to offer MOOCs as a mode of course delivery. For example, each MOOC offered in 2011 through Stanford University in the United States had a separate enrolment of over 100 000 students.[34] MOOCs represent unprecedented access to education, a potential solution for areas of need in workforce innovation and development, and a potential threat to traditional educational courses and institutions.

MOOCs have two consistent design features: (1) there are no limits on enrolments, due to the pre-prepared web-based curriculum, and (2) there are no restrictions to access, including that students are not being required to pay fees. MOOCs have the potential to become financially lucrative through students paying for examinations and credentialing.

MOOCs for health professional education?

So far MOOCs have not been applied to health professional education. Health professional education requires a complex interaction of knowledge with 'hands on' clinical skills and physical assessment. There are potential challenges in delivering and assessing clinical skill competency within an online environment. Health professional programmes typically utilise a component of clinical education within the health service, under the close supervision of qualified clinicians. In the interests of maintaining professional standards and in protecting health consumers, health professional programmes undergo immense scrutiny and accountability to retain their accreditation.

Key questions that arise in evaluating the feasibility of implementation of MOOCs within health professional education are as follows.

● *Can MOOCs feasibly deliver the skills and knowledge required for a student to become a healthcare professional?* Pedagogy research to date would indicate this is likely. Web-based delivery of practical skills training has been shown to be equally as effective as face-to-face learning when incorporating student self-video of performance, applied to falls prevention exercise prescription education to health professionals.[35] However, the information technology demand of these activities applied on such a large scale are sure to test students and academics alike.

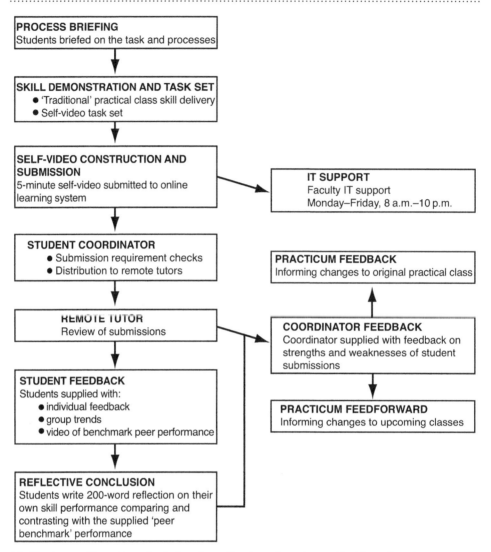

FIGURE 14.1 Flow chart depicting the utilisation of student self-video of performance within a clinical skills programmes curriculum[35]

- *Will MOOCs be an acceptable form of education from the perspective of the health service and professional registration bodies?* No published research is currently available to answer this question. It is conceivable that the protected nature of clinicians and professional associations towards their health professions, along with a rightly conservative approach to managing perceived risks to the quality of health professionals, could lead to difficulties in obtaining course accreditation for such a delivery mode.

● *Does the MOOCs model offer improved cost-effectiveness in comparison with traditional models of health professional education, improving workforce innovation and development?* At present, there are no published data on the cost-effectiveness of MOOCs for health professional education. However, economic analysis and quantitative head-to-head comparisons of teaching methods and their role in choice of pedagogy requires further discussion.

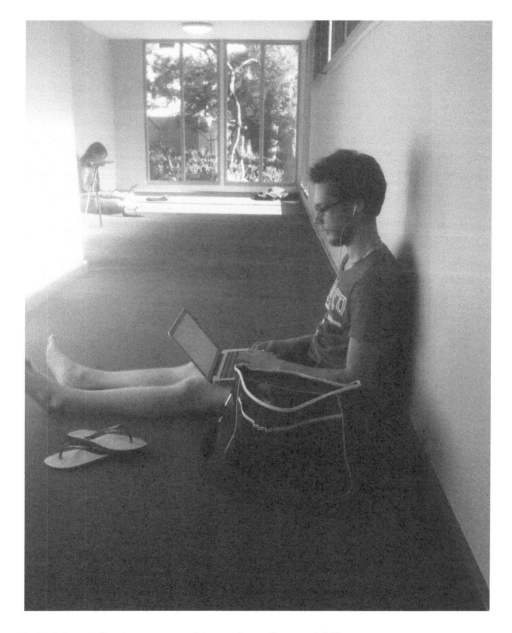

FIGURE 14.2 Students engaged in a web-conferenced CBL

EVALUATION METHODS: QUANTITATIVE EVIDENCE?

Level-one evidence investigating best evidence in educational techniques, obtained through RCTs of high scientific rigour, are relatively uncommon.[36,37] Reasons for this include perceived difficulties with establishing causation, relatively little opportunity for project funding,[38] and that RCTs are not the prevailing methodology in medical or health professional education research – particularly when focused on the qualitative human elements of both the learner and the patient, including the learning narrative and experience.[39] Although RCTs are limited by their rigid structure, their use still provides an important research perspective, which in conjunction with results from other more inclusive review designs may develop a more complete picture of the impact of teaching methods for health professionals.

It is important to acknowledge that there are a large number of factors that contribute to a valuable learning experience and which are not measured within the quantitative limitations of an RCT.[40] The combination of both high-quality qualitative and quantitative research methods is required to assist the transition of medical and health professional education from hearsay and strong opinion to evidence-based teaching methods.[41,42] However, for now, the contribution from quantitative methods has been comparatively lacking.[36] As health professional education continues to develop into an evidence-based discipline, it needs to foster a culture of self-scrutiny and accountability of its effectiveness, including economic evaluations, to begin making convincing arguments to research funders.[43]

A number of reviews have looked at quantitative learning outcomes in medical education literature,[10] but these commonly focus on a single professional discipline[11,44] or incorporate non-clinical elements within their outcome measures, such as general knowledge tests or changes in attitude.[45] For example, no review has yet investigated what level-one evidence exists for comparing the efficacy of teaching and learning of health professional clinical skills, as measured through authentic assessment contexts, to capture the quality of the performance at the patient–client interface. A common limitation of head-to-head comparisons of mode of education delivery is that the activities are not matched for duration. For example, teaching method A may be utilised for 4 hours of student education, compared with the alternative method that is used for only 2 hours. This limitation alters whether the effect is the duration or the quantity of education, rather than the quality of the method of delivery (see Figure 14.3). Another limitation is comparing learning outcomes with no education, or delayed education, rather than a direct comparison of the two techniques.

The level-one evidence for informing teachers on the best evidence approaches for the teaching and learning of clinical skills to health professional students and clinicians is, at best, underwhelming. Aside from moderate evidence for avoiding a traditional didactic lecture approach, all other approaches to clinical skill teaching methods, from student role-play to high-fidelity simulation, produced relatively equal quantitative learning outcomes – meaning that although they may be effective techniques in their own right, no delivery technique proved superior. The results may encourage new educators to question, experiment and measure the impact of their teaching methods.

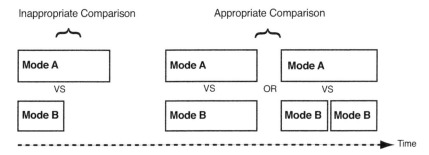

FIGURE 14.3 Visual representation of appropriate and inappropriate assessment of pedagogy evaluation, versus time, within quantitative health professional education literature

Evaluating the effectiveness of modes of pedagogy continues to evolve, assisting the decision-making of academics involved in the design and delivery of education. These evaluations require both qualitative and quantitative methods for creating a broader view of the benefits, risks and challenges. Teachers need to continue to focus on the quality of the learning experience, but they must also factor in the perspectives of the educational institution and workforce, which may have varying demands for efficiency, accountability and sustainability of the mode of pedagogy.

CONCLUSION

This chapter has explored a number of different modes of pedagogy for health professional education. The chapter has briefly examined the evidence-based education on a number of different pedagogies and alternative modes of delivery such as near-peer teaching, student self-review videos, web-conferencing in CBL and small group learner activities, and MOOCs; finally, the chapter explored the best evidence in educational techniques. The chapter has attempted to highlight a number of alternative approaches and evidence-based methods, providing (hopefully) teachers with important pragmatic and contemporary points of reference in their teaching journeys.

SUMMARY POINTS

- The mode of pedagogical delivery requires modernising.
- Near-peer teaching is a largely very positive experience for both peer teachers and peer learners.
- Student self-review performance shows very promising results and is likely to be replicated across all health professional groups.
- Web presence in different modes of delivery requires targeted and sustained support for short- and long-term success.
- MOOCs offer international health professional programmes with capacity for international attention and potential growth.
- Evaluating and measuring educational research requires mixed methodologies.

REVIEW QUESTIONS

- What are the key characteristics to traditional versus alternative modes of pedagogical delivery?
- If teaching is a key health professional competency, why isn't it more formally addressed in health professional curricula?
- Could student self-video reviewed performance be used in other elements of student learning?
- Are MOOCs the next panacea in offering different modes of pedagogical delivery?

REFLECTIVE QUESTIONS AND EXERCISES

- Why is the mode of delivery so important in curricula design?
- Why are traditional approaches to teaching health professionals still widespread in teaching institutions?
- Can alternative modes of pedagogical delivery facilitate the transition from novice to expert?
- Does your education institution have the strategic plan and support in place to integrate web presence through different modes of pedagogical delivery?
- What is meant by high-level evidence, evaluation and measurement in educational research?

REFERENCES

1. Henning JM, Weidner TG, Marty MC. Peer assisted learning in clinical education: literature review. *Athletic Train Educ J.* 2008; **3**(3): 84–90.
2. Topping KJ. The effectiveness of peer tutoring in further and higher education: a typology and review of the literature. *High Educ.* 1996; **32**(3): 321–45.
3. Field M, Burke JM, McAllister D, *et al.* Peer-assisted learning: a novel approach to clinical skills learning for medical students. *Med Educ.* 2007; **41**(4): 411–18.
4. Hill E, Liuzzi F, Giles J. Peer-assisted learning from three perspectives: student, tutor and co-ordinator. *Clin Teach.* 2010; 7(4): 244–6.
5. McKenna L, French J. A step ahead: teaching undergraduate students to be peer teachers. *Nurse Educ Pract.* 2011; **11**(2): 141–5.
6. Peets AD, Coderre S, Wright B, *et al.* Involvement in teaching improves learning in medical students: a randomized cross-over study. *BMC Med Educ.* 2009; **9**: 55.
7. Christiansen A, Bell A. Peer learning partnerships: exploring the experience of pre-registration nursing students. *J Clin Nurs.* 2010; **19**(5–6): 803–10.
8. Silbert BI, Lake FR. Peer-assisted learning in teaching clinical examination to junior medical students. *Med Teach.* 2012; **34**(5): 392–7.
9. Weyrich P, Celebi N, Schrauth M, *et al.* Peer-assisted versus faculty staff-led skills laboratory training: a randomised controlled trial. *Med Educ.* 2009; **43**(2): 113–20.

10. Grimshaw JM, Shirran L, Thomas R, *et al.* Changing provider behavior: an overview of systematic reviews of interventions. *Med Care.* 2001; **39**(8 Suppl. 2): 112–45.
11. Davis D, O'Brien MA, Freemantle N, *et al.* Impact of formal continuing medical education: do conferences, workshops, rounds, and other traditional continuing education activities change physician behavior or health care outcomes? *JAMA.* 1999; **282**(9): 867–74.
12. Hewson MG, Little ML. Giving feedback in medical education: verification of recommended techniques. *J Gen Intern Med.* 1998; **13**(2): 111–16.
13. Emmen H, Wesseling L, Bootsma R, *et al.* The effect of video-modelling and video-feedback on the learning of the tennis service by novices. *J Sports Sci.* 1985; **3**(2): 127–38.
14. Noordman J, Verhaak P, van Dulmen S. Web-enabled video-feedback: a method to reflect on the communication skills of experienced physicians. *Patient Educ Couns.* 2011; **82**(3): 335–40.
15. Hill J. Overcoming obstacles and creating connections: community building in web-based learning environments. *J Comput High Educ.* 2002; **14**(1): 67–86.
16. Oblinger D. *Space as a Change Agent.* Washington, DC: Educause; 2006.
17. Barker SP. Comparison of effectiveness of interactive videodisc versus lecture-demonstration instruction. *Phys Ther.* 1988; **68**(5): 699–703.
18. Coffee J, Hillier S. Teaching pre-cursor clinical skills using an online audio-visual tool: an evaluation using student responses. *J Online Learn Teach.* 2008; **4**(4): 469–76.
19. Coffee J. Using an on line audio visual aid to facilitate the teaching and learning of clinical reasoning. *Focus Health Prof Educ.* 2007; **9**(3): 89–91.
20. Salyers VL. Teaching psychomotor skills to beginning nursing students using a web-enhanced approach: a quasi-experimental study. *Int J Nurs Educ Scholarsh.* 2007; **4**: Article 11.
21. Biggs J. What the student does: teaching for enhanced learning. *High Educ Res Dev.* 1999; **18**(1): 57–75.
22. Shepard K, Jensen G. *Handbook of Teaching for Physical Therapists.* 2nd ed. Boston, MA: Butterworth–Heinemann; 2002.
23. Donaghy M, Morss K. An evaluation of a framework for facilitating and assessing physiotherapy students' reflection on practice. *Physiother Theory Pract.* 2007; **23**(2): 83–94.
24. George JH, Doto FX. A simple five-step method for teaching clinical skills. *Fam Med.* 2001; **33**(8): 577–8.
25. Kruger J, Dunning D. Unskilled and unaware of it: how difficulties in recognizing one's own incompetence lead to inflated self-assessments. *J Pers Soc Psychol.* 1999; **77**(6): 1121–34.
26. Gordon MJ. A review of the validity and accuracy of self-assessments in health professions training. *Acad Med.* 1991; **66**(12): 762–9.
27. Schwan S, Riempp R. The cognitive benefits of interactive videos: learning to tie nautical knots. *Learn Instruct.* 2004; **14**(3): 293–305.
28. Mayer RE. The promise of multimedia learning: using the same instructional design methods across different media. *Learn Instruct.* 2003; **13**(2): 125–39.
29. Aspegren K. BEME Guide No. 2: Teaching and learning communication skills in medicine; a review with quality grading of articles. *Med Teach.* 1999; **21**(6): 563–70.
30. Boyer E, Miltenberger RG, Batsche C, *et al.* Video modeling by experts with video feedback to enhance gymnastics skills. *J Appl Behav Anal.* 2009; **42**(4): 855–60.
31. Maloney S, Storr M, Morgan P, *et al.* The effect of student self-video of performance on clinical skill competency: a randomised controlled trial. *Adv Health Sci Educ Theory Pract.* 2013; **18**(1): 81–9.
32. Maloney S, Storr M, Paynter S, *et al.* Investigating the efficacy of practical skill teaching: a pilot-study comparing three educational methods. *Adv Health Sci Educ Theory Pract.* 2013; **18**(1): 71–80.

33. Maloney S, Haas R, Keating JL, *et al.* Breakeven, cost benefit, cost effectiveness, and willingness to pay for web-based versus face-to-face education delivery for health professionals. *J Med Internet Res.* 2012; **14**(2): e47.

34. Pérez-Peña R. Top universities test the online appeal of free. *New York Times.* 17 July 2012.

35. Maloney S, Haas R, Keating J, *et al.* The efficacy of web-based versus face-to-face delivery of falls prevention exercise prescription education to health professionals: a randomised trial. *J Med Internet Res.* 2011; **13**(4): e116.

36. Harden M, Grant J, Buckley G, *et al.* BEME Guide No. 1: best evidence medical education. *Med Teach.* 1999; **21**(6): 553–62.

37. Cook DA, Beckman TJ, Bordage G. Quality of reporting of experimental studies in medical education: a systematic review. *Med Educ.* 2007; **41**(8): 737–45.

38. Majumder MA. Issues and priorities of medical education research in Asia. *Ann Acad Med Singapore.* 2004; **33**(2): 257–63.

39. Greenhalgh T. Narrative based medicine: narrative based medicine in an evidence based world. *BMJ.* 1999; **318**(7179): 323–5.

40. Hoepfl M. Choosing qualitative research: a primer for technology education researchers. *J Technol Educ.* 1997; **9**(1): 47–63.

41. Newman I, Ridenour C. *Qualitative-Quantitative Research Methodology: exploring the interactive continuum.* Carbondale: Southern Illinois University Press; 1998.

42. Smith J, Heshusius L. Closing down the conversation: the end of the quantitative-qualitative debate among educational inquirers. *Educ Res.* 1986, **15**(1): 4–12.

43. Walsh K. Defining and costing educational interventions. *Med Educ.* 2011; **45**(10): 1063.

44. Bloom BS. Effects of continuing medical education on improving physician clinical care and patient health: a review of systematic reviews. *Int J Technol Assess Health Care.* 2005; **21**(3): 380–5.

45. Coomarasamy A, Khan KS. What is the evidence that postgraduate teaching in evidence based medicine changes anything? A systematic review. *BMJ.* 2004; **329**(7473): 1017.

CHAPTER 15

Educating healthcare professionals

From novice to expert

....

Arthur M Guilford, Sandra V Graham
and Jane Scheurele

OVERVIEW

Evidence-based education is presented through a model of progressing from the novice healthcare professional to the expert. A review of research identifying the characteristics of individuals considered to be experts is discussed for a variety of healthcare disciplines including curriculum and instructional methodologies that promote outcomes for students and patients or clients; challenges to programmes achieving established learning outcomes; gaps between theory and practice; and readiness of graduates to successfully practise and meet employer expectations. Models for experiential-based learning and methods of self-evaluation are explored as we monitor the developmental sequence of moving from a novice practitioner to an expert in healthcare. Attaining the level of expert indicates that an individual can perform complex tasks in his or her domain and accurately solve problems with greater ease than novices. Expertise, regardless of healthcare profession, is dependent on detailed knowledge basis, problem-solving abilities and the expert's specialised memory abilities and inference patterns.

CHAPTER OBJECTIVES

Upon completion of this chapter, the reader will be able to:

● describe how competence and expertise are features of a healthcare professional

● outline what the traits of a health professional novice are

● describe what the traits of a health professional expert are

● articulate how the curriculum of a health professional education programme provides the foundation skill development of students so they can move from being a novice to developing more expertise.

KEY TERMS: expertise, competence, healthcare education programmes, practice gaps

---

INTRODUCTION

The previous chapters have discussed thoroughly the need for evidence-based education within healthcare profession programmes of study. Through this text, educators in pre-professional and professional programmes have brought together a substantial body of evidence of standards of effective teaching across several disciplines and have affirmed our common goal of achieving competency in evidence-based practice. In addition, both students and professional programmes are accountable to external regulatory bodies, accreditation agencies and patients or clients deserving of the best possible outcomes.[1]

Meeting these needs and achieving designated outcomes requires the entire professional community to contribute to the development of health professionals. This community-wide effort includes the participation of the students, educators, preceptors, professional mentors, administrators and potential employers.[2] It is a massive undertaking to educate and train healthcare professionals – an undertaking that, to promote success in the practice of the professions, necessitates evidence of successful achievement of the targeted knowledge and skills, and provides reliable methods of benchmarking the achievement of professional training milestones. The combination of personal attributes, knowledge and skill development and professional attitude provide the foundation for the level of competence of the novice professional and the foundation for continued professional development throughout the career. Those contributing to the education and training of healthcare professionals must look beyond immediate learning objectives and consider the potential of each professional in training in order to promote the development of professional expertise.

While the healthcare profession encompasses many disciplines, the challenges to achieving educational outcomes are strikingly similar across disciplines. In the current educational climate, professional programmes cope with:

● unstable budgets and resources

● expanding learning objectives to meet accreditation requirements and consumer expectations

● successful recruitment, admission and retention of well-qualified students

- greater variability in student learner attributes and styles
- attrition and shrinking numbers of qualified candidates for academic positions
- expanding knowledge base(s) as a result of research endeavours
- broadening scope of practice for each discipline
- fluctuating healthcare costs and reimbursement formulas that affect the need for future professionals and the opportunity for collaborative educational experiences (practicum) in service provider settings
- increasing professional liability during practical experiences on and off campus.

Out of necessity, the curriculum must expand to respond to these demands and yet maintain reasonable breadth and scope to comply with university guidelines for maximum number of credits per degree, anticipated time to graduation following admission to a programme and graduation rates. Kevin *et al.*,[3] in summarising a literature review of nursing programmes, stated that the key issue in programme design is the preparation of graduates for practice of the profession and, graduates' readiness and ability to practise in the clinical environment after graduation. Holland *et al.*[4] indicated that for occupational therapy novices, 'Professional confidence is a dynamic personal belief that matures over time. It is closely linked to both competence and professional identity ensuring fitness for practice.'[(p106)]

HEALTHCARE PROFESSION CURRICULUM: THE FOUNDATION OF PROFESSIONAL COMPETENCE AND EXPERTISE

In a model of clinical expertise for the profession of speech-language pathology, knowledge and experience represent the foundation for the beginning professional. This foundation is essential as the basis for future professional growth and development as the professional moves from novice to expert within the discipline. Curriculum development encompasses not only the prerequisite content and skill knowledge (what to teach) but also considerations of the timing of courses and practicum experiences (when to teach), and emphasis on the most efficient and effective means for teaching (how to teach). Each discipline must draw upon general and profession-specific research to design the optimal curriculum to move students along the novice-to-expert continuum.[2]

Leffler *et al.*[5] reviewed models for teaching and training effective healthcare professionals across levels of professional development. They found commonalities among mental health programmes that included individualised approaches to training, incorporation of active learning strategies and methods for accurately measuring students' achievement of learning outcomes. The focus was to identify those programmatic components that would produce skilled clinicians who would competently meet the needs of clients and/or patients. This is the target for most, if not all, healthcare profession programmes. Attention must be focused on not only the courses and course content but also the sequencing of courses and practicum in order to reach this target.

Because of the influences of (a) teacher education research, (b) the medical model most often used in healthcare education and (c) the nature of professional programme design, a great deal of attention in research is focused on the clinical or practicum experiences of students as pre-professionals and novices. These experiences may be completed in on-campus facilities and/or off-campus settings that function as service providers for the discipline and are referred to as practicum, internship, externship, fellowship, fieldwork, residency and work-integrated learning (WIL). These components of the curriculum provide guided, practical educational experiences typically under the direct instruction and supervision of programme faculty and qualified practitioners from the designated profession who are employed by the setting providing the experience. 'Communities of practice' is a concept that refers to the continuum of experience. Nistor and Fischer[6] have indicated that the communities of practice lead to (a) experience, (b) stimulation of social knowledge and (3) expertise.[7,8]

Students report that the clinical or practicum experience or experiences are the most important part of their professional preparation. The study by Ralph et al.[9] suggests that students' perception of this portion of the curriculum were similar across the disciplines studied (nursing, engineering and education). They acknowledge that this type of educational experience is a key component of all professional education programmes. Even though feedback from participants is typically both positive and negative, research suggests that the positive comments outweigh the negative comments and the overall value of the educational experience is evident. The authors supported previous findings that a major feature of this common experience is the mentoring of qualified students to promote the development of their professional knowledge, skills and values.[10]

Weeks et al.[1] found that training in environments that utilised evidence-based practice increased the likelihood of professional development and growth for nursing students. Clinical settings have been characterised as 'learning workplaces' with the ability to produce 'knowledge in action' by stimulating alternative ideas and perspectives on common issues.[11,12] Duhamel[12] suggests that these types of experiences ensure the link between knowledge and the application of knowledge in clinical practice, foster knowledge exchange and provide opportunities to challenge the linear perspective between scientific and practice knowledge in order to appreciate how they complement each other.

Experiential learning and practice-based education are hallmarks of programmes of study for healthcare professions. These experiences offer the student the opportunity to connect theory and practice. The nature of practicum provides the student with real-time learning moments and requires rapid interpretation of situations to correctly apply principles of evidence-based practice across a range of settings and patient services. While these skills are essential for even the novice to be deemed 'competent', the level of functioning becomes highly skilled for the expert.

The effective use of student feedback following clinical and practicum experiences can provide programmes with opportunities to evaluate the effectiveness of the curriculum and instructional methods, and identify areas for improvement. Such mechanisms for programme improvement are typically required by accrediting bodies. This information can also assist programmes to identify and reward deserving supervisors and preceptors.

In order to constantly improve curriculum and the reputation of the programme, individual departments must frequently review and carefully consider feedback from employers of their graduates, departmental needs when hiring, the methods utilised to mentor doctoral students and new faculty, and the criteria for promoting effective teachers. The knowledge store of a programme cannot be utilised optimally if the content and skill knowledge cannot be successfully communicated to the students enrolled in the programme to the end that the student is successful in meeting the needs of the patient or client. The successful completion of programmatic outcomes and accomplishments can seem overwhelming for both student and teacher. Both must be fully engaged in activities that will enable the novice (pre-professional or professional in training) to meet universal standards of care required by the profession(s), patients or clients, and future employers.

The ultimate goal would be to graduate outstanding, well-qualified novices with the potential to self-propel themselves along the continuum of professional development after graduation and, in the end, become experts who will carry the profession forward.[7,8] Healthcare professions cannot meet this goal if graduates are typically minimally competent novices. Programmes must recruit well-qualified students, achieve learning outcomes, train highly competent professionals, and promote and inspire an attitude of excellence. Educators of future healthcare professionals must incorporate teaching methodologies that intrinsically promote decision-making and problem-solving, objective self-reflection and self-evaluation and which participate in lifelong professional growth. Evidence-based education becomes the path for accomplishing the goal.

MOVING FROM NOVICE TO EXPERT

Research in a variety of disciplines related to the development of clinical competence reflects the premise that a 'professional' demonstrates a set of basic competencies. The professional organisations and accrediting bodies for healthcare professions provide comprehensive sources of information related to the competencies for knowledge and skills that must be demonstrated by each programme graduate. In addition, regulatory and certification agencies designate the qualifications for professionals who apply for a healthcare provider licence and/or certificate. However, little research addresses the influence of the professional's level of competence on patient or client outcomes. Although specific competencies may be identified for each healthcare profession discipline, *degrees* of competence are less easily defined as the professional moves from novice to expert, and the effects on overall treatment outcome may be unclear or not documented.

Novice typically refers to individuals who are relatively new to their practice. In medical education, for example, novices are often seen as fourth-year medical students who have not as yet done their internships or clerkships.[13] Most typically, the novice has obtained the classroom instruction but has obtained little, if any, clinical training and experience regardless of the health-related area of practice.[2]

GENERAL CHARACTERISTICS OF THE EXPERT

Much of the seminal research which defined and described expertise has been drawn from the field of education and a variety of health professions including clinical psychology, medicine, nursing, social work and speech-language pathology. Ericsson *et al.*[14] described studies of experts in selected endeavours as attempts to understand and account for the features (described as inherited or acquired stable characteristics) that distinguish outstanding individuals in a specified field from others in the same occupation and from people in general. They concluded that the characteristics that differentiated experts from their colleagues are (a) acquired rather than inherited, (b) are occupation specific and (c) take a long time to acquire.

Further research provided evidence that when individuals present with the combination of innate ability and sufficient deliberate practice, training and feedback on performance, these individuals show few limitations to their development of expertise.[14] Jacobs[15] suggests that training can help individuals achieve a certain level of competence, but the individual must make the effort through controlled creativity and focused insight to achieve, over time, higher levels of development.

Experts are those most capable in specified areas of human endeavour; only individuals who possess the highest levels of competence are recognised as experts.[15] Assessing the presence or absence of knowledge and skills can be achieved through a variety of methods. Assessing levels of competence and expertise, however, is relatively arbitrary, because the levels of ability occur along a hypothesised continuum for which agreement can vary greatly depending on the perspective and skill of the observers.

Within professions, 'expertise' denotes exceptional or extreme performance and achievement of intended outcomes at the upper end of a normal distribution. Early research endeavoured to identify the distinguishing features of the expert. Attaining the level of expert means that an individual can perform complex tasks in their domain much more accurately and can solve problems with greater ease and automaticity than novices. Experts function with higher analytical perspectives when faced with novel characteristics and complex situations. They are more successful at perceiving patterns and utilising task-related cues. They have a greater sense of what is relevant and demonstrate greater self-confidence when making decisions. Experts are skilled in communication and are better able to handle adversity.[16,17] Experts, when compared with novices, demonstrate superior memory for information related to their occupation or discipline. As a result, expertise increases steadily with practice and is highly occupation or discipline specific.

More recent evidence specific to the profession of speech-language pathology indicates that expertise includes not only the intellectual factor but also intrapersonal, interpersonal and attitudinal factors. These factors influence clinical decision-making, clinician–client interaction and, ultimately, treatment outcomes. Achieving professional expertise presents anticipated benefits to professional effectiveness. Developing expertise requires identifying and describing important skills and behaviours. Such efforts also affect clinical practice efficacy and outcomes.[18,19]

Expertise has been found to be dependent on (a) the detailed knowledge base for a specific discipline, (b) the problem-solving abilities of the individual considered to be an expert and (c) the individual's specialised memory abilities and inference patterns. Clinical and applied research has focused more on the technical and procedural aspects of treatment protocols than the level of competence along the novice–expert professional continuum. Knowledge of expertise specific to healthcare professions can enhance the effective application of evidence-based education methodologies to improve learning outcomes, especially in the practical aspects of professional training.

THE FIRST STEPS TO EXPERTISE: THE PRE-PROFESSIONAL STUDENT AND NOVICE HEALTHCARE PROFESSIONAL

For the novice or beginning professional to move towards expertise, the novice must apply considerable attention and energy to 'how' to practise the profession (knowing the theoretical foundations and incorporating appropriately the technical aspects of the profession). Each novice practitioner must discover his or her strengths and weaknesses, analyse each and diminish the weaknesses while increasing the strengths. As he or she learns the practice parameters of the profession, the individual practitioner develops insight into interpersonal interactions, clinical practice and outcomes.

Proven academic activities that target the acquisition of knowledge and skills are enhanced by including opportunities for developing self-knowledge, self-evaluation, the ability for rapid recognition of situations for applying knowledge and skills, and the relationship of each to positive outcomes. The beginning professional must become aware of the relationship between his or her level of competence and clinical outcomes for the client or patient.

Monrouxe,[20] Monrouxe and Rees,[21] and Rees and Monrouxe[22] have indicated that *identity* (self-definition) is essential to medical education. It was also emphasised that there is *self-identity* and *client-identity* back to the medical student which changes one's perceptions of one-self. Monrouxe and Rees[21] have consistently stated that understanding the process of self-identify will greatly facilitate educational strategies for medical students. They view students' identification as a medical practitioner at the core of medical education and it certainly is an attribute of developing expertise.

As noted earlier, achieving expertise requires extensive practice over time. Bathgate *et al.*[23] remind us that 'not all practice yields good progress'[(p403)] and to enhance the efficacy of instructional practices, we must utilise methods that ensure that learners practise effectively. They attribute this lack of effective practice among novices to the rare use of frequent and explicit metacognitive strategies during practice as are observed with experts. The repetition of systematic errors and ineffective techniques negatively impacts the practice effect. Their study provided supportive evidence of the effectiveness of providing direct instruction on the use of metacognition when teaching novice music students. The authors concluded that having students explicitly verbalise and reflect on the learning process resulted in more efficient practice and improved performance for the task.

Fischer[24] reminds us that practice performance may not fully reflect the amount of learning that is occurring. Rather than providing for successful practice, the 'route from novice to expert' must incorporate challenges in order to optimise learning. In addition, meeting with challenges during the experience can stimulate and increase learning. Such experiences provide professional activities that promote competence (the integration of knowledge, skills and attitudes). Years of experience as teachers provide us with numerous examples of anecdotal information from students who report that they were terrified when faced with their first clinical experience but that it was the most rewarding experience and an invaluable learning opportunity. Utilising supervised reflection and introspection can provide support for students through their education, provide a sense of security during the learning process, enable students to accept criticism in a positive way and help bridge the gap between theoretical and practical knowledge.[25]

Carey and Colby[26] documented the successful use of quality improvement principles and procedures in their model curriculum for medical fellows. The intent was to utilise quality improvement methods to teach and evaluate residents during a practice-based learning experience that targeted specific competencies. Interpretation of the outcomes indicated that the curriculum provided fellows with a variety of means to demonstrate competence. In addition, there were immediate and meaningful improvements in observed patient care.

Similarly, Jones[27] and Manthorpe[28] reviewed the use of WIL applied to social work field education. WIL experiences in social work education are also viewed as promoting collaboration and utilising the expertise of practitioners within the discipline. Harris et al.[29] reported that WIL programmes offer opportunities for universities to participate in community engagement and benefit from the knowledge generated by these collaborations as a means of enhancing student educational experiences. Care must be used when designing WIL programmes in order to maximise the benefits and promote the efficacy of such programmes. Evaluation of these programmes and measurement of outcomes can add to the evidence for effectiveness as a teaching method. Smith[30] provides a model for evaluating a variety of WIL curricula. Such models may be useful to programmes when developing methods for outcomes measurement.

While experiential learning and practice-based education during practicum and clinical assignments are considered core educational experiences in healthcare profession programmes,[31] Fortune and McKinstry[32] support the implementation of a project-focused fieldwork as part of a capstone subject for masters level occupational therapy students. The rationale for the experience was that project placements enable students to learn and utilise macro-level strategies during the development of clinical skills required for contemporary occupational therapy practitioners. Results of the project yielded positive outcomes for students and fieldwork settings beyond those competencies targeted for the novice. Students benefitted from the opportunities to work collaboratively with supervisors. Specific skill sets that developed included advanced communication skills and ability to navigate the politics of the workplace. The researchers viewed the findings as support for the importance of WIL that enabled pre-professionals to cope with the complex issues of the workplace.

WIL curriculum components for professional healthcare programmes can be a challenge to secure for students, especially if there is a high degree of competition for these placements between programmes and if the community resources are limited.

As a result, programmes must be innovative in developing clinical experiences that will promote the development of required skill sets. Hill *et al.*[33] have explored the use of a standardised patient programme in speech-language pathology similar to those used in medicine and nursing.

Within the healthcare professions education programmes, there is great diversity in programme content, programme design, attributes of students enrolled and targeted outcomes. While the novice often asks to be told what to do, programmes seek to utilise teaching strategies that facilitate students' learning styles and promote problem-solving skills and independent thinking. Trying to teach every scenario related to the vast list of tasks that healthcare professionals must successfully perform does not encourage the development of competence and expertise. Programmes strive to teach students how to think critically.

The tenets of evidence-based education can contribute to the success of healthcare profession programmes in their endeavours to graduate competent, motivated beginning or novice professionals. Programmes must utilise the components of evidence-based education that are feasible; tailor these principles to the needs of their programme and students; align programme goals and learning outcomes with professional roles and responsibilities; facilitate students' goals for professional development; monitor the effectiveness of results; and revise accordingly. One such method is the scholarship of learning and teaching, which provides direction for teachers specific to how to teach novice students, how to enable their learning relevant to disciplinary standards and how to incorporate effective teaching methods.

PROGRESSING ALONG THE NOVICE–EXPERT CONTINUUM: EMPLOYABILITY OF THE BEGINNING AND PRACTISING HEALTHCARE PROFESSIONAL

Earlier, we discussed the difficulty of measuring levels of competence and the lack of evidence of the impact on patient or client outcomes. These levels of competence are also considered to affect the professionals' employability. Healthcare professions may benefit from a review of this issue in other fields such as business. Freudenberg *et al.*[34] found that WIL was a means of improving employment readiness and the development of generic skills for students. Rao *et al.*[35] conducted exploratory research to study employer requirements for skill levels of graduates seeking employment. The researchers proposed that this information could be helpful in filling the gap between the competence of graduates and the employer requirements.

Resulting recommendations included designing student programmes of study (curricula) to reflect the current market demand. The authors also recommended that teachers should be aware of the requirements of potential employers in order to enhance the preparation of students. It was noted that effective models of instruction included WIL programmes, opportunities for cooperative learning and professional mentoring programmes. For health professions, this would need to be an additional consideration following the compliance with requirements of accrediting and credentialing agencies. Some factors that contribute to the difficulty of preparing work-ready healthcare professionals include typically broad knowledge base and scope of practice; limited opportunities for repeated clinical practice; varying levels of competence, which create ethical dilemmas; availability of field placements; degree of collaboration between the academic programme and the site or preceptor; and specialisation of practising professionals serving as preceptors, which can limit the variety of clinical experiences.

Before the move to evidence-based practice, allied healthcare professionals relied on advice from supervisors and colleagues, theoretical knowledge, textbooks providing information on practice procedures and personal experience when making decisions about professional practice. These methodologies can represent barriers to eliminating the research–practice gap. Professional training programmes must incorporate both training of discipline-specific skills and training that will develop an interprofessional or team focus, research competence and work-ready professionals who can provide evidence-based care. Asokan[36] describes this as the challenge of the student-to-professional transition. Often there is a disconnect between educational experiences that taught and promoted the use of evidence-based practice and the realities of practice in the work place. Using an evidence-based curriculum promotes evidence-based practice after graduation. The curriculum may help to avert this disconnect by preparing beginning professionals for the different career stages and incorporating information about the preparation for the practice of the health profession and continuing professional development beyond the completion of the degree.[37]

Experience with field-based educational placements tells us that preceptors often report learning from the students. This can be a successful avenue for bridging the gap between academia and clinical practice, as well as reducing the barriers to implementation of evidence-based practice.[38,39] These experiences provide practising professionals with opportunities and incentives to participate in lifelong learning and refine their developing professional expertise.

Experts are proactive in their quest to improve and develop professional knowledge and skills. They know that successful professionals cannot practise in isolation. They stay connected through professional organisations and effectively engage in evidence-based practice using strong research evidence to support clinical decisions and practice. Activities for developing expertise include utilising opportunities for repeated practice, use of professional networking, participation in meaningful continuing education to keep up with professional advances, the review and application of quality research, and collaboration with university professional programmes. Scarvell and Stone[31] encourage interprofessional collaboration as an underlying philosophy for WIL programmes in healthcare profession education. By establishing formal plans for collaboration between university supervisors and field preceptors, offering workshops to preceptors and presenting at professional conferences, 'collaborative synergies' can enhance the WIL programme design and content as well as enhance the experience for students and preceptors.

CONCLUSION

In this chapter we have provided a review of the essential features of expertise and how they relate to the principles of evidence-based education in healthcare professions. These features tend to be common across disciplines and areas of expertise. These features are also evident in others' perceptions of individuals as expert in their field.[20,40–42] Experts objectively self-evaluate and formulate plans for developing the desired level of expertise, which in turn reflects positively on their own professional reputation and their value to employers. The foundation for this attitude for learning is often established during the educational experience, if not intrinsic to the student. Programmes and teachers must incorporate mechanisms in the curriculum that model and promote the adoption of a lifelong and life-wide concept of learning. Mechanisms for encouraging, supporting and recognising these efforts and achievements are reinforcing of this attitude of learning.[43] The tenets of evidence-based education can assist healthcare profession programmes to graduate competent, motivated professionals who will continue to grow professionally and develop their own expertise.

RECOMMENDATIONS FOR FUTURE RESEARCH

- Continue to define expertise in healthcare practice and its role in intervention processes
- Analyse the relationship between expertise and treatment outcomes
- Complete a longitudinal study of the development of professional skills and progress towards professional expertise after graduation
- Research to develop and assess effective educational models featuring collaboration between academic programmes and off-campus or WIL clinical experiences
- Continue to research the concept of self-identity as proposed by Monrouxe[20] across all healthcare-related disciplines

---

SUMMARY POINTS

- A professional's combination of personal attributes, knowledge and skill development, and professional attitude provide the foundation competencies required for the individual to move from being a novice professional to an expert.
- The health professional education curriculum provides the prerequisite content and skill knowledge (what to teach), but also considerations of the timing of courses and practicum experiences (when to teach) to lay the foundation for the novice.
- A 'community of practice' is a concept that refers to the continuum of experience and assists a healthcare professional move from being a neophyte to an experienced, confident clinician.
- Characteristics that differentiate experts from their colleagues (a) are acquired rather than inherited, (b) are occupation specific and (c) take a long time to acquire.

- Research indicates that health professionals who are 'experts' present with the combination of innate ability and sufficient deliberate practice, training and feedback on performance.
- Clinical and professional expertise has been found to be dependent on (a) the detailed knowledge base for a specific discipline, (b) the problem-solving abilities of the individual considered to be an expert and (c) the individual's specialised memory abilities and inference patterns.
- Rather than providing for successful practice, the 'route from novice to expert' must incorporate challenges in order to optimise learning. In addition, meeting with challenges during the experience can stimulate and increase learning.

REVIEW QUESTIONS

- What are the traits of a health professional novice?
- What are the traits of a health professional expert?
- How can the curriculum of a health professional education programme provide the foundation skill development of students so that they have the innate skills to move from being a novice to developing more expertise?
- What have clinical and professional expertise been found to be dependent on?

REFLECTIVE QUESTIONS AND EXERCISES

- Think about the feature of a health professional curriculum that would facilitate the development of a student's skills at the novice level.
- What traits do you associate with someone who is an expert?
- What strategies could new graduates utilise to promote their skill development so that they move from being a novice towards being an expert?

RECOMMENDED RESOURCES

- http://en.wikipedia.org/wiki/Scholarship_of_Teaching_and_Learning
- www.cebm.utoronto.ca
- www.cebm.net
- http://guideline.gov
- www.ebtn.org.uk
- www.guides.lib.unc.edu

REFERENCES

1. Weeks SM, Moore P, Allender M. A regional evidence-based practice fellowship : collaborating competitors. *J Nurs Adm.* 2011; **41**(1): 10–14.
2. Guilford AM, Graham SV, Scheuerle J. *The Speech-Language Pathologist from Novice to Expert.* Upper Saddle River, NJ: Pearson; 2007.
3. Kevin J, Callaghan A, Driver C, *et al.* A possible alternative model of clinical experience for student nurses. *J Nurses Staff Dev.* 2010; **26**(5): E5–9.
4. Holland KE, Middleton L, Uys L. Professional confidence: conceptions held by novice occupational therapists in South Africa. *Occup Ther Int.* 2013; **20**(3): 105–13.
5. Leffler JM, Jackson Y, West AE, *et al.* Training in evidence-based practice across the professional continuum. *Prof Psychol Res Pract.* 2013; **44**(1): 20–8.
6. Nistor N, Fischer F. Communities of practice in academia: testing a quantitative model. *Learn Culture Soc Interact.* 2012; **1**(2): 114–26.
7. Lave J, Wenger E. *Situated Learning: legitimate peripheral participation.* Cambridge, UK: University Press; 1991.
8. Wenger E. *Communities of Practice: learning, meaning, and identity.* Cambridge, UK: University Press; 1999.
9. Ralph E, Walker K, Wimmer R. Practicum and clinical experiences: postpracticum students' views. *J Nurs Educ.* 2009; **48**(8): 434–40.
10. Rose M, Best D. *Transforming Practice through Clinical Education, Professional Supervision and Mentoring.* New York, NY: Elsevier Churchill Livingstone; 2005.
11. Van de Ven AH. *Engaged Scholarship: a guide for organizational and social research.* Oxford, UK: Oxford University Press; 2007.
12. Duhamel F. Implementing family nursing: how do we translate knowledge into clinical practice? Part II: the evolution of 20 years of teaching research, and practice to a center of excellence in family nursing. *J Fam Nurs.* 2010; **16**(1): 8–25.
13. Verkoeijen PP, Rikers RM, Schmidt HG, *et al.* Case representation by medical experts, intermediates and novices for laboratory data presented with or without a clinical context. *Med Educ.* 2004; **38**(6): 617–27.
14. Ericsson KA, Krampe RT, Tesch-Romer C. The role of deliberate practice in the acquisition of expert performance. *Psychol Rev.* 1993; **100**(3): 363–406.
15. Jacobs RL. *Structured On-the-Job Training: unleashing employee expertise in the workplace.* San Francisco, CA: Berrett-Koehler; 2003.
16. Hoffman K. A comparison of novice and expert nurses' cue collection during clinical decision-making: verbal protocol analysis. *Int J Nurs Stud.* 2009; **46**(10): 1335–44.
17. Calkins S, Silva F, Tihan T. The role of pathology experts in defining practice gaps in continuing pathology education: what do we need to know and how can we find them? *Adv Anat Pathol.* 2012; **19**(3): 187–90.
18. Kamhi AG. Toward a theory of clinical expertise in speech-language pathology. *Lang Speech Hear Ser.* 1994; **25**(2): 115–88.
19. Graham SV. *Quality Treatment Indicators: a model for clinical expertise in speech-language pathology* [doctoral dissertation]. Tampa: University of South Florida; 1998.
20. Monrouxe, LV. Identity, identification and medical education: why should we care? *Med Educ.* 2010; **44**(1): 40–9.
21. Monrouxe LV, Rees CE. Picking up the gauntlet: constructing medical education as a social science. *Med Educ.* 2009; **43**(3): 196–8.
22. Rees CE, Monrouxe LV. Theory in medical education research: how do we get there? *Med Educ.* 2010; **44**(4): 334–9.
23. Bathgate M, Sims-Knight J, Schunn C. Thoughts on thinking: engaging novice music students in metacognition. *Appl Cogn Psychol.* 2012; **26**(3): 403–9.

24. Fischer MR. Challenging the challenge point framework. *Med Educ.* 2012; **46**(5): 442–4.

25. Holst HE, Hörberg U. Students' learning in an encounter with patients: supervised in pairs of students. *Reflect Pract.* 2012; **13**(5): 693–708.

26. Carey WA, Colby CE. Educating fellows in practice-based learning and improvement and systems-based practice: the value of quality improvement in clinical practice. *J Crit Care.* 2013; **28**(1): 112e1–5.

27. Jones M. Review of work integrated learning: a guide to effective practice. *Aust Soc Work.* 2012; **65**(2): 267–8.

28. Manthorpe J. Review of work integrated learning: a guide to effective practice. *Soc Work Educ.* 2012; **31**(4): 533–4.

29. Harris L, Jones M, Coutts S. Partnerships and learning communities in work-integrated learning: designing a community services student placement program. *High Educ Res Dev.* 2010; **29**(5): 547–59.

30. Smith C. Evaluating the quality of work-integrated learning curricula: a comprehensive framework. *High Educ Res Dev.* 2012; **31**(2): 247–62.

31. Scarvell JM, Stone J. An interprofessional collaborative practice model for preparation of clinical educators. *J Interprof Care.* 2010; **24**(4): 386–400.

32. Fortune T, McKinstry C. Project-based fieldwork: perspectives of graduate entry students and project sponsors. *Aust Occup Ther J.* 2012; **59**(4): 265–75.

33. Hill AE, Davidson BJ, Theodoros DG. A review of standardized patients in clinical education: implications for speech language pathology programs. *Int J Speech Lang Pathol.* 2010; **12**(3): 259–70.

34. Freudenberg B, Brimble M, Cameron C. Where there is a WIL there is a way. *High Educ Res Dev.* 2010; **29**(5): 575–88.

35. Rao AA, Shah SS, Aziz J, *et al.* Employability in MNCs: challenge for graduates. *Int J Contemp Res Bus.* 2011; **3**(4): 189–200.

36. Asokan GV. Evidence-based practice curriculum in allied health professions for teaching-research-practice nexus. *J Evid Based Med.* 2012; **5**(4): 226–31.

37. Taylor S, Allen D. Visions of evidence-based nursing practice. *Nurse Res.* 2007; **15**(1): 78–83.

38. Peck S, Lester J, Hinshaw G, *et al.* EBP partners: doctoral students and practicing clinicians bridging the theory-practice gap. *Crit Care Nurs Q.* 2009; **32**(2): 99–105.

39. Tart RC, Kautz DD, Rudisill KD, *et al.* Bridging the theory-practice gap: a practice-relevant research course for RN to BSN students. *Nurse Educ.* 2011; **36**(5): 219–23.

40. Enskär K. Being an expert nurse in pediatric oncology care: nurses' descriptions in narratives. *J Pediatr Oncol Nurs.* 2012; **29**(3): 151–60.

41. Morton JL, Hyrkas K. Management and leadership at the bedside. *J Nurs Manage.* 2012; **20**(5): 579–81.

42. Barnoy S, Ofra L, Bar-Tal Y. What makes patients perceive their health care worker as an epistemic authority? *Nurs Inq.* 2012; **19**(2): 128–33.

43. Jackson NJ. From a curriculum that integrates work to a curriculum that integrates life: changing a university's conceptions of curriculum. *High Educ Res Dev.* 2010; **29**(5): 491–505.

PART III

Key approaches and related evidence to health professional education

CHAPTER 16

e-Learning and use of technology in health professional education

Wikis, chat rooms, blogs, social network tools, clickers, video conferencing, podcasting and other emerging technologies

....

Andre Kushniruk, Elizabeth Borycki
and Mowafa Househ

OVERVIEW

This chapter examines the use of social media and related emerging technologies in health professional education and explores the benefits and challenges of the use of social media from an educational perspective. Technologies ranging from wikis and blogs to social networking tools, video conferencing and a range of other tools have emerged and have been employed in medical, nursing and allied professional education. The review of the evidence in the current literature indicates that effectively bringing social media into health professional education requires an understanding of the range, functions and limitations and potential of these technologies. This should include a strategy for evaluating the effectiveness of social media as well as perceived student and faculty satisfaction. Ideally learning outcomes using social media technologies should be considered before embarking on widespread deployment of the technologies in educational settings. Although there is a body of evidence to indicate that social media can increase the effectiveness of health professional education, improved evaluation and further studies providing evidence regarding the impact of social media on education are needed as current research has focused somewhat on the isolated use of a particular type of social media. More work is needed in describing effective strategies for integrating social media in online, blended and face-to-face learning. Along these lines, exploration of combinations of teaching methods and social media tools in healthcare are needed, including evaluations of the integration and use of social media within health professional learning and teaching.

CHAPTER OBJECTIVES

Upon completion of this chapter, the reader will be able to:

- describe the range and nature of social media applications in health professional education
- identity the strengths and weaknesses of using social media in health professional education
- outline future directions for the application of social media in health professional education
- make recommendations for future evaluation and research in this area.

KEY TERMS: social media, health professional education, learning management systems, YouTube, blogs, Twitter, Facebook, Second Life, podcasts, clickers, wikis, simulations, gaming

INTRODUCTION

Health professional education is being transformed through use of new and emerging technologies. One of the most promising and interesting ways in which education is being changed is through the use of social media. Social media are online tools that are designed to support collaboration, social activity and community building. Social media tools that support the social process of learning are making their way into education in general and are being applied in various ways in health professional education.[1,2] In addition to this, Web 2.0 tools have emerged to support networks and communities, allowing for more active student and faculty participation, and as such are rapidly making their way into health education.[3] In conjunction with these emerging trends, the understanding that learning is an active and social process has become increasingly recognised in the education of health professionals. Along these lines, problem-based learning and the use of technologies such as simulated patients for training groups of medical and nursing students how to interact in real collaborative settings have now become standard approaches in North America.[4]

With the advent of mobile devices and new forms of learning applications that are centred around social interaction, there are a whole new range of possibilities that are emerging for improving health professional education. In health professional education there has been a movement away from traditional teaching models where the instructor 'imparts' or 'transfers' their knowledge to the student, to a more active role for the learner.[5] In contrast, the instructor is considered a facilitator of the student's own learning process. With this move, there has also been recognition that the learner must collaborate not only with the instructor but also with other students. This is also being recognised in the trend towards interdisciplinary health professional education, where social interaction among nurses, doctors and other health professionals has become a focus. Emerging tools that support learning in a collaborative and social context are therefore promising and in recent years considerable interest has been shown in their application in health professional education in particular, given the collaborative and social nature of health professional work. These technologies have been touted by some as radically changing health professional education, while others have seen them as adjuncts to traditional teaching and learning methods. In addition, the body of evidence is unclear regarding the effectiveness of employing social media in terms of leading to significantly improved learning outcomes, despite a growing number of studies indicating that student and faculty have positive perceptions regarding use of the technology.

In this chapter we will review trends involving the use of social media technologies such as web-based video conferencing, wikis, chat rooms, podcasting, clickers and other forms of social media. For example, in the area of distance health professional education, the use of learning management systems (LMSs) has become common. Many of these tools support asynchronous interactions, such as Moodle, while an array of tools that support live synchronous education have also appeared. This review will begin by discussing the use of web-conference tools used in health professional education and then move to a discussion of related tools including use of YouTube videos, blogs and other social media tools. In addition, issues and questions related to how effective the use of social media is for health professional education will be explored. Evidence regarding the effectiveness of various approaches will be presented along with a discussion of strategies for integrating social media into health professional education. How social media is brought into health professional education needs to be considered, from stand-alone application to a variety of strategies for integrating social media in online approaches, blended learning environments, and face-to-face interactions, making a 'one size fits all' approach to the use of social media in healthcare impractical. Along these lines, there is increasing evidence that adopting effective strategies to such integration is essential and this will also be discussed in this chapter.[6]

LEARNING MANAGEMENT SYSTEMS AND WEB-BASED VIDEO CONFERENCING

In health professional education, perhaps the most transforming technology that has appeared and been adopted on a wide scale is web-based LMSs. As Chu et al.[7] describe, an LMS can be thought of as a virtual classroom that 'stays open 24 hours a day and seven days a week'.[(p28)] There are numerous commercial examples of LMSs, including WebCT, as well as open source LMSs such as the widely used Moodle. Such systems allow instructors to post, track and facilitate the delivery of course content over the World Wide Web (WWW). They allow for posting of lectures, slides, learning materials, chat facilities and discussion rooms. Both the advantages and the disadvantages of LMSs have, and continue to be, discussed in the literature. On the positive side, this technology allows for geographical and temporal flexibility and the ability for instructors to archive lectures and for students to search lectures. LMSs also provide ease of implementing and using the technology to support teaching and learning over the WWW. On the other hand, issues reported in the literature include the failure of students to watch lectures or participate in online distance courses in a meaningful way, as well as resistance from staff and students in the move from face-to-face to distance web-based educational formats using LMSs.[7] Furthermore, a continuing challenge has been the need to get both students and faculty familiar with the tools available through LMSs. This may include use of online tutorials or specially scheduled synchronous sessions at the beginning of a term or course where the instructor steps students through the use of the LMS and its features. However, effectively setting up and using LMSs can be a labour intensive process, with need for content specialists working together with information technology specialists to ensure a high-quality course.[6]

It is important to note that some of the most promising and innovative health professional educational programmes are using both asynchronous features and the capabilities of LMSs in conjunction with scheduling of live virtual classroom sessions (using a variety of web-based video conferencing tools such as Blackboard Collaborate). This application ranges from graduate programmes in nursing to medical and health informatics education delivered over the WWW.[8] Such tools allow for setting up of live classes where students can interact in real time from various geographical locations, and they include features such as sharable whiteboards (where PowerPoint slides can be presented in virtual classes), polling of students, shared chat boxes and ability for students to ask questions and engage in live discussions.[8] In areas such as education of health professionals about new drugs and medication practices, there is documented research showing that such tools are not only cost-effective but also may lead to increased uptake of research findings.[8] Such environments can also incorporate and be integrated with many of the features and technologies described in the rest of this chapter, such as live chat rooms, blogging and wikis. However, research has indicated that use of such tools does not mirror live face-to-face teaching interactions, but rather new social norms and methods for interacting develop and evolve for using these systems.[8] Using both asynchronous and synchronous LMSs, a wide variety of health professional educational programmes have been offered internationally, and use of these learning environments is rapidly increasing in areas such as nursing and health informatics education.[9]

YOUTUBE

YouTube is a website that allows users to upload and share videos and it has become extremely popular as an example of 'crowd' created content.[10] Since YouTube was introduced in 2005, it has been used in a variety of ways for health professional education. Even though there still remains a lack of research evidence supporting the use of YouTube as a medium for teaching health professionals, it continues to be used by faculty for teaching and by students for learning. In 2009, a pilot survey study was conducted to assess faculty usage of YouTube as a teaching resource for health professional education.[11] The study reported that, in general, faculty found the use of YouTube to be an effective method for teaching health education courses for students. The study concludes that YouTube may be a viable and innovative option for teaching health professional students. Burke *et al.*[11] discuss the benefits and challenges to using YouTube as a resource for college health education courses. The authors discuss the increasing number of health education YouTube videos that are becoming available by the American Red Cross, the Centers for Disease Control and Prevention, and the World Health Organization. The authors claim that these videos can be used in the classroom for teaching and can be of great benefit for students to generate discussion and to have different perspectives brought into the classroom, especially for students living in rural areas. The authors also suggest that the uses of YouTube videos are not a substitute for teaching but, rather, they should be used to generate discussion and debate within the class.

Within the literature, there have been various research publications around pro-fessional health education and the use of YouTube; these have primarily focused on nursing, with little focus on other health professional disciplines such as medicine, pharmacy, dentistry and the general health sciences. Various papers have been pub-lished around the use of YouTube in nursing education. Agazio and Buckley[12] discuss the use of YouTube in nursing education, describing theoretical nursing concepts and integrating student participation. The authors discuss the various YouTube videos that focus on describing the life and various theories of well-known nurses such as Nightingale, Rogers and Orem. The authors also report on various YouTube videos where individuals discuss their health problems and how they are used in class as case studies for nursing education. An example used by the authors was the use of YouTube videos to provide highlights from a conference around the principles of cultural and linguistic competence in health promotion training, hosted by the Center for Cultural Competence at the Georgetown University Center for Child and Human Development. The students listened to YouTube videos to hear personal sto-ries of families and health professionals from various ethnic backgrounds discussing issues around the delivery of health promotion programmes within their respective communities. Without YouTube, such information would have been difficult for the students to be exposed to.

YouTube has also been used to enhance clinical skills. Duncan *et al.*[13] conducted a study on how YouTube can help nurses enhance their clinical education. The authors found that even though there are many useful videos that can enhance the clinical knowledge of nurses, many of these videos need to be evaluated for credibility prior to their introduction to nursing students. The authors recommend that lecturers use appropriate video for students to watch that has been evaluated for credible content.

BLOGS

Blogs refer to sites that allow for sharing of individuals' thoughts, reflections, news and ideas, with the latest information usually appearing at the top of the blog (e.g. with entries in chronological order). In recent years, the literature shows an increasing use of blogs in professional medical education.[14] They have been used by medical, nursing, dental, public health and other healthcare professionals. In nursing, blogs have been used in a variety of settings and contexts. Lin and Shen[14] report on a study conducted in Taiwan examining nursing student attitudes towards using blogs in a nursing clinical practicum. One hundred and seventy-nine nursing students participated in the study by using a blog platform to write their reflection notes and obtain feedback from their peers around their observations. Results indicated that 90% of the blogs allowed them to share their experiences with other colleagues and that blogs provided them with emotional support and encouragement from their peers. The participants also noted that the blogs helped their professional development.

In another educational intervention using blogs, Reed[15] conducted a study where undergraduate nursing students, in a simulated laboratory environment, were asked to share their experiences of living with an ostomy. The 134 participants were asked to work in a small group and were asked to share their experiences through blogging while wearing an ostomy bag, which contained simulated faecal material, overnight. The results showed that the impacts of the experiential learning activity can have an impact on health professional education, especially around cognitive and psychomotor skills. Other studies around the use of blogging in professional health education have been used in medicine. Bogoch et al.[16] studied the use of a blog where the chief medical resident would write about relevant topics relating to medicine with links to journal articles and medical images, which he or she would disseminate to other hospital residents. The study evaluated the educational impacts of blogging and found that the blog was perceived to complement the medical residents' case-based education.

Chretien et al.[17] conducted a study with the aim of improving medical student professional development using blogs. The students were asked to place two reflective postings on the class blog throughout their rotation. Other students, as well as the instructor, were able to comment on the postings. With a total of 177 posts placed by 91 students, results showed that blogs promoted student reflection and professional development.

Studies around the use of blogs have also been conducted in dentistry. One example of a study conducted by El Tantawi[18] on the use of a blog in a dental terminology course reports that the use of blogs helped enhance student learning by understanding the dental terminology material and communicating with their colleagues. In the study, the instructor provided students with true or false question exercises and multiple-choice questions, and students were encouraged to answer them and comment on the course. The students also reported that the blog, although helpful in learning, was time-consuming because of the interactions required between students and instructors.

Issues with the use of blogging in health professional education include maintaining the appropriateness and credibility of blog content, confidentiality of information from student experiences (e.g. with patients) and the time and effort taken due to the interaction time required by students and faculty in blogging. On the other hand, blogs can be used to record evolving thoughts of student and faculty throughout a course, with the blog essentially becoming an artefact or record of student reflections on their learning that has taken place over time.

TWITTER

Twitter refers to a simple technology that allows for 'tweeting' – composing and sending messages of fewer than 140 characters that can be shared by others.[10] This simple yet powerful technology has become popular in general use; however, Giordano and Giordano[19] report that few health professional students use Twitter in educational programmes. The studies found relating to the use of Twitter have been primarily conceptual in nature, discussing the potential use of Twitter within professional health education. Of the studies found, they appear to be primarily focused on medical education relating to critical care, pharmacy, and ophthalmology, emergency medicine and other medical domains. In 2012, Bahner *et al.*[20] conducted a study on the supplementation of a medical education curriculum by sending daily tweets to students via their mobile phones.[20] Daily tweets were posted with a total of 87 followers. The authors showed that Twitter can offer educational content to students, which can enhance and complement the traditional educational approach.

Fox and Varadarajan[21] studied the impacts of Twitter to facilitate faculty, guests and student interaction and education in a multi-campus pharmacy management course. All participants were asked to tweet a minimum of 10 times, and over 1800 tweets were collected and analysed for the study. The results showed that 71% of students found Twitter to be distracting because it prevented them from taking notes during the class. However, over 80% of the students indicated that Twitter helped improve class participation by helping the students voice their opinions. The authors conclude that Twitter can be used positively to increase class interaction, but that it has a negative impact with regard to the large number of distracting tweets that occur during the class.

Another study, on critical care training, used Twitter with a group of 12 learners registered in a critical care course.[22] The students were asked to use Twitter to comment and discuss patient clinical videos and to respond to tutor questions and interact with other students. The study concludes that the use of Twitter is promising for group interaction and reflective learning.

How to effectively integrate Twitter within health professional courses is still an open question, with use of Twitter during lectures or conferences often involving display of ongoing Twitter conversations displayed to the audience on a second screen or display. Although this may allow for students and faculty to reveal their evolving thoughts of members of the audience during a face-to-face presentation or lecture (and may allow for those attending from a distance to participate), this type of use of Twitter can also potentially become a distraction.[21] Use of Twitter outside of classroom presentations does provide a way for students and faculty to provide real-time ideas and insights that are easily broadcast and can reach distance students in real time as well. Further work on how Twitter can be effectively integrated into health professional education is needed.

FACEBOOK

Facebook has allowed millions of people to create their own web pages, upload photos, make announcements and invite 'friends' to view their Facebook page.[10] According to Giordano and Giordano's[19] research, the majority of health professional students use Facebook at an educational, personal and professional level. A recent survey of health professional students in pharmacy, medicine, nursing, dentistry, speech and language pathology, physical therapy and medical laboratory sciences also found that over 77% of the students had Facebook accounts that were used for educational, personal and professional purposes.[23] Still, despite the high number of health professional students using Facebook for personal, professional and academic purposes, the evidence around the impact of Facebook on professional health education remains unclear, as more studies are needed to explore Facebook's potential.

Of the studies found, Facebook has mainly been used to facilitate learning through student–student and student–faculty interaction. Mena et al.[24] conducted a study on the willingness of medical students to use Facebook as a training channel for professional habits in influenza vaccination. The study asked 410 students to search Facebook for influenza vaccination of healthcare workers and their willingness to use Facebook as a method to search for such information and interaction. A high number of users were willing to search for influenza vaccination through Facebook. The study also reported that the students were more willing to engage in less formal Facebook pages than Facebook pages that were highly technical.

Another study, conducted by DiVall and Kirwin,[25] focused on the use of Facebook to facilitate course-related discussion between pharmacy students and faculty members. A Facebook page was created and students' course coordinators encouraged students to 'like' pages, read study tips and interact with other students and faculty. Over 57% of the students enjoyed the interaction and recommended that it be used in subsequent pharmacy courses because it enhanced their learning.

Cain and Policastri[26] conducted a study on the use of Facebook to expose pharmacy students to experts and thought leaders external to the university, which would provide complementary information to their course materials. The researchers used an informal learning strategy where participation by the students was optional. The results found that students enjoyed the informal learning strategy for exposing students to educational information that was brought to them by experts and grounded in real-world issues.

One of the major challenges moving forward with the use of Facebook for health professional education is the appropriate use of Facebook by students. Essary[27] notes that a number of medical students failed to distinguish between personal and professional use of Facebook and were dismissed from their university. The author states that clear policies and procedures by universities should be developed around the use of Facebook in the educational process, especially for health professional students, where many issues around ethics, and privacy and confidentiality are apparent.

SECOND LIFE

Second Life is a virtual environment where users create avatars and through their avatars they interact with other users in their virtual environment.[10] These virtual environments can be designed to visually simulate real-life health professional settings (such as hospitals and clinics) using game-like video and animation. Thus, the virtual world looks like the real one and users can create objects that can be customisable (e.g. their avatars are used to represent the student). In a number of examples, nursing and other health professional programmes have created replicas of their schools within Second Life. The purpose of such simulation is to add more realism to distance inter-actions than would be otherwise possible using conventional web-based conferencing and LMS tools, allowing students to gain an idea of differing healthcare contexts. For example, Johnson *et al.*[5] and colleagues have created a virtual nursing school, complete with virtual classroom environments, labs and meeting rooms. In their evaluation of use of the environment for teaching online nursing courses, measures included both close- and open-ended survey questions of nine learning and instructional domains (from the Student Assessment of Learning Gains course evaluation instrument). This included overall assessment of the learning environment, perceived quality of education, self-rated gains in content comprehension and perceived quality of class resources. After exposure to teaching using the Second Life environment, students rated all nine domains highly. However, several issues were identified from the open-ended questions, including lack of interaction with classmates, use of discussion boards potentially being intimidating and a potential decrease in spontaneity and lively discussion. Furthermore, technical difficulties were encountered related to managing multiple activities taking place at the same time, such as instant messaging and discussions.

Other examples of use of Second Life in health professional education include work at Imperial College London, where a virtual hospital was created that allowed students to perform a range of tasks such as interacting with patients, consulting with colleagues, ordering and reviewing X-rays and other medially related tasks.[28] The virtual environment includes operating rooms and a recovery area and requires that all the steps needed in surgery are performed by students through their avatars (e.g. wearing a mask and scrubbing before entering the operating room). Another example of using Second Life in healthcare education is work being done at the University of North Carolina's Eschelman School of Pharmacy, where parts of the pharmacy school have been replicated and students can visit (using their avatars) replicas of actual clinics and centres they will encounter in real life and do role-playing in real time.[29] In addition, replicas of medical devices (e.g. drug-dispensing devices) were made available through Second Life for students to train on. However, to date, evaluations of the effectiveness of these environments have been limited and more research is needed to determine their benefits as well as areas that need improvement.

Although use of simulations such as Second Life is promising, there are a number of issues with their use in health professional education. These include issues with user interfaces to these simulations and more specifically usability problems (as the interaction is more complex than with conventional web-based learning tools and resources). Furthermore, instructors developing such environments must be computer literate and tools such as Second Life may be restrictive in terms of what type of interactions can be created in the simulations.

PODCASTS

Podcasts have already become popular in education, allowing students to play back both audio and video segments of lectures and other pre-recorded educational material. For example, Heydarpour et al.[30] describe the use of podcasts for pharmacy education in medical school based on lectures. They conducted an evaluation of student perception of the usefulness of the podcasting and found that the perception of those who used it was high (96% of students who downloaded the podcasts perceived that podcasting had a positive impact on learning); however, usage was more limited, with only 46% of the students downloading the audio podcasts. In another study, Narula et al.[31] describe the use of video podcasts in a '5 Minute Medicine' series of video podcasts. Evaluation of this deployment of podcasts showed that the students almost unanimously perceived that the podcasts were effective learning tools and the majority of the students (who were clinical clerks) preferred the '5 Minute Medicine' videos to their previously preferred educational resources, such as textbooks and conventional online resources.

In another study, where podcasts were made available to clerks in general surgery, it was found that 84% of clerks listening to the podcasts highly agreed the recordings helped them to learn core topics, with 80% of listeners reporting that they found the recordings interesting and engaging.[23] Furthermore, it was noted that work in developing podcasts can be leveraged by wide-scale access, with the 'Surgery 101' podcast series being downloaded worldwide over 160 000 times. Podcasting has been found to be an effective adjunct when used in conjunction with other online and blending learning tools and techniques and is a relatively cost-effective approach to providing content to a potentially large and dispersed student audience.

CLICKERS

Clickers are classroom response systems that allow students to interact with instructors during lectures and other teaching contexts. Clickers have become widely used in health professional programmes in a number of countries. Using clickers (distributed to students) during lectures, health professional students can be presented with problems and polled as a group in real time for the correct answer. The instructor can then immediately present the class responses as a summarised histogram, which can be used both to elicit class discussion and to guide the instructor to modify teaching to address obvious weaknesses or misconceptions as identified from these real-time in-class assessments of knowledge. Using clickers in this way, a number of studies have shown they can be used to help teach problem-solving skills after allowing students to solve problems during class, either independently or in small groups. Although one study did not find a correlation between clicker participation by students and final exam performance, another study, conducted at the University of Colorado, found a number of positive benefits from use of clickers in seminar-style biology courses.[32,33] These included an increased chance students would do readings before class, increased ability to engage the entire class and the ability to give students a focused opportunity to share their thinking and learn from peers. Along these lines, in a study of the introduction of clickers in a medical-surgical nursing course (employing a quasi-experimental approach, with one group of students receiving clickers and the comparison group receiving only traditional teaching), although clickers were not found to improve learning outcomes (as measured by objective testing), students clearly indicated a perceived increase in the degree of engagement in the classroom. From a practical perspective, new approaches to using clickers encourage the use of the concept of 'bring your own device', where rather than providing clickers in classrooms, students can use their own mobile devices and smart phones to engage in the class. However, the issue of how to best integrate the use of clickers within the flow of a lecture or seminar is an issue, with the need to use them at key points to obtain live feedback from students while not distracting from the main intent of the lecture or seminar.

WIKIS

With the advent of Wikipedia, the concept of the wiki as a repository of knowledge that can be created and edited anonymously by multiple contributors (e.g. an example of crowd-created content) has emerged as one of the best-known Web 2.0 examples.[10] It has both been considered from the positive perspective by allowing for social interaction in co-creation of knowledge bases that facilitate the active learning processes of contributors and those accessing the wiki. In medical education, there have been a number of wiki projects – for example, the Massachusetts General Hospital's pathology informatics curriculum wiki – which can serve as an intelligence-sharing tool built up by multiple collaborators. Therefore, wikis can serve as an educational group's 'collective memory'. Students may be required to find, annotate and critique the reliability of resources that can be put in the wiki. For medical education this has included an expert-based peer-review model for controlling content generation to ensure content put on the wiki is reliable and correct.[34]

On the potentially negative side, the risk of having unreliable or incorrect information posted on a wiki is a real possibility and creates a problematic situation for health professional education if information is not properly vetted and reviewed before being posted. This concern has emerged from debate regarding Wikipedia, which currently has grown to over 3.8 million articles on a wide range of topics. However, the educational accuracy and reliability of information posted in Wikipedia has been hotly debated since its inception, and health professional educational applications have usually involved some kind of review process to ensure materials in the wiki are accurate and reliable.[35] However, wikis, if developed under the auspices of health professional faculty, and with their oversight, can form an effective adjunct to online, blended or face-to-face learning, with development of a wiki being a potential component of class group activities.

EDUCATIONAL GAMING

A promising and exciting approach to social media in health professional education involves games and simulations that involve role-playing and team-building collaborative skills. For example, use of games for teaching nurses how to interact with patients has been incorporated into gaming software. In Canada the SAGE (Simulation and Gaming in Education) project focused on healthcare applications of gaming and included a number of projects focused on group and collaborative use of games to instil health professional skills and competencies.[36] In the area of nursing, a number of studies employing games have been undertaken. For example, simulation games have been used to teach both cognitive and affective knowledge and have led to role-playing simulations as educational tools for healthcare professionals.[37] Use of information technology in such role-playing games and simulations has allowed for remote interactions, with students interacting collaboratively from various locations. In a study by Libin *et al.*,[37] a multimedia educational tool for healthcare professionals used a virtual experience immersive learning simulation, or VEILS, technology. It was found that the approach was partially effective in improving the learners' decision-making skills; however, a more individualised strategy was recommended for future applications. Furthermore, related studies have indicated that there must be an appropriate fit between instructional objectives and simulations or games.

DISCUSSION

Social media and Web 2.0 technologies have a huge potential to improve and facilitate health professional education. As described in this chapter, many of these technologies are already fundamentally changing health professional education in potentially profound ways, in particular LMSs and associated technologies. Advances such as web-conferencing have changed mainstream health professional education and this trend continues. Advantages include ability to provide education without geographical constraints, provide training using simulations that allow students to experience situations they would otherwise not encounter (e.g. using tools such as Second life), and the ability to leverage effort in creating such educational tools and resources by allowing widespread access throughout a country, region and the world. However, as described, each of the technologies that have been highlighted in this chapter have encountered a number of issues that need to be better understood and ultimately resolved. These include issues around the following areas: (a) concerns about quality of education and educational outcomes in moving from face-to-face to online distance learning formats; (b) concerns about the correctness and appropriateness of content and information in tools such as wikis and blogs; (c) technological and usability issues encountered in more complex applications, such as the simulated environments of Second Life; (d) potential for decreased student and instructor interaction in purely asynchronous modes of interaction (in particular as courses in many health professional programmes move from purely face-to-face to distance modes); (e) need for teaching health professionals about privacy and confidentiality when using social media, both in educational settings and for later use in practice.

It is recommended that research be conducted on a number of fronts, including evaluating the effectiveness of these new technologies, not only from evaluation of student and instructor perceptions but also in terms of studies of learning outcomes. Furthermore, usability evaluations are recommended for formative evaluation and piloting of learning tools and content prior to widespread release in health professional educational programmes.[38] Formative evaluation will be necessary for improving the chance of integrating these technologies successfully into health professional education.

RECOMMENDATIONS

From a practical perspective, recommendations for bringing the type of technologies described in this chapter into health professional education include the following: (a) understanding of the range, functions and limitations and potential of each of the technologies is an important basis for selecting and implementing the technology into health professional courses; (b) the insertion points into which exercises, class activities and student and faculty can be facilitated by social media need to be carefully considered; (c) a plan for evaluating the effectiveness, perceived student and faculty satisfaction and ideally learning outcomes using the technologies should be put into place before embarking on any major use of the technologies; and (d) piloting the use of the technologies in small-scale trial runs will often prove to be worth the effort in fine-tuning educational interventions involving them and increasing the chance of successfully introducing the technology into health professional education. In addition, a number of recommendations for engaging students can be made, including making students fully aware of the tools and capabilities of social media (including training them on their effective use) and carefully integrating the technology into courses using a strategy aimed at building relationships among students and faculty through the information-sharing capabilities of social media.

From this chapter it can be observed that there is variable evidence from current studies as to effectiveness of social media in health professional education. Although many studies have included an evaluation component where faculty and students have been asked if they felt that use of social media had been a positive experience or if it had improved their learning experience, fewer studies have been conducted that objectively measure learning outcomes. Some 'pre- and post-test' study designs have been employed (where learning outcomes have been measured before and after an intervention involving social media); however, fewer studies involving control groups and objective outcome measures have been reported. Furthermore, use of social media is not a 'one size fits all' proposition and the context of its application has to be considered as well as strategies for integrating it into health professional education in an effective way. Social media can be integrated with online, blended and classroom learning, as the studies in this review have shown. As such, more work into how to best combine different forms of social media within different teaching and learning formats is needed.

In particular, there is a need for improved evaluation of social media and Web 2.0 technologies in health professional education, and it is essential that their integration be based on sound curricular and pedagogical principles. As has been shown repeatedly in other areas of health information technology, technology itself can only lead to improvements in education when it is carefully inserted into the educational process, along with a clear understanding of both the positive and the negative aspects of its introduction and the technology's potential as well as limitations. Regarding future directions, there are a number of exciting developments that involve integration of the technologies described in this chapter with other emerging approaches, such as advanced educational simulations using computer-supported collaborative systems. This includes the integration of the type of educational tools described in this chapter with advanced clinical simulators that allow students to interact with computer-controlled manikins (representing patients) and educational electronic health record systems. Such systems are designed to closely resemble both the physical environment of the practising health professional and the emerging health information technologies that are becoming used throughout healthcare by nursing, medical and allied health professionals.[4] In addition, work at the intersection of gaming and simulation using social media is another emerging direction that is incorporating aspects of social media.

SUMMARY POINTS

- Social media is becoming increasingly incorporated into health professional education.
- There is a wide range of social media tools and technologies.
- The integration of specific social media technologies requires careful consideration of their role within online, blended and face-to-face educational formats.
- Evidence of the effectiveness of social media in improving educational outcomes is mixed; however, the majority of studies indicate student and faculty perceptions of social media are positive.
- Improved educational evaluation methods are needed to provide objective evidence for their effectiveness.
- Work is needed in developing strategies for combining different forms of social media in integrating them into health professional education.

REVIEW QUESTIONS

- What do you think the effect of social media will be on health professional education?
- How can such tools best be evaluated, in terms of (a) usability, (b) learner satisfaction and (c) learning outcomes?
- What are the major drawbacks to use of social media such as Facebook?
- What type of materials lend themselves to recording using podcasts?
- How can YouTube be incorporated into health professional education?
- How can the types of social media and teaching tools discussed in this chapter be integrated with traditional classroom teaching in health professional education?
- How can the types of social media and teaching tools discussed in this chapter be integrated with health professional teaching methodologies such as problem-based learning and small group teaching?

REFLECTIVE QUESTIONS AND EXERCISES

- Create an exercise for health professional education using one or more of the social media discussed in this chapter. Carefully select a technology and plan out how you would integrate the technology into health professional learning.
- Compare and contrast the potential strengths and limitations of the various types of social media as they can be incorporated into health professional education.

REFERENCES

1. Paton C, Bamidis P, Eysenbach G, *et al.* Experience in the use of social media in medical and health education. *Nursing and Health Professions Faculty Research.* Paper 6. Available at: http://repository.usfca.edu/nursing_fac/6 (accessed 15 January 2014).
2. Clauson KA, Singh-Franco D, Sircar-Ramsewak F, *et al.* Social media use and educational preferences among first-year pharmacy students. *Teach Learn Med.* 2013; **25**(2): 122–8.
3. Hollinderbäumer A, Hartz T, Ückert F. Education 2.0 – how has social media and Web 2.0 been integrated into medical education? A systematic literature review. *GMS Z Med Ausbild.* 2013; **30**(1): Doc 14.
4. Borycki E, Joe R, Armstrong B, *et al.* Educating health professionals about the electronic health record (EHR): removing barriers to adoption. *Know Manage E-learning.* 2011; **3**(1): 63–71.
5. Johnson CM, Corazzini KN, Shaw R. Assessing the feasibility of using virtual environments in distance education. *Know Manage E-learning.* 2011; **3**(1): 5–16.
6. Kipp K. *Teaching on the Education Frontier: instructional strategies for online and blended classroom.* San Francisco, CA: Jossey-Bass; 2013.
7. Chu LF, Young CA, Ngai LK, *et al.* Learning management systems and lecture capture in the medical academic environment. *Int Anesthesiol Clin.* 2010; **48**(3): 27–51.

8. Househ M, Kushniruk A, Maclure M, *et al.* Virtual knowledge production within a physician educational outreach program. *Know Manage E-learn.* 2011; **3**(1): 24–34.

9. Kushniruk A, Lau F, Borycki E, *et al.* The School of Health Information Science at the University of Victoria: towards an integrative model for health informatics education and research. *Yearb Med Inform.* 2006: 159–65.

10. Kelsey T. *Social Networking Spaces: from Facebook to Twitter and everything in between.* New York, NY: APress; 2010.

11. Burke S, Snyder S, Rager R. An assessment of faculty usage of YouTube as a teaching resource. *Internet J Allied Health Sci Pract.* 2009; **7**(1): 1–8.

12. Agazio J, Buckley K. An untapped resource: using YouTube in nursing education. *Nurse Educ.* 2009; **34**(1): 23–8.

13. Duncan I, Yarwood-Ross L, Haigh C. YouTube as a source of clinical skills education. *Nurse Educ Today.* 2013; **33**(12): 1576–80.

14. Lin K, Shen Y. The nursing students' attitude toward using blogs in a nursing clinical practicum in Taiwan: a 3-R framework. *Nurse Educ Today.* 2013; **33**(9): 1079–82.

15. Reed K. Bags and blogs: creating an ostomy experience for nursing students. *Rehab Nurs.* 2012; **37**(2): 62–5.

16. Bogoch I, Frost DW, Bridge S, *et al.* Morning report blog: a web-based tool to enhance case-based learning. *Teach Learn Med.* 2012; **24**(3): 238–41.

17. Chretien K, Goldman E, Faselis C. The reflective writing class blog: using technology to promote reflection and professional development. *J Gen Intern Med.* 2008; **23**(12): 2066–70.

18. El Tantawi M. Evaluation of a blog used in a dental terminology course for first-year dental students. *J Dent Educ.* 2008; **72**(6): 725–35.

19. Giordano C, Giordano C. Health professions students' use of social media. *J Allied Health.* 2011; **40**(2): 78–81.

20. Bahner D, Adkins E, Patel N, *et al.* How we use social media to supplement a novel curriculum in medical education. *Med Teach.* 2012; **34**(6): 439–44.

21. Fox BI, Varadarajan R. Use of Twitter to encourage interaction in a multi-campus pharmacy management course. *Am J Pharm Educ.* 2011; **75**(5): 88.

22. Mistry V. Critical care training: using Twitter as a teaching tool. *Br J Nurs.* 2011; **20**(20): 1292–6.

23. White J, Sharma N, Boora P. Surgery 101: evaluating the use of podcasting in a general surgery clerkship. *Med Teach.* 2011; **33**(11): 941–3.

24. Mena G, Llupià A, García-Basteiro AL, *et al.* The willingness of medical students to use Facebook as a training channel for professional habits: the case of influenza vaccination. *Cyberpsychol Behav Soc Netw.* 2012; **15**(6): 328–31.

25. DiVall MV, Kirwin JL. Using Facebook to facilitate course-related discussion between students and faculty members. *Am J Pharm Educ.* 2012; **76**(2): 32.

26. Cain J, Policastri A. Using Facebook as an informal learning environment. *Am J Pharm Educ.* 2011; **75**(10): 207.

27. Essary AC. The impact of social media and technology on professionalism in medical education. *J Physician Assist Educ.* 2011; **22**(4): 50–3.

28. Bradley J. Can Second Life help doctors to treat patients? CNN; 30 March 2009. Available at: http://edition.cnn.com/2009/TECH/03/30/doctors.second.life/ (accessed 15 January 2014).

29. Lee A, Berge Z. Second life in healthcare education: virtual environment's potential to improve patient safety. *Know Manage E-learn.* 2011; **3**(1): 17–23.

30. Heydarpour P, Hafezi-Nejad N, Khodabakhsh A, *et al.* Medical podcasting in Iran: pilot, implementation and attitude evaluation. *Acta Med Iran.* 2013; **51**(10): 59–61.

31. Narula N, Ahmed L, Rudkowski J. An evaluation of the '5 Minute Medicine' video podcast series compared to conventional medical resources for the internal medicine clerkship. *Med Teach.* 2012; **34**(11): e751–5.

32. Sterberger C. Interactive learning environment: engaging students using clickers. *Nurs Educ Perspect.* 2013; **33**(2): 121–4.

33. Smith M, Trujillo C, Su T. The benefits of using clickers in small-enrollment seminar-style biology courses. *CBE Life Sci Educ.* 2011; **10**(1): 14–17.

34. Park S, Parwani A, Macpherson T, *et al.* Use of a wiki as an interactive teaching tool in pathology residency education: experience with a genomics, research, and informatics in a pathology course. *J Pathol Inform.* 2012; **3**: 32.

35. Thompson C, Schulz W, Terrence A. A student authored online medical education textbook: editing patterns and content evaluation of a medical student wiki. *AMIA Annu Symp Proc.* 2011; 1392–401.

36. Sauve L, Renaud L, Kaufman D, *et al.* Distinguishing between games and simulations: A systematic review. *J Educ Technol Soc.* 2007; **10**(3): 247–56.

37. Libin A, Lauderdale M, Millo Y, *et al.* Role-playing simulation as an educational tool for health care personnel: developing an embedded assessment framework. *Cyberpsychol Behav Soc Netw.* 2010; **13**(2): 217–24.

38. Kushniruk AW, Patel VL. Cognitive and usability engineering approaches to the evaluation of clinical information systems. *J Biomed Inform.* 2004; **37**(1): 56–76.

CHAPTER 17

Use of e-Portfolios in health professional education

Application and evidence

· ·

Trudi Mannix and Kate Andre

OVERVIEW

In education, an e-Portfolio is a digitised collection of artefacts for teaching and learning purposes, made up of text-based, graphic or multimedia elements, archived and organised in a coherent manner for the purposes of enhancing and demonstrating performance and reflection. Students can independently store their academic and private work in the e-Portfolio over the course of their study. At a time and manner of their choosing, students can seek peer and academic review, or showcase items as formative and summative assessments and performance exemplars applying for employment after graduation. This chapter explores the possibilities of the e-Portfolio using contemporary examples from educationalists engaged in evidence-based education. The ECAR (EDUCAUSE Center for Analysis and Research) annual survey of 112 000 undergraduate students found seven times more students using e-Portfolios in 2012 than in 2010.[1] When the same survey was repeated in 2013, the use of e-Portfolios had plateaued, and this chapter also explores some of the impediments that may explain why e-Portfolios are not the runaway success that may have been anticipated. Hence this chapter is timely, as it offers strategies to facilitate the uptake of e-Portfolios in tertiary settings that deal with faculty and student issues.

CHAPTER OBJECTIVES

Upon completion of this chapter, the reader will be able to:

- provide an applied understanding of e-Portfolios as an educational and professional tool
- illustrate the diversity of applications with the e-Portfolio, using exemplars from educational specialists
- explore some of the enablers and barriers to the implementation of e-Portfolios in evidence-based education.

KEY TERMS

- *e-Portfolio*: an e-Portfolio is a purposeful aggregation of digital items – ideas, evidence, reflections, feedback, and so forth, that 'presents' a selected audience with evidence of a person's learning and/or ability.[2]
- *Digital repository*: a 'digital repository' stores, maintains and disseminates digital materials for a given community. Some communities are organised by subject (e.g. archaeological data, historical analyses, chemistry data) while others are organised by institution (e.g. materials from members of a university, usually focused on publications and theses rather than data).[3]
- *Personal learning space*: the nexus between the personal learning environment and the institutional learning environment. This space is institutionally provided but is under the control of the learner and is populated with personal content. Here individuals can learn at their own pace using a range of inbuilt scaffolding tools and templates.[4]
- *Lifelong learning*: the provision or use of both formal and informal learning opportunities throughout people's lives in order to foster the continuous development and improvement of the knowledge and skills needed for employment and personal fulfilment.[5]

INTRODUCTION

In a digital world, evidence fuels innovation and makes improvement possible. Evidence is what separates real advances from mere novelties, enhanced learning from mere entertainment.[6] Education can capitalise on the capacity for new technologies to collect and organise large amounts of data, and, if planned and managed appropriately, it can contribute to the evidence that informs our practice. e-Portfolios, in particular, have considerable potential in providing evidence about our students' performance outcomes applied to practice.

The concept of the e-Portfolio can be interpreted quite differently depending on the intended purpose and approach undertaken in its application. The purpose of this chapter is to provide exemplars of e-Portfolio use to illustrate its diverse applications in evidence-based education. We focus on the use of e-Portfolios as a reflective learning space that can be used individually and collectively to develop, store and retrieve learning and performance items in digital forms. As the exemplars demonstrate, however, the educationalists using e-Portfolios value their use beyond this to include the achievement of concepts such as collaboration, lifelong learning, independent learning and capstone experiences. Uptake and issues of e-Portfolio use will also be addressed from the perspective of providing ideas and approaches in use to attend to these.

WHAT IS AN E-PORTFOLIO?

Professional portfolios have long been used by photographers, architects and other professional groups to provide evidence of their achievements to entice potential clients or apply for positions and or promotions. It is therefore no wonder that many of us will automatically associate the term portfolio with a compilation of documentary evidence to support a curriculum vitae or suchlike. As an extension of this, the term *e-Portfolio*, with the inclusion of the prefix 'e', is commonly interpreted as a portfolio with digital evidence such as audio, video, websites and other technologies beyond the traditional documentary evidence. Certainly there is some basis for this perspective, particularly given that many of these digital technologies enhance the diversity, authenticity and quality of the evidence on display. However, as many authors have explained,[7,8] the reflective and analytical potential of portfolios is also enhanced by the move to digital technologies that support and demonstrate personal introspection and collaborative interaction.

A personal reflective journal for instance may become a blog that provides the user with extended options such as audio files, links to search repositories and dictionaries and the possibility to invite comment from others. Blogs, websites and the like can demonstrate the real-time contribution of individuals to online communities of practice, providing an individual with an opportunity to both develop and demonstrate process skills such as collaboration and problem-solving. Educationalists using e-Portfolios should keep in mind that any proposed innovation should align with deeper learning objectives and should incorporate sound learning principles.

So what is the range of possibilities of e-Portfolios and how will this influence the definition of this term? The following categories describe the major possibilities and opportunities of e-Portfolios.

A digital repository

Much of the literature is at pains to stress the potential value of the portfolio to extend beyond a repository and support reflection and analysis. However, the importance of keeping evidence of performance outcomes in a repository that accommodates digital formats, has tagging and search functions and can potentially be accessed at a range of locations is clearly a valuable aspect of e-Portfolios.[9] Hence most definitions of the term e-Portfolio will include reference to a digital repository. This is not to say that this negates the concepts of reflection; rather, the selection of items and decisions of how these are displayed – for instance, within a web page – provides the necessity for at least some reflection and analysis about how these meet the relevant criteria and needs of the intended audience. Importantly, the value of a digital repository should not be underestimated, as it provides an opportunity to store evidence of our various achievements so that we can search and access information readily and then present it in a manner that addresses a specific need.[10] An example of this is described by Garrett *et al.*[8] in a Bachelor of Science in Nursing programme, where the students' record of achievement is integrated throughout the e-Portfolio using hyperlinks between journal entries, learning plans and competencies. As students develop and store their assessments and items of evidence, they are required to apply a series of tags to each of the items. As a consequence, all items are stored in a single large repository, as opposed to folder systems, and items are then accessed using a search function for the various tags. This use of multiple tags avoids the need for replicas of items being stored in multiple folders.

Authentic and diverse evidence

The attention that the definition of e-Portfolios provided in the introduction to this chapter gives to the authenticity and diversity of the evidence is significant. The ability to record a range of our educational and professional activities in digital form is becoming increasingly available and mainstream. Podcasts, YouTube recordings and professional blog sites are increasingly being used to record performances in a manner that not only depicts theoretical and practical application but also often requires the performer to be present in the depiction, thus reducing concerns of plagiarism or outside assistance. Online clinical practice assessment tools that include the use of electronic signatures are now becoming available, thus allowing students to have staff sign off on their achievements in the practice setting. Similarly, using links to externally validated sites to support performance claims within personal websites, portfolios of curriculum vitae are becoming more commonplace. For instance, it is now relatively common for universities to require academics to have their publications recorded with facilities such as Google Scholar Citations and to include a link within their university web page, thus reducing the risk of fallacious claims of achievement.

Partly as a consequence of having access to digital forms of evidence, but also due to the emerging expectations of educationalists to support work integrated learning, the emphasis of e-Portfolios is increasingly being associated with performance outcomes with clear relevance to the workplace.[11] Increasingly, students are able to use their portfolios within the fieldwork education context or practicum workplace, with supervisors, academics and others able to provide feedback in both formative and summative forms. While there is a risk that the assessment and accreditation aspects of students' portfolios will become overly represented as a consequence of this move, there is a clear link between continued uptake of portfolios and the perception of the portfolio having professional and educational value.

Gordon and Campbell[12] provided a useful exemplar of the use of e-Portfolios in work settings in their article describing how physicians and surgeons used a personalised dashboard system linked to external sources to allow external validation of continuing professional development (CPD) activities. Their system also consisted of a 'holding area', where users are able to store questions to pursue, articles to review, assessments to complete and learning projects. They also had access to search engines and other online external resources from within the e-Portfolio system. In addition to having user buy-in because of the convenience of a tool such as this, the need for authenticity and validation of CPD activities with professional registration boards is also relevant here.

Students, while completing fieldwork placements or in a simulated practice environment, are increasingly being required to accumulate genuine artefacts of their practice assessment items. For instance, nursing students at Edith Cowan University in Western Australia are required to submit and comment on a digital recording of a time management exercise within a simulated ward environment. Similarly, it is now common practice for other health professional students to photograph, scan or replicate products of their practice as part of their portfolio submissions. Pharmacy students from Keele University in Staffordshire in the United Kingdom, for instance, are required to include evidence such as scanned copies of scripts, worksheets and further readings, the commentary of which is then commented upon by their professional mentors (K Maddock, personal communication, 28 August 2013). The clinical application, and where possible the validation of performance by others, supports the authenticity of these products and also demonstrates the educational potential.

Facilitates self-awareness, reflection and analysis

Portfolios have long been recognised as important educational and professional opportunities to engage in and demonstrate reflective and analytical activities and hence generate rather than merely record learning. Traditionally this has been undertaken via journal activities and other approaches where students reflect upon their personal performances to make sense of the experiences and potentially understand how such a performance might rate within professional standards. e-Portfolios have provided extended opportunities whereby platforms or mechanisms are integrated into the activities to direct and structure this reflection. Tasks that track students through the reflective process, at times restricting their progress until earlier tasks are successfully achieved, are features of some but not all e-Portfolio platforms. Given that this is the very essence of a portfolio, even without a set structure, students will need to achieve these skills in order to successfully achieve a quality outcome.

An exemplar that demonstrates the reflective aspect of portfolios well is described by Hall *et al.*[13] Teachers and coaches provide medical students with opportunities for debriefing challenging events within their e-Portfolios and address what they describe as the 'hidden curriculum – norms, values and socialisation issues associated with medical practice.'[13(p745)]

Personal learning space

There has been much discussion in the literature about the value of e-Portfolios being under the students' control and transitioning with them both over time and within the differing study, personal and professional contexts. This personal ownership enables students to work independently and, if appropriate, invite others in to interact, review and provide feedback. Extending on this concept of students having control over the access of others, some platforms also include learning platform structures to support students' engagement in reflection and critique. This follows on from the development of learning management systems such as Blackboard and Moodle, which provide tools to support a structure to enable learning. PebblePad, a commercial e-Portfolio company, assert that their product is more than an e-Portfolio and includes, for instance, inbuilt tools and functions that generate learning as distinct from simply recording and evidencing learning.[14] This is not necessarily a facility of all e-Portfolio platforms, and it may not necessarily be required if the students develop these skills external to the platform.

Collaborative practice

Collaborative practice and contributing to communities of practice are increasingly becoming important professional and educational performance outcomes. With the advent of e-Portfolios, students can now be provided with user-friendly online activities whereby they can collaborate with others. Through the provision of professional social media opportunities, students can present their work to others, engage with feedback and collaborate with others to achieve shared outcomes. While all of these activities can be achieved outside of an e-Portfolio, having these activities stored within a single repository is very convenient.

EXEMPLARS

As Garrett[15] identified, e-Portfolios are a widespread and popular educational technological approach, and while there are many claims about the varied possibilities of e-Portfolios, commonly in practice this is subverted by the focus being solely on assessment outcomes. This is not to say that assessment is not an important stimulus for learning; however, the quality and potential of the learning needs also to be central to portfolio activities. Hence within the responses that inform this chapter, health educationalists were asked to detail how they supported students in achieving outcomes such as collaborative and lifelong learning, higher order thinking and problem-solving, including reflective practice and critical thinking. Exemplars were provided by academics and clinicians in a variety of health professional courses including radiography, dentistry, nursing, midwifery, pharmacy and biomedical science. Access to these professionals was gained through an email invitation placed with the Association for Authentic, Experiential and Evidence-Based Learning; JISCmail listserv (formerly the Joint Information Systems Committee); PebblePad Google Groups; 'The Flinders Plus Group' (Flinders University); and EPAC listserv on Electronic Portfolios. In view of word limitations, for further detail about the survey questions, please contact the corresponding author. Contact details of the corresponding author are located at the beginning of the book under 'contributing chapter authors'.

Achievement record

G Colalillo (personal communication, 3 May 2013) describes how nursing students at the Queensborough Community College in New York select artefacts from their e-Portfolio of coursework, employment and personal experiences to present to the college and healthcare community partners as evidence of their achievements and accomplishments in a showcase awards ceremony on graduation. Reflecting on their e-Portfolio and their educational and personal journey helps students form an identity as a professional nurse. The e-Portfolio developed by nursing students of the Three Rivers Community College in Norwich, Connecticut, has served as a showcase portfolio for employers and continued education (L Rafeldt, personal communication, 4 June 2013). Students are given 'credit' towards being advanced technology users in the workforce and accepted into doctoral programmes that also use an e-Portfolio system. Students in the Operating Department Practice programme of the Buckinghamshire New University in Uxbridge, Middlesex, in the United Kingdom, scan and upload evidence of achievement supported by progress charts (B Nicols, personal communication, 28 June 2013). By reflecting on development and achievements the candidate has a substantial understanding of his or her own growth. If clinical instructors have access to nursing students' e-Portfolios in the clinical setting, they can document achievement of clinical competencies as they are achieved, a convenient way to consolidate learning.[8]

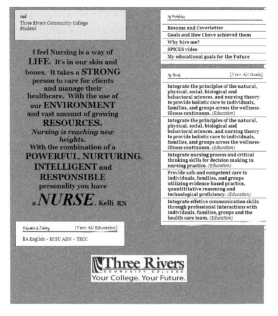

FIGURE 17.1 Example of an introduction to a student's e-Portfolio from Three Rivers Community College (reproduced with permission)

Reflection

Using an e-Portfolio approach has been shown to be effective in assisting students to reflect on their learning achievements at various levels and over time.[15-18] Reflection can be woven throughout a curriculum or positioned at specific times throughout a course of study. In the undergraduate radiography programme at the University of Derby in the United Kingdom, students use the blog tool in PebblePad to keep a reflective diary while completing their clinical placements. Kolb's reflective cycle is used to guide the students' weekly or twice weekly reflective posts, which form part of their formative assessment in third year. E Hyde (personal communication, 27 April 2013) has found that students who use this blog well tend to achieve higher grades in the summative piece of work for the module.

Similarly, Colalillo (personal communication, 3 May 2013) asks nursing students to reflect on their clinical placement experiences to facilitate the development of sound clinical decision-making skills, utilising the DEAL (Describe, Examine, Articulate, Learning) model.[19] Within the e-Portfolio, students debrief after a clinical activity, describe the activity or action objectively in detail, examine the experience with reflection and articulate the learning. They describe how they learned, what they learned and how it is important for their actions and critical thinking skills in the future. Colalillo believes that this process prompts personal growth, civic engagement and/or academic enhancement, and that the use of narrative pedagogy is becoming more recognised by healthcare professionals and healthcare institutions as a tool for critical thinking and decision-making.

The activities within the e-Portfolio can be structured to facilitate the capacity of the learner to move from simple to complex reflection while weaving connections and deeper understanding within and between courses. By example, Colalillo (personal communication, 3 May 2013) explained how, in the first year of the nursing course conducted at the Queensborough Community College in New York, students list their goals and create a profile about themselves as a learner, what they expect to gain from the course and why they chose nursing as a career. As the programme proceeds, reflective prompts and postings in the e-Portfolio allow students to create links with prior learning and experiences, to new and sometimes more complex experiences. The recursive process of revising writing using the scaffolded reflective prompts connects the college experience to prior learning, the coursework to a sense of identity as a learner, and learning to a stronger sense of the strategies and steps that are taken to complete the final product. The elements that make this practice particularly effective are the time and practice that are given to students to develop self-awareness and make the connections to their learning.

Students of the nursing course at the Three Rivers Community College in Connecticut share their reflections of competency achievement with their tutors and peers, a systematic approach to thinking that can be interpreted as critical thinking. Comments as feedback in the e-Portfolio are encouraged to develop inquiring minds leading to learning communities and collaborative working (Rafeldt, personal communication, 4 June 2013).

Collaboration and feedback

Collaborative learning fosters positive interdependence, individual accountability, group processing and social skills[7] and can be enabled using an e-Portfolio. This type of learning may seem at odds when the e-Portfolio is the student's own personal space, yet sharing aspects of an e-Portfolio has multiple benefits. Nursing students at the Three Rivers Community College in Connecticut share their work with faculty and peers when appropriate. Principles of confidentiality are maintained for all patients and clinical settings. Rafeldt describes how students can choose to share personal or sensitive stories with faculty only (personal communication, 4 June 2013). Skills development such as information literacy activities are shared with staff, faculty and peers using the e-Portfolio. Students use a collaborative versus cooperative approach in the hybrid Leadership and Management course for the online discussions; each student researching and posting individual solutions and then the clinical group revising to produce a final group post. A blog assessment held towards the end of the course, where students comment or respond to other students' blogs, allows students to collaborate in one another's professional development.

Garrett *et al.*[8] described how nursing students share aspects of their e-Portfolio with clinical instructors who assess their reflections of the achievement of the nursing competencies. In this situation, when clinical instructors have access to the students' e-Portfolio and are responsible for formative and summative evaluations of the reflective posts, Garrett *et al.*[8] believe it is important that instructors value the use of reflection as a learning tool, and that they agree to confidentiality requirements. Learning is enhanced through social experiences, and for students of the twenty-first century this is especially true. Colalillo describes the use of the Epsilen platform, which has a social learning wiki space where students can freely exchange ideas (personal communication, 3 May 2013). The role of the wiki space can be strengthened if students are able to give feedback to one another. As students are exposed to one another's perspectives and opinions, they are helped to become more tolerant and accepting. Students can serve as models for other learners. In addition, having a peer-review process with students reflecting on one another's work is good practice for developing students' reflection and writing skills. Expanding the wiki space of e-Portfolios to include a vertical learning model, where students in the upper semester share practical tips, knowledge and experiences on difficult concepts with beginning students, is another practice employed in the nursing programme at Queensborough Community College in New York.

Lifelong learning

One of the most significant drivers for e-Portfolios has been lifelong learning. There are expectations that students will continue to use an e-Portfolio after graduation, especially when the associated professional body requires evidence of CPD activities to maintain practitioner registration, such as the Health and Care Professions Council require of radiographers in the United Kingdom (Hyde, personal communication, 27 April 2013). Using the same recording templates required by the professional body during the student's studies, as in the Master of Pharmacy conducted at Keele

University in the United Kingdom, increases the possibility that students, once registered, will continue to use the e-Portfolio to collect evidence of their CPD (Maddock, personal communication, 30 April 2013). Colalillo believes that employers are beginning to recognise the e-Portfolio as a valuable tool in the selection process (personal communication, 3 May 2013). Nicols (personal communication, 28 June 2013) believes that when students own the e-Portfolio, as students in the Diploma in Higher Education in Operating Department Practice do, and can design and individualise the look, they are more likely to 'buy in' to the e-Portfolio as a lifelong learning tool.

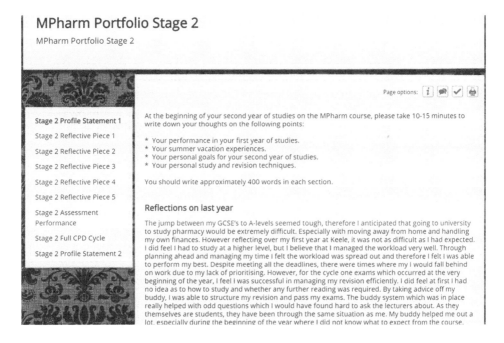

FIGURE 17.2 Screen shot from an e-Portfolio demonstrating reflection (Keele University Master of Pharmacy; reproduced with permission)

Independence from institutionally driven learning

The student owns the e-Portfolio, not the institution. Maddock explains how Master of Pharmacy students from Keele University are mentored by a registered pharmacist or registered pharmacy technician for the first 2 years of their portfolio work (personal communication, 30 April 2013). They are encouraged to reflect upon situations that happen in any area of their life, rather than just the academic environment, to demonstrate that professional development occurs in all aspects of life, not just in academia or the pharmacy practice environment. Rafeldt believes that those students who realise the potential to discover what they want to pursue when they graduate can use the e-Portfolio to gain independence from institutional learning, but many students with numerous outside responsibilities are prevented from putting increased focus on the use of the e-Portfolio beyond the learning assignments (personal communication, 4 June 2013).

A capstone experience bringing the components of a course together as a whole

A culminating experience that draws together an array of student learning in a holistic manner, and hence gives meaning and application to various components of a programme, is referred to as a capstone experience. These activities potentially enhance students' understanding of what they have learned and hence are important strategies in preparing students for postgraduate performance. As Maddock (personal communication, 30 April 2013) identified, when students use their e-Portfolios to reflect on their goals and achievements at the beginning and end of each year of a programme, or a whole programme, this activity can provide a useful capstone experience. Karsten[20] described how nursing students are required to develop a capstone or advanced e-Portfolio in their last semester of the course that documents achievement of all six final nursing competencies, allowing them to 'showcase academic achievement, clinical competence, and critical and analytical thinking ability in an innovative and technologically advanced manner'.[(p26)]

In the case of the undergraduate radiography course at the University of Derby in the United Kingdom, students who develop their e-Portfolio throughout the 3 years of the programme are encouraged to produce a suitable portfolio for job interviews – this portfolio is to represent all they have learned during their programme of study (Hyde, personal communication, 27 April 2013). In doing so, students are able to not only relate their learning outcomes to their career requirements but also reflect on the relevance of their course. Similarly, Raefelt recommended the use of e-Portfolios to assist students to identify, describe and begin to implement their continued education plans after graduation (Rafeldt, personal communication, 4 June 2013). In doing so, students are able to reflect on current skill sets and apply the principles of professional capacity building for future career objectives.

Learner mobility

Being a paperless system enhances the online usability of the e-Portfolio (M Twigger, personal communication, 29 April 2013). This usability is further enhanced when the learning system is independent of the learning platform belonging to the institution offering the educational programmes (Maddock, personal communication, 30 April 2013). This means that students can access their work from anywhere in the world, at any time. They can also share their e-Portfolio with potential employers, along with any attached evidence. When students are not able to use the e-Portfolio platform after graduation, they can be provided with flash drives upon which to copy the learning achieved over time to reinforce the philosophy and pedagogy of looking at learning over time as an iterative process (Rafeldt, personal communication, 4 June 2013).

Learner mobility was a key motivator for the midwifery programme at Edith Cowan University in Western Australia to develop a PebblePad application allowing students to keep records of their clinical activities while on placement. The paper-based portfolio previously used was cumbersome and provided a security risk if left unsecured. The system currently under development is designed to allow students to record information on their smartphones or tablets, thus reducing the need to carry bulky documents while also allowing security lock-out systems (E. Godwin, personal communication, 28 August 2013).

Obstacles and enablers to achieving aims associated with the use of e-Portfolios

As is evidenced in a range of reports about e-Portfolios, uptake and continued use within higher education in Australia and elsewhere has been described as 'flakey'[21] – although increasingly they are being implemented within university units or subjects and as institutional-wide initiatives.[22] Although the use of institutional licensing and specific software is not a focus of this chapter, it is relevant to note that there has been a consistent increase in universities purchasing or accessing licensing agreements with companies such as PebblePad and Mahara, and to a lesser degree with other providers such as Vumi, Adobe ePortfolios, and Chalk and Wire.[14] Recently, employers have started requesting e-Portfolio submission from graduating students applying for positions, and increasingly students are expecting an e-Portfolio as part of a standard university resource on offer. It is reasonable to expect that this will act as a further stimulant for students and universities to adopt e-Portfolios. The following section will provide a brief overview of some of the obstacles and enablers for institutions and staff in adopting e-Portfolios.

It has been well acknowledged both in the literature and anecdotally that problems arise when the strategic intent of the academic institution does not provide adequate support for the implementation and use of the e-Portfolio.[21-23] When an e-Portfolio is unambiguously linked to a university's strategic direction, explicitly accepted as an integral part of a university course, and woven overtly throughout a curriculum and topic assessment, its chances of success are significantly increased. Similarly, when the pedagogy of the e-Portfolio (social, reflective, collaborative, transparent and iterative synthesis on who you will become, and meeting the programme outcomes) is emphasised and faculty understand it, its use continues to grow (Rafeldt, personal communication, 4 June 2013).

Colalillo expresses the common complaint that if faculty do not embrace the e-Portfolio themselves, it reduces student motivation and the staff skills to assist (personal communication, 3 May 2013). As Colalillo explained, when she began developing her own teaching e-Portfolio, it enabled her to understand both the amount of work required and the value of reviewing, revising and evaluating achievements and accomplishments (personal communication, 3 May 2013). In her example, faculty and students have presented at conferences, and enthusiasm has spurred growth and pilots by other departments. Similarly, Rafeldt described how the first-year nursing students were excited to use an e-Portfolio but faculty were hesitant or resistant. Then with continued use, inclusion in syllabi and outlines and awarding points for work in some courses, the use of the e-Portfolio as a learning tool increased (personal communication, 4 June 2013).

Offering rewards and recognition for the efforts of faculty members to use an e-Portfolio, such as an honorarium and letter of appreciation from the dean, have been successful in facilitating the success of the system across a medical campus.[13] It is also helpful when a departmental decision to use e-Portfolio in all courses or units is made, and when an incremental course implementation plan is in place across all courses (Rafeldt, personal communication, 4 June 2013). Hall *et al.*[13] described how the success of their e-Portfolio programme with medical students was enhanced when students were invited to be members of the e-Portfolio faculty committees, and involved in decisions about how the e-Portfolio was presented to and used by students. Twigger (personal communication, 29 April 2013) believes that good teamwork and the ability to be open in discussion enables the success of the use of e-Portfolio.

Tying the use of the e-Portfolio together with a compulsory pass or fail element of each year of the degree course has been shown to enhance student engagement with the activities it promotes (Rafeldt, personal communication, 4 June 2013). It is recommended that e-Portfolio exercises and assignments be integrated across the whole curriculum, with faculty developing their own teaching e-Portfolio as role models for students. Incorporation of assessment using e-Portfolio as a part of teaching and learning can be promoted to the faculty through professional development days and committee meetings, reports and presentations (Rafeldt, personal communication, 4 June 2013). Similarly, this mandatory nature of e-Portfolio has been found by Hall *et al.*[13] to facilitate uptake and ongoing commitment. Indeed, results from a student survey and an analysis of e-Portfolio server data in a study by von Konsky and Oliver[23] demonstrated that the e-Portfolio uptake and use was 'driven largely by assessment requirements'.[(p68)]

Hyde (personal communication, 27 April 2013) explains how, in an undergraduate radiography course, there has been a lack of support from clinical partners to embed the portfolio into all aspects of students' clinical work. To overcome this she has supplemented it with a paper-based version for some aspects. Hyde also believes that an environmentally friendly argument can be used with students if they are encouraged to use the e-Portfolio as a backup to the paper parts of their portfolio. Clinicians and students need easy access to the e-Portfolio via the Internet while on clinical placements. Hyde explains that when Internet access on clinical placement is an issue, students are advised to think ahead about how they can access the e-Portfolio on placement (personal communication, 27 April 2013).

When students are first introduced to using the e-Portfolio, it is easy to underestimate the workload associated with providing them with individual feedback (J. D'Souza, personal communication, 30 April 2013). To overcome this, biomedical science students attended several workshops to assist them and provide generic feedback to enable progress. It is anticipated that employing peer reviewers will alleviate the lack of feedback received, as this should be more timely and the guidance written now for students is much more comprehensive in format. The positive outcome was to have 100% e-Portfolio submission at the deadline.

Maddock has concerns that students not having access to an e-Portfolio after graduation act as a disincentive for students during the course, and an impediment to allowing the e-Portfolio to contribute to lifelong learning (Maddock, personal communication, 30 April 2013). While this may appear to be an insurmountable problem if your institution lacks this resource, Hyde addressed this through introducing the class of radiology students to the publicly available versions of the tool (personal communication, 27 April 2013). Finally, the issue of long-term commitment to e-Portfolio to ensure its success means that institutions need to provide the necessary policies, funding and support structures to enable its success. Since a centralised model is more successful than topic or course-based implementation, it is recommended that funding for resources should be quarantined with this objective in mind. Similarly, it is recommended that organisational policies that support e-Portfolio be implemented in a top-down approach. In the national audit of e-Portfolio practice undertaken by the Australian Learning and Teaching Council in 2008, they surveyed academic managers who cited teaching and learning policy as the most important driver for e-Portfolio implementation.[17]

CONCLUSION

There is no doubt that implementation of e-Portfolios into health professional education can be challenging. But these challenges also represent opportunities! Integrating e-Portfolios into our curricula allows us to develop our students into highly skilled individuals with a personal commitment to lifelong learning. Many pedagogically sound principles of learning and teaching can be reinforced as students build and create their own learning spaces, respond to constructive feedback and engage with technology. Faculty in organisational settings can learn from one another as they share their personal and student-related e-Portfolio experiences. This strengthens collegial bonds and enhances their working life.

SUMMARY POINTS

- Electronic portfolios have become increasingly popular in universities in recent years to promote the collection of, and reflection on, evidence of learning.
- The uptake of e-Portfolios has plateaued recently, however, with evidence suggesting that this is in part due to inevitable implementation difficulties, from both a technological and an educational perspective.
- There are some potential pitfalls of implementing e-Portfolios.
- The exemplars and reflections of successful users are intended to provide genuine insights and advice to those wanting to enhance or commence their use of e-Portfolios.
- e-Portfolios have the potential to contribute to the educational repertoire by providing students with resources to record their achievements in a secure manner; engage in reflection, collaboration and peer feedback; and more broadly stimulate lifelong learning that transitions between personal, professional and formal learning.

REVIEW QUESTIONS

- How can we best use e-Portfolios to understand and enhance students' emerging sense of professional identity?
- The use of e-Portfolios as a peer-review tool in the development and dissemination of research initiatives is on the horizon. How might this best be facilitated?
- How might we best evaluate the effectiveness of e-Portfolios in enhancing student learning?
- What are some ways to assess students' e-Portfolios effectively and efficiently?
- How might you use an e-Portfolio across a programme of study to scaffold and enhance learning?

REFLECTIVE QUESTIONS AND EXERCISES

- You would like to recommend the implementation of an e-Portfolio in your faculty or organisation. What support systems need to be in place to ensure your success?
- How might you use an e-Portfolio for yourself? When addressing this question, consider a broad range of applications including your research, community engagement and teaching roles.

REFERENCES

1. Dahlstrom E, Walker JD, Dziuban C. *ECAR Study of Undergraduate Students and Information Technology, 2013.* Louisville, CO: EDUCAUSE Center for Analysis and Research; 2013. Available at: https://net.educause.edu/ir/library/pdf/ERS1302/ERS1302.pdf (accessed 3 February 2014).
2. Jisc. *e-Portfolios – An Overview.* www.jisc.ac.uk/whatwedo/programmes/elearning/eportfolios.aspx (accessed 3 February 2014).
3. University of Cambridge. *Digital Repositories.* www.lib.cam.ac.uk/dataman/pages/repositories.html (accessed 3 February 2014).
4. Sutherland S, Brotchie J, Chesney S. *Pebblegogy: ideas and activities to inspire and engage learners.* Telford, UK: Pebble Learning; 2011.
5. *Collins English Dictionary.* Complete and unabridged 10th ed. Glasgow: HarperCollins; 2009.
6. US Department of Education, Office of Educational Technology. *Expanding Evidence Approaches for Learning in a Digital World.* Washington, DC: US Department of Education; 2013. Available at: http://apo.org.au/files/Resource/usgov_expanding-evidence-approaches_2013.pdf. (accessed 12 October 2014).
7. Johnson DW, Johnson F. *Joining Together: group theory and group skills.* 10th ed. Boston, MA: Allyn & Bacon; 2009.
8. Garrett BM, MacPhee M, Jackson C. Evaluation of an ePortfolio for the assessment of clinical competence in a baccalaureate nursing program. *Nurse Educ Today.* 2012; **33**(10): 1207–13.
9. André K, Heartfield M. *Nursing and Midwifery Portfolios: evidence of continuing competence.* Chatswood, NSW: Churchill Livingstone/Elsevier Australia; 2011.

10. Hartnell-Young E, Morris M. *Digital Portfolios: powerful tools for promoting professional growth.* Thousand Oaks, CA: Corwin Press; 2007.

11. Simmons C, Williams A, Sher W, *et al. Work ready: e-Portfolios to support professional placements.* Sydney, NSW: Office of Teaching and Learning; 2012.

12. Gordon JA, Campbell CM. The role of ePortfolios in supporting continuing professional development in practice. *Med Teach.* 2013; **35**(4): 287–94.

13. Hall P, Byszewski A, Sutherland S. Developing a sustainable electronic portfolio (ePortfolio) program that fosters reflective practice and incorporates CanMEDS competencies into the undergraduate medical curriculum. *Acad Med.* 2012; **87**(6): 744–51.

14. PebblePad. *About PebblePad.* www.pebblepad.com.au/l/pebblepad.aspx (accessed 12 October 2014).

15. Garrett N. An ePortfolio design supporting ownership, social learning, and ease of use. *Educ Technol Soc.* 2011; **14**(1): 187–202.

16. Chen HL, Light TP. *Electronic Portfolios and Student Success: effectiveness, efficiency, and learning.* Washington, DC: Association of American Colleges and Universities; 2010.

17. Hallam G, Harper W, McCowan C, *et al. Australian ePortfolio Project. ePortfolio use by university students in Australia: informing excellence in policy and practice.* Brisbane, QLD: Queensland University of Technology; 2008.

18. Joyes G, Gray L, Hartnell-Young E. Effective practice with e-Portfolios: how can the UK experience inform implementation? *Aust J Educ Technol.* 2010; **26**(1): 15–27.

19. Ash SL, Clayton PH, Moses MG. *Schematic Overview of the DEAL Model for Critical Reflection: teaching and learning through critical reflection; an instructors' guide.* Sterling, VA: Stylus Publishing; 2007.

20. Karsten K. Using ePortfolio to demonstrate competence in associate degree nursing students. *Teach Learn Nurs.* 2012; **7**(1): 23–6.

21. Jisc. *Crossing the threshold: moving e-Portfolios into the mainstream.* Bristol: Jisc; 2012. Available at: www.jisc.ac.uk/publications/programmerelated/2012/crossingthethreshold.aspx (accessed 12 October 2014).

22. Hallum G, Harper W, McAllister L, *et al. Australian ePortfolio Practice – Supplementary Report. E-Portfolio use by university students in Australia: informing excellence in policy and practice.* Brisbane, QLD: Queensland University of Technology; 2010.

23. Von Konsky BR, Oliver B. The iPortfolio: measuring uptake and effective use of an institutional electronic portfolio in higher education. *Aust J Educ Technol.* 2013; **28**(1): 67–90.

CHAPTER 18

Simulation in health professional education

Application and evidence

....

Tracy Levett-Jones

OVERVIEW

The use of simulation in health professional education has evolved at an unprecedented pace. However, similar to many other teaching and learning innovations, the evidence base for simulation has not kept up with its rapid expansion and utilisation. Multimillion-dollar investments in infrastructure and simulation equipment have been made, too often with limited evidence of effectiveness or utility. There is some evidence suggesting that exposure to simulation, irrespective of the level of fidelity and modalities in use, is likely to have a positive impact on learner satisfaction and confidence. There is also increasing research claiming that simulation improves learners' knowledge, clinical reasoning, communication and teamwork skills, although these remain somewhat contested areas. While there has undoubtedly been an increase in the quality and amount of simulation research in recent years, important questions of transferability to practice and improved patient outcomes are yet to be convincingly addressed.

This chapter outlines and critiques the current evidence base for the use of simulation as a teaching and learning strategy for health professional students. Simulation best practice is discussed and recommendations for future research are offered.

CHAPTER OBJECTIVES

Upon completion of this chapter, the reader will be able to:

- discuss the current use of simulation in health professional education
- discuss the evidence base for the use of simulation in health professional education
- identify the research gaps that currently exist in simulation research
- recommend opportunities for future research
- propose research projects to address identified knowledge gaps.

KEY TERMS: simulation, evidence, transferability, quality, best practice

INTRODUCTION

'What's wrong with me? I can't get my breath. I'm scared … can't you do something?' 'Jack', a SimMan 3G™ manikin, gasps. Disbelief immediately suspended and fully immersed in the unfolding scenario, the students begin to take control. One responds, hesitantly at first, and others soon join in. 'Sit him up,' one person says, 'and get some oxygen … quickly!' Some students stand back, overwhelmed, unsure. One wants to make a rapid response call; another begins to auscultate Jack's lungs …

One group of students after another complete the simulation session, followed by a debriefing. 'That was amazing', one student says. Another laments, 'I had no idea what to do … I made so many mistakes.' All agree that the experience has been valuable, that they 'learned so much' and they 'feel more confident now'.

Few educators who have observed or been involved in a simulation session would disagree that this teaching and learning approach appears to be effective. However, the evidence base for simulation is limited and further research to validate such interventions and to add to the tacit knowledge that underpins this educational strategy is imperative. Additionally, in a time of economic rationalisation, the significant investment of time and money required for simulation experiences must be justified by evidence of effectiveness. This chapter discusses what we know and what we are still learning about the use of simulation as a teaching and learning strategy for health professional students. Simulation best practice is discussed, the quality of the current body of evidence for simulation outcomes is considered, and recommendations for future research are provided.

THE DEFINITION, EVOLUTION AND IMPETUS FOR THE USE OF SIMULATION

Simulation is broadly defined as an educational strategy in which elements of the real world are appropriately integrated to achieve specific goals related to learning or evaluation.[1] While this chapter, and indeed most of the current simulation research, focuses primarily on the use of human patient simulation manikins, it is acknowledged that there are many other less-technical simulation modalities, including actors, standardised patients and virtual worlds, to name just a few. While fascination with high-technology and high-fidelity simulation approaches is understandable, the type of equipment or technology used (as well as all other educational decisions) should be driven by desired learning outcomes and evidence of effectiveness (*see* Table 18.1 for fidelity descriptions).

TABLE 18.1 Levels of simulation fidelity

Term	Description
Fidelity	How authentic or lifelike the manikin and/or simulation experience is (sometimes referred to as the technological level)
Low fidelity	Simple task trainers such as intravenous arms and resuscitation torsos, and anatomically correct full-body static manikins that replicate the external anatomy and joint movement of humans but which have no interactive capacity
Medium fidelity	Full-body manikins, usually with embedded software; they are controlled by an external, handheld or wireless device and have limited physiological responses, such as palpable pulse and blood pressure on one arm, and verbal noises limited to breath sounds, coughing, vomiting, groaning and one syllable words
High fidelity	Actors, standardised patients or lifelike manikins with embedded software that can be remotely controlled by computer (usually in a separate control room), enabling individualised, programmed scenarios that allow the operator to set physiological parameters and respond to learners' interventions with changes in voice, heart rate, respiratory rate, blood pressure, oxygen saturation level and other physiological signs

The use of simulation has advanced at an exponential rate over the last decade.[2] DeVita,[3] in advocating for the increased use of simulation in health professional education, argued that simulation should be a core education strategy because it is 'measurable, focused, reproducible, mass producible, and importantly, very memorable.'[3(p46)] However, the evidence base for simulation has not kept pace with the increasing investment in resources and equipment. In nursing,[4] pharmacy[5] and medicine,[6] for example, there has been an ongoing quest for rigorous and valid ways to evaluate the outcomes of simulation sessions. While there has been some growth in the quality and maturity of simulation research and related simulation evaluation instruments in recent years,[7] questions of transferability to practice and improved patient outcomes are yet to be convincingly addressed. Later in this chapter, these issues are discussed with reference to Kirkpatrick's[8] levels of evaluation.

Simulation provides authentic and meaningful opportunities for students to engage in experiential learning.[9] Multiple benefits of simulation for students include opportunities (a) for active involvement in challenging clinical situations that involve unpredictable simulated patient deterioration; (b) for exposure to time-sensitive and critical clinical scenarios that, if encountered in a 'real' clinical environment, students could normally only passively observe; (c) to integrate clinical skills and content knowledge in realistic but non-threatening environments; (d) to develop both technical and non-technical skills; and (e) to make mistakes and learn from them without risk to patients.[9,10] There are also assertions that simulation benefits students by improving their confidence, competence, clinical reasoning and problem-solving skills.[11] Limited availability and questions about the quality of some clinical placements has also been cited as rationale for increasing students' exposure to simulation experiences, and simulation has been used both to prepare students for clinical placements and as remediation.[12] Perhaps most important, some studies have shown that simulation may have the potential to affect patient safety positively and to reduce clinical errors.[13,14]

SIMULATION BEST PRACTICE

Two important studies sought to identify the factors that define quality in terms of simulation education. Issenberg *et al.*[15] undertook a systematic review of 109 studies and developed a list of conditions that facilitate learning in simulation. These conditions, which are in many respects a synthesis of educational models and theories, include:

- the provision of timely feedback
- opportunities for repetitive practice
- curriculum integration of simulation
- provision of increasing levels of difficulty
- clearly defined and measurable outcomes
- ensuring validity of the simulation scenario and experience.

Arthur *et al.*[16] used a modified Delphi technique to achieve consensus of international expert opinion regarding quality use of simulation. The Delphi method involves the systematic solicitation and collection of expert opinions on a particular topic through sequential questionnaires interspersed with feedback derived from earlier responses. After three survey rounds, a set of quality indicator statements was agreed upon (*see* Table 18.2).

TABLE 18.2 Quality indicators for the use of simulation

Quality indicator	Description
Pedagogical principles	Simulation experiences should be aligned with the curriculum and course objectives. Scaffolding of learning experiences should occur and the required knowledge, psychomotor skills, clinical reasoning skills, reflective thinking skills and use of healthcare technologies should be taught prior to the simulation experience. Simulation, in some form, should be integrated into all clinical courses and should progress in complexity throughout the programme. Learning objectives should guide all aspects of the simulation.
Fidelity	The range of simulation approaches used should be consistent with learning objectives, resource availability and cost-effectiveness. Environmental fidelity (e.g. clinical documentation and equipment) is as important as scenario and simulation fidelity.

(continued)

Quality indicator	Description
Student preparation and orientation	A structured orientation should be provided for students prior to the simulation session.
Debriefing	A structured debriefing should be provided immediately following the simulation to facilitate students' reflection on practice, self-evaluation and feedback on their perceptions of the experience. Depending on the simulation objectives, opportunities for discussion of students' non-technical skills such as clinical reasoning, situation awareness, communication, leadership and teamwork should be included in the debrief.
Staff preparation and training	Staff who design scenarios, conduct the simulation sessions, facilitate debriefing and manage the technology should have each undertaken appropriate training.

THE EVIDENCE BASE FOR SIMULATION

A useful framework for considering the outcomes and impact of simulation is Kirkpatrick's[8] levels of evaluation (*see* Table 18.3). This framework highlights how the vast majority of simulation research is still of a relatively low level. Without doubt, attitudes and perceptions are still the 'low-hanging fruit' of simulation evaluation,[7] with minimal evidence demonstrating the transferability and sustainability of simulation outcomes to clinical practice. While on face value this may seem to cast doubt on the utility and effectiveness of simulation, this lack of evidence is more because of a lack of rigorous evaluation than evidence of ineffectiveness. As is the case with many educational activities, evaluation of simulation-related learning outcomes is fraught with conceptual and practical difficulties. That said, educators involved in simulation research should be encouraged to use evaluation instruments with strong evidence of psychometric integrity, and to consider approaches that strengthen the evidence base for simulation by turning their attention to Kirkpatrick's[8] levels 3 and 4.

TABLE 18.3 Kirkpatrick's[8] model of evaluation of educational outcomes

Level	Description
1: Reaction	Learners' perceptions of value or degree of satisfaction with the simulation experience
2a: Modification of attitudes and perceptions	Changes in learners' attitudes, perceptions or confidence
2b: Acquisition of knowledge and skills	Evidence of cognitive changes or improvement in skills or knowledge
3: Behavioural change	Sustained changed (in knowledge, abilities or behaviours) over time and transfer of learning to clinical practice
4a: Change in organisational practice	Wider changes in the organisation and delivery of care
4b: Benefits to patients or clients	Improved patient outcomes and patient safety

Kirkpatrick's[8] four levels of educational outcomes delineate the types of evidence produced by different simulation evaluations. Most instruments currently in use tend to focus on participant satisfaction, confidence, attitudes and knowledge acquisition. These outcomes correspond to levels one and two of Kirkpatrick's[8] model (*see* Table 18.3).

KNOWLEDGE ACQUISITION

In a systematic review of 23 studies undertaken by Laschinger *et al.*,[17] assessment of knowledge acquisition was identified as the most common approach used to determine the effectiveness of simulation sessions, with the use of multiple-choice questions (MCQs) evident in 18 of the studies reviewed. 'Pre- then post-test' MCQs are convenient to administer and are relatively uncomplicated to analyse. However, to date, the results have been variable and inconclusive. Educators are sometimes surprised and disappointed by results of 'pre- then post-tests' that use MCQs to evaluate the effectiveness of simulations. In fact, many studies have shown a deterioration in knowledge following the simulation experience, suggesting the need for repetition and reinforcement of students' learning.[18-19]

A systematic review by Lapkin *et al.*[20] identified five studies that demonstrated a statistically significant difference in knowledge acquisition when using high-fidelity manikins.[21-25] However, each of these studies had methodological shortcomings, with the use of convenience samples and small sample sizes being a feature of many. In addition, only one of the studies[23] examined whether knowledge remained stable over time. Most of the studies in this review used MCQs developed by academics or taken from an item bank.[26]

Two studies[19,27] explored and compared knowledge acquisition in students exposed to medium- and high-fidelity manikins. In a study by Kardong-Edgren *et al.*,[19] MCQs were used to assess knowledge levels before and 2 weeks and 6 months after the intervention. Results indicated significant increases in knowledge for all groups at post-test 1 but significant decreases in knowledge for all groups at post-test 2, 6 months later. The authors of this paper acknowledged that an MCQ test may not have been a valid tool to evaluate the potential higher-order thinking benefits of simulation activities. In a study by Levett-Jones *et al.*,[27] a quasi-experimental design was used to evaluate the effect of the level of manikin fidelity on knowledge acquisition using a 'pre- then post-test' design. Although there was some improvement in knowledge scores in both the control group (medium fidelity) and the experimental group (high fidelity), this was not significant. No statistically significant difference was identified between groups in test 1 (prior to the simulation), test 2 (before the debrief) or test 3 (2 weeks later).

While the results outlined here should be factored into decision-making, they do need to be considered with a degree of caution, as the validity and appropriateness of using MCQs as a method of assessing the effectiveness of simulation experiences is questionable. Although the most common form of assessment in undergraduate programmes, few academics have adequate experience and training in developing quality MCQs,[28] and questions taken from commercial test banks, including those taken from textbooks, are not without problems. Additionally, the equivocal results from these studies suggest that assessment of knowledge acquisition using MCQs, although relatively convenient, may not be an appropriate method for measuring the effectiveness of simulation experiences. Levett-Jones *et al.*[27] proposed that, in seeking to validate the effectiveness of simulation sessions, it may be counterintuitive to use MCQs that focus most often on lower-order cognitive skills, as simulation experiences are designed to promote higher-order thinking skills such as critical thinking, clinical judgement and clinical reasoning. There is a real need for further evaluation using more in-depth and holistic approaches for assessing knowledge acquisition and cognitive abilities as outcomes of simulation – for example, objective structured clinical examinations and verbal protocol analysis.

SATISFACTION

Student satisfaction is accorded a lot of weight and it significantly influences if and to what extent educational activities are integrated into university curricula. Although student satisfaction is one of the lower-level learning outcomes of Fitzpatrick's model, it is nevertheless important, as there is evidence that it facilitates active and purposeful participation in learning experiences.[29] There are also suggestions that student satisfaction may have some correlation with performance, with educational psychologists identifying that satisfaction helps to build self-confidence, which in turn helps students develop skills and acquire knowledge.[30]

A number of studies have reported on the levels of satisfaction with simulation experiences, and results consistently indicate that, overall, students tend to be highly satisfied with this type of learning activity.[30–32] Such studies include the use of high-fidelity manikins for mock cardiac arrest training, and when lectures or tutorials are supplemented with simulation sessions.[33,34] The impact of manikin fidelity on student satisfaction is less clear, however. In studies by Levett-Jones *et al.*[35] and Kardong-Edgren *et al.*,[19] no statistically significant difference was found between students exposed to either medium- or high-fidelity manikins. Similarly, no statistically significant differences were found in student satisfaction when comparing high- and low-fidelity manikins for life support training in a study by Hoadley.[36] By contrast, in a study by Jeffries and Rizzolo,[25] student satisfaction was higher when using high-fidelity manikins than when using either low-fidelity manikins or a paper-based case study. These contradictory findings have important cost-benefit implications and indicate the need for further research, particularly as there is currently an impetus to invest in high-fidelity manikins despite the increasing fiscal constraints being experienced by many universities and health services.

CONFIDENCE

Another frequently evaluated outcome of simulation is confidence. This is appropriate, given that clinicians with adequate knowledge and skills may be reluctant to take appropriate actions unless they are confident in their abilities.[37] Evaluating self-confidence following simulation experiences has most often used 'pre- then post-test' designs. Examples of studies focusing on self-confidence include confidence in caring for a patient experiencing pain,[38] confidence working in a highly technological environment;[21] self-perception of ability to lead a cardiopulmonary arrest;[39] and confidence in communication and teamwork during a simulated emergency situation.[40]

The majority of the papers report that students participating in a simulation session are more confident following the simulation. However, few studies reported statistically significant results using valid and reliable instruments.[22,41] Additionally, it should be noted that confidence is not necessarily commensurate with competence, and care should be taken that newfound confidence does not lead learners to adopt inappropriate behaviours in the workplace.

CLINICAL REASONING

The dynamic nature of contemporary healthcare settings requires health professionals to assume more complex roles, which, in turn, necessitates the acquisition of a requisite level of critical thinking and clinical reasoning (sometimes referred to as clinical judgement or decision-making) abilities during their undergraduate education. Clinical reasoning is a process that involves both cognition and metacognition (or reflective thinking) and which is dependent upon a critical thinking 'disposition'. Development of critical thinking and clinical reasoning skills enhances the clinician's ability to build on previously acquired knowledge and past experiences in order to address new or unfamiliar situations. Clinical reasoning is an essential component of competence, and clinicians with effective clinical reasoning skills have a positive impact on patient outcomes; conversely, those with poor clinical reasoning skills often fail to detect impending patient deterioration, thus compromising patient safety and resulting in a 'failure to rescue'.[42] Simulation has been increasingly advocated as a method of enhancing health professionals' clinical reasoning and critical thinking skills.

A systematic review by Lapkin *et al.*,[20] which included randomised and quasi-randomised controlled trials, identified only seven studies that examined the effectiveness of simulation in terms of improved clinical reasoning skills. Five of these studies[21,43–46] compared exposure to high-fidelity manikins with exposure to usual nursing courses. One study compared the outcomes between students exposed to manikins of different levels of fidelity.[25] Another study compared outcomes between undergraduate nursing students exposed to simulation and those exposed to a written case study only.[24]

The results of the systematic review were inconclusive. Although one study[45] reported a statistically significant increase in the ability of students to identify deteriorating patients, most of the studies evaluated only critical thinking abilities[24,45,46] or simply knowledge acquisition.[22,25] While knowledge and critical thinking inform clinical reasoning,[47,48] the results of these studies are inconclusive in regard to the effectiveness of simulation on clinical reasoning skills.

Many of the studies that featured in the review had weak designs and small sample sizes, and a number were missing important details regarding the research methods utilised. These issues, along with the lack of unequivocal evidence on the effectiveness of simulation in the teaching of clinical reasoning skills, calls for further research using larger sample sizes and more rigorous 'pre- then post-test' multi-site experimental studies with reliable and valid instruments.

COMMUNICATION AND TEAMWORK

In a landmark study examining sentinel events in healthcare settings, communication errors were implicated in over 70% of cases.[49] Healthcare is becoming increasingly complex; this complexity coupled with inherent human performance limitations – even in experienced, skilled and committed health professionals – means that errors will inevitably happen. However, patient-safe communication and effective teamwork can help prevent these errors from becoming consequential and harming patients.[50] Simulation provides a wealth of opportunities for students to practise and develop their communication and teamwork skills. In simulation, students can practise the language of effective communication in a realistic setting. Additionally, simulation experiences provide opportunities to record, review and repeat communication scenarios and can be used to identify and thereby avoid common communication errors within and across professional groups.[51]

Standardised communication tools such as ISBAR (Identify, Situation, Background, Assessment and Recommendation) and IMIST-AMBO (Identification, Mechanism, Injuries, Signs, Treatment and Trends, Allergies, Medications, Background, Other issues) can be practised safely in the simulation environment without risk to patients.[52] Although few studies have focused on this aspect of the simulation, Marshall et al.[53] found a statistically significant difference between medical students exposed to ISBAR training prior to participating in a simulation scenario and those who were not exposed to the training.

Actors or standardised patients are often used in communication skills training for medical students and less often for nursing students. While inconsistent results are evident, the majority do point to improvements in performance in students exposed to simulation experiences as opposed to lectures, role plays and videos.[54-56] However, issues of transferability to practice and potential impact on patient care remain less well understood.

CONCLUSION

The multiple diverse studies outlined in this chapter bear testament to the impact that simulation has, and will continue to have, on health professional education. What is equally apparent is that the body of research underpinning simulation is growing in both quantity and quality. There is unequivocal evidence attesting to the fact that exposure to simulation, irrespective of the level of fidelity and modalities in use, is most likely to have a positive impact on learner satisfaction and confidence. There is also increasing evidence supporting the premise that simulation improves learners' knowledge, clinical reasoning, communication and teamwork, although these remain somewhat contested areas. To date, there are few studies that demonstrate evidence of transferability to practice and improved patient outcomes. Despite the inherent challenges and complexity, educators should seek to address these issues with rigorous research designs and evaluation instruments that have strong evidence of psychometric integrity.

SUMMARY POINTS

- The use of simulation in health professional education has grown at an unprecedented pace.
- The investment of time and money required for simulation must be justified by evidence of effectiveness.
- Although improving, the current evidence base for simulation is limited in depth and quality.
- Simulation is said to enhance learner satisfaction and confidence and to improve learners' knowledge, clinical reasoning, communication and teamwork skills.
- Questions of the transferability of learning from simulation to clinical practice are yet to be convincingly addressed.

REVIEW QUESTIONS

- What are some of the challenges associated with implementing a simulation programme for health professional students?
- What are some of the challenges associated with simulation research?
- Why is there limited evidence of transferability of learning from simulation to clinical practice?
- What types of patient outcomes are potentially enhanced through the learner's exposure to simulation?

REFLECTIVE QUESTIONS AND EXERCISES

- Is the improvement in confidence that is said to arise from exposure to simulation always a positive learning outcome? Why?
- What well-substantiated arguments could you use to support your organisation's investment in simulation?
- How might you design a research project that evaluates the effectiveness of simulation in improving the non-technical skills of health professional students? How would you address questions of reliability and validity?
- Meta-analyses provide a higher level of evidence. What is needed in order for a meta-analysis of the effectiveness of simulation to be undertaken?

REFERENCES

1. Gaba D. The future vision of simulation in healthcare. *Simul Healthc.* 2007; **2**(2): 126–35.
2. Health Workforce Australia. *Simulated Learning Environments Program.* www.hwa.gov.au/work-programs/clinical-training-reform/simulated-learning-environments-sles (accessed 15 May 2013).
3. DeVita M. Society for simulation in healthcare presidential address, January 2009. *Simul Healthc.* 2009; **41**(1): 43–8.
4. Davis A, Kimble L. Human patient simulation evaluation rubrics for nursing education: measuring the essentials of baccalaureate education for professional nursing practice. *J Nurs Educ.* 2011; **50**(11): 605–11.
5. Bray B, Schwartz C, Odegard P, *et al.* Assessment of human patient simulation-based learning. *Am J Pharm Educ.* 2011; **75**(10): 208.
6. Kogan J, Holmboe E, Hauer K. Tools for direct observation and assessment of clinical skills of medical trainees. *JAMA.* 2009; **302**(12): 1216–326.
7. Adamson K, Kardon-Edgren S, Willhaus H. An updated review of published simulation evaluation instruments. *Clin Simul Nurs.* 2012; **9**(9) e393–400.
8. Kirkpatrick D. *Evaluating Training Programs: the four levels.* San Francisco, CA: Bennett-Koehler; 1994.
9. Jeffries P, Rizzolo M. *Designing and Implementing Models for the Innovative Use of Simulation to Teach Nursing Care of Ill Adults and Children: a national, multi-site, multi-method study.* New York, NY: National League for Nursing; 2006.
10. Larew C, Lessans S, Spunt D, *et al.* Innovations in clinical simulation: application of Benner's theory in an interactive patient care simulation. *Nurs Educ Perspect.* 2006; **27**(1): 16–21.
11. Rudd C, Freeman K, Smith P. *Use of Simulated Learning Environments in Paramedicine Curricula.* Canberra, ACT: Health Workforce Australia; 2010.
12. Ward-Smith P. The effect of simulation learning as a quality initiative. *Urol Nurs.* 2008; **28**(6): 471–3.
13. Boyle M, Williams B, Burgess S. Contemporary simulation education for undergraduate paramedic students. *Emerg Med J.* 2007; **24**(12): 854–7.
14. Croskerry P, Wears R, Binder L. Setting the educational agenda and curriculum for error prevention in emergency medicine. *Acad Emerg Med.* 2000; **7**(11): 1194–200.
15. Issenberg S, McGaghie W, Petrusa E, *et al.* Features and uses of high fidelity medical simulation that lead to effective learning: a BEME systematic review. *Med Teach.* 2005; **27**(1): 10–28.
16. Arthur C, Kable A, Levett-Jones T. Quality indicators for the design and implementation of simulation experiences: a Delphi study. *Nurse Educ Today.* 2013; **33**(11): 1357–61.
17. Laschinger S, Medves J, Pulling C, *et al.* Effectiveness of simulation on health profession students' knowledge, skills, confidence and satisfaction. *Int J Evid Based Healthc.* 2008; **6**(3): 278–302.
18. Bruce S, Scherer Y, Curran C, *et al.* A collaborative exercise between graduate and undergraduate nursing students using a computer assisted simulator in a mock cardiac arrest. *Nurs Educ Perspect.* 2009; **30**(1): 22–7.
19. Kardong-Edgren S, Lungstrom N, Bendel B. VitalSim versus SimMan: a comparison of BSN student test scores, knowledge retention and satisfaction. *Clin Simul Nurs.* 2009; **5**: e105–11.
20. Lapkin S, Fernandez R, Levett-Jones T. The effectiveness of using human patient simulation manikins in the teaching of clinical reasoning skills to undergraduate nursing students: a systematic review. *Joanna Briggs Institute Library of Systematic Reviews* (JBI000287). 2010; **8**(16): 661–94.
21. Alinier G, Hunt B, Gordon R, *et al.* Effectiveness of intermediate-fidelity simulation training technology in undergraduate nursing education. *J Adv Nurs.* 2006; **54**(3): 359–69.
22. Brannan J, White A, Bezanson J. Simulator effects on cognitive skills and confidence levels. *J Nurs Educ.* 2008; **47**(11): 495–500.

23. Hoffmann R, O'Donnell J, Kim Y. The effects of human patient simulators on basic knowledge in critical care nursing with undergraduate senior baccalaureate nursing students. *Simul Healthc.* 2007; **2**(2): 110–14.

24. Howard V. *A Comparison of Educational Strategies for the Acquisition of Medical-Surgical Nursing Knowledge and Critical Thinking Skills: human patient simulator vs. the interactive case study approach.* Pittsburgh, PA: University of Pittsburgh; 2007.

25. Jeffries P, Rizzolo M. *NLN/Laerdal Project Summary Report: designing and implementing models for the innovative use of simulation to teach nursing care of ill adults and children; a national multi-site study.* New York, NY: National League for Nursing; 2006.

26. Cant R, Cooper S. Simulation-based learning in nurse education: systematic review. *J Adv Nurs.* 2009; **66**(1): 3–15.

27. Levett-Jones T, Lapkin S, Hoffman K, *et al.* A comparison of knowledge acquisition in students exposed to medium versus high fidelity human patient simulation manikins. *Nurs Educ Pract.* 2011; **11**: 380–3.

28. Tarrant M, Knierim A, Hayes S, *et al.* The frequency of item writing flaws in multiple choice questions used in high stakes nursing assessments. *Nurs Educ Today.* 2006; **26**(8): 662–71.

29. Prion S. A practical framework for evaluating the impact of clinical simulation experiences in prelicensure nursing education. *Clin Simul Nurs.* 2008; **4**(5): e69–78.

30. Bremner M, Aduddell K, Bennett F, *et al.* The use of human patient simulators: best practice with novice nursing students. *Nurs Educ.* 2006; **31**(4): 170–4.

31. Schoening A, Sittner B, Todd M. Simulated clinical experience: nursing students' perceptions and the educator's role. *Nurs Educ.* 2006; **31**(6): 253–8.

32. Williams B, Dousek S. The satisfaction with simulation experience scale: a validation study. *J Nurs Educ Pract.* 2012; **2**(3): 74–80.

33. Bruce S, Scherer Y, Curran C, *et al.* A collaborative exercise between graduate and undergraduate nursing students using a computer-assisted simulator in a mock cardiac arrest. *Nurs Educ Res.* 2009; **30**(1): 22–7.

34. Sinclair B, Ferguson K. Integrating simulated teaching/learning strategies in undergraduate nursing education. *Int J Nurs Educ Scholarsh.* 2009; **6**(1): Article 7.

35. Levett-Jones T, McCoy M, Lapkin S, *et al.* The development and psychometric testing of the Satisfaction with Simulation Experience Scale. *Nurs Educ Today.* 2011; **31**(7): 705–10.

36. Hoadley T. Learning advanced cardiac life support: a comparison study of the effects of low- and high-fidelity simulation. *Nurs Educ Res.* 2009; **30**(2): 91–5.

37. Lyles D. Use of human patient simulators and perceived self-efficacy of nursing skills in associate degree nursing students [unpublished thesis]. 3379891. Minneapolis, MN: Capella University; 2009.

38. Alfes C. Evaluating the use of simulation with beginning nursing students. *J Nurs Educ.* 2011; **50**(2): 89.

39. Andreatta P, Saxton E, Thompson M, *et al.* Simulation-based mock codes significantly correlate with improved pediatric patient cardiopulmonary arrest survival rates. *Pediatr Crit Care Med.* 2011; **12**(1): 33–8.

40. Gordon C, Buckley T. The effect of high-fidelity simulation training on medical-surgical graduate nurses' perceived ability to respond to patient clinical emergencies. *J Cont Educ Nurs.* 2009; **40**(11): 491–8.

41. Curran V, Aziz K, O'Young S, *et al.* Evaluation of the effect of a computerized training simulator (ANAKIN) on the retention of neonatal resuscitation skills. *Teach Learn Med.* 2004; **16**(2): 157–64.

42. Aiken L, Clarke S, Cheung R, *et al.* Educational levels of hospital nurses and surgical patient mortality. *JAMA.* 2003; **290**(12): 1617–23.

43. Banning M. Clinical reasoning and its application to nursing: concepts and research studies. *Nurs Educ Pract*. 2008; **8**(3): 177–83.

44. Radhakrishnan K, Roche J, Cunningham H. Measuring clinical practice parameters with human patient simulation: a pilot study. *Int J Nurs Educ Scholarsh*. 2007; **4**(1): 1–11.

45. Ravert P. Patient simulator sessions and critical thinking. *J Nurs Educ*. 2008; **47**(12): 557–62.

46. Schumacher L. The impact of using high-fidelity computer simulation on critical thinking abilities and learning outcomes in undergraduate nursing students. *Diss Abs Int*. 2004; **65**(10b).

47. Alinier G, Hunt W, Gordon R. Determining the value of simulation in nurse education: study design and initial results. *Nurs Educ Pract*. 2004; **4**(3): 200–7.

48. Levett-Jones T, Hoffman K, Dempsey Y, *et al.* The 'five rights' of clinical reasoning: an educational model to enhance nursing students' ability to identify and manage clinically 'at risk' patients. *Nurs Educ Today*. 2012; **31**(6): 587–94.

49. Leonard M, Graham S, Bonacum D. The human factor: the critical importance of effective teamwork and communication in providing safe care. *Qual Safe Health Care*. 2004; **13**(Suppl. 1): i85–90.

50. Levett-Jones T, editor. *Critical Conversations for Patient Safety: an essential guide for health professionals*. Sydney, NSW: Pearson; 2014.

51. Riley R, editor. *Manual of Simulation in Healthcare*. New York, NY: Oxford University Press; 2008.

52. Iedema R. Handover. In: Levett-Jones T, editor. *Critical Conversations for Patient Safety: an essential guide for health professionals*. Sydney, NSW: Pearson. pp. 62–73.

53. Marshall S, Harrison J, Flanagan B. The teaching of a structured tool improves the clarity and content of interprofessional clinical communication. *Qual Safe Health Care*. 2009; **18**(2): 137–40.

54. Moulton C, Tabak D, Kneebone R, *et al.* Teaching communication skills using the integrated procedural performance instrument (IPPI): a randomized controlled trial. *Am J Surg*. 2009; **197**(1): 113–18.

55. Schlegal C, Woermann U, Shaha M, *et al.* Effects of communication training on real practice performance: a role-play module versus a standardized patient module. *J Nurs Educ*. 2012; **51**(1): 16–22.

56. Siassakos D, Draycott T, O'Brien K, *et al.* Exploratory trial of hybrid obstetric simulation training for undergraduate students. *Simul Healthc*. 2010; **5**(4): 193–8.

CHAPTER 19

Peer-assisted learning in health professional education

·························

Allen Thurston

OVERVIEW

There are many forms of peer-assisted learning (PAL), and there are well-established theoretical models as to why PAL is proven to be effective across educational sectors. To maximise gains from PAL, careful consideration needs to be given to the roles of peers. Evidence suggests that PAL projects with clearly defined roles for interaction result in the strongest outcomes. Meta-analyses of PAL indicate effect sizes of between 0.25 and 0.50. Outcomes can be social and emotional as well as academic. PAL generally requires adaptation of existing resources and can be cost-effective to implement in comparison with other educational developments.

CHAPTER OBJECTIVES

Upon completion of this chapter, the reader will be able to:
- describe the different forms that PAL can take
- discuss the benefits of PAL
- explore the theoretical models that underpin PAL
- report findings of previous literature reviews of PAL from across the education sector
- examine evidence for the effectiveness of PAL from the health education sector
- recommend what the health professional educators may need to consider if planning to implement PAL in their education setting.

KEY TERMS: peer, learning, health, work, effectiveness, theory, organisation

PEER-ASSISTED LEARNING

There is strong evidence from across the education sectors that peer-assisted learning (PAL) can be an effective means of learning. PAL is the acquisition of knowledge, understanding, skill and socio-emotional development during a process of working with peers in a cooperative manner. PAL strategies are generally characterised as belonging to one of the classifications identified in Table 19.1.[1]

TABLE 19.1 Classifications and characteristics of peer-assisted learning types

Classification of peer learning	Characteristics
Peer tutoring	Characterised by specific role taking as tutor or tutee, with high focus on curriculum or skills content and usually specific procedures for interaction, in which participants are trained
Cooperative learning	Typically the participants are working in small heterogeneous groups with various role specification or job division towards some common goal, performance or output, rather than primarily and consciously helping one another's learning
Collaborative learning	Typically the participants are ability-peers working in small groups in parallel towards some common goal
Peer assessment	Peers formatively and qualitatively evaluating the products or outcomes of learning of others in the group
Peer mentoring	Typically one-to-one interaction with a focus on aspirational, social, motivational or organisational issues; the helpers themselves are more experienced and are usually older, and they are usually not expected to gain from the process
Peer education	Peers offering credible and reliable information about sensitive life issues and the opportunity to discuss this in an informal peer group setting
Peer counselling	Peers helping clarify general life problems and identify solutions by listening, feeding back, summarising and being positive and supportive
Peer modelling	The provision of a competent exemplar of desirable learning behaviour by a member or members of a group with the intention that others in the group will imitate it
Peer monitoring	Peers observing and checking the process learning behaviours of others in the group with respect to appropriateness and effectiveness

THE BENEFITS OF PEER-ASSISTED LEARNING

PAL provides learners with a context through which to practise, develop and consolidate new and existing knowledge, understanding, ways of thinking and behaving. There are a number of reasons why it is repeatedly shown by research to be successful in healthcare professions. These include the time spent on task by peers as they learn together. The level of one-to-one interactions during PAL greatly increases the actual time being spent on learning. The frequency of feedback is higher than the feedback that peers normally get from teachers and lecturers. It must be acknowledged that the quality of dialogue and feedback may not be as great as that from a skilled professional; however, the intensity and frequency seems to outweigh the perceived pitfalls of such interactions. A number of factors may be responsible for this. First, the fact that things are explained in a language and level of understanding closer to the current understanding of the peer, as compared with that which a skilled professional may offer, and this could help the learner reshape his or her thinking. Second, through the act of helping a peer, a learner first has to clarify exactly how he or she knows something to be true. The learners have to unpack their learning and analyse their thinking. This metacognitive approach enables learners to self-regulate their own learning. Third, it is possible that there may be less anxiety in disclosing patterns of thinking in small peer groups than to the teacher. The power relationships between peers are not as dichotomous as those between learners and skilled teachers and lecturers. This might also facilitate the disclosure and exploration of faulty or flawed thinking without fear of ridicule or judgement by someone who may be the source of summative assessment at some later point in the learning process. This is explained in more depth in the theoretical model of peer learning proposed in the next section of this chapter.

THEORY OF PEER-ASSISTED LEARNING

Piaget[2] proposed that understanding develops in learners through the processes of assimilation and accommodation, associated with the construction of internal schemas for understanding the world. This has been termed cognitive constructivism. Piagetian thought would suggest that PAL could provide the right balance between the disequilibrium caused through cognitive challenge and social exchanges between peers for effective learning to take place.[3] Vygotsky[4] placed greater emphasis on the role of social interaction, language and discourse in the development of understanding, allowing learners to scaffold one another's learning and co-construct new knowledge and understanding. This has been termed social constructivism. Vygotskian PAL offers more possibility of congruence between cognitive structures of the learner (and therefore a greater likelihood of understanding the difficulties the learner may experience). This is reported to allow peers to engage in effective dialogue.[5] Fantuzzo and Ginsburg-Block[6] reported that Vygotskian PAL offered learners opportunities to explain concepts to their peers and practise these academic skills. Despite the apparent differences between the theories, both require peer interaction.[7] The essential difference between the techniques is that Piagetian tutoring involves cognitive challenge and post-interactive reflection and restructuring, whereas Vygotskian tutoring involves leading or support, and co-constructing during activities to promote cognitive growth. Peer tutoring based on one or the other of these theoretical models has been reported to promote gains in students in a wide range of subject disciplines including mathematics, science and reading.[8-10]

These models can be summarised in Figure 19.1, which shows the learning cycles of two peers engaged in PAL. Interaction brings about perturbation of existing cognitive structures. In forms of PAL more akin to peer tutoring, where a peer at a higher level of ability tutors a peer of lower ability, one might imagine the predominate driver of perturbation to be cognitive conflict. In more cooperative forms of PAL it would be reasonable to conclude that each peer might contribute more equally towards the perturbation of existing thought. This is more likely to result in co-construction of new ways of thinking. Whether peer tutoring or a more cooperative form of PAL is being used, each will still require new ways of thinking that need to be addressed by each peer. During the perturbation, compensation and regulation processes that take place both during and after PAL, there is the opportunity for metacognitive understanding to be achieved by learners. Not only understanding what they know but also being able to justify what they know, why they know it and how they know it.[11] Acquiring this metacognitive understanding should lead to self-regulation of knowledge by each learner, and this in turn should lead to the associated affective gains as an individual masters these concepts. In this manner the metacognitive understanding, self-regulation processes and affective responses to new learning are interlinked.[12]

An important part of the process is that peers must be dependent upon one another in order to succeed. Unless each peer fulfils his or her role independently within the process of PAL, then it is not possible for all of the peer(s) to gain maximum benefit from the interactive processes. All peers involved in the PAL process have to

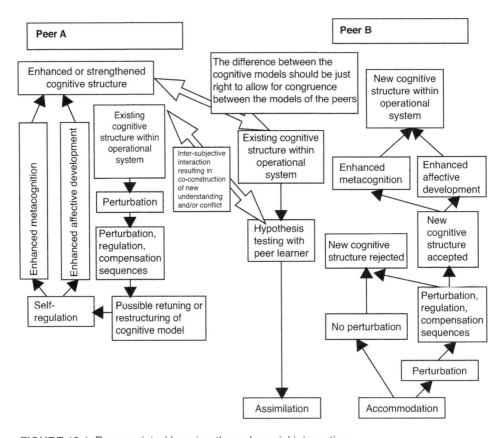

FIGURE 19.1 Peer-assisted learning through social interaction

fulfil their roles effectively. This creates a social interdependence among peers. Their individual success is linked through common goals and mutual dependence on one another for gains in the PAL process to accrue. Without all peers performing their roles in accordance with prescribed patterns for interaction, none can gain benefit from the interaction. Theories describing social interdependence have been substantively developed and described by social interdependence theory.[13,14] For cooperative learning to be present during PAL then social interdependence must be present in the form of:

- goal structure (the peers work together with the aim of solving questions)
- positive interdependence (in the PAL process, clear patterns for interaction need to be defined)
- individual accountability (all peers have responsibilities, and each must reflect on his or her own performance and the performance of his or her peer partner)
- interaction patterns (the PAL process must be structured to stimulate promotive interaction, group processing and enhanced social skills).

THE EFFECTIVENESS OF PEER-ASSISTED LEARNING

The idea of formal PAL is a very old one, first noted hundreds of years ago. In Britain, Bell and Lancaster used PAL about 200 years ago.[15] By 1816, 100 000 students were learning in this way. As more and more schools for everyone were set up, publicly funded rather than private or charitable, PAL was used less and less. The job of helping students to learn was taken over by paid adult teachers. However, in the 1960s PAL began to be used on a large scale again, especially in the United States. Teachers came to grasp that PAL was a great 'boost' or extra help for all students. Today, PAL is again spreading rapidly in many parts of the world.[15] The increased interest in PAL means that it is now one of the best-evidenced methods in education, consistently showing not only high effectiveness in a number of areas of learner functioning but also very high cost-effectiveness. There is a great deal of good-quality research on the subject of PAL, but less on PAL beyond schools.

Cohen *et al.*[16] located more than 500 titles relating to tutoring, and carried out a quantitative synthesis, or meta-analysis, of them. However, only 65 studies fully reported quantitative outcomes for both the tutored and a non-tutored control group and had no serious methodological flaws. In 45 of 52 studies, tutored learners outperformed control learners in attainment, while in six studies control learners did better and in one study there was no difference, with a mean effect size (ES) of 0.40. Larger ESs were associated with cross-age tutoring, structured tutoring, training for tutors, tutees of *low* ability, short-term projects, mathematics projects, locally developed tests (compare with nationally standardised tests) and published journal papers (compare with dissertations and other reports). Tutoring programmes had a positive effect on the tutees' attitudes towards the curriculum area being tutored. Seven out of nine studies found the self-concept of tutees improved, but the average ES was small. Learners who served as tutors performed better than control learners in attainment in the tutored curriculum area in 33 out of 38 studies. Four out of five studies found improved tutor attitudes towards the tutored subject, and 12 out of 16 studies found the self-concept of tutors improved.

Research has continued to accumulate and reinforce earlier findings of the effectiveness of PAL. The scope of PAL has continued to widen, particularly with respect to extension to younger learners, equal opportunity class-wide programmes, peers who themselves have special needs, and combining PAL with peer formative assessment. Scruggs and Mastropieri[17] reviewed the literature on peer tutoring (a specific form of PAL) with special needs learners and concluded that learners with special needs benefit academically whether tutees or tutors; tutors benefit less academically if there is no cognitive challenge for them; participants benefit more if carefully selected and trained; participants benefit more if progress is continuously monitored; improved attitudes to the curriculum area are frequent; improved interactions with partners outside tutoring sessions are frequent; and more generalised attitudinal or interactive gains are less consistent.

Reviews of the effectiveness of PAL continue to be conducted. Rohrbeck et al.[18] offered a meta-analytic review of group comparison design studies evaluating PAL interventions. The meta-analytic review of PAL produced positive ESs, indicating increases in achievement (unweighted mean ES = 0.59, standard deviation = 0.90; weighted ES, d = 0.33, p < 0.0001, 95% confidence interval = 0.29–0.37). ESs were strongest for studies with younger, urban, low-income, ethnic minority students. In addition, PAL that used interdependent reward schemes and ipsative evaluation and which provided learners with more autonomy also had greater ESs.

A literature review on PAL in clinical education reviewed 40 articles that spanned the time period from 1980 to 2006. Articles were included from nursing, physical therapy, occupational therapy, medicine and higher education.[19] The review concluded that PAL could provide a good supplement to clinical training. However, the review highlighted that more research was required to quantify the benefits of PAL and to establish which forms of PAL would provide the greatest enhancement to learning and teaching.

Roseth et al.[20] conducted a meta-analysis of 148 independent studies comparing the relative contribution of cooperative, competitive and individualistic goal structures on outcomes in learning and achieving positive peer relationships. The studies reviewed included data from 8 decades of research, 17 000 research participants and 11 different countries. Studies showed clearly that pedagogies that adopted PAL strategies with cooperative structures showed significantly higher gains than those using competitive or individualistic goal structures. On attainment measures, ESs were generally 0.46 and 0.55 standard deviations higher for achievement over competitive and individualistic goal structures respectively. On social measures (termed forming effective peer relationships) ESs were 0.48 and 0.42 standard deviations higher for cooperative structures than for competitive and individualistic goal structures.

PEER-ASSISTED LEARNING IN HEALTH PROFESSIONAL EDUCATION

Peer learning initiatives have been successfully implemented in a number of work-based health education settings, although the literature in this sector is not extensive and the quality of studies is generally not high. Most of the published work has included medical and nursing students[21-27] and, more recently, paramedics.[28-30] Examples include a peer learning initiative that was reported in a group of 10 young disabled adults aged 18–27 years.[31] The programme involved peer mediation and collaborative group work based on Feuerstein's theory of mediated learning and instrumental enrichment programme, and it was reported to have positive cognitive benefits. The participants' learning self-concept increased and their reflections on how they had changed as a result of their involvement in the programme showed deepened levels of cognitive, emotional and social development.[31] Peer learning was also reported to be effective during health counselling sessions in a health centre in Hong Kong. Small health counselling groups led by volunteer nurses focused on hypertension, diabetes mellitus, high serum cholesterol and obesity. Patients responded well to the peer learning initiative and the results indicated that clients felt empowered.[32]

Peer learning was used in a women's health initiative to promote health and social justice in communities in California. Graduates were encouraged to engage in peer learning via a network using peer learning techniques to mobilise trained grassroots leaders who could influence policy decisions and provide technical support and resources to local communities.[33]

The Public Health Leadership Institute developed a peer learning programme to expand and enhance the leadership skills of senior public health officials. Participants were supported by face-to-face peer learning and through electronic conferencing. The programme was effective at developing leadership skills, and participants reported favourably on the positive effects of peer learning.[34] Despite the variability of this literature, it seems that peer learning in health workplace settings is certainly possible – but how should it be organised?

A group of 27 entry-level students enrolled in a doctorate degree in physical therapy programme and who were engaged in peer tutoring in a practical laboratory setting were reported to develop better 'study habits' and an improved attitude towards their subject matter than a comparator group of 21 students who did not engage with PAL.[35] Another study reported that a group of 14 medical students acting in the role of clinical skills teaching assistants to 113 other undergraduate students felt more confident in their ability to give and receive feedback. They also reported that acting in this role improved their own clinical knowledge.[36]

In a study of 50 nursing students undertaking a baccalaureate in nursing, a volunteer group of 25 students undertook PAL and 15 undertook individual teaching. It was reported that students who had been engaged with PAL significantly improved their psychomotor test scores and overall clinical knowledge. The study also reported favourable attitudes to PAL compared with previous experiences of teaching and learning.[37]

Yu et al.[38] completed a systematic review of the evidence on peer-teaching effectiveness and affects on objective learning outcomes of medical students. A total of

127 citations were found and, upon closer review, 19 studies were selected for the systematic review. Ten studies utilised random allocation.

> Overall, results suggested that peer-teaching, in highly selective contexts, achieves short-term learning outcomes that are comparable with those produced by faculty-based teaching. Furthermore, peer-teaching has beneficial effects on student-teacher learning outcomes ... There is evidence that participating student-teachers benefit academically and professionally.[38(p157)]

However, despite the substantive evidence from the small-scale studies on PAL mentioned here, there remains the need for additional work. In other sectors of education, large-scale randomised controlled trials and/or design experiments have been run on PAL. These have helped establish the efficacy and generalisability of PAL techniques. Evidence of this nature is still required within the health sector. Although a number of studies report evidence of the effectiveness of PAL, then large-scale RCTs are conspicuous by their absence. The health professional education sector needs to consider how to address this issue.

TYPOLOGY OF PEER-ASSISTED LEARNING

If a health education professional wanted to implement a PAL project, what factors would he or she need to consider during the planning process? Given the variety of forms of PAL and the different ways in which PAL groups could be constructed, there are a number of factors that need to be taken into account. Thurston and Topping[1] reported that the methods for PAL can vary in a number of different organisational dimensions.

- *Curriculum content:* knowledge or skills or combination to be covered. The scope of PAL is very wide and projects are reported in the literature in virtually every imaginable subject.
- *Contact constellation:* some projects operate with one peer taking a role as a 'tutor' and working with a group of peers, but the size of a group can vary from 2 to 30 or more. Sometimes groups will be organised into groups of up to six peers. In these more cooperative or collaborative forms of PAL it is best to have clear roles for each group member to avoid 'free-rider' effects, where one or more peers become inactive within the group.
- *Contact frequency:* thought needs to be given to frequency of contact. Should this be once a week for a set time period (many studies tend to do once a week for 12 weeks or more)?
- *Within or between institutions:* while most PAL takes place within the same institution, it can also take place between different institutions, as when young people from a high school tutor in their neighbourhood primary school, or university students help in regular schools.

- *Year of study:* helpers and helped may be from the same or different years of study, and/or be the same or different ages.
- *Ability:* while many projects operate on a cross-ability basis (even if they are same-age peers at the same stage of study), there is increasing interest in same-ability peer tutoring. In this, the peers might have superior mastery of only a very small portion of the curriculum, or all might be of equal ability but working towards a shared, deeper and hopefully correct understanding. 'Meta-ignorance' can be a problem – peers do not know that they don't know the correct facts.
- *Role continuity:* especially in same-ability projects, roles need not be permanent. Structured switching of roles at strategic moments can have the advantage of involving greater novelty and a wider boost to self-esteem, in that all participants get to be helpers.
- *Time:* PAL might be scheduled in regular class contact time, outside of this or in a combination of both, depending on the extent to which it is substitutional or supplementary for regular teaching.
- *Place:* correspondingly, PAL can vary enormously in location of operation – during class time or in time away from the formal classroom?
- *Peer characteristics:* if groups are made up of peers who are performing at average (or even less) levels, all peers need to find some challenge in their joint activities.
- *Characteristics of the peers:* projects may be for all or a targeted subgroup (e.g. the especially able or gifted; those with disabilities; those considered at risk of underachievement, failure or dropout; or those from ethnic, religious and other minorities).
- *Objectives:* projects may target intellectual (cognitive) gains, formal academic achievement, affective and attitudinal gains, social and emotional gains, self-image and self-concept gains, or any combination of these. Organisational objectives might include reducing dropout, increasing access, and so on and so forth.
- *Voluntary or compulsory:* some projects require participation, while in others peers self-select. This can have marked effects on the quality of what ensues.
- *Training:* there is strong evidence to suggest that training is essential for PAL to be successful. Students need good information on how they should interact. This requires training and normally needs specific materials to develop the skills needed for successful peer interaction (those of interaction patterns, communication and social skills).
- *Reinforcement:* some projects involve extrinsic reinforcement for the helpers (and sometimes also the helped), while others rely on intrinsic motivation. Beyond simple social praise, extrinsic reward can take the form of certification, course credit or more tangible reinforcement such as money. Extrinsic reward is much more common in North America than elsewhere, and this has led to some debate about possible excess in this regard. Availability of extrinsic reinforcement can have effects on recruitment in voluntary projects, which might be good or bad.
- *Monitoring and feedback:* thought needs to be given to feedback for peers. Should this be given by peers only or is there a role for the educator in this process? Should

it be qualitative or quantitative? Either way, it needs to tell peers how to improve their interactions and the processes they are using to work together.

CONCLUSION AND IMPLICATIONS FOR PRACTICE AND RESEARCH

There is a growing evidence base regarding the benefits of PAL in health professional education.[19-38] PAL is used to support vulnerable as well as regular learners. Pre-service and continuing professional development opportunities focused on PAL are needed for those engaged in health professional education and work-based contexts. It will be essential that researchers work closely with health education providers to ensure that this potential is maximised.

It is now generally accepted that there is excellent evidence for the effectiveness of PAL.[39-41] However, much of this research has been in schools, and rigorous research in health professional education settings is limited. Peer assessment is a more recent development and seems very promising. The range of contexts for peer assessment needs to be broadened. There is a growing literature regarding peer counselling in health education; however, much of the literature reports only small-scale studies. The evidence for the effectiveness of peer modelling and monitoring is not as strong, and comes from a narrow range of contexts. There is a need to test the effectiveness of PAL in health professional education in a more rigorous and scientific manner.

The challenge for those working in health professional education is to develop a research base in peer learning that is specific to the context of the sector – exploring the constraints and affordances. Future research should be rigorous, it needs to include the use of properly scaled RCTs and it should be informed by theoretical models such as the one presented in this chapter. Once the effects and potential of PAL in health professional education are fully explored and established, there needs to be effective knowledge transfer between health professional researchers and practitioners, to ensure the potential of the techniques is fully realised in the sector. Although this is a major challenge, it has been achieved in other educational sectors.

SUMMARY POINTS

- Peer learning can be an effective means of raising attainment levels in health education settings.
- Peer interactions are seldom as complex and carefully structured as teacher–student interactions; however, they are more frequent and more immediate.
- Peer learning can promote effective learning when there is:
  - goal structure (the peers work together with the aim of solving questions)
  - positive interdependence (in the PAL process clear patterns for interaction need to be defined)
  - individual accountability (all peers have responsibilities, and each must reflect on his or her own performance and the performance of his or her peer partner)

— interaction patterns (the PAL process must be structured to stimulate pro-motive interaction, group processing and enhanced social skills).
- PAL can be an effective pedagogy in health education.
- Outcomes from peer learning can be socio-emotional as well as cognitive.
- Educators should carefully plan and structure PAL to maximise learning potential.
- Further research is required in the health education sector to explore the potentials of PAL.

REVIEW QUESTIONS

- What are some types of PAL?
- How can PAL assist in promoting effective education in health professional student education?
- What are three components of the PAL typology?
- What features can promote PAL?

REFLECTIVE QUESTIONS AND EXERCISES

- What topic areas in your teaching might lend themselves to peer learning?
- What form of peer learning (*see* Table 19.1) might be most beneficial to your students?
- Reflect on the typology of PAL. Which of these aspects would be important for you to address before implementing a PAL initiative?
- What challenges might you face if implementing a PAL project? How might you overcome them?

REFERENCES

1. Thurston A, Topping K. Peer tutoring in schools: cognitive models and organizational typography. *J Cogn Educ Psychol.* 2007; **6**(3): 356–72.
2. Piaget J. *The Development of Thought: equilibration of cognitive structures.* Oxford, UK: Basil Blackwell; 1978.
3. Palincsar AS. Social constructivist perspectives on teaching and learning. *Annu Rev Psychol.* 1998; **49**: 345–75.
4. Vygotsky LS. *Mind in Society: the development of higher psychological processes.* Cambridge, MA: MIT Press; 1978.
5. Bruner JS. Vygotsky: a historical and conceptual perspective. In: Wertsch JW, editor, *Culture, Communication, and Cognition: Vygotskian perspectives.* Cambridge, UK: Cambridge University Press; 1985. pp. 21–34.
6. Fantuzzo JW, Ginsburg-Block M. Reciprocal peer tutoring: developing and testing effective peer collaborations for elementary school students. In: Topping KJ, Ehly S, editors. *Peer-Assisted Learning.* Mahwah, NJ: Erlbaum; 1998. pp. 121–44.

7. Blatchford P, Kutnick P, Baines E, et al. Changes in grouping practices over primary and secondary school. *Int J Educ Res.* 2003; **39**(1): 9–34.
8. Howe CJ, Tolmie A, Greer K, et al. Peer collaboration and conceptual growth in physics: Task influences on children's understanding of heating and cooling. *Cognition Instruct.* 1995; **13**(4): 483–503.
9. Robinson D, Schofield J, Steers-Wentzell K. Peer and cross-age tutoring in math: Outcomes and their design implications. *Educ Psychol Rev.* 2005; **17**(4): 327–62.
10. Webb N. Peer interaction and learning in small groups. *Int J Educ Res.* 1989; **13**(1): 21–39.
11. Woolfolk A. *Educational Psychology.* 8th ed. Boston, MA: Allyn & Bacon; 2001.
12. Eggen P, Kauchak D. *Educational Psychology: windows on the classroom.* 3rd ed. Upper Saddle River, NJ: Prentice Hall; 1997.
13. Johnson DW, Johnson RT, Roseth C. Cooperative learning in middle schools: interrelationship of relationships and achievement. *Middle Grades Res J.* 2010; **5**(1): 1–18.
14. Johnson DW, Johnson RT. Restorative justice in the classroom: necessary roles of cooperative context, constructive conflict, and civic values. *Negotiation Conflict Manage Res.* 2012; **5**(1): 4–28.
15. Thurston A. *Learning Together in Maths.* London: Times Educational Supplement; 2012.
16. Cohen PA, Kulik JA, Kulik C-LC. Educational outcomes of tutoring: a meta-analysis of findings. *Am Educ Res J.* 1982; **19**(2): 237–48.
17. Scruggs TE, Mastropieri MA. Tutoring and students with special needs. In: Topping KJ, Ehly S, editors. *Peer-Assisted Learning.* Mahwah, NJ: Lawrence Erlbaum Associates, 1998. pp. 165–82.
18. Rohrbeck CA, Ginsburg-Block MD, Fantuzzo JW, et al. Peer-assisted learning interventions with elementary school students: a meta-analytic review. *J Educ Psychol.* 2003; **95**(2): 240–57.
19. Henning JM, Weidner TG, Marty MC. Peer assisted learning in clinical education: literature review. *Athl Train Educ J.* 2008; **3**: 84–90.
20. Roseth CJ, Johnson DW, Johnson RT. Promoting early adolescents' achievement and peer relationships: the effects of cooperative, competitive, and individualistic goal structures. *Psychol Bull.* 2008; **134**(2): 223–46.
21. Glass N, Walter R. An experience of peer mentoring with student nurses: enhancement of personal and professional growth. *J Nurs Educ.* 2000; **39**(4): 155–60.
22. Arnold L, Shue CK, Kritt B, et al. Medical students' views on peer assessment of professionalism. *J Gen Intern Med.* 2005; **20**(9): 819–24.
23. Aviram M, Ophir R, Raviv D, et al. Experiential learning of clinical skills by beginning nursing students: 'coaching' project by fourth-year student interns. *J Nurs Educ.* 1998; **37**(5): 228–31.
24. Yates P, Cunningham J, Moyle W, et al. Peer mentorship in clinical education: outcomes of a pilot programme for first year students. *Nurse Educ Today.* 1997; **17**(6): 508–14.
25. Christiansen A, Bell A. Peer learning partnerships: exploring the experience of pre-registration nursing students. *J Clin Nurs.* 2010; **19**(5–6): 803–10.
26. Glynn LG, MacFarlane A, Kelly M, et al. Helping each other to learn: a process evaluation of peer assisted learning. *BMC Med Educ.* 2006; **6**: 18.
27. Saunders C, Smith A, Watson H. The experience of interdisciplinary peer-assisted learning (PAL). *Clin Teach.* 2012; **9**(6): 398–402.
28. Williams B, Winship C. Psychometric examination of the modified Clinical Teaching Preference Questionnaire (CTPQ). *J Peer Learn.* 2013; **6**(1): 19–29.
29. Williams B, Fellows H, Eastwood K, et al. Peer teaching experiences of final year paramedic students: 2011–2012. *J Peer Learn.* 2015; in press.
30. Fox M, Winship C, Williams W, et al. Peer-assisted teaching and learning in paramedic education: a pilot study. *J Paramed Pract.* 2015: in press.
31. Kaufman R, Burden R. Peer tutoring between young adults with severe and complex learning difficulties: the effects of mediation training with Feuerstein's Instrumental Enrichment programme. *Eur J Psychol Educ.* 2004; **19**(1): 107–17.

32. Ma S, Chi I. Health counselling for older people in Hong Kong. *Educ Gerontol.* 1995; **21**(5): 515–28.

33. Littlefield D, Robison CC, Engelbrecht L, *et al.* Mobilizing women for minority health and social justice in California. *Am J Public Health.* 2002; **92**(4): 576–9.

34. Scutchfield FD, Spain C, Pointer DD, *et al.* The public health leadership institute: leadership training for state and local health officers. *J Public Health Policy.* 1995; **16**(3): 304–23.

35. Hendelman WJ, Boss M. Reciprocal peer teaching by medical students in the gross anatomy laboratory. *J Med Educ.* 1986; **61**(8): 674–80.

36. Weyrich P, Schrauth M, Kraus B, *et al.* Undergraduate technical skills training guided by student tutors: analysis of tutors' attitudes, tutees' acceptance and learning progress in an innovative teaching model. *BMC Med Educ.* 2008; **8**: 18.

37. Iwasiw CL, Goldenberg D. Peer teaching among nursing students in the clinical area: effects on student learning. *J Adv Nurs.* 1993; **18**(4): 659–68.

38. Yu TC, Wilson NC, Singh PP, *et al.* Medical students-as-teachers: a systematic review of peer-assisted teaching during medical school. *Adv Med Educ Pract.* 2011; **2011**(2): 157–72.

39. Topping KJ. *Thinking, Reading, Writing: a practical guide to paired learning with peers, parents & volunteers.* New York, NY: Continuum International; 2001.

40. Topping K. Peer assessment between students in colleges and universities. *Rev Educ Res.* 1998; **68**(3): 249–76.

41. Topping KJ, Ehly S. *Peer-Assisted Learning.* Mahwah, NJ: Lawrence Erlbaum Associates; 1998.

CHAPTER 20

Interprofessional education

Application and evidence

....

Sharla King and Sam Magus

OVERVIEW

Health professionals of the twenty-first century not only require the skills, knowledge and attitudes to work in their profession, but also they must master how to collaborate across professions in order to provide effective and efficient patient care. Interprofessional education (IPE) is seen as a means to enhance collaborative practice (CP). Post-secondary institutions are increasingly developing IPE opportunities for their students; however, the specific empirical evidence is lacking to determine the most effective IPE experiences to strengthen specific competencies that lead to CP and improved patient care. The 3P model[1] provides a framework to assist with *developing* interprofessional (IP) learning experiences, and Barr *et al.*[2] outline models for the *delivery* of IP learning experiences. IPE occurs in the classroom, in simulation-based environments, online, in clinical learning units and in the clinical setting. The evidence that currently exists examines the learners' perceptions about the experience and attitudes towards IPE. Opportunities for students to reflect on their clinical or community placements before and after the experiences are critical. The preparation of preceptors and facilitators must not be overlooked in the development of IP learning experiences, as modelling for students' effective CP skills is critical. To best support the transition of learners from the classroom into the workplace, health workforce planners and health professional educators must work together.

CHAPTER OBJECTIVES

Upon completion of this chapter, the reader will be able to:
- describe the existing evidence for IPE in several types of learning environments, including simulation-based, online and clinical environments
- outline a model or approach for the development of IPE experiences
- identify further educational research required to advance the field of IPE with pre-licensure health professionals.

KEY TERMS: collaborative practice, interprofessional learning, competency-based education

INTRODUCTION

This chapter provides the key essentials to developing, and implementing evidence-based interprofessional education (IPE) experiences for pre-licensure health professional learners. The chapter begins with a brief introduction to IPE and then provides a description of a model for the development of interprofessional (IP) learning experiences; the chapter then outlines curricula models and, finally, highlights the evidence for IP in a variety of learning environments.

Health professionals of the twenty-first century require the skills, knowledge and attitudes to adapt to the increasing complexity of healthcare issues they must manage now and in the future. Unfortunately, health professional education has not evolved or kept pace with this increasing complexity of healthcare issues, and the 'fragmented, outdated and static curricula'[3(p1923)] produces graduates ill-equipped to manage these complexities. However, one change occurring with health professional education is the move towards IPE to enhance collaborative practice (CP). Effective CP is viewed as critical for optimal patient health outcomes and it provides a greater personal satisfaction for health workers.[4] IPE is when two or more learners from different professions 'learn with, from and about each other.'[5] This classic definition has been adopted at a global level and has come to represent the essence of IPE.

Despite the recognition of the value of CP to improve patient care,[6-8] struggles exist around developing meaningful educational experiences at both the educational institutional level and the health organisational level that focus on IPE. At the practice level, issues around role clarity, hierarchy, poor communication and conflict resolution strategies, all a reality in healthcare, are often ongoing barriers to successful implementation of CP approaches. Simultaneously, but for different reasons, such as the efficiency of individualised programmes, health professional students are educated in institutional silos. Health professional students are competent in their own uni-professional role upon graduation; however, they are not always ready to work well in teams.

GUIDING DOCUMENTS TO SUPPORT INTERPROFESSIONAL EDUCATION AND COLLABORATIVE PRACTICE

As the field of IPE has evolved, key guiding documents and frameworks have been created to support the development and implementation of IPE and CP. These documents include frameworks for how to implement IPE and the necessary competencies for IPE. The World Health Organization[8] developed a global strategy to help aid the creation of shared information required to move CP forward. The *Framework for Action on Interprofessional Education and Collaborative Practice*[9] provides strategies at both educational and organisational levels to best support and enhance IPE for CP.

INTERPROFESSIONAL COMPETENCY FRAMEWORKS

IP competency frameworks have emerged in various countries to support IPE and the development of CP at both a pre-licensure and a postgraduate level. A competency-based model or framework allows educational institutions to integrate IPE experiences into their curricula, with the ultimate goal of students graduating with the knowledge, skills and attitudes necessary to work with other professionals in a collaborative manner once in the health sector.[10] Student competencies may be tracked and measured, in order to document the development of the appropriate skills.

In the United Kingdom, an IP Capability Framework[11] was developed that articulates the learning outcomes that students need to achieve and continue to develop in order to become capable IP health providers. The four key domains in which the framework outlines the capabilities and associated learning levels are (1) knowledge in practice, (2) ethical practice, (3) IP working and (4) reflection. In 2010, the Canadian Interprofessional Health Collaborative published a National IP Competency Framework.[12] This framework identified six domains for IPE and CP for both pre-licensure and continuing professionals: (1) IP communication; (2) patient-, client-, family-, community-centred care; (3) role clarification; (4) team functioning; (5) collaborative leadership; and (6) IP conflict resolution. As outlined in the framework document, the set of competencies provides both students and practitioners with the ability to learn and apply the competencies, no matter their level of skill or the context. More recently, the Interprofessional Education Collaborative – comprising the American Association of Colleges of Nursing, American Association of Colleges of Osteopathic Medicine, American Association of Colleges of Pharmacy, American Dental Education Association, Association of American Medical Colleges and Association of Schools and Programs of Public Health – published the *Core Competencies for Interprofessional Collaborative Practice*[12] in order to guide the development and evaluation of IPE and CP in the United States. This document outlines four competency domains: (1) values/ethics for interprofessional practice; (2) roles/responsibilities; (3) interprofessional communication; and (4) teams and teamwork. These four competencies are linked to the Institute of Medicine's core competencies for all health professionals.

Each competency framework includes the patient, or client, either as a key consideration within a set of principles that helped guide the development of the competencies,[12] embedded within some of the competencies,[10] or as their own standalone competency.[11] What is the impact of this difference across the frameworks, with respect to IPE and the development of CP practice skills? At this time, that is unknown. Within educational institutions, the competency frameworks are linked to accreditation for health professional programmes and therefore are both context and content specific.

THE EVIDENCE FOR INTERPROFESSIONAL EDUCATION

The growth of IPE in health professional education programmes has resulted in an increase in the number of publications focused on IPE. However, these publications are mainly descriptions of IP programmes and learning experiences that may or may not have methodological rigour or be supported by sound evidence. In other words, strong evidence for IPE may still be anecdotal rather than empirical. Several systematic reviews have been conducted over the past 10 years[13-15] indicating mixed outcomes to support IPE. For example, a recent review by Lapkin *et al.*[14] examined the effectiveness of IPE in university-based health professional programmes. Out of 4217 studies initially retrieved, only nine were included in the review. Of these nine, six evaluated educational outcomes such as knowledge, skills and attitudes using pre-validated IP instruments using the Interdisciplinary Education Perception Scale, the Readiness for Interprofessional Learning Scale and the Student Stereotypes Rating Questionnaire.[15-19] The outcome of the systematic review indicated that students' attitudes towards collaboration may be enhanced by IPE; however, the evidence is lacking with respect to the duration that these positive changes are sustained for. This outcome is consistent with other reviews of the literature. Despite the lack of strong evidence and methodological rigour in evaluation studies of IP educational experiences, models to guide the development and implementation of experiences have evolved.

DEVELOPING INTERPROFESSIONAL LEARNING EXPERIENCES: THE 3P MODEL

The development of planned and relevant IPE must consider the components and dynamics of the learning experience. The 3P model[1] supports the development of IP learning experiences. The Ps stand for *presage, process* and *product*. *Presage* means the factors providing the context for the learning experience, including the characteristics of teachers, facilitators, programme developers and learners; *process* outlines the approaches to teaching and learning; *product* refers to the collaborative competencies. The 3P model[1] provides educators and IP programme developers with a useful tool or approach to support the development of IP learning experiences. An in-depth explanation of this model can be found in Freeth and Reeves[1] and Freeth *et al.*[20]

INTEGRATING INTERPROFESSIONAL EDUCATION INTO CURRICULA

Barr et al.[2] outlined two models for delivery of IPE. The first is an extracurricular or co-curricular model. This model is the result of limited curricular time due to very full academic schedules. Finding the time to integrate IPE into discipline-specific curricula is challenging. One option to circumvent this challenge is to provide IPE outside regular curriculum time. This model provides a relatively easy way to implement small-scale IPE experiences. However, students may believe that IPE is less important than mainstream professional studies if it is only offered outside of regular curricula. The second model is the crossbar model. This is a more integrated model that introduces one or more shared learning sequences across programmes. The IPE may include themes such as ethics or geriatrics. Deutschlander et al.[21] identified a third model, the IP enhancement approach, which takes advantage of pre-existing courses and clinical placements. IP activities were offered during clinical placements, including face-to-face and online discussions, in order to develop a student community of practice. IP mentoring was also incorporated into this model. The purpose of the IP mentoring was to engage individual students with staff of varying professional backgrounds.[22]

The debate as to when IPE should be offered in a pre-licensure programme, either early before professional identities are formed or later once the professional knowledge and skill set is more solid, is ongoing. Research has indicated that even upon entry into health professional programmes, students already possess stereotypes about other health professionals.[2] Additionally, the readiness of students for IPE was found to be high at entry but declined over time.[23] Based on these outcomes, the focus of when to provide IP experiences should shift to early, regular and sustained IPE for pre-licensure students, rather than either an early or a late conversation.[15]

Barr et al.[2] outlined the type of educational approach that best supports the development of IP competencies. The interactive approaches highlighted include exchange-based learning (seminar discussions), observation-based learning (joint visits to patients). action-based learning (problem-based learning), simulation-based learning, practice-based learning and e-Learning. The key for any successful type of learning approach is the relevance or authenticity of the experience for the student.[13] Focusing on the principles of adult learning is a key mechanism for positive learning experiences, which takes into account the learners' needs and the learning context.[13] As identified earlier, IPE must reflect the reality of practice for specific groups of IP learners.

CLASSROOM-BASED INTERPROFESSIONAL EXPERIENCES

Published evaluations of IPE experiences are often classroom-based rather than clinically based;[14] however, strong empirical evidence does not exist for classroom-based IP experiences. The classroom experiences often involve discussion of case scenarios or other interactive group activities for the purpose of role clarification and communication. The majority of evaluations focus on student satisfaction with the experience, rather than examining behavioural changes, short- or long-term.

Due to the commonality of case-based discussions in IP learning experiences, Packard et al.[24] developed the Interprofessional Team Reasoning Framework to assist student teams with case study analysis. In a pilot study of three student IP teams, two of which used the framework to structure their discussion, Packard et al.[24] reported a significant improvement in perceived IP skills. The one team that did not use the framework did not report a significant improvement in perceived IP skills. The authors suggested that this framework may be useful in the early stages of student learning and that it should be embedded in future coursework throughout their programme. However, this framework and its appropriate use within curricula needs further examination.

An IP programme at any institution should not involve classroom-based experiences alone. As suggested by Lapkin et al.,[14] the classroom-based IPE experiences should be supported by intentional opportunities for IPE during experiential learning that occurs during clinical placements, providing support for the idea of early, regular and sustained IPE.

SIMULATION-BASED INTERPROFESSIONAL EXPERIENCES

Simulation is a standard instructional strategy in health science education, particularly in medicine and nursing.[25,26] IP simulation learning experiences are becoming increasingly common, with a focus on enhancing non-technical skills such as communication and collaboration.[15,25,27–31] Brief and intense simulation-based scenarios can increase perceived confidence in communicating and working in impromptu teams of pre-licensed students from multiple health science disciplines.[32]

The majority of IP simulation studies have focused on enhancing communication and team skills between nurses and physicians (pre-licensed and postgraduate), residents and specialists,[29] typically in urgent care situations. Teamwork knowledge and attitudes significantly improved after medical and nursing students participated in one of four different modalities, including high-fidelity simulation.[33] Unfortunately, details are lacking with respect to the type of simulations.

A comprehensive study on the use of IP simulation with undergraduates from medicine, nursing, physiotherapy, radiography and operating department practice from four different institutions was conducted.[32] The IP simulation intervention consisted of half-day sessions with 'pre- then post-test' assessment of student perceptions of learning and attitudes to IP. Overall the findings demonstrated positive improvements on students' perceptions after the intervention. Working with other institutions allowed them to share expertise, effectively model complex teamwork and increase the range of professions. Although five disciplines were represented, medicine and nursing students accounted for 82% of the participants. More recently, Garbee et al.[34] used a quasi-experimental design to evaluate the efficacy of using crisis resource management principles for IP team training with undergraduate students from nursing, nurse anesthesia, medicine and respiratory therapy. Student IP teams participated in two simulations in an emergency room setting in both the autumn and spring semesters. Team performance was measured using the Communication and Teamwork Skills assessment, while the Teamwork Assessment Scale and the Mayo High Performance Teamwork Scale were used to measure crisis resource management skills. With a sample of 40 students, improvements were demonstrated with the subscales of the Teamwork Assessment Scale from the autumn to the spring simulation sessions.

INTERPROFESSIONAL EDUCATION AND COLLABORATION IN CLINICAL EXPERIENCES

As students wind down their classroom and laboratory work and enter into their clinical practicum, the variety and complexity of learning experience increases. In order for optimal IP learning to occur, students should acquire the necessary background information prior to entering their clinical experience, where they will be expected to practise and refine IP collaboration.[35] However, this kind of ideal preparation is not always possible and is not absolutely necessary, as some collaborative learning and IP competencies can be achieved with no formal preclinical IPE.[36] Well-planned IPE can increase student IP collaboration, especially when clinical sites and practitioners within those sites vary greatly as to their level of working collaboratively.[37] IP tools of communication, learning about others' roles and exploring the concept of culture all make excellent focal points for bringing students together for preclinical IPE.[36] Didactic learning prior to student clinical practice of an evidence-based collection of team-based concepts also has the potential to improve student team performance upon graduation.[38] Every clinical placement has the potential for IPE or CP learning. Determining when and where students will encounter these opportunities – and how they will integrate classroom knowledge into practice – should be thoroughly explored by school practicum coordinators prior to clinical placements.

INTERPROFESSIONAL CLINICAL LEARNING UNITS

Interprofessional clinical learning units first emerged out of Sweden[39,40] as IP training wards, where IP groups of students worked on a designated unit with real patients in a clinical setting. The course outcomes included learning to work together, enhancing understanding of the other students' professions and developing one's own professional role and function as a team member. Elsewhere, specialised learning units have emerged[41] that have not only supported the development of IP competencies with students but also enhanced the IP knowledge and CP skills of clinicians.

DURING THE CLINICAL EXPERIENCE

The amount of IP collaboration existing in clinical practice varies widely between countries, and even between institutions right across the street from each other. Therefore, the amount of CP that students witness and experience on their clinical practicums will also vary. In an effort to reduce the harm that a non-collaborative clinical practicum environment may inflict on student attitudes and outcomes, didactic and clinical instructors should thoroughly prepare students for this inevitability by discussing potential emotions that the students may experience. There can be a resistance to students having competency requirements focusing on collaborative care, especially in a clinical setting that is not practised in this model. Often, this lack of exposure and understanding of CP may hamper both the student learning and the preceptor's ability to provide this exposure, especially if these circumstances are not anticipated and mitigated.

It is necessary to 'set the practicum stage' in order for a positive and truly collaborative clinical experience to occur. To begin with, there needs to be clear and consistent references to an existing list or group of IPE or CP clinical objectives or competencies. A framework such as that developed by the Canadian Interprofessional Health Collaborative[11] is helpful to ensure that common knowledge and the common language of IPE is established. Only then will students and preceptors have the shared required direction to move student learning forward. With complete and clear guidelines for achievement, the IPE or CP competencies can be treated as equivalent to mandatory uni-professional competencies.

Many models of student exposure to IPE concepts exist in the clinical setting. IP peer-assisted learning, as described by McLelland et al.,[42] can be used clinically to expose students to such competencies as role clarity and IP communication. Other clinical models have students experience work-shadowing with a preceptor from their own or another profession. When shadowing another profession it has been demonstrated that students develop role clarity (knowledge and appreciation of that profession's roles and abilities). Regardless of the exact student–clinician working relationship, one must keep in mind that this partnership will only propel the student towards IPE learning as much as the preceptor is collaborative in his or her own work.[36]

'Clinical capacity' is a term sometimes used to describe the number of available practicum openings or spots for students. In the health evidence-based literature, clinical capacity – both for the purpose of experiencing uni-professional and for IP competency – can be increased through alternative supervision models, such as pairing novice students with senior students,[43] or having one preceptor work with multiple students at a time.[44] Often initiatives that improve student IPE and CP concurrently report to have increased clinical capacity.[45]

For the most meaningful collaborative student experience, it is recommended to have a rich variety of activities, assignments and simulations to complement the clinical experience. Although becoming competent in uni-professional skill sets is essential to the student becoming a capable professional, IPE and CP skills should have the same level of importance and can also be directly related to health outcomes for the patients and their caregivers and families. Measuring the effectiveness or determining a score in the difficult skill of collaboration can be challenging and difficult to determine. The evidence-based literature has determined that reflecting on practice can be appropriate for individual[37] and group formative and summative assessment.[36] Facilitated debriefing of CP by the preceptor and/or school clinical faculty has been evaluated in simulation[46] and should translate as an effective tool for clinical assessment.

The clinical setting provides opportunities for students to observe and work in existing health teams, giving the students a sense of their own role in teams upon graduation. Students may be lucky enough to experience true collaborative patient-centred care. However, in a team environment, not every interaction is a happy or completely positive experience. Nonetheless, a chance to learn from team dysfunction and conflict resolution should be an intentional part of student clinical experience.

E-LEARNING

e-Learning or online learning has been suggested as a solution to overcoming the logistical challenges of implementing IPE within the educational sector.[47] Despite this suggestion, there is a dearth of published literature on the outcomes of and evidence for IPE in an online or blended setting. Carbonaro et al.[48] redesigned an IP course from a face-to-face, small group learning course to a blended learning course with 70% of the class time delivered online. The student teams in the blended course were compared with the student teams in the traditional face-to-face course in terms of the development of the IP competencies of communication, collaboration and role clarification. No differences were reported between the groups of students on self-report measures of teamwork and communication skills or an observed team interaction.

PREPARATION OF PRECEPTORS OR CLINICAL EDUCATORS

Ideally, students arrive in the healthcare setting IPE ready, and it is the staff and preceptors who assist in the translation of theory into practice. Assumptions are often made that healthcare providers work together and therefore are readily prepared to involve students in CP. This may not be correct; therefore, the educational institution will find it necessary to, at the very least, establish and share common IPE and CP language, and ideally provide education in these concepts for clinical educators, preceptors and anyone working with students. Healthcare providers may fundamentally understand the importance of patient-centred CP, but they may not observe collaboration in their own work environment or feel empowered to foster collaboration themselves. Empowering the preceptors' ability to assist the students can be thought of as the responsibility of the school, or the health provider, or ideally a synergistic process involving educational institutions, health service providers and the bodies or colleges that regulate health professions.

SYSTEMS PLANNING FOR A COLLABORATIVE PRACTICE MODEL

We would be remiss if we overlooked the importance of culture to support IPE and CP within not only the health sector but also the educational sector. As with any change in the culture or direction in health education, a systematic approach is important for successful implementation. It is possible for an educational institution to catalyse change in a clinical environment towards IP care and create a clinical experience for students,[49] but circumstances where and when this can be realised are few and far between. When the administration, leadership and management teams within the educational institution make a commitment to support CP, developed initiatives will be well on their way towards implementation. A strategic approach can then be developed to engage educators in a plan that calls for the valuation of an IP approach to health education.

Without true commitment to patient-centered CP on multiple fronts – within the governments responsible for health and education, within educational institution administration and within the leadership of the healthcare system – we cannot expect front-line staff to adopt a CP model. An effective way to maximise engagement is to involve all stakeholders in an education and collaboration exercise.[43] Role-modelling collaboration as one develops a plan for CP will further illustrate the value of collaboration. A plan to sustain collaboration is necessary to further garner support within all participating organisations and will allow for ongoing allocation of resources.[38] A systems approach is essential for continuous improvement and refinement of CP. Finally, ongoing evaluation and research are vital to keep practice collaborative.

CONCLUSION

As has been identified in this chapter, the lack of empirical rigour in IPE evaluation studies does not translate to lack of support. This situation can be viewed as an opportunity to enhance the quality of educational research within the IPE and CP context. Another gap is in the lack of evidence and understanding about the transferability of the IP knowledge, skills and attitudes gained in post-secondary education to the clinical or community practice. The majority of the published studies describe and evaluate the development of skills over the short term; therefore, an examination of the long-term impact of IPE experiences on key behaviours required for CP as a health professional are essential. In this age of accountability, determining what learning experiences best support the development of specific competencies and how long the duration of the 'effects' is are questions that must be pursued within IPE. Finally, there is a need for a greater understanding of CP in the practice setting.

SUMMARY POINTS

- Empirical evidence for IPE affecting student learning and student outcomes is limited, although it is slowly developing as the field matures.
- Simulation-based education is increasingly used to support the development of teamwork and communication skills, particularly in urgent care settings. The clinical environment holds the most promise for providing relevant IP learning experiences for students; however, not all clinicians are prepared for or capable of adequately modelling CP.
- IP learning experiences should be introduced early in professional programmes, with the appropriate support for early learners.
- Integration throughout the professional programme in simulation-based environments, online learning and clinical environments will continue to enhance the IP competencies and reinforce the knowledge, skills and attitudes required for collaborative practice.
- IP competencies are best learned in authentic and relevant experiences that focus on active or experiential learning approaches embedded in curriculum throughout all years of a professional programme.

REVIEW QUESTIONS

- How can the World Health Organization's Framework for Action[9] and competency or capability frameworks guide the development of IP learning experiences at post-secondary institutions?
- Integrating IP learning experiences into curricula is often impeded by logistical barriers. What are specific strategies to overcome the common barriers to integration?
- How can educators in post-secondary institutions and clinical environments support one another to model CP behaviours for pre-licensure students and prepare (create) a positive learning environment?
- List the models or approaches to exposing students to CP in the clinical setting.
- The 3P model (presage, process and product) provides an approach to support the development of IP learning experiences. Highlight the relevant factors from the three components of this model to develop an IP learning experience at your own institution.

REFLECTIVE EXERCISES AND QUESTIONS

- Think of specific strategies to overcome the logistical challenges of developing and integrating IPE into formal curricula.
- Identify the key strategies to support the development of clinical preceptors (educators) who will effectively model collaborative practice behaviours for students on clinical placements. What can educators do to prepare students for collaborative practice in a clinical setting?
- What types of learning environments work best to develop the IP competencies?
- IP learning experiences should be integrated early and repeated throughout the pre-licensure students' programme. Thinking of your own environment, how would this educational model be supported?

REFERENCES

1. Freeth D, Reeves S. Learning to work together: using the presage, process, product (3P) model to highlight decisions and possibilities. *J Interprof Care.* 2004; **18**(1): 43–56.
2. Barr H, Koppel I, Reeves S, *et al. Effective Interprofessional Education: argument, assumption and evidence.* Oxford: Blackwells; 2005.
3. Frenk J, Chen L, Bhutta ZA, *et al.* Health professionals for a new century: transforming education to strengthen health systems in an interdependent world. *Lancet.* 2010; **376**(9756): 1923–58.
4. Health Council of Canada. *Health Care Renewal in Canada: accelerating change.* Toronto, ON: Health Council of Canada; 2005.
5. http://caipe.org.uk/about-us/defining-ipe/
6. Canadian Health Services Research Foundation (CHSRF). *Teamwork in Healthcare: promoting effective teamwork in healthcare in Canada.* Ottawa, ON: CHSRF; 2006. Available at: www. CHSRF.ca/Migrated/PDF/ResearchReports/CommissionedResearch/teamwork-synthesis-report_e.pdf (accessed 10 September 2010).
7. Committee on Quality of Health Care in America, Institute of Medicine. *Crossing the Quality Chasm: a new health system for the 21st century.* Washington, DC: The National Academies Press; 2001.
8. World Health Organization (WHO). *Global Consultation: the contribution to primary health care and the global health agenda.* Geneva: WHO; 2009.
9. Health Professions Network Nursing and Midwifery Office, Department of Human Resources for Health. *Framework for Action on Interprofessional Education and Collaborative Practice.* Geneva: World Health Organization, Department of Human Resources for Health; 2010.
10. Walsh CL, Gordon MF, Marshall M, *et al.* Interprofessional capability: a developing framework for interprofessional education. *Nurse Educ Pract.* 2005; **5**(3): 230–7.
11. Canadian Interprofessional Health Collaborative (CIHC). *A National Interprofessional Competency Framework.* Vancouver, BC: CIHC; 2010. Available at: www.cihc.ca/files/CIHC_IPCompetencies_Feb1210r.pdf (accessed 15 January 2014).
12. Interprofessional Education Collaborative (IPEC) Expert Panel. *Core Competencies for Interprofessional Collaborative Practice: report of an expert panel.* Washington, DC: Interprofessional Education Collaborative; 2011.
13. Hammick M, Freeth D, Koppel I, *et al.* A best evidence systematic review of interprofessional education: BEME Guide No. 9. *Med Teach.* 2007; **29**(8): 735–51.

14. Lapkin S, Levett-Jones T, Gilligan, C. A systematic review of the effectiveness of interprofessional education in health professional programs. *Nurse Educ Today*. 2013; **33**(2): 90–102.

15. Reeves S, Lewin S, Espin S, *et al. Interprofessional Teamwork in Health and Social Care*. New York, NY: Wiley-Blackwell; 2010.

16. Becker EA, Godwin EM. Methods to improve teaching interdisciplinary teamwork through computer conferencing. *J Allied Health*. 2005; **34**(3): 169–76.

17. Goelen G, De Clercq G, Huyghens L, *et al*. Measuring the effect of interprofessional problem-based learning on the attitudes of undergraduate health care students. *Med Educ*. 2006; **40**(6): 555–61.

18. McFadyen AK, Maclaren WM, Webster VS. The Interdisciplinary Education Perception Scale (IEPS): an alternative remodelled sub-scale structure and its reliability. *J Interprof Care*. 2007; **21**(4): 433–43.

19. Ateach CA, Snow W, Wener P, *et al*. Stereotyping as a barrier to collaboration: does interprofessional education make a difference. *Nurse Educ Today*. 2011; **31**(2): 208–13.

20. Freeth D, Hammick M, Reeves S, *et al. Effective Interprofessional Education: development, delivery, and evaluation*. Oxford: Blackwell Publishing; 2005.

21. Deutschlander S, Suter E, Grymonpre R. Interprofessional practice education: is the 'interprofessional' component relevant to recruiting new graduates to underserved areas? *Rural Remote Health*. 2013; **13**(4): 2489.

22. Lait J, Suter E, Arthur N, *et al*. Interprofessional mentoring: enhancing students' clinical learning. *Nurse Educ Pract*. 2011; **11**(3): 211–15.

23. Coster S, Norman I, Murrells T, *et al*. Interprofessional attitudes amongst undergraduate students in the health professions: a longitudinal questionnaire survey. *Int J Nurs Stud*. 2008; **45**(11): 1667–81.

24. Packard K, Chelal H, Maio A. Interprofessional team reasoning framework as a tool for case study analysis with health professions students: a randomized study. *J Res Interprof Pract Educ*. 2012; **2**(3): 250–63.

25. McGaghie W, Issenberg SB, Petrusa ER, *et al*. A critical review of simulation-based medical education research: 2003–2009. *Med Educ*. 2009; **44**(1): 50–63.

26. Reznek M, Smith-Coggins R, Howard S, *et al*. Emergency medicine crisis resource management (EMCRM): pilot study of a simulation-based crisis management course for emergency medicine. *Acad Emerg Med*. 2003; **10**(4): 386–9.

27. DeVita MA, Schaefer J, Lutz J, *et al*. Improving medical emergency team (MET) performance using a novel curriculum and a computerized human patient simulator. *Qual Safe Health Care*. 2005; **14**(5): 326–31.

28. Shapiro MJ, Morey JC, Small SD, *et al*. Simulation based teamwork training for emergency department staff: does it improve clinical team performance when added to an existing didactic teamwork curriculum? *Qual Safe Health Care*. 2004; **13**(6): 417–21.

29. Jankouskas T, Bush MC, Murray B, *et al*. Crisis Resource Management: evaluating outcomes of a multidisciplinary team. Empirical Investigations. *Simul Healthc*. 2007; **2**(2): 96–101.

30. Shoemaker MJ, Beasley J, Cooper M, *et al*. A method for providing high-volume interprofessional simulation encounters in physical and occupational therapy education programs. *J Allied Health*. 2011; **41**(3): e15–21.

31. King AEA, Conrad M, Ahmed RA. Improving collaboration among medical, nursing and respiratory therapy students through interprofessional simulation. *J Interprof Care*. 2013; **27**(3): 269–71.

32. Buckley S, Hensman M, Thomas S, *et al*. Developing interprofessional simulation in the undergraduate setting: experience with five different professional groups. *J Interprof Care*. 2012; **26**(5): 362–9.

33. Hobgood C, Sherwood G, Frush K, *et al*. Teamwork training with nursing and medical students: does the method matter? Results of an interinstitutional, interdisciplinary collaboration. *Qual Safe Health Care*. 2010; **19**(6): e25.

34. Garbee DD, Paige J, Barrier K, *et al*. Interprofessional teamwork among students in simulated codes: a quasi-experimental study. *Nurs Educ Perspect*. 2013; **34**(5): 339–44.

35. Bandali KS, Craig R, Ziv A. Innovations in applied health: evaluating a simulation-enhanced, interprofessional curriculum. *Med Teach*. 2012; **34**(3): e176–84.

36. Salm T, Greenberg H, Pitzel M, *et al*. Interprofessional education internship in schools: jump starting change. *J Interprof Care*. 2010; **24**(3): 251–63.

37. Russel L, Nyhof-Young J, Abosh B, *et al*. An exploratory analysis of an interprofessional learning environment in two hospital clinical teaching units. *J Interprof Care*. 2006; **20**(1): 29–39.

38. Dow A, Blue A, Konrad SC, *et al*. The moving target: outcomes of interprofessional education. *J Interprof Care*. 2013; **27**(5): 353–5.

39. Lidskog M, Lofmark A, Ahlstrom G. Learning through participating on an interprofessional training ward. *J Interprof Care*. 2009; **23**(5): 486–97.

40. Ponzer S, Hylin U, Kusoffsky A, *et al*. Interprofessional training in the context of clinical practice: goals and students' perceptions on clinical education wards. *Med Educ*. 2004; **38**(7): 727–36.

41. Sommerfeldt SC, Barton SS, Stayko P, *et al*. Creating interprofessional clinical learning units: Developing an acute-care model. *Nurse Educ Pract*. 2011; **11**(4): 273–7.

42. McLelland G, McKenna L, French J. Crossing professional barriers with peer-assisted learning: undergraduate midwifery students teaching undergraduate paramedic students. *Nurse Educ Today*. 2013; **33**(7): 724–8.

43. Missen K, Jacob ER, Barnett T, *et al*. Interprofessional clinical education: clinicians' views on the importance of leadership. *Collegian*. 2012; **19**(4): 189–95.

44. O'Connor A, Cahill M, McKay EA. Revisiting 1:1 and 2:1 clinical placement models: student and clinical educator perspectives. *Aust Occup Ther J*. 2012; **59**(4): 276–83.

45. Smith P, Seely J. A review of the evidence for the maximization of clinical placement opportunities through interprofessional collaboration. *J Interprof Care*. 2010; **24**(6): 690–8.

46. Marken PA, Zimmerman C, Kennedy C, *et al*. Human simulators and standardized patients to teach difficult conversations to interprofessional health care teams. *Am J Pharm Educ*. 2010; **74**(7): 120.

47. Luke R, Solomon P, Baptiste S, *et al*. Online interprofessional health sciences education: from theory to practice. *J Cont Educ Health Prof*. 2009; **29**(3): 161–7.

48. Carbonaro M, King S, Taylor E, *et al*. Integration of e-Learning technologies in an interprofessional health science course. *Med Teach*. 2008; **30**(1): 25–33.

49. Lam W, Chan EA, Yeung K. Implications for school nursing through interprofessional education and practice. *J Clin Nurs*. 2013; **22**(13–14): 1988–2001.

CHAPTER 21

Problem-based learning

Best evidence in health professional education

....

Lisa O'Brien

OVERVIEW

Problem-based learning (PBL) is a major education model that originated in medical schools and has since expanded to fields including health, science, engineering, economics and architecture. Its four key components are (1) ill-structured problems or scenarios, (2) a student-centred approach, (3) teachers acting as facilitators (not lecturers) and (4) authentic and applicable problems or scenarios. Proponents claim that integrative learning engages students in higher-order thinking, prepares them for similar situations in the future, and builds communication and collaboration skills. Detractors point out that the cost and effort associated with its delivery are unwarranted, given the small effects on students' knowledge and clinical performance. While there is no conclusive evidence that PBL is more effective than traditional didactic education for nursing or entry-level therapy professions, research in this field is particularly challenging. Improvements are required in both study design and reporting to minimise the uncertainty in the evaluation of educational interventions.

CHAPTER OBJECTIVES

Upon completion of this chapter, the reader will be able to:
- define the term 'problem-based learning'
- expand on the six core characteristics of PBL
- describe the PBL process
- summarise the evidence for PBL in allied health and nursing curricula on students' knowledge, clinical skills and approaches to learning
- identify key challenges to research in this field, and suggest ways of strengthening the quality of evidence.

KEY TERMS: problem-based learning (PBL); case-based, inquiry-based or scenario-based learning; student-centred approach; self-directed learning; constructivist education theory

---

INTRODUCTION

In the 1990s, evidence-based practice was introduced in the teaching of medical students and it soon become the dominant paradigm in clinical practice and clinical decision-making.[1] After spreading across all health fields, it was applied, inevitably, to education. The push for evidence-based education arose in the United Kingdom and the United States at the start of this century. Robert Coe,[2] from the Curriculum Evaluation and Management Centre at the University of Durham in the United Kingdom, argued in 2000 that

> the ease with which politicians, policy makers – and even teachers – have been able to get away with implementing their prejudices without even token consideration of the evidence, let alone engaging in a serious and informed debate about its quality and importance, is a disgrace.

One of the major education models introduced in the last century was problem-based learning (PBL). It grew from constructivist education theory, which contends that 'learning is a process in which the learner actively constructs knowledge'[3(p13)] and that not only is problem-solving a stimulus for learning but also it determines the nature and organisation of what is learned.[4]

PBL was originally implemented in a new medical school at Canada's McMaster University, which graduated its first class in 1972.[5] It was developed as an alternative to the traditional educational model of passive learning of vast quantities of information, which was not always perceived as relevant by students and could quickly become outdated. PBL emphasised integrative learning in small self-directed groups working on an authentic problem or scenario. The tutor role became that of facilitator rather than an expert lecturer.[6] Its introduction resulted in major, complex and widespread change in educational practice within higher education, especially in health professional education. Since the 1970s it has been adapted and applied across many health curricula and has since spread to science, architecture, economics, education and engineering. Its proponents argue that it promotes active learning, engages learners in higher-order thinking (such as analysis and synthesis), and helps learners to identify key elements of a problem or situation so that they are better prepared for similar situations in the future.[7] In addition, the process of working through a problem in a small group enables growth in discipline or context-specific terminology, as well as improved skills in communication and collaboration.[7]

Despite its common use, debate still rages about its effectiveness and whether the cost and effort associated with its delivery is warranted. While much of the PBL literature relates to its use in medicine, the primary focus of this chapter is on allied health and nursing education.

DEFINITION OF PROBLEM-BASED LEARNING AND ALTERNATIVE TERMS

Defining PBL can be confusing and contentious, although one agreed definition is 'an instructional method characterised by the use of patient problems as a context for students to acquire knowledge about the basic and clinical sciences'.[8(p53)] Based on the original McMaster description, Howard Barrows[5] identified six central characteristics that define PBL in its purest form (*see* summary in Table 21.1).

The term PBL, however, does not refer to a specific educational method. Although the use of problems may be a common denominator in the instructional sequence, PBL may have many different meanings depending on the curriculum design employed and the skills of the facilitator or teacher. To assist in defining it further, and to clarify its various forms, Barrows[9] published a taxonomy in 1986. This defined the terms *lecture-based cases, case-based lectures* and *case method* and the terms *modified case-based, problem-based* and *closed loop or reiterative problem-based learning* based on the degree to which the education methods address specific objectives.[9] Other terms in frequent use, and which may be considered adaptations or hybrids of PBL, are *case-based, inquiry-based* or *scenario-based learning.*

For the purposes of this chapter, the following four key components constitute the minimum standards of PBL: (1) *ill-structured problems* (these require students to generate multiple ideas on how to solve them); (2) a *student-centred approach* (in which students decide what they need to learn); (3) *teachers acting as facilitators* (not lecturers); and (4) problems are selected based on *authenticity* or professional *real-world* applicability.[10]

THE PROBLEM-BASED LEARNING PROCESS

As stated earlier, students work in small groups that are facilitated by a tutor. Problems or cases are prepared by a panel of experts in a particular field and are highly structured. According to Sibley,[11] the six criteria that should be met in the development of the problem are as follows.

TABLE 21.1 Six core characteristics of problem-based learning

Characteristic	Summary
1 Learning is student centred	Under the guidance of a tutor, students: • take responsibility for their own learning • identify what they need to know to better understand and manage the problem • determine where they will get that information (e.g. books, journals, expert opinion)
2 Learning occurs in small student groups	• Ideally, groups are made up of five to nine students • At the end of the unit, groups are randomly reallocated into new groups with a new tutor, to allow practice in working with a variety of different people
3 Teachers are facilitators or guides	The group facilitator (or tutor): does not – • give students a lecture or factual information • tell the students whether they are right or wrong • tell them what they ought to study or read does – • ask students questions that they should be asking themselves to improve understanding of the problem • encourage students to take on this role themselves, including challenging one another
4 Problems form the organising focus and stimulus for learning	• A patient or community health problem is presented in some format, such as a written case, a simulated patient or videotape, which represents a challenge students may face in practice • Gives a focus for integrating information from many disciplines • Facilitates later recall and application to future patient problems
5 Problems are a vehicle for the development of clinical problem-solving skills	The problem format: • presents the patient problem in the same way that it occurs in the real world (e.g. presenting complaints or symptoms) • permits students to ask the patient questions, conduct further assessment (e.g. physical examinations, laboratory tests) and receive the results of these enquiries as they work their way through the problem
6 New information is acquired through self-directed learning	Students are expected to: • learn from the world's knowledge and expertise by virtue of their own study and research (just as real practitioners do) • work together, discussing, comparing, reviewing and debating what they have learned

Note: adapted from Barrows[5]

1. *Prevalence:* the problem should be relatively common
2. *Treatability:* evidence exists for intervention/s
3. *Prototype value:* this allows for the inclusion of experimental or poorly understood problems for more advanced groups later in the curriculum
4. *Interdisciplinary input:* the inclusion of specialised knowledge from several different sciences (e.g. anatomy, psychology, human development, medicine or neurology) and disciplines (the roles of different professions in the management of the problem should be explored)
5. *Length:* the problem should have sufficient depth, focus and complexity to challenge the group for the duration of the problem's cycle, but it should not be so long that it causes students to feel overwhelmed or they are unable to solve it
6. *Format:* this is *how* the problem is presented to students and can include a variety of media such as case histories, reports by practitioners and videotaped or simulated patients and cases

The execution of PBL varies in practice, but the typical tutorial group usually meets twice a week, with sessions running for 1–3 hours.[12] At the commencement of the problem or case, groups are given a 'trigger', which may be a simulated patient or client or a brief written referral. The process then follows a specific sequence, such as the Maastricht 'seven jump' sequence, named after a Dutch children's song (*see* Box 21.1). The first five of these jumps, or steps, occur in the first tutorial. At its conclusion, students agree on a set of learning objectives and then enter a self-directed learning phase, which may include lectures, practicums and independent research. At the second tutorial (usually 2–4 days later), students present the new learning to one another, conclude the case discussion, identify unanswered questions and evaluate the group's performance.

BOX 21.1 Maastricht 'seven jump' sequence for problem-based learning[13]

1. Clarify and agree working definitions and unclear terms and concepts
2. Define the problems; agree which phenomena need explanation
3. Analyse the problem (brainstorm)
4. Arrange possible explanations and working hypotheses
5. Generate and prioritise learning objectives
6. Research the learning objectives
7. Report back, synthesise explanations and apply newly acquired information to the problem

---

THE USE OF PROBLEM-BASED LEARNING IN HEALTH PROFESSIONAL EDUCATION

PBL has experienced growing popularity in health professional education and has been implemented in professional entry-level or postgraduate curricula of nursing,[14–16] physiotherapy,[17–21] occupational therapy,[22–24] speech pathology and language therapy,[25,26] podiatry,[27] dietetics,[28,29] chiropractic[30] and respiratory therapy.[31,32] This choice to apply this approach is not surprising, as problem-solving skills are considered essential for therapists in daily clinical practice, and PBL is thought to assist students to develop these along with clinical reasoning and communication skills.[6,33] A review of educational approaches and teaching methods in occupational therapy found

> a trend to endorse educational approaches believed to help students develop higher-order thinking, collaboration with others, civic responsibility and clinical reasoning, among other capacities deemed important for a professional. Examples included PBL, service learning and interprofessional learning.[34(p14)]

The purported benefits, however, need to be weighed against the costs of PBL, as it comes with substantial resource requirements including start-up costs in curriculum development, increased demands on teaching and assessment time,[35] and the maintenance of tutorial teaching rooms and equipment.[12]

HOW EFFECTIVE IS PROBLEM-BASED LEARNING OVERALL?

Given the inconsistencies in PBL definition and implementation, comparison of the effectiveness of traditional and problem-based curricula has been difficult. Despite extensive research on PBL over the last 40 years, there is still robust debate regarding its efficacy. In 1993, three comprehensive reviews of PBL in medical education were published in the same journal with varying findings. Two meta-analyses[8,36] concluded that graduates of traditional curricula performed better in tests of factual knowledge, and PBL students tended to engage in less-desirable backward reasoning strategies; however, PBL students and educators generally enjoyed PBL more than traditional curricula. The third review, a narrative review, concluded that there was no distinguishable difference between PBL and traditional graduates, that PBL can be stressful for student and faculty, and that it is unreasonably costly.[37]

The debate continued in 2000, when a new review of the medical education literature on the effectiveness of PBL found 'no convincing evidence that PBL improves knowledge base and clinical performance, at least not of the magnitude that would be expected given the resources required'.[38(p259)] A rebuttal by Norman and Schmidt[39] argued that the small effect sizes and inconclusive findings are not the result of inadequate theory behind PBL but, rather, they reflect

> the futility of conducting research on interventions which are so complex and multifactorial, with so many unseen interacting forces, using

outcomes so distant from the learning setting, that any predicted effects would inevitably be diffused by myriad unexplained variables.[(p722)]

Norman and Schmidt[39] contend that the significant effects reported *are* evidence of the effectiveness of PBL, as it is able to show differences *despite* the impediments noted.

A major meta-analysis published by Walker and Leary[10] in 2009 analysed the effectiveness of PBL across disciplines (specifically, medical education, teacher education, science, engineering, business, social science and allied health), problem types, the PBL approach employed and the level of assessment. Across 82 studies and 201 outcomes (which included written and oral exam results, employer or supervisor ratings, and measures of problem-solving, critical thinking and clinical reasoning), they concluded that across almost all analyses, 'PBL students either did as well as or better than their lecture-based counterparts, and they tended to do better when the subject matter was outside of medical education'.[10(p24)] In fact, their regression analysis found that PBL performed best *outside* of medical education and allied health, when assessment is at the application rather than the concept level and when the intervention uses the full closed-loop approach. The authors, however, cautioned that a lack of homogeneity warranted closer examination of moderating factors.[10]

HOW EFFECTIVE IS PROBLEM-BASED LEARNING IN HEALTH PROFESSIONAL EDUCATION?

It is important to note that most of the studies included in Walker and Leary's[10] meta-analysis were of medical students, as there is limited research in allied health that could meet the quality criteria required for inclusion. For a review in 2011 of the effectiveness of PBL in professional entry-level therapy education, O'Donoghue *et al.*[33] searched the following databases: ERIC (Education Resources Information Center), Academic Search Premier, PsycINFO, Embase, PubMed, CINAHL (Cumulative Index to Nursing and Allied Health Literature), Scopus and Web of Science. Subject headings and keywords based on 'problem-based learning' were combined with the various therapy professions, and studies that utilised solely qualitative designs were excluded. Other inclusion criteria encompassed study design (randomised controlled trials, controlled trials, interrupted time series analyses, controlled before-and-after studies), types of intervention (the presence of the six central characteristics identified by Barrows[5]) and outcome measures (accumulation of knowledge, improved performance, improved approach to learning, student satisfaction). The authors found only six studies that met their inclusion criteria. Three were from physiotherapy,[18,19,40] and there was one each from occupational therapy,[41] dietetics[28] and podiatry.[27] Outcome measures were students' knowledge, clinical performance, approaches to learning and satisfaction.[33] An updated search by the author of this chapter revealed no new studies meeting the inclusion criteria.

Student knowledge

In terms of student knowledge, one high-quality study of podiatry students[27] found that PBL students had significantly higher levels of knowledge acquisition (as measured by exam results). However, there were no significant differences between groups in a high-quality study of dietetics students[28] and between groups in a lower-quality study of occupational therapy students.[41]

Clinical performance

Only two studies[18,40] included measures of clinical performance (the American Physical Therapy Association's Clinical Performance Instrument), but neither of these studies found a significant difference in performance between PBL and control groups.

Approaches to learning

Results for student approaches to learning were more encouraging. One high-quality study[27] found that PBL students performed significantly better in tests of deeper understanding and patient treatment-related cognitive skills, and another found greater gains in reflective thinking, suggesting improved critical thinking skills.[28] Of the lower-quality studies, however, one found no difference[41] and the other, a longitudinal comparative study of physiotherapy students in two different schools,[19] found students in the subject-centred curriculum were adopting significantly more desirable study approaches than the problem-based students were at the end of their second year.

HOW EFFECTIVE IS PROBLEM-BASED LEARNING IN NURSING EDUCATION?

Two major systematic reviews of nursing education have been conducted in the last 2 years: one by Thompson and Stapley,[42] examining the impact of educational approaches on judgement and clinical decision-making; the other by Kong et al.,[43] specifically focused on PBL's effectiveness in developing critical thinking skills. Both reviews had exhaustive search strategies, both rated study quality against specific criteria published by the Cochrane Collaboration[44] and both only included randomised controlled trials; Thompson and Stapley[42] included both undergraduate and postgraduate nursing students, while Kong et al.[43] included only undergraduates.

Critical thinking skills

The review by Thompson and Stapley[42] only included three studies that measured PBL's effectiveness in improving critical thinking skills. One of these studies showed higher scores for comprehension, application, analysis, synthesis and evaluation skills but not overall critical thinking;[45] one study showed no difference in critical thinking between groups;[46] and one study showed no immediate effect but reported significant differences between groups on subscales of the California Critical Thinking Disposition Inventory at 1- and 2-year follow-up.[47] Nine articles representing eight studies were included in the more recent review by Kong *et al.*[43] Six of these were published in English, two were in Chinese and one was in Korean. A pooled meta-analysis found that PBL was able to improve nursing students' critical thinking (overall critical thinking scores: standard mean difference = 0.33; 95% confidence interval = 0.13–0.52; p = 0.0009) when compared with traditional lectures. This indicates a relatively small effect size but it supports the findings of an earlier review.[48]

Student knowledge and motivation

There are limited high-quality studies conducted that compare PBL with other teaching methods in nursing. One quasi-experimental study compared pre- and post-test scores for Korean nursing students enrolled in a cardiorespiratory subject and allocated to either a PBL group or traditional lectures based on year of enrolment.[49] The authors found that the PBL students scored higher on an objective test of knowledge and were more motivated to learn, according to the Instructional Materials Motivation Survey. A similar quasi-experimental study of midwifery students conducted in Iran also found higher motivation and better performance on a student learning progress test.[50] It must be noted, however, that both studies only applied PBL for a specific subject, not for the entire duration of the course, and both had small sample sizes.

CONCLUSIONS

The development and evaluation of education approaches for health practitioners is not always supported by sound educational theory. Gibbs *et al.*[51] point out that

> practicing physicians and researchers base their decisions on research evidence, (whereas) medical teachers frequently rely on tradition and intuition rather than explicit theory-driven activities, and many such assumptions are eventually proven wrong when subjected to scrutiny.[(p183)]

A review of physiotherapy research into the effectiveness of PBL concluded that 'literature evaluating PBL and PT [physiotherapy] is still in its infancy'.[21(p47)] Similarly, a systematic mapping review of educational approaches in occupational therapy[34] found that most researchers chose to measure student perceptions of the learning activity, often using customised assessment tools, rather than the more important measures of changes in student behaviour or skills. Finally, it is important to acknowledge that the implementation of PBL involves substantial resource requirements over and above the traditional curriculum, in terms of student contact hours, teacher-to-student ratios and assessment methods.[35] These issues can become critical in class sizes greater than 100.

RECOMMENDATIONS FOR BUILDING THE BODY OF EVIDENCE IN ALLIED HEALTH EDUCATION

Research into the effectiveness of PBL should include:

- some form of randomisation of students – for example, the randomised facto-rial block design used by Lohse *et al.*[28]
- clear descriptions of both the experimental (PBL) and the control interventions – this will enable distinctions between different types of PBL and between PBL and other educational interventions
- valid and reliable measures, such as objective structured clinical examina-tions, portfolios, observation checklists, logbooks, and interviews or written feedback from fieldwork educators
- a cost-benefit analysis.

SUMMARY POINTS

- There is limited evidence to support PBL for improving students' approaches to learning in allied health and nursing education.
- A major problem with determining the effectiveness of education approaches in allied health and nursing is the difficulty in applying a rigorous research design. It is almost impossible to randomise students to a specific curriculum, as the students themselves select which course they want to enrol in. Future studies could address this by randomising students *within* a curriculum.
- Another issue is the variability of implementation of PBL in different environ-ments. The process described earlier this chapter is not always adhered to, and group size, number of meetings per week and the intensity of supple-mentary teaching (lectures, practicums) can differ vastly between courses and schools.
- Research to date has also been constrained by poor choices of outcome measures.
- Compared with traditional lecture-based curricula, PBL is highly resource-intensive and it may become unwieldy in larger class sizes.

REVIEW QUESTIONS

- List the six core characteristics of PBL.
- Which educational theory underpins PBL?
- How does the Maastricht 'seven jump' sequence contribute to the construc-tion of new knowledge in the student group?
- Give one example each of an ill-defined and a well-defined problem.
- List two key challenges to research comparing educational approaches, and suggest ways of addressing these.

REFLECTIVE QUESTIONS AND EXERCISES

- Why are ill-defined problems so important in PBL?
- Discuss the advantages and disadvantages of PBL in comparison with lecture-based models of teaching.
- Define 'critical thinking', and identify how this could be elicited or assessed in classroom activities.

REFERENCES

1. Biesta G. Why 'what works' won't work: evidence-based practice and the democratic deficit in educational research. *Educ Theory.* 2007; **57**(1): 1–22.
2. Coe R. *A Manifesto for Evidence-Based Education: an essay which presents a particular view of evidence-based education and why we need it.* Durham, UK: Evidence-Based Education Network, University of Durham; 1999.
3. Gijselaers WH. Connecting problem-based practices with educational theory. *New Direct Teach Learn.* 1996; **1996**(68): 13–21.
4. Savery JR, Duffy TM. Problem based learning. an instructional model and its constructivist framework. *Educ Technol.* 1995; **35**(5): 31–8.
5. Barrows HS. Problem-based learning in medicine and beyond: a brief overview. *New Direct Teach Learn.* 1996; **1996**(68): 3–12.
6. Walton HJ, Matthews M. Essentials of problem-based learning. *Med Educ.* 1989; **23**(6): 542–8.
7. Savery JR. Overview of problem-based learning: definitions and distinctions. *Int J Problem Based Learn.* 2006; **1**(1): 3.
8. Albanese MA, Mitchell S. Problem-based learning: a review of literature on its outcomes and implementation issues. *Acad Med.* 1993; **68**(1): 52–81.
9. Barrows HS. A taxonomy of problem-based learning methods. *Med Educ.* 1986; **20**(6): 481–6.
10. Walker A, Leary H. A problem based learning meta analysis: differences across problem types, implementation types, disciplines, and assessment levels. *Int J Problem Based Learn.* 2009; **3**(1): 12–43.
11. Sibley JC. Toward an emphasis on problem solving in teaching and learning: the McMaster experience. In: Schmidt H, Lipkin M, de Vries M, *et al.*, editors. *New Directions for Medical Education.* New York, NY: Springer-Verlag; 1989. pp. 147–56.
12. Brown GT, Ebden M. The efficacy of problem-based learning: what does the research evidence say? *Philippine J Occup Ther.* 2006; **2**(1–2): 5–17.
13. Spencer JA, Jordan RK. Learner centred approaches in medical education. *BMJ.* 1999; **318**(7193): 1280.
14. Biley FC, Smith KL. Making sense of problem-based learning: the perceptions and experiences of undergraduate nursing students. *J Adv Nurs.* 1999; **30**(5): 1205–12.
15. Wong FKY, Lee WM, Mok E. Educating nurses to care for the dying in Hong Kong: a problem-based learning approach. *Cancer Nurs.* 2001; **24**(2): 112–21.
16. Baker CM. Problem-based learning for nursing: integrating lessons from other disciplines with nursing experiences. *J Prof Nur.* 2000; **16**(5): 258–66.
17. Eksteen C, Slabbert J. Problem based curricula and problem based learning in physiotherapy: a critical review. *S Afr J Physiother.* 2001; **57**(4): 23–9.
18. Kaufman R, Portney L, Jette D. Clinical performance of physical therapy students in traditional and problem-based curricula. *J Phys Ther Educ.* 1997; **11**(1): 26–31.

19. Titchen AC, Coles CR. Comparative study of physiotherapy students' approaches to their study in subject-centered and problem-based curricula. *Physiother Theory Pract.* 1991; **7**(2): 127–33.

20. Van Langenberghe HV. Evaluation of students' approaches to studying in a problem-based physical therapy curriculum. *Phys Ther.* 1988; **68**(4): 522–7.

21. Solomon P. Problem-based learning: a review of current issues relevant to physiotherapy education. *Physiother Theory Pract.* 2005; **21**(1): 37–49.

22. Busuttil JA. Problem based learning occupational therapy course: the second year. *Br J Occup Ther.* 1988; **51**(11): 8–10.

23. McCarron KA, Amico FD. The impact of problem-based learning on clinical reasoning in occupational therapy education. *Occup Ther Health Care.* 2002; **16**(1): 1–13.

24. Royeen CB. A problem-based learning curriculum for occupational therapy education. *Am J Occup Ther.* 1995; **49**(4): 338–46.

25. Whitworth A, Franklin S, Dodd B. Case-based problem solving for speech and language therapy students. In: Brumfitt S, editor. *Innovations in Professional Education for Speech and Language Therapy.* London: Whurr Publishers; 2004. pp. 29–50.

26. Mok CK, Whitehill TL, Dodd BJ. Problem-based learning, critical thinking and concept mapping in speech-language pathology education: a review. *Int J Speech Lang Pathol.* 2008; **10**(6): 438–48.

27. Finch PM. The effect of problem-based learning on the academic performance of students studying podiatric medicine in Ontario. *Med Educ.* 1999; **33**(6): 411–17.

28. Lohse B, Nitzke S, Ney DM. Introducing a problem-based unit into a lifespan nutrition class using a randomized design produces equivocal outcomes. *J Am Diet Assoc.* 2003; **103**(8): 1020–5.

29. Terry PH, Seibels DR. Incorporating problem-based learning into an undergraduate community nutrition class. *J Nutr Educ Behav.* 2006; **38**(2): 121–2.

30. Bovee ML, Gran DF. Comparison of two teaching methods in a chiropractic clinical science course. *J Allied Health.* 2000; **29**(3): 157–60.

31. Ceconi A. *Influence of Problem-Based Learning Instruction on Decision-Making Skills in Respiratory Therapy Students* [dissertation]. South Orange, NJ: Seton Hall University; 2006.

32. Beachey WD. A comparison of problem-based learning and traditional curricula in baccalaureate respiratory therapy education. *Respir Care.* 2007; **52**(11): 1497–506.

33. O'Donoghue G, McMahon S, Doody C, *et al.* Problem-based learning in professional entry-level therapy education: a review of controlled evaluation studies. *Int J Problem Based Learn.* 2011; **5**(1): 5.

34. Hooper B, King R, Wood W, *et al.* An international systematic mapping review of educational approaches and teaching methods in occupational therapy. *Br J Occup Ther.* 2013; **76**(1): 9–22.

35. Koh GC-H, Khoo HE, Wong ML, *et al.* The effects of problem-based learning during medical school on physician competency: a systematic review. *CMAJ.* 2008; **178**(1): 34–41.

36. Vernon DT, Blake RL. Does problem-based learning work? A meta-analysis of evaluative research. *Acad Med.* 1993; **68**(7): 550–63.

37. Berkson L. Problem-based learning: have the expectations been met? *Acad Med.* 1993; **68**(10): S79–88.

38. Colliver JA. Effectiveness of problem-based learning curricula: research and theory. *Acad Med.* 2000; **75**(3): 259–66.

39. Norman GR, Schmidt HG. Effectiveness of problem based learning curricula: theory, practice and paper darts. *Med Educ.* 2000; **34**(9): 721–8.

40. Van Duijn A, Bevins S. Clinical performances of physical therapist students in problem-based, mixed-model, and traditional curricula. *J Phys Ther Educ.* 2005; **19**(2): 15.

41. Liotta-Kleinfeld L, McPhee S. Comparison of final exam test scores of neuroscience students who experienced traditional methodologies versus problem-based learning methodologies. *Occup Ther Health Care.* 2002; **14**(3–4): 35–53.

42. Thompson C, Stapley S. Do educational interventions improve nurses' clinical decision making and judgement? A systematic review. *Inter J Nurs Stud.* 2011; **48**(7): 881–93.

43. Kong L-N, Qin B, Zhou Y-Q, *et al.* The effectiveness of problem-based learning on development of nursing students' critical thinking: a systematic review and meta-analysis. *Inter J Nurs Stud.* 2014; **51**(3): 458–69.

44. Higgins JP, Green S, editors. *Cochrane Handbook for Systematic Reviews of Interventions. Version 5.1.0.* The Cochrane Collaboration, 2011. Available: www.cochrane-handbook.org.

45. Jones M. Developing clinically savvy nursing students: an evaluation of problem-based learning in an associate degree program. *Nurs Educ Perspect.* 2008; **29**(5): 278–83.

46. Yuan H, Kunaviktikul W, Klunklin A, *et al.* Improvement of nursing students' critical thinking skills through problem-based learning in the People's Republic of China: a quasi-experimental study. *Nurs Health Sci.* 2008; **10**(1): 70–6.

47. Tiwari A, Lai P, So M, *et al.* A comparison of the effects of problem-based learning and lecturing on the development of students' critical thinking. *Med Educ.* 2006; **40**(6): 547–54.

48. Oja KJ. Using problem-based learning in the clinical setting to improve nursing students' critical thinking: an evidence review. *J Nurs Educ.* 2011; **50**(3): 145.

49. Hwang SY, Kim MJ. A comparison of problem-based learning and lecture-based learning in an adult health nursing course. *Nurse Educ Today.* 2006; **26**(4): 315–21.

50. Sangestani G, Khatiban M. Comparison of problem-based learning and lecture-based learning in midwifery. *Nurse Educ Today.* 2013; **33**(8): 791–5.

51. Gibbs T, Durning S, Van Der Vleuten C. Theories in medical education: towards creating a union between educational practice and research traditions. *Med Teach.* 2011; **33**(3): 183–7.

CHAPTER 22

Case-based learning

Application and evidence in health professional education contexts

....

Jill E Thistlethwaite

OVERVIEW

The patient case is the basis of the practice of healthcare delivery and cases have been used for the education of health professionals for many decades. This chapter considers the nature of 'cases' and defines case-based learning (CBL), an educational strategy that is more formal than but has many similarities to problem-based learning (PBL). The characteristics of good cases have been defined and they should have the following attributes: relevance, realism, engagement, challenge and instructional ability. I discuss the evidence for the effectiveness of CBL, drawing on a recent BEME (Best Evidence Medical Education) review of CBL and updating this with more recent publications. The literature shows that learners like CBL and that CBL helps them apply knowledge to clinical experience, thus enhancing its relevance.

CHAPTER OBJECTIVES

Upon completion of this chapter, the reader will be able to:
- define the terms 'case' and 'case-based learning'
- understand the similarities and differences between CBL and PBL
- describe how to use cases through experiential learning
- outline the characteristics of good cases
- summarise the evidence for CBL
- explain the BEME process and reviews.

KEY TERMS: case-based learning, case method, problem-based learning, BEME (Best Evidence Medical Education)

INTRODUCTION

Professor David Irby, the distinguished health professional educator with more than 40 years' experience, wrote in an essay in 1994: 'Clinical teaching in medicine takes place in the discourse surrounding particular cases.'[1(p947)] In the context of health professional practice, a 'case' generally refers to a patient's (or client's) episode of a condition affecting health in some way. It may be short term (she had shingles) or occur over a longer time (he has bowel cancer). In a more derogatory fashion, some patients may be referred to as 'the case of diabetes in bed 3'. Particularly in hospital settings 'the case' is time-limited, a single occurrence in the professional's work, although obviously for the patient the 'case' started before that admission and may last long after discharge. A patient's (hi)story is captured in the medical records or 'case notes'; these records may be scattered across several settings so that only with the patient is the complete case or history combined.

Other professions besides health also use the discourse of cases – in particular, law and business. Indeed, the Harvard Business School (HBS) was one of the pioneers of what the HBS faculty called the case method. The method was adopted by the HBS in 1920, just over a decade after the school's foundation, and is still in use there today. In the context of the case method, a case was defined by the HBS in 1975 as a description of a management situation. The cases can be up to 25 pages long (much longer than those used in health professional education) and are 'not written to illustrate correct or incorrect handling of an administrative situation, nor is there an editorial bias that implies a particular conclusion.'[1(p947)] However, the success of the HBS was not repeated by the Harvard Graduate School of Education, which failed to introduce the case method into its programmes in the 1920s due to lack of resources, failure to articulate the conceptual orientation of the approach and its underlying philosophy, and case writing not being seen as a legitimate use of faculty time.[1]

So when the nature of, and evidence for, case-based learning (CBL) is considered, the definition of 'case' in the particular context in which the word is being used needs to be considered. There is as yet no one succinct and consensus definition of CBL.[2]

There are also a number of similar terms to CBL that have proliferated over the years (*see* Table 22.1). Some of these focus on 'learning', while other, usually older, methods stress 'teaching'. To complicate matters further, CBL is often compared with problem-based learning (PBL), with varying degrees of similarity and difference occurring between the two approaches.

TABLE 22.1 Variations on case-based learning

- Case-based learning
- Case study teaching
- Case study-based learning
- Case method learning
- Case method of teaching (dates back to 1912)
- Case-based problem-based learning
- Investigative case-based learning – combines PBL with investigative approaches in which students develop and test hypotheses
- Integrative, longitudinal case-based learning

Irby's[1] paper highlights the nature of the difficulties with 'case' against the background of traditional medical student teaching. He compares the use of cases as bedside teaching (a 'real' person – an inpatient), written mini-cases presented during interactive sessions, and iterative teaching in which small pieces of information pertinent to the case are disclosed gradually to facilitate clinical reasoning and management planning. Finally, he recommends that using cases in this way should be based on the five principles of experiential learning: (1) anchor teaching in cases, (2) actively involve learners, (3) model professional thinking and action, (4) provide direction and feedback and (5) create a collaborative learning environment.

CASE-BASED VERSUS PROBLEM-BASED LEARNING

It is important to consider the similarities and differences between CBL and PBL. Similar to CBL, PBL has been characterised by a widening of its definition in recent decades to a multiplicity of formats.[3,4] Barrows and Tamblyn[5] initially defined PBL as 'learning that results from the process of working towards the understanding of a resolution of a problem. The problem is encountered first in the learning process.'[(p74)] Thus the emphasis is on a 'problem' rather than a case, although, as the definition is in relation to medical education, the problems used are frequently discrete patient cases. CBL is frequently referred to as more structured than PBL, with defined learning outcomes rather than students having to set their own outcomes, as is recommended for PBL.[5] However, 'hybrid' models of PBL may also involve more structured teaching.

One such hybrid model is case-based problem-based learning (CBPBL), which is described as a variation of PBL and is

> the use of storytelling to engage students in the problems or dilemmas faced by the character(s) in the narrative, calling upon the students' use of

information gathering and decision-making skills in identifying key issues and postulating possible solutions.[5](p74)

Barrows and Tamblyn[5] claim that

> CBPBL tends to be more open-ended than the PBL designed for medical students, which of necessity guides students toward the solution of specific problems. CBPBL potentially guides learners to many problems and solutions that they define for themselves.(p74)

This chapter highlights the way in which terminology is used to establish a method without establishing in any great depth the differences between CBPBL, CBL and PBL. All approaches can be referred to as 'student centred', which is an overused phrase similar to patient centred and which also has multiple expressions. The CBPBL paper follows a common structure of definition of term, rationale for the approach, description of what was done, examples of cases, and advantages and disadvantages, without any evaluation data or discussion of what makes the approach effective in this context. The method is described as being implemented in a medical library with the librarian as facilitator, and the students working on the case in what is essentially (without being labelled as such) an evidence-based practice approach.

Both PBL and CBL are referred to as examples of student-centred learning, with its emphasis on active rather than passive learning, deep rather than surface understanding, student autonomy and responsibility, and a reflexive approach to teaching and learning.[6,7] However, CBL does not extend to the logical endpoint of student-centred learning, where students decide what they want to learn and how; instead, cases are written for students to facilitate learning in specific areas related to their health professional curricula, which are mandated ultimately by the relevant health professional accreditation bodies.

CHARACTERISTICS OF CASE-BASED LEARNING AND THE CASES

Nowadays, CBL usually refers to cases drawn from real life but not involving a living, 'real' person. They may feature paper-based 'people' or families, virtual (online) and/or simulated patients (real people role-playing). Cases used for CBL generally have several of the characteristics shown in Table 22.2 (many of which have been stipulated by the National Center for Case Study Teaching in Science). The main aims of CBL as stated in the literature are to facilitate the integration of theory with practice, link health sciences with clinical applications, and stimulate learners' interest through professional relevance.[4] The purpose of this chapter, therefore, is to appraise the evidence for the effectiveness of CBL in achieving these aims.

TABLE 22.2 Characteristics of 'good cases'[9]

Cases should:
- be based on real patient histories (e.g. they are authentic)
- involve common scenarios based on core learning outcomes
- tell a story and be logical
- have educational value
- be stimulating
- create empathy with the characters
- include patients' or clients' sayings (voices) that are credible and which add drama and realism
- facilitate inquiry and problem-solving
- promote decision-making
- link theory with practice

The integrative, longitudinal case-based learning approach[8] features cases that span generations through the use of family trees. The idea for the Indiana University Doctor of Physical Therapy Family Tree, an integrated case series, was developed during a faculty retreat. The additional features arising from the longitudinal nature of the case are consideration of the lifespan of clients, family relationships over time and the changing impact of illness on function and quality of life.

In 2006, Kim *et al.*[10] published a review of 'case-based teaching' including law, engineering and business as well as the health professions with the aim of defining a framework to assist with the development of cases. They identified five core attributes of cases: (1) relevance, (2) realism, (3) engagement, (4) challenge and (5) being instructional. While the framework is useful, the papers from which this is synthesised are not critically appraised but, rather, categorised under various headings. So without reading all the papers it is not possible to gain any sense of how the findings are achieved, and whether opinion is based on evaluation data. The teaching aids identified are interesting as a sign of the diversity of approaches and include branching diagrams to support decision-making, concept maps, questions, expert modelling of problem-solving approaches and teaching points.

THE EVIDENCE FOR CASE-BASED LEARNING: A BEME SYSTEMATIC REVIEW

Between 2010 and 2011, I was the lead reviewer of a research group based at the University of Warwick in the United Kingdom. Together we carried out a systematic review of the effectiveness of CBL[4] following a Best Evidence Medical Education (BEME) review process (*see* Table 22.3), following the submission of a standard review protocol (*see* Table 22.4). The aim was to explore, analyse and synthesise the evidence relating to the effectiveness of CBL as a means of achieving defined learning outcomes in health professional pre-qualification training programmes.[4]

TABLE 22.3 Stages of a BEME (Best Evidence Medical Education) review[11]

- Select a topic
- Form a review group (usually 6–10 members and involving two or more institutions)
- Register the topic
- Write the review protocol, submit for feedback and revise as necessary
- Pilot the review (scoping search)
- Undertake the main review
- Report on progress
- Submit completed review
- Revise review following feedback from four reviewers
- Once accepted, review is published on BEME website and in *Medical Teacher* journal

TABLE 22.4 The BEME (Best Evidence Medical Education) protocol[11]

- Cover sheet with title and members of topic review group
- Background to the topic (with references)
- Review questions and review objectives
- Study selection criteria (inclusion and exclusion)
- Procedure for extracting data and analysis
- How extracted data will be synthesised (theoretical framework for synthesis)
- Project timetable
- Plans for updating the review

One hundred and four papers were included in the review, which showed marked variation in the ways cases were defined and used to enhance learning. While medical students were the most frequently involved professional group (68 papers), there were also reports of CBL implementation with nursing (9), mixed (multi- or interprofessional) groups (7), psychology (9), veterinary science (5), dentistry (5), paramedicine (2), pharmacy (2) and one each from chiropractic, social science and speech pathology.[4] Papers included learning activities involving only one case and lasting 2 hours through to a CBL curriculum running over a whole year.

EVALUATION OF EDUCATION

To be eligible for inclusion in a systematic review of effectiveness, papers have to include evaluation data rather than be simple descriptions of learning and teaching activities and innovations. In this respect, evaluation is a 'systematic collection of information about the activities, characteristics and results of programmes to make judgments about the programme, improve or further develop programme effectiveness, inform decisions about future programming, and/or increase understanding'.[12(p39)]

BEME reviews in general highlight the diversity of approaches to evaluation. Most health professional education evaluation is outcomes focused: *Was the intervention effective?* Such a question is linked to the necessity of curricular innovations showing change for the better in terms of student satisfaction and learning. Funders want to know that learning activities are cost-effective, particularly with respect to what they are, or are potentially, replacing. However, few evaluations involve comparison of learning approaches – such comparison is costly and raises ethical issues around equity and assessment. Comparison, if attempted, may involve change within a particular cohort of students, or comparisons may be made, for example, with a control (without the intervention) or with another group (with a different intervention).

For larger-scale changes such as a new curriculum, there may be a 'historical control' – one whole year's cohort of students is compared with the previous year group. The gold standard of biomedical research, the double-blind randomised crossover trial, is not feasible for obvious reasons, although educators are frequently still encouraged to try some type of randomisation. Thus, CBL in small groups may be compared with traditional lectures; however, such methods have many confounding factors: we cannot be sure in this instance if any effect is due to the cases or the small group delivery method. CBL using paper cases may be compared with the same cases but online – this trial is then concerned with exploring the difference between the learning medium rather than the CBL itself.

The Kirkpatrick model is an example of an outcomes-based evaluation method for training programmes.[13] It was originally developed in 1959 for use in business organisations and was later adapted for use in health professional education – specifically, interprofessional education – by the Interprofessional Education Joint Evaluation Team in the United Kingdom.[14] This adapted model expanded the Kirkpatrick framework from four to six categories or levels, and it can be further adapted for use for any educational outcome (*see* Table 22.5). The outcomes are learner reaction (usually focusing on satisfaction), changes in attitudes, learning of knowledge and skills, change in behaviour and, for level 4, outcomes relating to patients and health service delivery.

TABLE 22.5 Classification of educational outcomes: modified Kirkpatrick framework

Level	Educational outcome
1: Reaction	Learners' views on the learning experience and its interprofessional nature
2a: Modification of perceptions and attitudes	Changes in reciprocal attitudes or perceptions between participant groups
2b: Acquisition of knowledge and skills	Learners gain new knowledge and skills
3: Behavioural change	Identifies individuals' transfer of learning to their practice setting and their changed professional practice
4a: Change in organisational practice	Wider changes in the organisation and delivery of care
4b: Benefits to patients or clients	Improvements in health or well-being of patients or clients

This modified model is used as part of the BEME process to categorise outcomes and therefore evidence of effectiveness, in relation to educational interventions and innovations. In health professional education the ultimate aim may be to improve patient health, patient safety and satisfaction as outcomes but, certainly for pre-qualification courses, this is almost impossible to do without long-term evaluation. As would be expected, most evaluation is at the level of student reaction – but this is still an important parameter to explore. Students are more likely to learn if they are engaged and motivated to turn up to activities. The BEME CBL review had 83% papers reporting on student reaction, 40% on changes in student knowledge, 9% on changes in student attitudes and none for levels 3 and 4.[4]

EVIDENCE: STUDENT REACTION TO CASE-BASED LEARNING

In terms of student feedback, common words mentioned in the papers included 'liked', 'highly satisfied', 'stimulated', 'motivated', 'challenged', 'helpful', 'valuable', 'appreciated' and 'fun'. Students also commented on the real-life relevance of cases, their improved confidence in planning patient management and that they felt they had achieved their objectives. CBL was stated as involving a deeper learning approach, facilitating the learning of factual material and bolstering personal interest and involvement in the subject matter. More negative reaction focused on workload and lack of structure, with some students struggling with the amount of self-direction required for some CBL activities.[4]

MOVING BEYOND OUTCOMES AND EFFECTIVENESS: HOW DOES CASE-BASED LEARNING WORK?

Outcomes-based evaluation does not tell us anything about how and why an intervention works. Educators want to know why some students enjoy CBL and others struggle; how to enhance any learning effect; why some students prefer online cases and others prefer paper-based cases in classrooms. This is a realist evaluation approach, as defined by Pawson and Tilley[15]: the exploration of what works for whom and in what contexts. In summary from the BEME review, the effectiveness of CBL appears to relate to the active learning undertaken by students and the application of knowledge acquired to different cases, thus enhancing its relevance.[4] Such active learning fits within the conceptual framework of inquiry-based learning as defined by Banchi and Bell.[16] Inquiry-based learning emphasises constructivist approaches to learning, with knowledge being acquired in a series of steps and through group processes. In the BEME review we concluded that of the four levels of inquiry-based learning (confirmation, structured, guided and open), CBL in most manifestations fits between structured and guided.

EXAMPLES OF MORE RECENT EVALUATIONS OF CASE-BASED LEARNING
Tutorial-based versus online case-based learning

A review published in 2011 focused on online CBL in higher education.[17] Of the 11 papers eligible for inclusion because they reported on empirical data, 3 were based on 'experimental design' and the remaining 8 had self-reported data such as surveys and interviews. It is hard to draw conclusions from this review and its papers, which compare CBL online with CBL in more traditional tutorials. Students reported learning with all interventions, which is not surprising.

Case-based learning compared with didactic lectures

CBL is often added to more didactic teaching formats to enhance interaction. In Pakistan one medical school changed from delivering only didactic lectures in pharmacology to lectures incorporating small group work (seven to nine students) on clinical case scenarios. Again evaluation was limited to students' attitudes. The 68 students surveyed were happy with the change and did feel a CBL approach could be used for other science subjects. Tayem[18] concluded that CBL is effective and improves learning skills.

Similarly, at the Karolinska Institutet in Sweden, 'case seminars' replaced the traditional Friday morning 3-hour surgery lectures.[19] These seminars were labelled as CBL based on the case method of the HBS, with the cases written from one perspective in the past tense. In each case there is one main character who encounters different forms of dilemmas or problems that he or she must consider and act upon. The educators at the Karolinska Institutet emphasise that the case story and the dilemma must always be open to different interpretations, as the HBS stipulates. The case is not supposed to be centred only on facts but should provide a social context as a backdrop for different professional dilemmas.[19] The focus is not on right or wrong answers but on a reflective learning process. Evaluation in this study focused on both student and faculty feedback through interviews, moving beyond outcomes to exploring what the mechanism of learning might be. However, only five students and five faculty members were interviewed. While the number of participants is not an indicator of the quality of research within a qualitative methodological approach, the inclusion of only five students in this study for such an evaluation process lacks credibility. These medical students had little or no previous experience of working with interactive methods and were initially concerned about the approach. They had to become familiar with the process as well as the content of the cases. The students did not know what was expected of them, as there was no specific orientation to the method. The facilitators also stated they needed professional development in the method. They found it difficult to engage students in discussion, as the students preferred to interact through a simple question-and-answer process directed via the teacher. The findings showed that students were critical, as the seminars were not rated as quality learning experience. As time went on, they stopped preparing for the sessions – mainly because their performance in the seminars was not being assessed. Nordquist *et al.*[19] concluded that the change was not a success and contributed this to poor implementation rather than the CBL approach itself.

In spite of the small numbers, this Swedish study does highlight a number of points about educational interventions and their evaluation. As with any change process and innovation, all participants need to be adequately prepared and not rushed. Lack of facilitator training can jeopardise results. The rationale for the change needs to be explained. In terms of cases, the case material must be well aligned with the rest of the rotation, and related learning material must fit the case. Moreover, it once again highlights the importance of aligning assessment with activities and the strategic nature of student learning in relation to what is or is not being assessed.

Learner preparation is an important part of the learning environment as students make the transition from secondary to higher education. In professional teacher education, for example, Baeten et al.[20] have shown that both students in a completely lecture-based learning environment and in a gradually implemented CBL environment (e.g. the proportion of CBL in the curriculum is gradually increased) performed better in assessment measuring the application of learned knowledge than those who undertake CBL alone.[20]

Upfront case delivery versus 'just in time' delivery

Ramaekers et al.[21] from Utrecht University have considered the timing of information release with cases. For example, in some CBL formats the students receive the whole case at the start of the learning session, whereas in other formats the information is given in chunks by the tutor (or equivalent) to mimic real-life practice. Thus, the tutor may be functioning in several roles: information giver, facilitator of problem analysis and solving, and possibly assessor of performance within the group session. In their study of veterinary medicine 'clinical lessons', Ramaekers et al.[21] explored how this requirement to fulfil multiple roles affected teacher behaviour. The clinical problems were designed to help students begin to reason clinically, transferring their knowledge from preclinical learning to clinical clerkships. An ethnographic process was used with observation and recording of 63 case discussions. Teachers were found to intervene in the learning process for three reasons: (1) for control, as in checking the students' knowledge, (2) to correct any misunderstandings and (3) to stimulate elaboration by raising the discussion to a higher level. Such scaffolding of learning was not always welcomed by the students, particularly if the teachers took over and became more didactic. However, they appreciated appropriate feedback and the chance to reflect. The optimum learning and teacher intervention was the 'just in time' provision of extra information limited to what was requested by the students rather than the teacher frequently interacting. This delayed scaffolding and facilitation of reflection enabled the students to practise clinical reasoning while obtaining patient information in a realistic time scale. This study is interesting for its methodology and its aim of teasing out the effects of different facilitator styles.[21]

CONCLUSION

Given the lack of consensus about the meaning and format of CBL, together with the diversity of application and delivery, it is difficult to draw firm conclusions about its effectiveness. However, taking all the evidence together, the following conclusions may be drawn: CBL complements other methods of learning and teaching for health professional students; students prefer explicit learning outcomes and some structure; when introduced as a new method, facilitators and students need orientation to what is expected of them. CBL appears to achieve the aim of linking theory with practice but there is unlikely to be one optimal way of delivering CBL. Its effectiveness is contextual and depends on a number of factors, including preparation, size of groups, learner and facilitator support and authenticity of cases.[22–24]

SUMMARY POINTS

- CBL is now frequently used in health professional education but there is a diverse range of methods and applications reported.
- The evidence for effectiveness of CBL shows a trend towards learner satisfaction and the ability of learners to apply knowledge to clinical experience through active learning.

AREAS FOR FURTHER RESEARCH

Key areas for further research into the effectiveness and process of CBL should include:
- an evaluation of how much structure is required
- an exploration of whether cases extend or limit students' clinical reasoning by suggesting a single diagnosis per case.

REVIEW QUESTIONS

- What features of cases are important for effective CBL?
- What are the advantages and disadvantages of (a) releasing the whole case at the beginning of a learning activity and (b) letting the case unfold during the activity with release of information 'just in time'?
- What preparation do learners and facilitators require before using CBL?

REFLECTIVE QUESTIONS AND EXERCISES

- Your institution is renewing its curriculum and is considering using CBL as a learning approach. The head of school asks your opinion about this proposed change and for the evidence relating to effectiveness of CBL. How would you reply?
- Design a case and decide on the mode of delivery of that case to help students achieve learning outcomes relating to one of your programme's first-year courses. How would you evaluate the activity?

REFERENCES

1. Irby D. Three exemplary models of case-based teaching. *Acad Med.* 1994; **69**(12): 947–53.
2. Shapiro BP. *Case studies for Harvard Business School.* Cambridge, MA: Harvard College; 1975. Available at: www.hbs.edu/faculty/research/Documents/Case%20Studies%20for%20Harvard%20Business%20School_Brochure.pdf (accessed 15 January 2014).
3. Merseth KK. The early history of case-based instruction: in-sights for teacher education today. *J Teach Educ.* 1991; **42**(4): 243–9.
4. Thistlethwaite JE, Davies D, Ekeocha S, *et al.* The effectiveness of case-based learning in health professional education: a BEME systematic review. *Med Teach.* 2012; **34**(6): e421–44.
5. Barrows H, Tamblyn R. *Problem-Based Learning: an approach to medical education.* New York, NY: Springer; 1980.
6. Srinivasan M, Wilkes M, Stevenson F, *et al.* Comparing problem-based learning with case-based learning: effects of a major curricular shift at two institutions. *Acad Med.* 2007; **82**(1): 74–82.
7. Hamdy H. The fuzzy world of problem-based learning. *Med Teach.* 2008; **30**(8): 739–41.
8. O'Neill G, McMahon T. Student-centred learning: what does it mean for students and lecturers? In: O'Neill G, Moore S, McMullin B, editors. *Emerging Issues in the Practice of University Learning and Teaching.* Dublin: All Ireland Society for Higher Education; 2005. pp. 27–36.
9. Herreid CF. What makes a good case? *J Coll Sci Teach.* 1997–1998; **27**(3): 163–5.
10. Kim S, Phillips WR, Pinsky L, *et al.* A conceptual framework for developing teaching cases: a review and synthesis of the literature across disciplines. *Med Educ.* 2006; **40**(9): 867–76.
11. www.bemecollaboration.org
12. Patton MQ. *Utilization-Focused Evaluation.* 4th ed. Los Angeles, CA: Sage; 2008.
13. Kirkpatrick DL. Evaluation. In: Craig RL, editor. *Training and Development Handbook: a guide to human resource development.* New York, NY: McGraw-Hill; 1987. pp. 301–19.
14. Barr H, Koppel I, Reeves S, *et al. Effective Interprofessional Education: argument, assumption and evidence.* Oxford: Blackwell Publishing; 2005.
15. Pawson R, Tilley N. *Realistic Evaluation.* London: Sage Publications; 1997.
16. Banchi H, Bell R. The many levels of inquiry-based learning. *Sci Child.* 2008; **46**(2): 26–9.
17. Saleewong D, Suwannatthachote P, Kuhraken S. Case-based learning on web in higher education: a review of empirical research. *Creat Educ.* 2012; **3**(8B): 31–4.
18. Tayem YI. The impact of small group case-based learning on traditional pharmacology teaching. *Sultan Qaboos Univ Med J.* 2013; **13**(1): 115–20.
19. Nordquist J, Sundberg K, Johansson L, *et al.* Case-based learning in surgery: lessons learned. *World J Surg.* 2012; **36**(5): 945–55.
20. Baeten M, Dochy F, Struyven K. Using students' motivation and learning profiles in in investigating their perceptions and achievement in case-based and lecture-based learning environments. *Educ Stud.* 2012; **38**(5): 49.
21. Ramaekers S, Keulen H-V, Kremer W, *et al.* Effective teaching in case-based education: patterns in teacher behavior and their impact on the students' clinical problem solving and learning. *Int J Teach Learn High Educ.* 2011; **23**(3): 303–13.
22. Sturdy S. Scientific method for medical practitioners: the case method of teaching pathology in early twentieth-century Edinburgh. *Bull Hist Med.* 2007; **81**(4): 760–92.
23. Carder L, Willingham P, Bibb D. Case-based, problem-based learning: information literacy for the real world. *Res Strat.* 2001; **18**(3): 181–90.
24. Loghmani MT, Bayliss AJ, Strunk V, *et al.* An integrative, longitudinal case-based learning model as a curriculum strategy to enhance teaching and learning. *J Phys Ther Educ.* 2011; **25**(2): 42–50.

CHAPTER 23

Team-Based Learning

Overview and best evidence

∙∙∙

Larry K Michaelsen, Dean X Parmelee,
Abbas Hyderi and Michael Sweet

OVERVIEW

This chapter describes the foundational practices of Team-Based Learning™ (TBL): strategically formed permanent teams; content coverage through pre-class, individual student study and an in-class individual and team Readiness Assurance Process; developing students' application skills through the use of in-class team application activities and the use of peer assessment to ensure that students are accountable to their teams. Also described in this chapter are the 'educational best practices' identified in evidence-based education (EBE) literature: cooperative learning, feedback (or assessment for learning), reciprocal teaching, whole-class interactive teaching, requiring concept-driven decisions and using visual presentations and graphic organisers. The chapter then discusses and provides medical education examples to highlight the relationship between foundational practices of TBL and the best practices identified in the EBE literature. Finally, the chapter provides a summary of the empirical evidence linking TBL to a wide variety of outcomes that are important in medical education settings.

CHAPTER OBJECTIVES

Upon completion of this chapter, the reader will be able to:

- articulate the relationship between the practices and principles that constitute TBL and the 'educational best practices' identified in EBE literature
- provide examples to illustrate how the EBE best practices regularly occur as a result of implementing standard TBL in medical education courses
- summarise the empirical evidence linking TBL to a wide variety of important educational outcomes.

KEY TERMS: small group learning, active learning, Readiness Assurance Process, Individual Readiness Assurance Test (iRAT), Team Readiness Assurance Test (tRAT), 4S applications

TEAM-BASED LEARNING™ AND EDUCATIONAL BEST PRACTICE: AN OVERVIEW

Team-Based Learning™ (TBL) is a specific and intensive form of small group-based learning (described in more detail later in this chapter) in which (a) the majority of class time involves students working in permanent, strategically formed teams; (b) concept coverage is achieved through students' pre-class individual self-study followed by an in-class Readiness Assurance Process that involves both individual and team tests; (c) the majority of class time is used for team assignments through which students help one another learn course material at an applied level; and (d) students are accountable to one another through the use of a peer-assessment and feedback process. Furthermore, TBL's unique sequence of individual and team activities, as well as its feedback rhythm and incentive structures, promote groups to evolve from collections of individuals into high-performance, self-managed learning teams.

In *Evidence Based Teaching: A Practical Approach*, Petty[1] built on a great deal of research – most notably, that of Bransford *et al.*[2] in *How People Learn*, and the meta-analyses of educational research by Hattie[3] and Marzano *et al.*[4] – to present the six best practices in evidence-based teaching. These six best practices and the effect sizes derived from the meta-analysis are reported in Table 23.1.

TABLE 23.1 Effect size for various educational interventions

Cooperative learning	0.75
Feedback or 'assessment for learning'	0.81
Reciprocal teaching	0.86
Whole-class interactive teaching	0.81
Requiring concept-driven decisions	0.89
Visual presentations and graphic organisers	1.30

As will be discussed in this chapter, when properly implemented, TBL includes many, if not all, of the common elements of these evidence-based education (EBE) best practices. For an earlier examination of the relationship between EBE and TBL, please refer to Michaelsen and Sweet.[5] To explain the how and why of TBL, a brief overview is in order.

The four foundational practices of TBL[6] are:

1. strategically forming permanent teams
2. ensuring student familiarity with course content by using a Readiness Assurance Process
3. developing students' critical thinking skills by using carefully designed, in-class activities and assignments
4. creating and administering a peer-assessment and feedback system.

In brief, the structure of a TBL module is as follows. After being oriented to the process of TBL, students are given a pre-class assignment through which they will be exposed to the key concepts for a unit of study. In class, students begin each unit of the

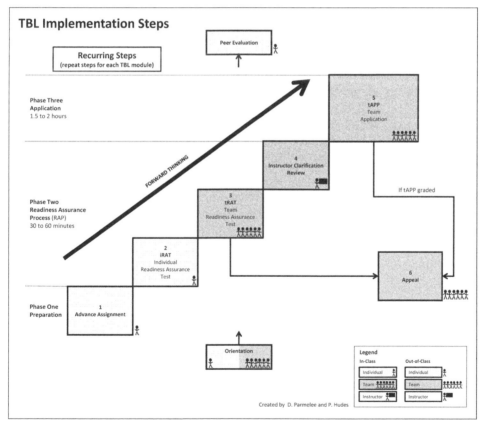

FIGURE 23.1 A typical Team-Based Learning™ module (reproduced with permission of the authors)

course taking a short test to assess their understanding of the assigned pre-readings. They then take that exact same test again as a team, getting immediate feedback on their team answers. This immediate feedback serves two functions: (1) confirming their content understanding (or alerting them to their lack of understanding) and (2) providing information that enables them to develop effective decision-making strategies as a team. Once the team test is completed, they can then write 'appeals' to reclaim credit for incorrect answers when they feel they can cite evidence from the reading to make a case for an 'incorrect' answer.

After this readiness-testing experience, the educator provides corrective instruction as needed. The class, while staying in their teams, then completes one or more activities in which they apply the concepts from the readiness tests by making decisions to complex problems or dilemmas posed by case studies. This process repeats for each unit of the course, with students filling out peer evaluations for the members of their team at least once during the unit or course and at the end of the term. A typical TBL module for one unit is illustrated in Figure 23.1.

This sequence of activities shifts the focus of class time away from content 'delivery' to the students working together, helping one another learn and applying the content. Evidence is rapidly mounting that by increasing pre-class learning and peer instruction, TBL enables instructors to achieve equal or better content coverage and still use 70%–80% of class time with students engaged in activities that deepen their understanding of how course content applies to real-life situations and problems.[7-9] In addition, TBL uses peer assessment and feedback both to increase team members' accountability to one another and to develop students' interpersonal and team skills.

EVIDENCE-BASED EDUCATION BEST PRACTICES AND THE FOUR FOUNDATIONAL PRACTICES OF TEAM-BASED LEARNING™

Now, the relationship between the four foundational practices of TBL and the approaches that have been identified by Petty[1] as EBE best practices will be described. The four TBL foundational practices are (1) using strategically forming permanent teams correlates with cooperative learning, albeit in a comprehensive, structured fashion; (2) using a Readiness Assurance Process (RAP) correlates with assessment for learning and reciprocal teaching; (3) using carefully designed, in-class activities and assignments correlates with the 'Decisions, Decisions' learning structure,[1] and when these activities involve visual aids such as concept maps this correlates with visual tools; and (4) peer evaluation helps bring accountability to help enhance assessment for learning and reciprocal teaching. This is in addition to the fact that the TBL strategy correlates with the practice of interactive teaching.

Strategically forming permanent teams

Although the first essential element of TBL is strategically forming permanent teams, TBL practitioners tend to be very wary of being grouped with those who practise 'cooperative learning'. This wariness stems from the fact that, although both TBL and cooperative learning use small groups and in-class group assignments, the similarities pretty much end there.[10] For example, many cooperative learning techniques such as the jigsaw or 'think-pair-share' are activities that can be used as a way to 'spice up' an otherwise traditional, lecture-based course. TBL, on the other hand, is *a comprehensive instructional strategy* that, when implemented correctly, builds groups into teams whose members' collective capability far exceeds that of even their very best member.[11]

However, using Petty's[1] definitions, TBL very clearly qualifies as an example of cooperative learning. Specifically, Petty[1] described the characteristics of cooperative learning as:

- groups sink or swim together
- students work interactively
- students have a goal to learn but also a goal to help others in their group
- students are held accountable by the teacher
- students learn how to cooperate effectively.

In TBL, the instructor organises permanent teams of five to seven students at the beginning of the term and uses group work *every* time the class meets for a TBL session. As a result, many of the differences between the two approaches stem from the fact that, with strategically formed, permanent teams working together in every class, the impact of each of the characteristics of cooperative learning is even more apparent than with the temporary groups that are typically used in cooperative learning.[10]

Ensuring student familiarity with course content by using a Readiness Assurance Process

The first in-class activity for each unit of the course is a four-step process: the RAP.

1. *Individual Readiness Assurance Test (iRAT):* short, basic, multiple-choice test over the key concepts in pre-class assignment.
2. *Team Readiness Assurance Test (tRAT):* once students turn in their individual tests, they then answer the exact same questions again but with their team, by reaching consensus on each answer, and they receive *immediate* feedback on each of the teams' choices (which, since the questions are exactly the same, also provides feedback on two other important things: (i) team members' individual choices on the iRAT and (ii) how effectively the team is using its pool of potential intellectual resources). This choice-by-choice feedback is best achieved by using 'scratch off' answer sheets – cards that students can scratch like lotto tickets to reveal their answer. These are called Immediate Feedback Assessment Technique (IF-AT) cards (*see* Figure 23.2); this immediate feedback is invaluable for both content learning and team development. When all teams have turned in their team test forms, the instructor reviews them to identify the most frequently missed questions and this informs the instructor what material needs to be clarified for the class in a follow-up lecture.
3. *Appeals:* when teams feel they can make a case for an answer marked as incorrect, they can reclaim credit by creating a written appeal based on either the content addressed by the question or the wording of the question. If their appeal is based on content, they must pull out their course materials and generate a written appeal

consisting of (a) a clear statement of argument and (b) evidence cited from the preparation materials. If their appeal is based on what they feel is an inadequacy of the question, they must provide an alternative wording that corrects the language that led them astray.

4. *Instructor clarification and review:* the final stage in each RAP is a tutorial in which the teacher provides corrective or clarifying instruction on concepts identified by students as being problematic or on questions that were missed by multiple teams. These 'lectures' are typically very short (5–10 minutes at most), because the process both pinpoints areas of concern and provides information so that corrective instruction can be framed using concepts that students already understand.

The RAP incorporates several of the best practices identified by EBE. The most obvious reason is that the process is designed to provide truly immediate *feedback* that both enhances content learning and enables an immediate awareness of how well members are expressing and listening to one another's point of view. This immediate feedback is the foundation that underlies both *assessments for learning* and *reciprocal teaching*. The purpose of the RAP is to motivate students to come to class prepared for the unit and to give them multiple forms of feedback – both on their grasp of the key concepts in the assigned material and, at least equally important, on the effectiveness of their team's use of its intellectual resources. The former, as with *assessment for learning* and *reciprocal teaching*, facilitates concept learning. The latter is a no-cost bonus, in that it enables team members to develop interpersonal and team interaction skills.

The key to the RAP's success is providing immediate feedback on the tRAT. The TBL literature strongly recommends providing this immediate feedback by using

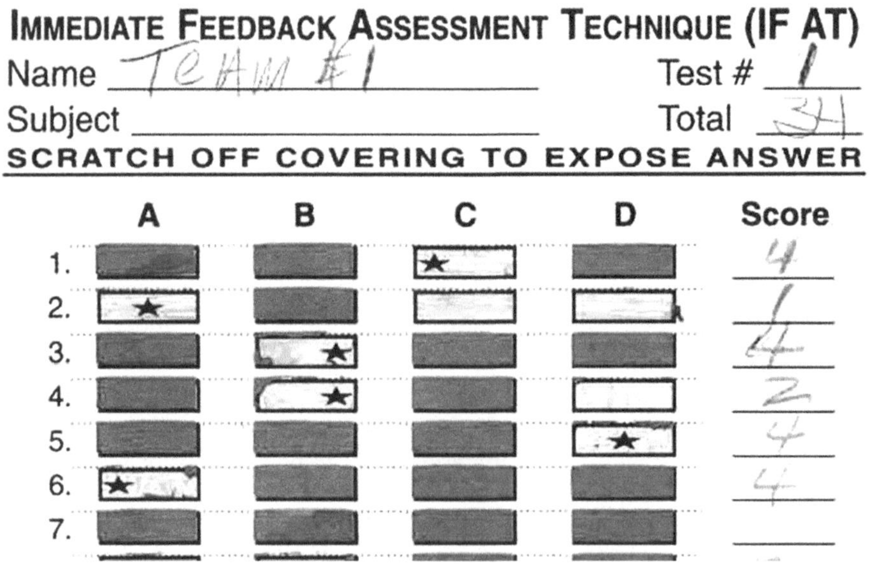

IMMEDIATE FEEDBACK ASSESSMENT TECHNIQUE (IF AT)

Name _TEAM #1_   Test # _1_

Subject _____   Total _31_

SCRATCH OFF COVERING TO EXPOSE ANSWER

	A	B	C	D	Score
1.			★		4
2.	★				1
3.		★			4
4.		★			2
5.				★	4
6.	★				4
7.					

FIGURE 23.2 Example of an Immediate Feedback Assessment Technique card (reproduced with permission of the author)

'IF-AT' cards when the team have agreed on an answer. If their answer is correct, their scratching on the card will reveal a star. If they are incorrect, the box revealed will be blank (*see* Figure 23.2). Using the IF-AT gives teams real-time feedback on every team decision, and it also enables teams to receive partial credit when they find the correct answer on a second or even a third scratch-off.

As was pointed out by Michaelsen and Sweet,[5] the value of using the IF-AT to provide immediate feedback is that, even though the teams are proceeding at their own pace, students receive many rounds of low-stakes, formative feedback in a very short period of time. What may not be so obvious is the extent to which the tRAT stimulates students to interact in much the same way as they would in a formal reciprocal teaching situation, in which the interaction is between the teacher and his or her students, *even though the educator is not actually present*. In their search for correct answers, students invariably alternate in and out of an educator's role by asking one another the kind of questions that would normally be asked by the educator. For example, on any given question, they might ask one another to make predictions, explain their rationales for those predictions and clarify their different understandings of the material. This interaction pattern is illustrated by the following excerpt from a recorded transcript during a tRAT in an undergraduate educational psychology class.[12]

Student 4:	I put A.
Student 6:	Well, I'd go with A. I put D but –
Student 1:	I put D too, but …
Student 2:	I put D.
Student 3:	I put D, but …
Student 4:	Well!
[group laughter]	
Student 4:	Well, then someone argue for D and then someone argue for A, and we'll figure it out.
Student 6:	I don't even have a good argument.
Student 1:	It just seems more logical to me, that's all. D sort of seems more logical, but …
Student 4:	Yeah, I just, I remember reading A and not D. That's the only thing why I would not change it.
Student 1:	Yeah, if you remember reading it. I would be willing to trust your reading it more than my logic.
Student 6:	Yeah, we're just trying to justify it.

In this excerpt, Student 4 was not assigned to play the role of the educator – TBL specifically advises against the assignment of group roles[10] – but she briefly assumed the teacher's role by proposing an inquiry-based task to the group: '*Someone argue for D and then someone argue for A, and we'll figure it out.*' In the next few statements, students evaluated their confidence in the sources of their opinions, with Student 1 stating, '*I would be willing to trust your reading it more than my logic*', and with Student 6 even stating that the purpose of this extemporaneous exercise is that '*we're just trying to justify it'*. Although these particular statements do not fall crisply into the categories of summarising, questioning, clarifying and predicting as outlined by Palincsar and Brown[13] in the initial description of reciprocal teaching, they nonetheless structure the interaction and help students co-regulate one another's learning in much the same ways by alternating teacher and student roles.[14]

The tRAT also serves one additional function: enabling the teacher to discover both what concepts need additional attention and what concepts have been mastered. These two pieces of information prepare the teacher to deliver a precisely targeted clarifying lecture, 'a teaching moment', which is the final step in the RAP. The feedback that is so critical to providing a truly targeted clarifying lecture comes from three sources: (1) observing which questions are being missed by multiple teams, (2) 'listening in' to the discussions that occur during the tRAT and (3) inviting students to identify issues about which they would like additional input.

Even in large classes, instructors are well aware when teams struggle with a particular concept, and he or she is able to engage in whole-class interactive teaching[1] for two reasons: first, students have been *primed* to listen actively by the feedback they have received from their peers and from the IF-AT cards; second, the instructor is able to zero in on exactly the parts of the content the students do not understand. At this point, the educator can do one of two things. The ideal strategy is to conduct a class discussion in which teams who correctly answered challenging questions can explain their answers. The other strategy is that, when students' explanations are inadequate, the educator is in a position to deliver a pinpointed, clarifying lecture.

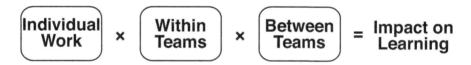

Maximum learning occurs when assignments at each stage are characterised by 4 Ss:

◆ **Significant problem** – problem involves issues that are significant to *students*.

◆ **Same problem** – individuals or groups are working on the same problem, case or question.

◆ **Specific choice** – individuals or groups are required to use course concepts to make a specific choice.

◆ **Simultaneous report** – individuals or groups report their choices simultaneously.

FIGURE 23.3 Effective group assignments

Developing students' critical thinking skills by using carefully designed, in-class activities and assignments

After completing the RAP and engaging in whole-class interactive teaching, and then receiving whatever clarifying instruction is needed, teams then engage in activities that enable students to practise applying their newly acquired knowledge. The key to creating and implementing effective team assignments is following what TBL users refer to as the '4 Ss': (1) assignments should always be designed around a problem that is **S**ignificant to students; (2) all of the students in the class should be working on the **S**ame problem; (3) students should be required to make a **S**pecific choice; and (4) groups should **S**imultaneously report their choices. Further, these procedures apply to all three stages in which students interface with course concepts: (1) individual work prior to group discussions, (2) discussions within groups and (3) whole-class discussion between groups (*see* Figure 23.3).

The '4 Ss', and 4S application activites, are explained in more detail in the following list.

1. *Significant [to students] problem.* Effective assignments must capture students' interest.[15] Unless assignments focus on what students see as a relevant issue, most students will view what they are being asked to do as 'busy work', referred to as 'exercising' by Fink,[16] and so they will make the minimum effort required to get a satisfactory grade. The key to identifying what will be significant to health professions students is using 'backwards design'.[17] Organising teaching around something you, as a medical practitioner, think your students should to be able to do by applying the content will have a very different impact than organising your teaching around what you think they should know. If you know what you want them to do and you create an activity that will give them the chance to try, it is very likely that your enthusiasm will carry over to your students in a way that rarely happens when the focus is on simply exposing them to the content.

2. *Same problem.* Group assignments only promote interactive teaching to the extent that they promote discussion. When groups work on different problems, students have to try to build inter-team discussions, even though they are faced with a comparison of 'apples and oranges'. By contrast, having all of the groups work on the same problem energises both the within-team and the between-team discussions. When all of the groups have a common frame of reference, within-team discussions tend to produce interactive teaching, because students realise they will be accountable for the quality of their thinking. This, in turn, provides an intellectual and emotional foundation for a more conceptually rich and energetic exchange when the results of teams' deliberations are made public.

3. *Specific choice.* In general, the best activity to challenge students to engage in higher levels of cognitive complexity is to require them to make a specific choice.[7,18] In the words of Roberson and Franchini,[8]

> The most clarifying action a student can take is a decision. Well-designed 'collective decisions' (e.g. focused team tasks) provide an opportunity

for students to practice the kind of thinking we want to promote in our courses and disciplines.

A well-constructed decision-based task integrates components of higher-order thinking: analysis of the particular situation to determine competing priorities, values and lines of reasoning; use of relevant concepts, principles, laws or other abstractions at play in the situation; reflective, critical thinking (*Are we sure of these facts? Are we sure we understand?*); and, ultimately, a judgement that is expressed in a visible, concrete outcome that can be evaluated. Team tasks need to point students consistently towards decisions, not simply rehashing information. In the classroom, the best way to promote content-related discussion is to use assignments that require groups to use course concepts to make decisions. For example:

a. What drug would you recommend to reduce the blood pressure of a patient who is/has [give list of potentially complicating factors]? Why?

b. Which physical finding in this patient is *most* confirmatory of the diagnosis? Which commonly used diagnostic study would confound making this diagnosis?

c. If untreated immediately, what do you predict the blood pressure will be in 6 hours?

4. *Simultaneous reports.* Once groups have completed their deliberations on questions such as those listed in the previous point, it is critical to have them simultaneously reveal their choices for three reasons. First, all of the groups get immediate feedback on how their choices compare with those from other teams. Second, having all of the choices visible at the same time and in a simple form highlights *differences* among them. Third, because their choice is clearly visible to the rest of the class, every team is then accountable to explain and defend their position. For a more detailed discussion of options for simultaneous reporting, see Sibley.[19] By contrast when teams report sequentially, the initial report sets a standard that influences all of the subsequent reports, because later-reporting teams usually emphasise the similarities and the downplay differences between their position and that reported by the initial team (e.g. 'answer drift' – Michaelsen *et al.*[7]). Unfortunately, the absence of differences tends to reduce both the amount and the intensity of the discussion about differences that is so critical to creating an environment in which whole-class and interactive teaching can occur.

Although the details of implementing 4S application activities are unique, based on factors such as the subject matter and the class size, the 4 Ss are wholly consistent with the best practices of EBE. For example, because every 4S application activity requires teams to make specific decisions, even though not all of them involve a card-sorting game, 4S application activities can be said to employ a general form of the 'Decisions, Decisions' learning structure.[1] That said, some 4S application activities do involve sorting cards. For example, King[20] distributed cards with pictures of an infant in various positions and required teams to sort the cards according to various criteria – the most basic being 'normal or abnormal?' (e.g. when lying on their backs, infants of a certain age should habitually face forward and keep their head in line with their body, whereas dropping their head and looking to one side or another is a sign of abnormal development).

Similarly, many teachers use 4S application activities that require teams to complete graphic displays of their 'thinking', hypotheses or commitments to a decision, thereby implementing the EBE practice of visual presentations or graphic organisers. One example is the 'gallery walk', for which students must first analyse, evaluate and synthesise complex data, zero in on their best guess or choice in response to a focused question and display their response using either large poster paper or one of the electronic-based display applications. Thereafter, the teams evaluate one another's responses. In one example of a TBL session on health issues in adolescence in the first year of medical school in MedEdPORTAL,[21] teams must specify two public health interventions for a particular town's increase in teen pregnancy and sexually transmitted diseases. The teams post their plans, then teams review and award 'stickies' to the ones that they feel have the greatest likelihood of success. In another example, also on MedEdPORTAL,[22] teams evaluate a complex and confounding neurological lesion presentation and free-hand draw a localisation image and write a hypothesis about the cause in just a few words. The instructor selects the five most plausible sets of images and hypotheses, and then teams vote on and defend their vote on one of the five.

Another popular form of visualising TBL course content in medical education is to ask teams to generate concept maps in response to a given prompt. For example, Thompson et al.[23] received the concept map shown in Figure 23.1 from a team diagramming the primary and secondary biochemical effects in the case of an

Content	All relevant concepts are included and are correct		Most relevant concepts and mechanisms are included and are correct		Few relevant facts or concepts are included or correct	
Points	6	5	4	3	2	1
Logic and understanding	Understanding of facts and concepts is clearly demonstrated by correct links and active verbs		Understanding of facts and concepts is demonstrated but with some incorrect links and/or missing active verbs		Poor understanding of facts and concepts with significant errors in links and active verbs	
Points	6	5	4	3	2	1
Presentation	Concept map is neat, clear, legible, has easy-to-follow links, and has no spelling errors		Concept map is neat, legible but with some links difficult to follow and some spelling errors		Concept map is untidy with links difficult to follow and spelling errors	
Points	3		2		1	

FIGURE 23.4 Rubric developed by Thompson et al.[23] to grade team-generated concept maps

18-month-old infant with medium-chain acyl-coenzyme A dehydrogenase deficiency. Using the 'gallery walk', teams then critiqued one another's concept maps, with different colours representing primary and secondary effects, and teams also critiqued and scored one another using the rubric shown to the right in Figure 23.1. The 4S application activities can be graded or ungraded, and they need not have a 'correct' answer. While it may seem difficult to grade a concept visualisation, Thompson *et al.*[23] developed an elegant rubric with which to grade team-generated concept maps.

Peer evaluation

Peer evaluation is the fourth and final practical element of TBL, providing students with both formative and summative feedback from their teammates about their contributions to the team and its success. Whereas members of a *group* feel mostly

TABLE 23.2 A sample Team-Based Learning™ peer evaluation feedback form

Team Reflection and Feedback	**Team #:** _____
Name: _____	

To help your team become more effective, give your teammates some *anonymous* feedback.

Consider such things as:
- *preparation* – were they prepared when they came to class?
- *contribution* – did they contribute to the team discussion and work?
- *gatekeeping* – did they help *others* contribute?
- *flexibility* – did they listen when disagreements occurred?

You have 25 points to distribute among your teammates. The results are anonymous, so be honest. :-)

1. Name of team member: Points

Things I appreciate about this team member:

Things I would like to request of this team member:

2. Name of team member: Points

Things I appreciate about this team member:

Things I would like to request of this team member:

accountable to an outside authority, members of a *team* also feel accountable to one another, and peer evaluation is a mechanism by which one can enhance *assessment for learning* and *reciprocal teaching*. As Petty[1] noted, the format of feedback is important: it should be informative and not judgemental. Therefore, many TBL teachers have their students fill out peer evaluation forms that ask students simply to express things they 'appreciate' about their teammates and things they 'request' (*see* Table 23.2). This language is carefully chosen so as not to stimulate attacks or judgements, but instead to promote constructive peer feedback. Students submit these forms to the teacher, who then processes the feedback and emails it to each student. Because the teacher knows who said what to whom (students do, too), the students tend to be civil and constructive. However, students receive the feedback as anonymous, so any one piece of feedback need not be received as too personalised.

EVIDENCE FOR THE EFFECTIVENESS OF TEAM-BASED LEARNING™

One strong, although indirect, set of evidence for the effectiveness of TBL is the extremely close fit between TBL and virtually all of the prescriptions common to the best practice approaches identified by Petty.[1] In fact, in many cases, TBL goes beyond the specific prescriptions in ways that promote consistency *across* the entire set of the best practice approaches. For example, a common practice of 'Decisions, Decisions'[1] involves assigning students to specific roles to ensure differences of opinion as they attempt to reach a decision that affects multiple parties. TBL also creates differences of opinion, but, instead of ensuring differences by assigning students to adopt different roles, TBL uses 4S application assignments that are specifically designed so that teams are likely to be highly committed to different choices, by requiring them to decide what they think is the best answer to a highly complex problem with multiple plausible answers. With TBL, students benefit in three ways. First, the positions they are defending are truly authentic. As a result, students are highly motivated to challenge other teams that have reached a conclusion different to their own. Second, and consistent with all of the best practice approaches, as long as the problem is not so difficult that they get discouraged and give up, students learn more as the questions they face become more difficult. Third, because TBL explicitly harnesses the power of real teams, teachers are able to give them decision tasks that would be overwhelming for individual students and which are too difficult for the majority of learning groups that lack team cohesion.

Given the consistency between TBL and the best practices of EBE, it is not surprising that TBL produces a wide range of positive outcomes. Since the initial studies nearly 30 years ago,[24] the volume of the literature about TBL's effectiveness has accumulated across a wide variety of disciplines, in dozens of countries worldwide, and it has grown too large to summarise in much depth here. Currently, the two best sources for a listing of empirical studies of TBL are Haidet *et al.*[25] and from the bibliography available on the Team-Based Learning Collaborative's website.[26]

For example, empirical studies of TBL have reported that improved academic outcomes in test performance,[27–32] self-efficacy,[33] retention,[24] attitudes towards group work,[34] student satisfaction with their learning experience[34,35] and co-regulated learning (also known as team 'synergy' in Watson *et al.*[36]) increase emotional intelligence[37] and show a long-term positive impact on team skills[38] and actual job performance.[39,40]

SUMMARY POINTS

- TBL involves a sequence of individual and team activities, feedback and incentive structures, and an evolution of student groups from collections of individuals into high-performance, self-managed learning teams
- The four foundational practices of TBL include: strategically forming permanent teams; ensuring student familiarity with course content by using a Readiness Assurance Process; developing students' critical thinking skills by in-class activities and assignments; and creating and administering a peer-assessment and feedback system
- The key to generating effective team assignments in the TBL context refers to the the '4 Ss': (1) assignments should be designed around a problem that is **S**ignificant to students; (2) all of the students should be working on the **S**ame problem; (3) students are required to make a **S**pecific choice; and (4) groups should **S**imultaneously report their choices.

REVIEW QUESTIONS

- Why does TBL use permanent groups?
- How is content coverage achieved with TBL?
- How do TBL instructors determine which topics need additional input?
- What is the instructor's role while teams are working on application activities?
- Why are the teams required to do 'simultaneous reports'?
- What should the instructor do after the reports have been made?

REFLECTIVE QUESTIONS AND EXERCISES

- What aspect of standard TBL practice contributes most to developing groups into effective, self-managed teams?
- What aspect of standard TBL practice is most consistent with feedback for 'assessment for learning'? What aspect is the least consistent?
- What aspect of standard TBL practice is most consistent with reciprocal teaching? What aspect is the least consistent?
- What aspect of standard TBL practice is most consistent with whole-class interactive teaching? What aspect is the least consistent?
- What aspect of standard TBL practice is most consistent with requiring concept-driven decisions? What aspect is the least consistent?
- What aspect of standard TBL practice is most consistent with visual presentations and graphic organisers? What aspect is the least consistent?

FURTHER READING

- Michaelsen LK, Knight AB, Fink LD. *Team-Based Learning: a transformative use of small groups in college teaching*. Sterling, VA: Stylus Publishing; 2004.
- Khogali SE. Team-Based Learning: a practical guide. Guide Supplement 65.1: viewpoint 1. *Med Teach*. 2013; **35**(2): 163–5.
- Parmelee DX, Michaelsen LK. Twelve tips for doing effective Team-Based Learning (TBL). *Med Teach*. 2010; **32**(2): 118–22.

REFERENCES

1. Petty G. *Evidence Based Teaching: a practical approach*. Glouchestershire, UK: Nelson-Thomas Publishing; 2006.
2. Bransford JD, Brown AB, Cocking RR. *How People Learn: brain, mind, experience and school*. Washington, DC: National Academies Press; 2000.
3. Hattie J. *Visible Learning: a synthesis of over 800 meta-analyses relating to achievement*. New York, NY: Routledge Publishing; 2009.
4. Marzano RJ, Pickering DJ, Pollock JE. *Classroom Instruction that Works: research-based strategies for increasing student achievement*. Alexandria, VA: Association for Curriculum and Development; 2001.
5. Michaelsen LK, Sweet M. Team-Based Learning. In: Buskist W, Groccia JE, editors. *Evidence-Based Teaching: new directions in teaching and learning*. San Francisco, CA: Jossey-Bass; 2011. pp. 41–52.
6. Michaelsen LK, Davidson N, Major C. Team-Based Learning practices and principles in comparison with cooperative learning and problem based learning. *J Excel Coll Teach*. 2014; **25**(4): in press.
7. Michaelsen LK, Parmelee DX, McMahon KK, *et al. Team-Based Learning for Health Professions Education: a guide to using small groups for improving learning*. Sterling, VA: Stylus Publishing; 2008.
8. Roberson B, Franchini B. Effective task design for the TBL classroom. *J Excel Coll Teach*. 2014; **25**(4): in press.

9. Michaelsen LK, Knight AB, Fink LD. *Team-Based Learning: a transformative use of small groups.* Westport, CT: Greenwood Publishing Group; 2002.

10. Fink LD. Beyond small groups: harnessing the extraordinary power of learning teams. In: Michaelsen LK, Knight AB, Fink LD, editors. *Team-Based Learning: a transformative use of small groups in college teaching.* Sterling, VA: Stylus Publishing; 2004. pp. 3–26.

11. Michaelsen LK, Watson WE, Black RH. A realistic test of individual versus group consensus decision making. *J Appl Psychol.* 1989; **74**(5): 834–9.

12. Sweet M, Pelton-Sweet L. The power of belonging: students accountable to students. In: Michaelsen LK, Sweet M, Parmelee D, editors. *Team-Based Learning: small group learning's next big step; new directions for teaching and learning.* San Francisco, CA: Jossey-Bass; 2008. pp. 29–40.

13. Palincsar AS, Brown AL. Reciprocal teaching of comprehension-fostering and comprehension-monitoring activities. *Cogn Instruct.* 1984; **1**(2): 117–75.

14. Michaelsen L, Sweet M, Parmelee D. *Team-Based Learning: small group learning's next big step; new directions for teaching and learning.* San Francisco, CA: Jossey-Bass; 2008.

15. Parmelee D, Michaelsen L, Hudes P. Team-Based Learning. In: Dent J, Harden R, editors. *A Practical Guide for Medical Teachers.* Edinburgh: Elsevier; 2013. pp. 173–82.

16. Fink D. *Creating Significant Learning Experiences: an integrated approach to designing college courses.* San Francisco, CA: Jossey-Bass; 2003.

17. Wiggins G, McTighe J. *Understanding by Design.* Columbus, OH: Merrill Prentice Hall; 1998.

18. Roberson B, Reimers C. TBL for critical reading and thinking in literature and 'great books' courses. In: Michaelsen L, Sweet M, editors. *Team-Based Learning in the Humanities and Social Sciences: group work that works to generate critical thinking and engagement.* Sterling, VA: Stylus Publishing; 2012. pp. 129–42.

19. Sibley J. Facilitating application activities. In: Michaelsen L, Sweet M, editors. *Team-Based Learning in the Humanities and Social Sciences: group work that works to generate critical thinking and engagement.* Sterling, VA: Stylus Publishing; 2012. pp. 33–50.

20. King MP. Successful application exercises: charting data and image sorting for an intra-professional group of graduate nursing students. *Poster presented at the Annual Meeting of the Team-Based Learning Collaborative.* 2010 March; New Orleans, Louisiana.

21. Neeley S, Roman B, Parmelee D. *Teenage Pregnancy: Team-Based Learning exercise.* MedEd PORTAL; 2013. Available at: www.mededportal.org/publication/9357 (accessed 15 January 2014).

22. Pearson J, Rich M, Parmelee D. *Neurologic Localizations.* MedEdPORTAL; 2012. Available at: www.mededportal.org/publication/7704 (accessed 15 January 2014).

23. Thompson KH, LeClair RJ, Winterson BJ, *et al.* Concept mapping as a Team-Based Learning application exercise in a first-year medical biochemistry course. *Poster presented at the Annual Meeting of the International Association of Medical Science Educators.* 2010 July; New Orleans, Louisiana.

24. Wilson WR. The use of permanent learning groups in teaching introductory accounting [unpublished doctoral dissertation]. The University of Oklahoma; 1982.

25. Haidet P, Kubitz K, McCormack WE. An analysis of the Team-Based Learning literature: TBL comes of age. *J Excel Coll Teach.* 2014; **25**(4): in press.

26. Team-Based Learning Collaborative. *Bibliography.* www.teambasedlearning.org/refs/ (accessed 15 January 2014).

27. Tan NCK, Kandiah N, Chan YH, *et al.* A controlled study of Team-Based Learning for undergraduate clinical neurology education. *BMC Med Educ.* 2011; **11**: 91.

28. Koles P, Stolfi A, Borges N, *et al.* The impact of Team-Based Learning on medical students' academic performance. *Acad Med.* 2010; **85**(11): 1739–45.

29. Zgheib NK, Ghaddar F, Sabra R. Teaching pharmacogenetics in low and middle-income countries: Team-Based Learning and lessons learned at the American University of Beirut. *Curr Pharm Pers Med.* 2011; **9**: 25–40.

30. Zingone MM, Franks AS, Guirgis AB, *et al.* Comparing team-based and mixed active-learning methods in an ambulatory care elective course. *Am J Pharm Educ.* 2010; **74**(9): Article 160.

31. Weiner H, Plass RM, Marz R. Team-Based Learning in intensive course format for first-year medical students. *Croat Med J.* 2009; **50**(1): 69–76.

32. Letassy NA, Fugate SE, Medina MS, *et al.* Using Team-Based Learning in an endocrine module taught across two campuses. *Am J Pharm Educ.* 2008; **72**(5): Article 103.

33. Macke C, Tapp K. Teaching research to MSW students: effectiveness of the Team-Based Learning pedagogy. *J Teach Soc Work.* 2012; **32**(2): 48–160.

34. Clark MC, Nguyen HT, Bray C, *et al.* Team-Based Learning in an undergraduate nursing course. *Nurs Educ.* 2008; **47**(3): 111–17.

35. Beatty SJ, Kelley KA, Metzger AH, *et al.* Team-Based Learning in therapeutics workshop sessions. *Am J Pharm Educ.* 2009; **73**(6): 100.

36. Watson WE, Michaelsen LK, Sharp W. Member competence, group interaction and group decision-making: a longitudinal study. *J Appl Psychol.* 1991; **76**(6): 801–9.

37. Borges NJ, Kirkham K, Deardorff AS, *et al.* Development of emotional intelligence in a Team-Based Learning internal medicine clerkship. *Med Teach.* 2012; **34**(10): 802–6.

38. Opatrny C, Michaelsen LK, McCord M. Can transferable team skills be taught? A longitudinal study. *Acad Educ Leader.* 2015; in press.

39. Considine J, Payne R, Williamson S, *et al.* Expanding nurse initiated X-rays in emergency care using Team-Based Learning and decision support. *Aust Emerg Nurs J.* 2014; **17**(2): 68–76.

40. Touchet BK, Coon KA. A pilot use of Team-Based Learning in psychiatry resident psychodynamic psychotherapy education. *Acad Psychiatry.* 2005; **29**(3): 293–6.

CHAPTER 24

Traditional didactic learning

Overview and evidence in health professional education environments

....

Francis Amara

OVERVIEW

Teaching is a complex process that involves many variable factors. Research on teaching and learning is providing useful information for instructors to enhance their teaching in ways to improve student learning. Because of increasing emphasis on active, interactive and electronicly-managed learning methods, one would expect that traditional lectures (didactic lectures) would soon disappear. However, the didactic lecture endures and is still one of the most popular teaching methods in universities. Despite the criticism about its effectiveness in promoting problem-solving skills and critical thinking, some learning objectives are best served by the appropriate use of the didactic lecture. This chapter discusses what we know of research studies in health and higher education literature on the effectiveness and limitations of the didactic lecture. Evidence-based recommendations on how to overcome the limitations of the didactic lecture are discussed. Research findings are discussed to resolve issues surrounding what the didactic lecture can and cannot achieve, when it is appropriate to use the didactic lecture, and how to effectively use the didactic lecture to facilitate student learning. The quality of research data on the didactic lecture's impact on learning, as well as future research on the integration of the didactic lecture with active learning strategies, is explored.

CHAPTER OBJECTIVES

Upon completion of this chapter, the reader will be able to:
- identify evidence in support of the appropriate purposes and attributes of the didactic lecture
- describe research findings of the impact of the didactic lecture on learning
- outline evidence on identifying the limitations of the didactic lecture
- describe evidence-based recommendations on how to effectively deliver the didactic lecture
- suggest future research studies that examine how to integrate the didactic lecture format with other teaching methods.

KEY TERMS: didactic lecture, traditional lecture, learning objectives, reflection, feedback, student engagement, active and cooperative learning

INTRODUCTION

The didactic lecture is broadly viewed across a range of subjects, including health professions education, as a direct teaching method for the transmission of knowledge in a monotone manner.[1] However, in practice, most didactic lecturing can involve various techniques: the use of multimedia, student questioning and limited note taking. The didactic lecture is a frequently used strategy for teaching,[2] one that still has strengths and value in attaining some educational goals.[3] However, the relevance of the didactic lecture as an instructional strategy that enhances learning is being challenged. There is an increasing body of evidence within scientific disciplines that supports and validates active learning. These data are reviewed here, and their applicability to health professions education is discussed. The aim of this chapter is to provide evidence for the purposes and attributes of the didactic lecture, and to provide evidence-based recommendations on how to deliver an effective didactic lecture. Where evidence for trials with experimental or quasi-experimental designs is lacking, interpretations and recommendations are based on recognised expert opinions from cognitive theory, educational psychology and educational models. Some of the evidence is expert opinions based on theories. Evidence that is based on experience outside of the health professions is extrapolated to the health professional studies. However, opinions that are not based on published work are excluded from the evidence. The quality of the evidence is based on the impact on students' approaches to learning, performance and evaluation of teaching.

In this chapter, future research is discussed and a summary of the important concepts about the didactic lecture is provided. Two case studies are provided as examples to demonstrate different approaches of lecturing to a large group; these formed the basis of the review and discussion questions. In the final section of this chapter, reflective exercises are included to prompt the reader to think critically about how to make changes to his or her didactic lectures, consequently improving student learning.

PEDAGOGICAL PRACTICE

The didactic lecture format is one of many teaching methods, but it must not be viewed as the answer to all learning problems. McLaughlin and Mandin[4] have proposed questions to consider when selecting the didactic lecture format, and these are based on several research studies of students' and teachers' views of effective lectures: (a) Is the didactic lecture format aligned with the curriculum and course objectives? (b) Does the lecturer have the content knowledge and attitude to teach the subject matter? (c) Does the lecturer have the skills and confidence to effectively use the didactic mode of teaching to enhance student learning? Brookfield[5] has elaborated on the effective didactic lecture as a suitable teaching method for specific purposes. These purposes, which are grounded in educational principles, include:

- providing expert knowledge of information unavailable to students
- enhancing comprehension of information
- reinforcing foundational knowledge
- preparing the class for a cooperative and active learning activity (induction)
- stimulating variation in cooperative and active learning activities.

If used appropriately, the didactic lecture can be as effective and interactive as any other instructional method. For example, introducing interactive techniques using the traditional lecture led to improved student participation and learning in a large class based on participants' self-report and observational data. The observational data includes the ability to explain difficult concepts, to apply those concepts and organise thinking to solve problems.[6] In an effort to build health capacity through education and training, two studies have identified common characteristics for effective didactic lectures that have implications for teacher training and future research. Sandhu *et al.*[7] analysed several studies and developed the characteristics of the effective and ineffective didactic lecture. Bligh[8] reviewed research that compared the effectiveness of lecture with that of other teaching methods and identified common characteristics of the effective didactic lecture. These characteristics, which are supported by educational and cognitive theories, emphasise that the effective didactic lecture:

- is aligned with the learning objectives, is well organised and is delivered with enthusiasm
- is oriented towards the learning process
- is supported by a variety of technology to focus attention on the topic
- activates prior knowledge
- encourages two-way communication through questioning skills and limited note taking
- provides opportunity for feedback and reflection.

IMPACT ON STUDENTS' APPROACHES TO LEARNING, PERFORMANCE AND EVALUATION OF TEACHING

Research findings offer mixed conclusions on the effectiveness of the didactic lecture compared with other methods of teaching. Some studies show positive effects of didactic lectures on student learning. For example, based on a large body of research and cognitive theory, McKeachie[9] argues that, in comparison with didactic lecture, active learning is inappropriate for large groups taking lower-level courses, where the classroom is too small for discussion groups and students lack a firmer grounding in comprehensive knowledge of the subject. Indeed, Lake[10] observed that even though 170 physical therapist students in a first-year physiology course had higher grades in the active learning sections than in the lectures, they perceived that they have learned less in active learning. They also had lower perceptions of the course and the instructor's quality in the active learning sections, and there were no differences between the lecture and active learning sections on the students' perceptions of the course difficulty. Merrill[11] demonstrated that students with less study time, especially part-time students, prefer lectures over active learning for obtaining concise information for essays, which makes a difference to their attendance in class and performance in examinations. Reports of analyses of problem-solving strategies in clinical reasoning reveal that successful problem-solvers must possess comprehensive knowledge. If done effectively, didactic lectures can be important in activation of prior knowledge during active learning.[12]

Other studies show no significant difference in learning outcomes between the traditional lecture and other teaching methods. For example, one study investigated the effect of teaching method on objective test scores of nursing students. In this study, two groups of students were taught the same content: one by problem-based learning and the other by traditional lecture method. A 'pre- then post-test' design was used to evaluate both groups, and no statistically significant difference was found in the scores of the two groups.[13] In another study, in order to determine the most successful method of teaching nursing students infection control, web-based learning was compared with traditional lectures, and it was concluded that the students were equally satisfied with both teaching approaches.[3] Vreven and McFadden[14] demonstrated that in large classes with compressed lecture time, cooperative-learning tasks had no effect on students. However, results of several studies that compared the effectiveness of the didactic lecture with those of active and interactive teaching methods showed that students' satisfaction, approach to learning and learning outcomes are significantly better following active and interactive teaching techniques.[15-17] For example, group discussions promoted deep learning and problem-solving skills when compared with lectures.[15] Another study showed that problem-based courses promoted better disposition to developing critical thinking skills than lecture-based courses.[16] These results indicate that students value a blend of traditional lecturing and active learning tasks, and that neither method on its own is the panacea for all learning objectives. Thus, the didactic lecture still has its place in enhancing learning.

LIMITATIONS

Although there are some advantages associated with the effective didactic lecture format, there are also some limitations that have to be resolved. For example, it does not practically reflect how knowledge is used in real life: students are expected to construct their thinking and compare themselves with others, as well as to consider different views and express their thoughts to one another, and try out their hypotheses by comparing and contrasting their views.[18] There are also concerns that the didactic lecture format does not model the practice of some competencies of the health professions, such as collaborative learning, the application of knowledge to clinical experiences and the ability to evaluate. Students can only master these competencies through active and cooperative learning. In nursing education, Young and Diekelmann[19] questioned the consequences of one-way communication of many facts that overwhelm nursing students and fail to engage them in critical thinking and problem-solving. The diversity of our students demands that we also use a variety of approaches to teaching and learning.[20] Students who are motivated enough can easily absorb didactic lectures, whereas other students cannot equally learn from didactic lectures. The lecture method is not inherently flawed, because ineffective didactic lecturing could be due to many other factors. These factors include unskilled teachers who deliver the didactic lecture poorly, misjudging the didactic lecture as a suitable format for the course objectives, and poor structure and organisation of the content.[4,5]

EVIDENCE-BASED RECOMMENDATIONS

Didactic lecturing, like all forms of teaching, should be oriented towards the learning process. Didactic lecturing continues to evolve to be more than just transmission of knowledge; students should be affected by the topic to become motivated.[21] The knowledge they receive should be important enough for them to be in class and should relate to their purpose for learning. It is worth noting that non-cognitive attributes of teachers promote student learning.[22]

Several studies suggest that it is very difficult to generate and maintain interest in particular tasks for a very long period of time.[23] After the first 15 minutes or so of a lecture, the attention level of most students decreases.[24] Therefore, it is important to capture the attention of the students and to generate and maintain their interests in the lecture, particularly during didactic lectures where the lecturer does most of the talking. Students' levels of attention, interests and performance can be maintained in a variety of ways. Two studies[22,25] involving a systematic review of the relevant literature on teaching methods led to the identification of conditions that contribute to effective didactic lecturing. These conditions include:
- opening the lecture with 'captivating' statements that stimulate the learners to be aware and receptive
- demonstrating the instructor's enthusiasm for the topic, rather than demonstrating of his/her expertise
- stating the relevance of the topic to the learners' expectations and connecting it to their prior knowledge

- providing opportunities for the learners to make personal connections to the topic at hand
- reviewing the learning objectives, so that the students know what is expected of them at the end of the lecture
- when appropriate, providing real-life illustrations and examples of the concepts or ideas that the students can relate to
- sharing key points to provide a clear road map of how to achieve the learning objectives; these are the main ideas, facts and concepts that the lecture hangs on
- using a variety of media to enable the students to use different senses to refocus their attention
- taking breaks in order for the students to take a short rest and help regain their attention.

The didactic lecture should be properly structured and organised in such a way as to enhance student learning.[25] The key to achieving this is to break the lecture into its constituent parts: opening, body and conclusion. The opening should include an 'attention-grabber' to capture the students' attention and excite them enough to maintain their interests throughout the lecture.[25] An attention-grabber could be a provocative statement, a rhetorical question, an analogy or an appropriate image. The opening can also serve to set up expectations for students, so that they are aware of their commitment to learn what is taught.[26] First impressions are important, so a good opening is critical to the success of the lecture. It must begin to connect the lecturer to the students through personal or topic-related experiences that both the student and lecturer have encountered.

The body is the main content of the lecture. It is the knowledge that the students should learn. This knowledge embodies the concepts, theories and principles that the topic covers. When selecting the content, it must be aligned with the course objectives, and the main ideas in the content must adhere to the objectives. There are some challenges that must be overcome in order to optimise the content. There is tension between the amount of curriculum material to be covered and the time available. Several strategies have been suggested to resolve such tensions.[27]

Another challenge is the sequencing between, and within, the key points, concepts or main ideas in the content.[28] The sequencing between the main ideas should reflect the order of the learning objectives, which reflects the connections throughout the content. This also represents a logical progression through the lecture, and it encourages deep learning and extension of knowledge. Sequencing within key points refers to the use of examples, illustration and making connections between ideas or facts that lead to a broader understanding of the topic, which could lead to higher-level learning. It allows for information to be presented in different contexts, allowing learning to be encoded in different ways. A lack of connections between main ideas is also another challenge that contributes to poor structure of lectures.

Summarising a previous idea and connecting it to the next main idea can make these linkages. The purpose of the conclusion is to bring closure to the lecture, with the view that students should leave the lecture with a clear understanding of the content materials, and that they should want to further explore the topic after class. The conclusion brings together the key points presented and it should be brief. In addition to a review of statements of the key points, several other approaches can be used to summarise a lecture. Asking questions of the students on the key points, allowing the students to ask questions in return, or administering quizzes will help clarify their understanding of the content.[29] Students' last memory of a lecture can be enhanced by questions. This also encourages curiosity about and ongoing interest in the topic.

The effective didactic lecture should be motivating and rewarding for both the student and the instructor. Students are more likely to be successful in attaining the learning outcomes and maintaining interest in the lecture if the instructor is not only knowledgeable about the topic but also enthusiastic and interested in the lecture.[30] A lecturer must also be able to relate to, and care about, the students by sharing personal experiences with them that are relevant to the topic.[31] The lecturing should not be about the teacher but, rather, the teacher should draw attention to the content so that the students feel that they are part of that content by relating their experiences to it; students should be emotionally activated to engage in learning.[32]

Several techniques that foster student engagement have been suggested that can be used effectively in the didactic lecture format. These techniques include:
- focusing attention on the content
- encouraging questions from students
- pausing after every 15 minutes with an activity, and varying the content presentation
- providing a positive learning environment and relationships with the students
- using effective communication skills
- asking questions of students – the questions can act as a cue for constructing missing pieces in their learning and can also help guide the teaching.[33–36]

FUTURE RESEARCH

Despite clear evidence regarding the effectiveness of active learning in comparison with didactic lectures in enhancing deep learning, it does not mean that students do not learn during didactic lectures. The implementation of active learning strategies can be difficult in large lecture groups. Also, there are potential disadvantages associated with active and interactive techniques, such as loss of time and content, which can be alleviated by the didactic lecture method. Thus, depending on the educational settings, both active learning and didactic lecture can be used to affect student learning and performance. Therefore, instead of discarding traditional lectures entirely, active learning methods can be selectively incorporated into traditional lectures to change the pace. The different interpretations of active learning, the evolution of the didactic lecture, and different measurements of effectiveness make it difficult to compare results. Therefore, there is still need for further investigation into some important questions: When are teaching strategies most effective? What are the specific nature and design of the teaching activities that make them effective? What factors, including the subject discipline, the experience level of students and educational settings, affect the effectiveness of different instructional strategies? How best to integrate active learning and cooperative activities into didactic lectures, or vice versa?

Addressing these questions is essential because of the concerns about the quality and transferability of the evidence on the effectiveness of different teaching strategies. These concerns are justifiable, as there are several reasons why conducting educational research has inherent difficulties: the student groups used in comparing different teaching methods may not be equally matched; variation in the knowledge and teaching skills between instructors; and differences in the abilities of an instructor to use a particular teaching method. In addition, it is difficult to isolate and change the independent variables such as experiences, expectations and maturation with respect to prior knowledge. There may also be problems with measuring the learning outcomes because different assessment tools may not be a valid measure of the learning outcomes. So, disagreements on the dependent variables are problematic too.

Furthermore, it is important to address these questions because the limitations posed on different instructional strategies can be amplified because of confounding factors such as the generational mix of students. Instructional techniques should take advantage of the diverse generational characteristics now present in our classrooms.[37] Another factor that has a profound influence on learning is the increasing popularity of web-based lectures, such as digital audio and video files to record and transmit lectures.[37] This type of learning requires further investigation into how it will affect the integration of lectures into active learning tasks, since there are concerns of the impact of technologies on lecture attendance.

CONCLUSION

The effective didactic lecture format will continue to be used as a teaching format, especially with increasing level of student population. Students should be productively engaged during didactic lecturing. Thus, didactic lectures will continue to be carefully designed and delivered in ways to positively influence learning. There has to be a balance between the effective didactic lecturing and active learning to address the conflict between the instructor covering enough content material and students' active engagement in learning.

SUMMARY POINTS

The didactic lecture can be highly effective when it:
- aligns with the learning objectives
- connects to prior knowledge
- involves a variety of activities and multimedia that promote learner and instructor interaction
- relates to real-life experiences
- concludes by reinforcing the main ideas
- is consistently improved through regular student and peer feedback, reflection and evidence-based practices.

REVIEW QUESTIONS

Read the following case study examples of different approaches to lecturing to large groups, and then discuss the questions provided.

Case study 1: Engaging students through storytelling
I teach the history leading up to the establishment of the College of Dental Hygienists of Manitoba, the regulatory body of our profession, to dental hygiene students at the University of Manitoba, Canada. Some would think such a 'lecture' would be dry and boring, but I saw it as an opportunity to tell the story of those who helped shaped the practice of the dental hygiene profession. The Imaginative Education Theory from the Imaginative Education Research Group in British Columbia, Canada, was used to conceptualise and create the session to capture attention and generate student interest. The theory suggests five means of understanding: (1) somatic, (2) mythic, (3) romantic, (4) philosophical and (5) ironic. With just over an hour to share the history, I provide the students with the chronology of significant events, but do so by presenting it as a fictional story based on true events. My colleague and I shared the task: she documented the chronology and key outcomes and I created the story. I learned that for a story to be a classic, it has to appeal to a wide audience and have universal attributes. I researched elements of a story: character, plot, part and whole, and cohesiveness. I stayed true to events but I created fictional characters who were blends of many real-life persons. I drew on the somatic, mythic, romantic, philosophical and ironic ways of knowing. The students in the class hear a story and not a lecture. Students actively engage in the story by responding to its elements (example: part and whole – what and why events happened), querying about factual events described through a combination of PowerPoint slides outlining key facts and hyperlinks to governmental documents, and listening with attentiveness and sometimes tears to the narrative fictional story woven into the session.

(Laura MacDonald, Associate Professor at the School of Dental Hygiene, University of Manitoba)

Case study 2: Engaging students through diverse strategies
I teach anatomy, physiology and pathophysiology courses designed for physician assistant and nursing students. The courses are divided into two three-credit hour-long blocks. At the beginning of every course the students are provided with a syllabus that clearly outlines the course objectives, class schedule, required reading and laboratory material, so that students are able to manage their time more effectively and properly prepare for classes. All material, including anything supplemental, is made available in the library or online. Notes are posted on the learning centre web page well in advance of the class. The lectures are either 2 hours long or include 2 hours of traditional classroom

lecturing followed by 2 hours of laboratory work that reflects the material covered in the class. The blocks are no longer than 50 minutes (20–25 PowerPoint slides, maximum) followed by 10-minute breaks between the blocks. The learning objectives are clearly stated at the beginning of every lecture and a short quiz is provided at the end of the lecture. The quiz reflects the materials covered in the lecture and is answered in class, followed by a summary with references.

A clinical case scenario is presented at the beginning of the lecture so that students immediately connect what they are learning with the practical application of that knowledge. Students are encouraged to actively participate in open discussion, either individually or as smaller groups, and to ask and answer questions of their colleagues. Every time the students solve a piece of the 'puzzle', more clues are added, until the case is solved. A PowerPoint lecture typically follows in which the students are welcome to ask questions at any time. A variety of media (video material, animations, models, diagrams and tables, and examples) are used to aid learning whenever applicable in order to make the lecture a more dynamic and interesting experience. Students' interests and questions help guide which media and methods will be used in order to keep them engaged. I find that this approach creates a relaxed atmosphere, helping to make learning as painless as possible.

> (Dr Deni Pirnat, Lecturer in the Physician Assistant Education
> Program, University of Manitoba)

Case study questions
- Which elements from the lists of the characteristics of an effective lecture were used in these case study examples?
- Which elements were used in these case studies that could hinder students' learning experiences?
- What do you understand by the Imaginative Education Theory?
- How does this theory enhance learning?
- Which elements of the Imaginative Education Theory are supported by evidence to enhance learning?

REFLECTIVE QUESTIONS AND EXERCISES
- Which characteristics of your lectures facilitate and which hinder student learning?
- What evidence from the literature can you provide in support of the effectiveness of the characteristics in your lectures that you think enrich students' learning experiences?
- What might you do to improve on your techniques that are consistent with the conditions of an effective lecture?

REFERENCES

1. Sutherland P, Badger R. Lecturers' perceptions of lectures. *J Furth High Educ.* 2004; **28**(3): 277–89.
2. Lammers WJ, Murphy JJ. A profile of teaching techniques used in the university classroom. *Act Learn High Educ.* 2002; **3**(1): 54–67.
3. Reime MH, Harris A, Aksnes J, *et al.* The most successful method in teaching nursing students infection control: E-learning or lecture? *Nurs Educ Today.* 2008; **28**(7): 798–806.
4. McLaughlin K, Mandin H. A schematic approach to diagnosing and resolving lecturalgia. *Med Educ.* 2001; **35**(12): 1135–42.
5. Brookfield SD. *The Skillful Teacher: on technique, trust, and responsiveness in the classroom.* 2nd ed. San Francisco, CA: Jossey-Bass; 2006.
6. Naismith L, Steinert Y. The evaluation of a workshop to promote interactive lecturing. *Teach Learn Med.* 2001; **13**(1): 43–8.
7. Sandhu S, Afifi TO, Amara FM. Theories and practical steps for delivering effective lectures. *J Community Med Health Educ.* 2012; **2**(6): 158.
8. Bligh DA. *What's the Use of Lectures?* San Francisco, CA: Jossey-Bass; 2000.
9. McKeachie WJ. *McKeachie's Teaching Tips: strategies, research, and theory for college and university teachers.* College Teaching Series. 11th ed. Boston, MA: Houghton Mifflin; 2002.
10. Lake DA. Student performance and perceptions of a lecture-based course compared with the same course utilizing group discussion. *Phys Ther.* 2001; **81**(3): 896–903.
11. Merrill B. Learning and teaching in universities; perspectives from adult learners and lecturers. *High Educ.* 2001, **6**(1). 5–18.
12. Mandin H, Jones A, Woloschuk W, *et al.* Helping students learn to think like experts when solving clinical problems. *Acad Med.* 1997; **72**(3): 173–9.
13. Beers GW. The effect of teaching method on objective test scores: problem-based learning versus lecture. *J Nurs Educ.* 2005; **44**(7): 305–9.
14. Vreven D, McFadden S. An empirical assessment of cooperative groups in large, time-compressed, introductory courses. *Innov High Educ.* 2007; **32**(1): 85–92.
15. Costa ML, Rensburg LV, Rushton N. Does teaching style matter? A randomised trial of group discussion versus lectures in orthopaedic undergraduate teaching. *Med Educ.* 2007; **41**(2): 214–17.
16. Tiwari A, Lai P, So M, *et al.* A comparison of the effectiveness of problem-based learning and lecturing on the development of students' critical thinking. *Med Educ.* 2006; **40**(6): 547–54.
17. Dunnington G, Witzke D, Rubeck R, *et al.* A comparison of the teaching effectiveness of the didactic lecture and the problem-oriented small group session: a prospective study. *Surg.* 1987; **102**(2): 291–6.
18. Herrington A, Herrington J. What is an authentic learning environment? In: Herrington A, Herrington J, editors. *Authentic Learning Environments in Higher Education.* Hershey, PA: Information Science Publishing; 2006. pp. 1–13.
19. Young P, Diekelmann N. Learning to lecture: exploring the skills, strategies, and practices of new nurses in nursing education. *J Nurs Educ.* 2002; **41**(9): 405–512.
20. Rogers MKA. A preliminary investigation and analysis of student learning style preferences in further and higher education. *J Furth High Educ.* 2011; **33**(1): 13–21.
21. Ten Cate O, Snell L, Mann K, *et al.* Orienting teaching toward the learning process. *Acad Med.* 2004; **79**(3): 219–28.
22. Sutkin G, Wagner E, Harris I, *et al.* What makes a good clinical teacher in medicine? A review of the literature. *Acad Med.* 2008; **83**(5): 452–60.
23. Matthews G, Davies DR, Holley PJ. Cognitive predictors of vigilance. *Hum Fact.* 1993; **35**(1): 3–24.
24. Young MS, Robinson S, Alberts P. Students pay attention! Combating the vigilance decrement to improve learning during lectures. *Act Learn High Educ.* 2009; **10**(1): 41–5.

25. Heitzmann R. Ten suggestions for enhancing lecturing. *Educ Digest*. 2010; **75**(9): 50–4.
26. Gump SE. Daily class objectives and instructor's effectiveness as perceived by students. *Psychol Rep*. 2004; **94**(3): 1250–2.
27. Gerald B. Content vs. learning: an old dichotomy in science courses. *J Async Learn Network*. 2011; **15**(1): 33–44.
28. Regehr G, Norman GR. Issues in cognitive psychology: implications for professional education. *Acad Med*. 1996; **71**(9): 988–1001.
29. Woodring BC, Woodring RC. Lecture: reclaiming a place in pedagogy. In: Bradshaw MJ, Lowenstein AJ, editors. *Innovative Teaching Strategies in Nursing and Related Health Professions*. 5th ed. Burlington, MA: Jones & Bartlett Learning; 2011. pp. 113–34.
30. Metcalfe A, Game A. The teacher's enthusiasm. *Aust Educ Res*. 2006; **33**(3): 91–106.
31. Goldstein G, Fernald P. Humanistic education in a capstone course. *Col Teach*. 2009; **57**(1): 27–36.
32. Gray JR. Integration of emotion and cognitive control. *Curr Direct Psychol Sci*. 2004; **13**(1): 46–8.
33. Lewis A. *The Art of Lecturing*. West Roxbury, MA: B & R Samizdat Express; 2011.
34. Cutting MF, Saks SN. Twelve tips for utilizing principles of learning to support medical education. *Med Teach*. 2012; **34**(1): 20–4.
35. Chin C, Osborne J. Students' questions: a potential resource for teaching and learning science. *Stud Sci Educ*. 2008; **44**(1): 1–39.
36. Goldman KD, Schmalz KJ. Builders, boomers, busters, bridgers: vive la (generational) difference! *Health Promot Pract*. 2006; **7**(2): 159–61.
37. McGarr O. A review of podcasting in higher education: its influence on the traditional lecture. *Aust J Educ Technol*. 2009; **25**(3): 309–12.

CHAPTER 25

Just-in-Time Teaching

Approach and evidence in health professional education settings

Gregor Novak and Dianna Tison

OVERVIEW

In this chapter, the Just-in-Time Teaching (JiTT) pedagogy is described, the education research that underpins it is summarised, and some examples of how one health professional educator has adapted the pedagogy to her field are outlined.

CHAPTER OBJECTIVES

Upon completion of this chapter, the reader will be able to:
- define the term 'Just-in-Time Teaching'
- explain the pedagogical concepts that underlie JiTT as an education approach
- articulate the current body of evidence that is available that underpins the JiTT approach
- describe how the JiTT approach can be applied to health professional education.

KEY TERMS: Just-in-Time Teaching, warm-up

INTRODUCTION

> There is abundant anecdotal evidence that much of what happens in school is driven by need to maintain bureaucratic and institutional norms rather than scholarly norms. Much research literature documents this interpretation; it is likely that many students hold similar views of schools and the instructional activities that take place there. To the extent that this is true then, it is unlikely that individual conceptual change will take place without restructuring classrooms and schools along lines that will foster the development of a community of intentional, motivated, and thoughtful learners.[1(p117)]

Allison is driving with her parents when they are involved in a serious car accident. At the emergency room, her doctor tells Allison that her mother is fine but that her father, Bob, has lost a lot of blood and will need a blood transfusion. Allison volunteers to donate blood for her father. She is told that her blood type is AB. Bob is type O.
- Can Allison donate blood to Bob? Why or why not?
- Allison, who is a biology student, begins to wonder if she is adopted. What would you tell her and why?

The questions quoted above are a pre-class assignment to prepare students for an interactive lesson on genetics in an introductory biology class. The teacher who assigned this question (Kathy Marrs at Indiana University–Purdue University Indianapolis) is practising *Just-in-Time Teaching* (JiTT), an interactive engagement pedagogical strategy, developed in the 1990s.[2]

To prepare for a JiTT lesson, students are asked to complete a web-based assignment, called a *warm-up*, and submit their responses electronically just hours before class time. The instructor looks at the online responses, or a subset of these, and adjusts the upcoming lesson activity accordingly. The warm-up assignments require that the student examines his or her prior knowledge about the upcoming topic, consults the textbook and other sources if necessary and answers the assigned question, which is often somewhat vague, requiring the student to make a judgement call, take a stand and defend it.

In a JiTT classroom, students construct the same knowledge as in a passive lecture, but with two important added benefits: first, having completed a web-based assignment (the warm-up) very recently, they enter the classroom ready to participate actively in the activities; second, students have a feeling of ownership because the interactive lesson is based on their own wording and understanding of the relevant issues. The March/April 2007 issue of the *Journal of College Science Teaching* lists JiTT as one of six inductive pedagogical techniques where

> the instructor begins by presenting students with a specific challenge, such as experimental data to interpret, a case study to analyse, or a complex real-world problem to solve. Students grappling with these challenges

quickly recognise the need for facts, skills, and conceptual understanding, at which point the teacher provides instruction or helps students learn on their own.[3(p14)]

Exactly what do JiTT questions look like? Below are seven examples of 'good' JiTT questions, spanning a variety of disciplines. In this context, 'good' infers that these questions have been proven to yield a rich set of student responses for classroom discussion.

1. What is the difference between a theory and a belief? You may want to look these terms up before answering. Be as specific as you can, and give an example of each. *(Educator, Introductory Biology)*

2. Please explain in your own words what a focal length is. Try not to use any equations or refer to a specific type of mirror or lens. *(Gavrin, Introductory Physics)*

3. Your everyday experience, common sense and mathematics classes all suggest to you that the shortest distance between two points in two-dimensional space is a straight line (unless, of course, you want to consider a warped space–time continuum!). Please describe how you would go about proving that this is true, using the methods of variational calculus. Don't actually do this, but describe in English the procedure you would follow. Please be specific in your steps. *(Educator, Advanced Mechanics)*

4. Explain in simple terms how you solved warm-up #1. In particular, what questions did you ask yourself and what conclusions did you draw from the answers? *(Educator)*

5. Estimate the probability that a North American male is precisely 6 feet tall. *(Educator, Statistics)*

6. Let's say you have a prescription for contact lenses of −2 diopters. If you accidentally get glasses (as opposed to contacts) made to the same strength, your prescription will be a bit off, and you won't be able to focus at infinity. Estimate how far you will be able to focus. *(Educator, Introductory Physics)*

7. In your opinion … do we need to save ancient Egyptian monuments? Why? What are the monuments worth – are they worth anything? *(Educator, Earth Science)*

These questions illustrate some of the pedagogical issues targeted by educators who utilise the JiTT approach, such as:

- preparing for a discussion of a complex, possibly controversial topic[1]
- creating a need to know, addressing motivation and sufficiently captivating students so that even weak students may be interested in the answer[2]
- going beyond the bare definition – for example, 'In your own words …' kind of questions[3,4]
- metacogniton – extending the understanding and applying the knowledge at the present level of understanding.[5,6]

JiTT had its origins in classrooms where teachers were looking for more effective ways to engage a particular audience – non-traditional students. Eventually it found its way into virtually all higher education environments. The pedagogy evolved mostly by trial and error, although many JiTT practitioners were paying attention to the education research literature. JiTT started in the physics community, which has a rich and much appreciated tradition of education research[4] and then spread to all STEM (science, technology, engineering and mathematics) disciplines and to many humanities.

Over the years the attention of JiTT practitioners has shifted to the broader questions: *Which aspects of the technique work well? Which aspects of JiTT do not work so well and why?* To answer these questions, it is necessary to examine the body of knowledge about teaching and learning that has accumulated over the past half century.[5]

To put JiTT into a broader teaching and learning perspective, the two broad JiTT goals are:

1. to encourage the students to construct and monitor their own learning experience
2. to create a learning environment where students are actually motivated to do just that, both in the classroom and away from the classroom.

PLANNING AND CONSTRUCTING JITT LESSONS

As mentioned earlier in this chapter, in preparation for a JiTT lesson activity students must complete a pre-instruction assignment (called a JiTT warm-up) hours before the lesson. Students submit their responses online where the assignments are available 24 hours a day. This must be done on a daily basis, a requirement that conflicts with the studying practices of many students. Most JiTT practitioners have found it essential to give the students a clear idea of the purpose of these assignments – where they fit into the teaching and learning scheme. Students tend to view any assignment as a summative assessment, ultimately related to the course grade rather than to learning objectives. If JiTT is initiated on a class without elaborate explanation and justification, many students walk away believing that they are required to self-teach. There is no guarantee that even the most careful explanation will shake many students' belief that to teach means to tell (e.g. lecture) and to learn means to pay attention and remember. Nevertheless, there is much anecdotal evidence that with time many students begin to understand what JiTT is all about and even perceive some of the benefits, despite the fact that they are often still bothered by the daily grind.

Here are a few 'frequently asked questions' (and accompanying answers) regarding JiTT, developed by Dr Mary Beth Camp from the Department of Economics, Indiana University.

Question 1. *What do we expect to accomplish with the warm-ups?*
Answer 1. We expect the students to survey the topic that is the subject of the upcoming lesson. There is new material in this and there may be review material. There may be real-world examples that make sense to the student but the analysis of which is new and will be taught in class or there may be unfamiliar examples. Students will not be rewarded for understanding (learning) the new material, but instead for being exposed to the jargon, recognising the familiar (e.g. there will be graphs to plot, equations to solve, 'things I'd better review before the lesson') and the unfamiliar (e.g. 'there

will be calculus operations involved that I don't remember or even don't remember seeing before. I'll have to ask the instructor what to do about that.')

Which of these issues gets how much emphasis will depend on at least two factors. First, where in the topic hierarchy is the upcoming lesson? This ranges from the first exposure introductory lessons to classes later in the sequence of course. The metacognitive exercise the students are rewarded for can be complex if they have to dig into their past experiences with subject matter prerequisites and ancillary prerequisites (e.g. mathematics background, computer skills from spreadsheet expertise to programming). It is helpful to state that students are *rewarded* for this work rather than formally *assessed* or graded. This kind of reward is the equivalent to the credit for *effort* in the elementary grades. Some higher education instructors have a hard time with the *reward for effort* concept, but the reality in most classrooms is such that, unless explicitly directed to do this, the majority of students will not monitor their own learning. Students will not be learning basic course content but instead will become conversant with *meta-content*.

The second factor is: what kind of knowledge best describes the new lesson? Some theorists distinguish between 'declarative knowledge' and 'procedural knowledge'. Declarative knowledge is facts and explanations (e.g. laws of physics, how many planets, what is gravity, what temperature water freezes at, the chemical structure of hydrogen) while procedural knowledge is skills and processing of observable data (e.g. calculus, graphing, measuring the distance between two points, determining the running spead of a person). Most academic subjects deal with both types of knowledge. The pre-class warm-up assignments have to take that into account. Thinking about the type, content and format of questions that best prepare students for each of these types of knowledge is at the heart of constructing quality warm-up assignments. The lesson preparatory work is to be done in parallel with *studying* the new material after instruction and completing the homework and laboratory exercises.

Question 2. *Are the warm-ups supposed to gauge what students understand about the lesson topic based on their reading or on what they knew before their reading?*
Answer 2. If the term 'understand' is interpreted as having learned the upcoming material on their own, then no, the warm-ups are not supposed to gauge what students understand about the lesson topic based on their reading. If this is made clear to students right from the start, and reinforced frequently, students will eventually accept it. Students will still be bothered by the fact that this implies that they will have to change their time management paradigm. They want to *surface learn* and *cram* before exams and tests, but educators want students to engage in *deep learning* so that the material will resonate with them for times to come.

Question 3. *How does a pre-class assignment fit into the JiTT process?*
Answer 3. The pre-class assignment helps the student get an overview of the upcoming lesson topic, sort out the familiar concepts and the new concepts and skills, connect topic to the real-world examples and, if possible, generate interest in the material. If student responses to warm-up exercises include statements like *'This looks interesting*

– too bad I'm not able to understand it better' or *'Too bad my maths skills are so poor that I expect the qualitative parts to be difficult'*, then the educator has at least the affective part under control. Also, the students are rewarded for sharing their perspectives on the topic being studied.

Question 4. *Is it or is it not expected that students will prepare for class? If it is, what is expected of that preparation? Is it expected that students will be confronted with new ideas and begin processing them before class?*

Answer 4. It has to be explained to the students in an explicit manner what the JiTT processing of new ideas is all about, what is expected of them and how they will be rewarded. They are not required to *learn* new material on their own; however, what is expected is that students will become familiar with the general outline of the upcoming lesson, to examine any prior knowledge they already have and try to relate this prior knowledge to the new. During the upcoming lesson activities they will be able to compare their knowledge status with that of their peers. With the help of the instructor they will begin to integrate the new material with the prior knowledge. This process will promote a deeper level of learning among students.

Question 5. *If so, what is this called if self-teaching is out?*

Answer 5. The answer to this question is largely a marketing issue. Educators teach; students learn. Educators give students tasks to do; educators talk, explain and model; and educators assess. In the JiTT process, students themselves perform the tasks and analyse their own work. To associate *teaching* with what the students do will cause confusion over the distinction between the role of the educator and the role of the student. Students might end up stating that 'you are paid to teach me and now you have me do your work'. So, it is suggested that educators stay away from the term *self-teach* and maybe use 'manage and supervise my own learning'.

Question 6. *Where, if at all, does the preparation fit into the warm-ups schedule? Is attempting to gauge what the students have learned and what they have not learned or what is clear and what is confusing inappropriate for warm-ups?*

Answer 6. It is all appropriate. Realising and confronting what is confusing and what is challenging is the initial step. Articulating it helps the student and the educator to look for the next step. (For example, it is sometimes easy – say, a mini lecture to help with a difficult test – and sometimes difficult – say, making up for inadequate algebra skills, or even reading skills.)

JiTT assignments can be described as formative assessment, enabling and forward-looking. They offer the class a chance to grapple with authentic tasks. 'Authentic assessments require students to be effective performers with acquired knowledge.'[7(p229)] When the students perceive the warm-ups as non-judgemental diagnostic tools, they become more willing to take risks and reveal the actual state of their knowledge. Warm-up assignments usually include a request for student comments. These comments often contain a wealth of helpful metacognitive observations.

JITT IN HEALTH PROFESSIONAL EDUCATION: DIANNA TISON'S PERSPECTIVE

My experience with JiTT started with my university adopting laptops for all students. Feeling laptops should be somehow utilised if the students were going to have them, I attended a JiTT workshop at the American Air Force Academy in 2000. My discovery was that JiTT offered much more than just a way to use the laptops. The method fit well with the challenges in teaching professional nursing students how to think critically and conceptually and how to recognise when to develop skills in seeking answers to questions presented about patients and their situations (in case studies or vignettes presented in JiTT exercises).

You may be thinking at this point, 'I *already* use case studies and vignettes in class and have students discuss them.' However, often you see students in the group who are not prepared to participate or who choose not to participate for whatever reason. Often they have not read the material before class and so depend on others in the group to carry the discussion. The JiTT exercise requires students to think about the upcoming topic and prepare and defend an *individual* response. The class is engaged when responses are then discussed together in class and the material is expanded. The first time I tried it, I was amazed that not one of the 40 students in the class was texting or using other social media – they were more engaged because they had participated in creating the class.

Since the case study and vignettes represent real-world situations and the kind of thinking they will be doing as graduates, the students are motivated to understand how the facts they are reading and studying translate into practice situations. I call it the 'so what for nursing' processing. My courses are fundamental nursing courses in the 'on the ground' and online course sequence for beginning nursing students and registered nurses returning for a baccalaureate degree. When simulation with manikins that sweat, speak and perform many other functions became popular for students to practise real-world nursing, I wondered if JiTT would still be relevant. Actually, when my students participated in simulation in another course, they commented to the faculty during the simulation debriefing that the JiTT exercises had prepared them for the kind of thinking they were required to do during the simulation.

One other benefit shared with students is that their thinking work in doing the JiTT exercises strengthens their ability to do the kind of thinking required to successfully answer application-level questions on exams. Recognition that knowledge is required to think and focus on detail helps them to be successful. The teacher is able to review each individual's answers in the JiTT exercises and is able to reach out and contact students who are really not grasping the material before lack of success is identified on an exam.

Classroom philosophies vary, so one can ask to know if the student received help in the assignment and from whom they received the help: another classmate, a tutor or a study group. The activities should be kept brief and focused on the important concepts of the lesson. This makes the activity helpful for students who have a variety of roles and demands on their time and it helps to focus them on the important material. A component of the activity should challenge students to apply the knowledge they have read about to the real-life situations they will encounter that will call upon them to use that information. This helps students to see that they are not just learning facts for facts but for lifelong application in their chosen career of nursing or other discipline.

It is important to remember that what happens in the classroom is an important part of the JiTT strategy. The classroom discussion of the warm-up assignment reveals much about the status of the student understanding of the lesson topic. The instructor knows what the class knows or understands, so he or she can reinforce, clarify and/or correct any misinformation. The classroom discussion of the warm-up also provides an opportunity to talk about answers where terminology is not clear to the students. In presenting the student responses, one can say: 'Some of you had this idea represented by this response.' It is important to not be judgemental in the approach, since the object is not to be punitive in judging responses but rather to be encouraging in order to continue to have students respond and be open to critique and assistance in applying information. For me, the fact that students collaborate with one another, as indicated in some of their responses, is a positive. Health professionals need to be able to communicate and problem-solve collaboratively.

I will now describe a case study that is the subject of a sample warm-up assignment. The warm-up assignment follows the description of the case study.

Case study of Ms RL: the subject of the warm-up

Ms RL is a 78-year-old white female. She has white hair, she weighs 63.5 kg and she is 158.8 cm in height. She is a widow of 1 year. She is in relatively good health except for the following medical problems: atrial fibrillation and hypertension.

Ms RL takes the following medications:
- furosemide 40 mg po qd
- KCl 20 mEq po qd
- Diltiazem 240 mg cap 1 cap po qd
- Lanoxin 0.125 mg po qd
- Coumadin 5 mg po qd; 2.5 mg on Mondays and Thursdays
- was recently put on propranolol hydrochloride 40 mg po bid
- multivitamin 1 cap qd
- calcium 600 mg and vitamin D 1 tab qd

Recent laboratory results:
- INR 6
- K 3.5 mEq/L.

Body changes related to ageing:
- she states she sometimes has stiffness in the morning, especially with cold or wet weather
- she has a low Na diet restricted to 2 g a day; she used to salt food before tasting it, and she likes sweets; she usually eats frozen dinners, such as the brand Healthy Choice – she tries to choose those with 500 mg or less sodium content
- but sometimes she just has to have her favourite potato chips and dip.

Health perception and health management:
- she describes her health state as good
- she has a flu shot every year; she had a pneumonia shot 2 years ago
- she gets exercise feeding her small terrier-type dog and taking her laundry out to the detached garage, where her washing machine and dryer are located
- she keeps her doctor's appointments; she is concerned about her high blood pressure
- general appearance – she has thick, white hair and wrinkles in her face; she states she has had some skin cancers, caused by time spent in the sun fishing with her husband when he was alive, removed from her face and arms; she does not have body odour; she bathes every few days, and her skin is thin.

Activity and exercise:
- she likes to attend the senior centre every Monday; recently she has had others pick her up and so has decreased her driving; she enjoys working outside with a few plants in her garden and in pots on her porch
- she states she fell recently – she got up from her recliner and the next thing she knew she was on the floor in the kitchen; she has a bruise on her forehead from the fall
- musculoskeletal – she has stiffness in the morning but this gets better during the day; she says she sometimes takes aspirin to help with the discomfort
- radial pulse is 80 beats per minute but is irregular (atrial fibrillation).

Nutrition and metabolic pattern:
- she states 'appetite is good', but she doesn't 'enjoy cooking much just for one person'
- no food intolerances or restrictions; she states she tries to eat a banana or orange since she is taking a water pill; she states she doesn't take water pill when she is going somewhere since she 'might not make it to a bathroom'
- she drinks water and has coffee every morning
- no cyanosis or jaundice; her skin is warm; 1+ dependent oedema in her ankles; she says she usually elevates her feet when sitting in her recliner watching television; she weighs herself at least twice a week.

Elimination pattern:
- has soft brown stool every morning
- she states she has no problems with urination; no escape of urine with coughing or sneezing
- bowel sounds are present in all quadrants
- no tenderness in her abdomen on palpation.

Cognitive and perceptual:
- she states she has 'no problems with memory'
- her hearing is good
- some impairment of vision due to cataracts.

Roles and relationships:
- widowed with no children, but she does have an uncle who lives a few miles down the road; occasional visits from nephews
- she wants to be independent
- she is unable to drive at night because of her cataracts, as the flare of oncoming headlights impairs her vision.

Coping and stress:
- she states she can tolerate a lot of pain, so when she says something hurts, it hurts
- she is concerned about living alone in the country
- she talks to two different neighbours almost daily.

Directions given to the students to prepare for a warm-up about the case study of Ms RL

Read the case study data provided as 'Case study of Ms RL'. Go to the warm-up questions to practise skills in analysing data and writing nursing diagnoses and outcomes. Remember to type in your name before each of your answers.

Here are some links to help you search for information, and you can also use your drug book or an electronic source:
- medical information link – www.nlm.nih.gov/medlineplus/encyclopedia.html
- laboratory test information link – http://labtestsonline.org/understanding/analytes/pt/tab/test

Warm-up questions for the case study of Ms RL
- What client strengths do you identify?
- Identify two nursing diagnoses, writing them in proper format and giving an outcome for each.
- Identify any potential complications for Ms RL. Be sure to write in the proper format for collaborative problems as described in the textbook

I review the student responses to the warm-up questions the evening before the class discussion. There are usually between 40 and 50 students in the class group, so it takes a while to review the responses and get a sense of where the class is in their understanding of the concepts taught and what they have read. I prepare a PowerPoint presentation to assist in conducting the discussion, using examples of the responses. Students like to have the PowerPoint file posted online after the discussion so they can go back and look over the responses again.

Although student names are not included with the examples shown in the PowerPoint file, the students are encouraged to prepare their responses in Microsoft Word and then copy and paste when posting the responses, as otherwise they can forget what they wrote by the time they get to the discussion! I do not strictly 'grade' the warm-ups. There is a rubric for what I look for and the warm-ups, along with other assignments in the course, are given points that contribute to 10% of their letter grade once they have achieved a 75% average on the major exams.

Rubric for grading warm-ups and assignments

Warm-ups and assignments are used as one of the teaching methods in this course. Students are expected to work on these independently, since the educator's review of all the assignment results helps to identify where knowledge about a topic has not been attained and therefore helps to guide the class. The rubric guides the faculty in grading and the student in knowing the expectations for the assignment.

The student is awarded points depending on the quality of his or her answers for assignments and nursing code preparations according to the criteria outlined here. Assignments must be completed on time in order to receive points according to quality of answer by the following rubric.

5 – Formal Understanding (Correct and Complete Applies Knowledge): the student answers the assignment or nursing code prep questions correctly and completely. The student incorporates information from the text or class notes or previous course knowledge into the answer.

4 – Intermediate Understanding (Moderate Accurate Knowledge): the student shows some accurate knowledge and may use correct terminology to answer the assignment or nursing code prep questions. The student does not use appropriate information from the text or lecture notes to answer the question. (The answer may be partially correct but still incomplete.)

3 – Elementary Understanding (Minimal Accurate Knowledge): the student tries to answer the assignment or nursing code prep questions but shows minimal accurate knowledge to assist in answering. The student shows significant misconceptions about concepts and uses inappropriate terminology. The student does not use any information from the text or other sources to answer the question. (The answer is incorrect.)

0 – No Demonstrated Understanding: the student may have logged onto the assignment but does not write his or her name on responses or there is a 'no response' answer. The student may say he or she did not know how to answer the assignment or warm-up questions.

GETTING COMFORTABLE WITH JITT: DEMANDS ON EDUCATORS – GREGOR NOVAK'S PERSPECTIVE

The transition from passive mode teaching to any interactive engagement approach requires time, reflection and practice. For most educators, this is not how they were taught. Some educators may even question the necessity for a change. Once the decision to go interactive is made, the transition has to be made deliberately, allowing the students to provide feedback. It is important that the students understand why the teaching strategy has been changed and what the new strategy is trying to accomplish. The students have to be told explicitly what will expected from them and from the educator as the new strategy is implemented.

Developing expertise in a profession is a process that has the attention of cognitive scientists. Particularly appropriate for our case may be the reflective practitioner model developed by Donald Schön in the 1980s.[6–9] Schön[8,9] proposed a developmental sequence that professionals pass through on the way to becoming experts.

1. First, we bring routinised responses to situations. These responses are based on tacit knowledge and are spontaneously delivered without conscious deliberation. The routines work as long as the situation fits within the normal range of familiar problems.
2. At some point, the routine response results in a surprise, an unexpected outcome, positive or negative, that draws our attention.
3. The surprise leads to reflection-in-action. We tacitly ask ourselves, 'What's going on here?' and 'What was I thinking that led up to this?'
4. Through immediate reflection, we re-examine assumptions or recast the problem in another way. We may quickly evaluate two or three new ways to frame the problem.
5. We engage in an on-the-spot experiment. We try out a new perspective or understanding of the situation and we carefully note its effects. The cycle of routine performance–surprise–interpretation–experiment is repeated as needed.[9]

These considerations should be kept in mind when switching to new and challenging teaching strategies such as JiTT.

JiTT has to be adopted, not adapted

It has become clear that there is no such thing as canonical JiTT, no 'one size fits all'. Just as educators demand that students construct their own version of the subject matter, interactive engagement pedagogies demand that a practitioner construct his or her own brand of the teaching tactics. Faculty reactions from JiTT classrooms range from euphoria to despair, largely dependent on whether JiTT was approached in an exploratory mode or adopted as a set of recipes. Cognitive science can shed light on this issue as well.[10] Putnum's[10] model of teaching uncovers a striking similarity to what is seen in JiTT workshops.

> As one participant said after a workshop on promoting organisational learning, 'If you could only give us a list of the eight things to say, that would be really helpful in getting started.' This person was not naive; he understood that a handful of recipes was not a substitute for genuine mastery. The difficulty is that a new theory of practice cannot be acquired whole. Yet if it is acquired piecemeal, the pieces are likely to be used in ways that violate the whole.[10(p145)]

Novices using JiTT often use recipes as 'one-liners' or invariant procedures.

> Lacking experience in the theory of practice from which the recipe was drawn, novices may get themselves in trouble they cannot get themselves

out of. Nevertheless, they may feel a sense of success at having done what they are 'supposed to do,' what they believe an expert might have done. At the same time they may feel some discomfort or chagrin at imitating or 'being a parrot'.[10(p145)]

The novice gradually shifts orientation from the recipe itself to broader strategies and concepts. Still,

learners may remain caught in a kind of tunnel vision, concentrating intently on the mechanics of implementing the new strategy. It is therefore difficult to respond flexibly to the [dynamic feedback] of the situation.[10(p145)]

Eventually, learners become able to

respond to surprising data by reframing the situation, stepping out of their original perspective to take account of another.[10(p145)]

Learners' attitudes about recipe-following also shift:

Rather than feeling successful simply by using a recipe, they may consider whether that usage was pro forma or genuine.[10(p145)]

CONCLUSION

JiTT has many potential applications in health professional student education. Although the evidence of JiTT as an education approach is still emerging, it appears to be promising. This chapter has provided an overview of the features of JiTT and included an example of the use of JiTT in nursing education.

SUMMARY POINTS

In summary, a teacher contemplating the use of JiTT must:
- be prepared for a trial-and-error period while adapting existing JiTT materials and creating one's own
- be sensitive to students' ideas, attitudes and state of knowledge, and constantly monitor the progress of their learning
- have a good grasp on the material and have a repertoire of conceptual pathways for the subject matter at hand to be able to appreciate and respond to students' ideas
- be creative and able to develop learning tasks to support this kind of learning
- be able to maintain a classroom climate where everybody is free to participate without the experience degenerating into frustrating chaos.

REVIEW QUESTIONS

- What are the main features of JiTT?
- What is the purpose of the warm-up in the JiTT context?
- Why is it important to make it explicit to students what the purpose of the JiTT process is?
- When do you provide feedback to students and how?

REFLECTIVE QUESTIONS AND EXERCISES

- What are the strengths and weaknesses of the JiTT approach to education?
- In your opinion, would the JiTT be a suitable approach to use with health professional students?
- What resources would be needed to implement the JiTT education approach?
- How would you ensure timely feedback to students if you implemented the JiTT approach?

REFERENCES

1. Pintrich PR. The dynamic interplay of student motivation and cognition in the college classroom. In: Ames C, Maehr M, editors. *Advances in Motivation and Achievement: motivation-enhancing environments.* Vol. 6. Greenwich: JAI Press; 1989. pp. 117–60.
2. Novak GM, Patterson ET, Gavrin AD, *et al. Just-in-Time Teaching: blending active learning with web technology.* Upper Saddle River, NJ: Prentice Hall; 1999.
3. Prince M, Felder R. The many faces of inductive teaching and learning. *J Coll Sci Teach.* 2007; **36**(5): 14–23.
4. Bransford JD, Brown AL, Cocking RR. *How People Learn: brain, mind, experience, and school.* Washington, DC: National Academies Press; 2000.
5. Arons AB. *Teaching Introductory Physics.* New York, NY: John Wiley & Sons; 1997.
6. Wilson B, Cole P. A critical review of elaboration theory. *Educ Technol Res Dev.* 1992; **40**(3): 63–79.
7. Wiggins GP. *Assessing Student Performance.* San Francisco, CA: Jossey-Bass; 1993.
8. Schön D. *The Reflective Practitioner.* New York, NY: Basic Books; 1983.
9. Schön D. *Educating the Reflective Practitioner: toward a new design for teaching and learning in the professions.* San Francisco, CA: Jossey-Bass; 1987.
10. Putnam RW. Recipes and reflective learning: 'What would prevent you from saying it that way?' In: Schön DA, editor. *The Reflective Turn: case studies in and on reflective practice.* New York, NY: Teacher College Press; 1991. pp. 145–63.

CHAPTER 26

Service-learning

Application and evidence in the education of health professional students

Barbara Gottlieb and Suzanne B Cashman

OVERVIEW

Service-learning, defined as a structured learning experience that combines community service with student preparation and reflection, has been used to educate health professions students across a broad array of content areas in the formal curriculum as well as in extracurricular learning activities. This chapter reviews the evidence for using service-learning pedagogy to instruct graduate health professions students. The review was structured according to twenty-first-century priority educational objectives – for example, discipline-specific clinical skills and knowledge, knowledge of broad contexts and concepts such as cultural competency, thinking skills, professionalism, and values and commitments. In this review, educational outcomes, including student satisfaction, acquisition of clinical skills and knowledge, promotion of critical thinking, professionalism, civic engagement and altruism were generally positive. However, much of the evidence for the effectiveness of service-learning pedagogy rests on small studies, based in a single course in a single institution, with short-term follow-up. Few studies employed sophisticated study designs; several lacked clear hypotheses and clearly delineated analytic methodologies. To strengthen the evidence for this promising pedagogy, a few studies used strategies that can be applied in future studies. These include mixed qualitative and quantitative methods to bolster findings through triangulation; clear hypotheses and measurable educational objectives; validated tools to measure outcomes; enlarged study size and scope through including several programmes within a school or collaborating across institutions; clear and replicable methods of data analysis, particularly in qualitative studies; and elements of experimental or quasi-experimental design, with clear description of baseline characteristics and careful pre- and post-intervention comparisons.

CHAPTER OBJECTIVES

Upon completion of this chapter, the reader will be able to:

- review the evidence base for effectiveness of service-learning pedagogy in health professions education
- become knowledgeable regarding evidence for using service-learning to ensure learners have command of each of five specific categorical educational objectives
- model ways in which educators should review health professions education service-learning literature
- identify areas that warrant further research.

KEY TERMS: service-learning, evidence-based education, health professions education

---

INTRODUCTION

Health professions educators must prepare their students to be practitioners, citizens and leaders who are competent to address the twenty-first century's global challenges. Health professionals are expected to master complex clinical and scientific knowledge and to embody humanistic values and characteristics. While health professions students acquire the attributes of professionals – for example, commitment to lifelong learning, capacity for teamwork and collaboration, altruism and dedication to their patients and the broader community – they must also learn to function in a world of rapidly evolving information and technology, instant, multidimensional communication and permeable disciplinary boundaries. Moreover, teaching methods must promote critical thinking and problem-solving skills, capacity to embrace ambiguity and the unknown, and awareness of and commitment to equity and social justice.

Service-learning offers great promise to promote many of these twenty-first-century skills and attributes, particularly those that are difficult to achieve in traditional classroom and clinical settings. Furthermore, service-learning offers developmentally appropriate channels for leadership as well as opportunities to develop relationships, and to participate in and contribute to communities outside of a relatively homogeneous peer group. Indeed, service-learning has played a valuable role in training health professionals in all fields; several actively promote or have an explicit service-learning requirement.[1]

In this chapter, the experience of service-learning in educating health professionals – including physicians, nurses, dentists, pharmacists, public health practitioners and physical and occupational therapists – are reviewed and analysed. This review

will be structured according to the categories of educational objectives that track with priority areas within the health professions. The assumption is that if service-learning can achieve any of these objectives, the pedagogy has merit. The categories are:
- clinical skills and knowledge relevant to the discipline (e.g. basic skills and applied skills for special needs individuals and populations)
- contextual and conceptual knowledge and skills (e.g. cultural competency and cultural humility; population health)
- thinking skills, approach to learning (e.g. critical thinking, embracing ambiguity, lifelong learning)
- professional conduct (e.g. teamwork, collaboration, interprofessionalism)
- values and commitments (e.g. civic engagement, altruism, advocacy, commitment to social justice).

Typical service-learning programmes incorporate the following: connecting classroom learning with community-based experience, addressing a community-identified and valued need or objective, fostering students' civic responsibility, providing an opportunity for deep learning through reflection, promoting partnership and collaboration. Given the vast spectrum of programmes that encompass service and learning in community settings, as well as variability in the definition of 'service-learning', a balance was struck between inclusivity and exclusivity. A definition of service-learning was used that explains it as 'a structured learning experience that combines community service with preparation and reflection'[2(p273)] and used the following minimum set of components for inclusion in the review: a structured learning experience that combines community service with student preparation and reflection,[2] graduate health professions students as the study population, stated learning objectives, and outcomes that can be linked to programme activities and learning objectives.

METHODS

This review involved a structured literature search using standard databases and search engines as well as an opportunistic 'hand search' of bibliographies from the initial sources and streams of citations noted in PubMed.

Focusing on service-learning in the twenty-first century, PubMed was searched for all citations between 2000 and 2013 using the search term service-learning. This yielded 889 English language publications. Of these, 46 were actually about service-learning and 18 met criteria for review. Discipline-specific search terms were added (medicine and service-learning, nursing and service-learning, etc.) This yielded an additional 345 English-language publications, 33 non-duplicates that were about service-learning and an additional three that met review criteria.

A series of searches through Google Scholar were conducted combining health professions with educational topics: cultural competence, professionalism, altruism, critical thinking, self-directed learning. This produced another 63 English-language publications, of which seven were non-duplicates and met review criteria. Four additional citations were added through hand searching bibliographies and citation streams.

The total sample included 32 papers referring to 29 studies. There were 24 studies from American-based institutions, three from Canada, and one each from Hong Kong and South Africa. Programmes typically served marginalised and/or special needs individuals and communities in urban and rural areas. Table 26.1 outlines the professional disciplines and Table 26.2 outlines the educational domains these studies represented.

TABLE 26.1 Health education disciplines represented in literature review

Medicine	Nursing	Pharmacy	Dental	Other	Interprofessional
8	3	6	3	3 (dental hygiene, physical therapy, public health)	6

TABLE 26.2 Primary educational domains represented in literature review

Acquisition of clinical skills, discipline-specific knowledge	Contextual and conceptual knowledge and skills	Thinking skills, orientations and habits of mind	Professional knowledge, attitudes and skills	Values and commitments
22	28	8	27	25

Each study was reviewed according to project description, educational or programme objective, explicit service objectives and outcomes, learning objectives, evaluation design and outcomes. Educational research covers a wide range of descriptive reports, small single-institution studies, studies with an experimental or quasi-experimental design, and statistical analyses. In order to fully represent this wide range, the minimum thresholds for inclusion were opted for. These included using the service-learning definition noted earlier; learner at the graduate health professions level; learning objectives explicitly stated or implicit, based on the programme description; and presentation of evidence (e.g. descriptive or quantitative data regarding outputs and/or outcomes that can be conceptually linked to programme activities and learning objectives). Additionally, the study's size, scope, design and outcomes, highlighting the use of standardised or validated measurement instruments, formal methods for qualitative analysis, or experimental design to strengthen findings were reported.

CLINICAL SKILLS AND KNOWLEDGE

Service-learning is often employed to teach clinical skills and population health. Population health has been defined as 'the health outcomes of a group of individuals, including the distribution of such outcomes within the group'.[3(p380)] Through service-learning, students engage directly with social determinants of health and begin to define their professional responsibility to improve individual and population health and reduce disparities. Service-learning experiences can also enhance skills, knowledge and confidence in standard curricular areas. The following examples high-light the skills and specialised knowledge taught through service-learning.

Johnson[4] described a capstone project in which pharmacy students spent 1 week at a camp for diabetic children, providing education and assisting campers in managing diabetes. Young et al.[5] documented a programme for medical students to learn health education and health promotion skills by providing sessions for elderly public hous-ing residents. Cox et al.[6] used service-learning to strengthen a third-year paediatric clerkship curricular element related to care of underserved populations.

Service-learning also provides opportunities for exposure to learning that is under-represented in the curriculum, such as caring for vulnerable populations. Brown et al.[7] described a project that exposed public health, medical and nursing students to the needs of homeless populations. Roche et al.[8] documented a pharmacy student elective on Native American health featuring classroom activities and a week-long service experience under the supervision of Indian Health Services pharmacists. Keselyak et al.[9] added a service-learning component to a required dental hygiene course on care of special needs patients. Leung et al.[10] developed an emersion course for medical and nursing students to learn about elders' health needs.

These programmes encompassed all health professions, elective and required courses, brief emersion and semester or year-long, and ranged from eight[4] to more than 400 participants.[7] Most described a single iteration of a course, while several described courses that evolved over several years. All were based in a single institution.

All claimed to enhance knowledge and skills. Students in the study by Young et al.[5] gained communication skills. Pharmacy students in the study by Johnson[4] learned to educate children with type 1 diabetes. Several enhanced interest and curiosity about the population;[8,9] others changed attitudes, understanding and empathy.[4-7,10] Knowledge and attitudinal changes were reinforced by the affective dimension of 'making a difference'.[6(p342)]

Most studies used convenience samples (students in required courses, self-selected students in electives), and a range of strategies to measure outcomes including students' post-experience comments,[7] course evaluations, exam performance, and pre- and post-test comparisons. Several studies were more rigorous: the study by Cox et al.[6] was a randomised controlled trial comparing three modalities of delivering curriculum. The two intervention groups with the service-learning component dem-onstrated statistically significantly greater knowledge and changes in attitudes towards vulnerable populations' needs versus the control group that received the established curriculum; the study by Leung et al.[10] measured the impact of a 10-week service-learning experience on knowledge of and attitudes towards the elderly. The study found statistically significant reductions in negative attitudes and greater knowledge about elder health in the intervention compared with the control group.

Qualitative studies ranged from informal representation of students' comments[5,8] to structured, formal qualitative analysis, multiple coders and other strategies to strengthen findings.[9] Despite positive findings, Leung et al.[10] appropriately raised the question of durability of effect. Most studies focused on short-term outcomes. Roche et al.[8] examined durability indirectly by looking into actions students took following the course, from seeking additional learning about Native American health to pursuing careers in the Indian Health Service.

Brush *et al.*[11] measured the correlation between level of service-learning involvement and indicators of academic achievement including class rank, Alpha Omega Alpha Medical Honor Society election, performance on clinical exams in years 3 and 4, professional outcomes, and choice of residency field. They found a statistically significant relationship between participation and class rank, with low participation correlating with relatively low rank and high participation correlating with high rank. There was a marginally significant relationship between service-learning participation and election to the Alpha Omega Alpha Medical Honor Society and no association with performance on clinical exams, election to the Gold Humanism in Medicine Society, or choice of residency field.

CONTEXTUAL AND CONCEPTUAL KNOWLEDGE AND SKILLS

Health professionals of the twenty-first century will be caring for increasingly diverse populations at home and abroad. Understanding populations' cultural contexts and beliefs is imperative for addressing medical and health issues. Service-learning pedagogy can contribute to the skills, attitudes and knowledge needed to work effectively in a multicultural society, providing opportunities to move from abstract classroom discussions to real-life experiences. Recognising that new knowledge does not necessarily lead to new behaviours, service-learning experiences can broaden the lens through which students see the world and allow them to practise new behaviours. Through experience, students can become aware of their own biases and learn to reflect upon the experience of 'being the one who is different'.

The following section highlights service-learning programmes where learning objectives include enhanced understanding of population health and/or cultural competence in real-world settings. Again, the studies encompass a spectrum of professional disciplines, a wide range of scope and sizes, and required and elective courses. In many cases, an elective service-learning component was added to a required course. Pharmacy students provided service to local community organisations to gain understanding of civic, cultural and social issues and health disparities.[12] A voluntary service-learning experience was added to a clinical practicum for nursing students to promote cultural competence, critical thinking and civic engagement.[13] Elam *et al.*[14] describe a similar elective community-based experience added to a required preclinical course. Medical students collaborated with community organisations on asset-needs assessments and service activities. Narsavage *et al.*[15] conducted a pilot study that linked nursing theory and clinical experience in the social environment, in which nursing students worked with community members and organisations to serve and learn in the 'real world'. Two other studies[16,17] described fully elective courses. The former, e.g. international service-learning, designed for medical students to learn about social determinants and explore their role as advocates in a low-income country; the latter for public health students to work with local communities on food and nutrition issues.

These studies involved primarily single institutions, although two[13,15] encompassed several programmes within their institutions. Numbers of participants ranged from three[16] through to 79.[14] With few exceptions, the studies were short-term and described a single iteration. Most authors reported positive findings: enhanced knowledge of cultural and social issues and health disparities,[12,14-16] as well as greater understanding of community issues, resources and needs.[12,15] Nokes et al.[13] however, reported that cultural competency scores decreased following the intervention. The authors suggest that the course raised participants' awareness of cultural competency and may have generated a more discerning and self-critical group of students.

Evaluation strategies ranged from programme output description to sophisticated statistical analyses.[12-15] The study by Nokes et al.[13] was a purely quantitative study using pre- and post-intervention surveys. Brown et al.,[12] Narsavage et al.[15] and Elam et al.[14] used mixed methods, including pre- and post-intervention surveys and analysis of reflective writings, triangulating to confirm and strengthen findings. The studies by Dharamsi et al.[16] and Love[17] were qualitative. Qualitative analyses ranged from informal analyses of students' reflective writings[17] to highly structured analyses, providing a description of strategies to strengthen findings.[14-16] In two studies, authors acknowledged potential bias in using self-selected participants.[12,13] Two studies considered baseline assessments of participants and non-participants in their interpretation of findings. There was no blinding of readers or coders in any of the qualitative studies.[14,15]

THINKING SKILLS AND APPROACH TO LEARNING

Developing and mastering critical thinking skills is foundational for health professionals, who must solve complex problems, think creatively and interpret data in order to function within their professional domains and address unfamiliar challenges.[18] Critical thinking can be defined as the ability to broaden and deepen one's thinking through systematic intellectual self-assessment, internal reflection and collaborative validation.[19-21] A critical thinker can define an issue, evaluate available evidence, acknowledge assumptions[22] and tolerate ambiguity.[23] Through experiencing the realities and ambiguities of people's lives, students in service-learning courses can practise critical thinking. By sharing responsibility for the learning process, students learn *how* to think, rather than *what* to think.[24] Learning to value experience as a teacher is a step towards becoming a lifelong learner.

Several studies included critical thinking learning objectives. Kabli et al.[25] aimed to enhance pharmacy students' thinking skills in a drug misuse and addiction course. Keselyak et al.[9] explored the impact on thinking strategies among dental hygiene students who interacted with special needs populations. Two studies included critical thinking modules in required courses' service-learning enhancements: Brondani et al.[26] for preclinical dental students; Nokes et al.[13] for nursing students.

Most course evaluations demonstrated a positive impact on thinking skills. Kabli et al.[25] asked students to rank effective learning strategies. In the pre-course survey students reported learning most effectively by 'relating to the educational content', 'discussing the material' and 'attending lectures'.[25(p8)] Following the course, rankings shifted to 'learning through writing' and 'group work'.[25(p8)] Analysis of reflections demonstrated evolution from narrowly articulated scientific questions to questions about science in a social context. The authors believe that service-learning – including peer learning, group experiences and written reflections – allowed students to make explicit connections among course content, placement experiences and their own beliefs and values.

In the study by Keselyak *et al.*,[9] student reflections showed a positive impact on interpretation, analysis and manipulation skills: students reported that they learned to find new and creative solutions to problems and developed flexibility in their thinking in order to apply knowledge to new circumstances and new populations. Brondani[27] found that students' reflections ranged from descriptive to metacognitive, demonstrating that they learned to reconsider their first reactions and observations, and to propose alternative ways of responding to and observing phenomena. Reflection activities encouraged students to seek extra learning and to think critically, and they promoted personal growth. Only the study by Nokes *et al.*[13] did not yield positive results. Parallel to the decline in cultural competence scores, students' self-rated critical thinking scores declined at the end of the course. Here, also, authors suggest that the intervention may have created a more discerning group of participants whose self-assessment skills became more self-critical.

Studies used a range of methods and designs: pre- and post-intervention survey,[13,25] validated tools[13] and mixed methods.[9,25–27] All qualitative studies used carefully described methods for analysing data: one study used multiple strategies to triangulate and confirm findings, including obtaining data from multiple sources, member checking and peer debriefing to confirm data interpretations.[9] Another study's approach was structured and theory-driven,[27] using Witmer's[28] conceptual LEARN framework. Use of validated tools, transparent data analysis methods and multiple data sources, added weight to the studies' rich descriptive data.

PROFESSIONALISM

In exchange for respect, authority and autonomy, professionals commit to a social contract to provide service and value social good over individual gain. Sullivan[29] defines professionalism as 'the moral understanding … that gives concrete reality to this social contract'.[(p673)] Coulehan[30] promotes developing 'narrative competence',[(p892)] 'the ability to acknowledge, absorb, interpret, and act on the stories and plights of others',[(p892)] advocating that

> medical curriculum include socially relevant service-oriented learning. Interaction with patients in the hospital or office setting is insufficient to provide students and young physicians with narratives of interdisciplinary practice, biopsychosocial modelling and social responsibility.[(p892)]

Dose must be 'sufficiently large for students to view it as integral to the culture of medical education.'[31(p1897)] Masella[32] echoes this view in a commentary on dental education. Along with attitudes, professionalism encompasses team work and inter-professional collaboration skills that service-learning can foster through experiential learning and role-modelling.

Studies with explicit professionalism learning objectives included: a medical student 'professionalism attitudes-in-action' project that encompassed a summer internship, a clinical clerkship and a curriculum that covered service, community assessment, advocacy and ethical behaviour;[33] an interprofessional health educa-tion programme to reduce childhood obesity[34] a dental student Professionalism and Community Service course promoting social awareness and global responsibility and values of a civil and sustainable society;[26] a nutrition education service-learning component added to a required pharmacy course;[35] a course combining classroom learning with family-based projects for medical, nursing, dental, pharmacy, physical therapy and clinical psychology students to promote professionalism and interprofes-sional care;[36] an elective that combined classroom preparation and a 1-week emersion, during which teams of nursing, physical and occupational therapy students provided supervised health services;[37] and participation in a student-run medical clinic that reinforced altruism, advocacy and humanism.[38]

Outcomes were largely positive. Using an open-ended survey, O'Toole et al.[33] found that students articulated factors influencing professional behaviour, highlighted the importance of physician advocacy on behalf of patients, and expressed strength-ened commitments to vulnerable populations. The authors concluded that 'basing a curriculum in community organisations that care for indigent and marginalised populations is effective in grounding professionalism and professional behavior in a real-world context.'[33]

While there was no formal measurement of professionalism objectives, student feedback and course evaluations in the Brondani[27] project indicated that the course allowed students to 'develop comprehensive knowledge and awareness of the needs and dynamics of a community as they collaboratively interact'.(p636) In the study by Falter et al.,[35] pre- and post-intervention surveys demonstrated enhanced communi-cation, a sense of 'taking responsibility as a health care provider and feeling a sense of community responsibility'.(p85)

Informal analysis of reflections in the study by Batra et al.[38] indicated that students benefitted from opportunities to express altruism, patient and community advocacy, and humanism in the context of hands-on activities. Using formal content analysis of reflective writings, Fries et al.[37] determined that the course enhanced collaboration and trust across disciplines and enhanced students' understanding and appreciation of their own and other professions' roles.

From faculty and client evaluations of students and student course evaluations, Davidson and Waddell[36] concluded the service-learning component of the course met its objectives. The vast majority of students endorsed that the interprofessional experience enhanced their professional education, understanding of barriers to health promotion and wellness, and provided a broader perspective on healthcare.

While most studies were small, several spanned multiple disciplines,[36,37] mul-tiple years and hundreds of students,[36] and multiple institutions.[33] All studies use convenience samples, including self-selected students.[33,34,37,38] While one study[35] used pre- and post-intervention comparisons, others used post-experience surveys without baseline assessments.[33,34,36] No study was blinded or had a comparison group. Qualitative studies ranged from informal student feedback and reflections[38] to rigorous qualitative analysis.[37]

VALUES AND COMMITMENTS

Disparities of economic, social and health status are widening. Indeed, inequality itself is a leading contributor to poor health. Dharamsi et al.[39] state that social responsibility is a moral commitment, part of a professional's social contract that encompasses accountability, altruism, ethical behaviour and commitment to advance the common good. Because these are not easily taught in the classroom, the authors conclude, 'a curriculum focused on developing social responsibility … will require pedagogical approaches that are innovative, collaborative, participatory and transformative.'[39(p1108)] Through community engagement, students can learn to become citizens of the world, gain appreciation of the challenges that communities face, learn to value community members' voices, develop altruistic attributes and commitment to social justice.[40]

Examples in this domain include a service-learning enhancement to an ethics course for dental hygiene students,[41] a social justice curriculum for nursing students,[42] a community and social determinants of health course for dental students,[43] a voluntary civic engagement component in a clinical nursing course,[13] curricular and extracurricular components in a faculty-medical student-led free clinic for patients,[44] and an elective international service-learning experience to promote altruism and advocacy.[16]

Findings were generally positive: in the study by Gadbury-Amyot et al.,[41] pre- and post-intervention assessment found a statistically significant positive change in perception of volunteering. Qualitative analysis of reflection papers noted rich and thoughtful insights regarding privilege, teamwork and interprofessional learning. Students were motivated to seek additional experiences and knowledge about access to care. A retrospective evaluation of the impact of this course on students determined that they articulated deep learning across several domains, including understanding the needs of underserved populations and cultural diversity.[45] In the Redman and Clark[42] study, while students articulated that service experiences placed them outside of their comfort zone, qualitative findings indicated that students' civic engagement experience enhanced their sense of responsibility and shaped their professional careers.

Rubin's[43] analysis of students' reflections found positive attitude shifts, demonstrating greater empathy for diverse and vulnerable populations, enhanced communication skills and understanding of social determinants. He concluded that an early service experience promotes 'the development of culturally competent, community-minded, and reflective dental health professionals.'[43(p460)] In the study by Nokes et al.,[13] civic engagement scores showed statistically significant increases among nursing students following their field experience. A study by Jimenez et al.[44] measured programme outputs and indirect indicators of student interest and satisfaction – for example, high rates of student participation.

Educational interventions in this domain included elective courses or course enhancements,[13,16] required courses,[41–43,45] and highly structured extracurricular activities for course credit or other formal recognition.[44] Courses ranged in size, from three people[39] through to 129.[44] Evaluation methods included process measures (e.g. student demand for the course and service outputs),[44] and qualitative evaluations ranging from informal[42] to highly structured analyses using multiple reviewers and formal methods.[39,43] Nokes *et al.*[13] used validated tools for pre- and post-intervention surveys, including a tool to measure civic engagement. Gadbury-Amyot *et al.*[41] and Aston-Brown *et al.*[45] used mixed methods including advanced statistical analyses, tests of significance and structured qualitative review.

Dharamsi *et al.*[16] quoted one student as follows:

> my experience … taught me that social responsibility is about building strong relationships, witnessing and giving voice to those who are stifled by the social burdens that seem impossible to overcome because of poverty and vulnerability. It is not about creating a dependency relationship. It is about developing relationships based on mutual respect, care and compassion … being a facilitator toward achieving what communities feel is best for them.[(p980)]

While these words capture students' spirit and voice, the impact of these studies is weakened by absence of experimental or quasi-experimental design, lack of triangulation, reliance on informal methods to analyse qualitative data[42] and lack of clearly articulated educational outcomes.[44] It was recognised, however, that it is within the capacity of even small studies to use stronger designs and evaluation strategies.

AREAS FOR IMPROVEMENT AND FURTHER RESEARCH

As health professions educators, it is important to remain cognisant of the social contract that exists between health professionals and society, and to design educational programmes to meet this expectation. Expecting a single educational intervention to produce the desired outcomes in prospective learners, and to expect that these attributes be sustained, may be asking too much. However, limited resources and curricular time should be devoted to interventions that are supported by solid evidence. Education is not alchemy – as educators it is important to apply scientific principles to designing and evaluating one's pedagogy. Based on this review, the following paragraphs highlight opportunities and strategies for improvement and identify additional areas for further research.

Size and scope

Most of the studies were conducted in a single institution, involved a single experience with a single course, and involved a small number of participants. Size and scope can be enlarged by including several programmes and disciplines within an institution, collaborating with other institutions, and reporting on data from several years of implementation.[4,5,7,45]

Minimum standards for descriptive data

Rich and detailed description of context, intervention and outcomes is valuable, but it cannot stand on its own. In order to generate verifiable data and advance knowledge, data collection methods must be transparent and guided by theory, with clear hypotheses or previous evidence.[46]

Qualitative methods

Studies using qualitative data must clearly describe and justify decisions regarding choice of methodology, approach to data analysis, data integrity and 'reflexivity' (the influence of the researcher's presence and stance on the study).[47] Moreover, they must validate and authenticate their findings. Keselyak *et al.*,[9] Elam *et al.*[14] and Fries *et al.*[37] demonstrated that this is within the scope of educational research.

Choice of instruments

Regardless of sample size, educators should select validated tools and measures where they exist. The use of validated instruments in combination with qualitative data can provide findings that are rich and compelling, with nuance and specificity to guide local programming.[13]

Study design

Few of the studies cited employ a sophisticated experimental design. As long as hypotheses, methods and findings are clearly reported and limitations acknowledged, they can contribute to the evidence. However, in the absence of an experimental or quasi-experimental design, it is difficult to attribute changes in learning outcomes to service-learning. Pre- and post-intervention measurements, historical controls, other quasi-experimental designs and even a comparison group are feasible in most settings, even when numbers are small. Reporting baseline characteristics and measurements should be a minimum requirement. Two studies employed randomised controlled trials,[6,10] demonstrating that this level of rigour is not only desirable but also possible in educational research.

Recommendations: strengthening the evidence

Service-learning appears to show promise of having an impact on complex and subtle habits of thinking and learning, students' values, professional attributes and, by extension, on health outcomes and healthcare delivery more broadly. However, service-learning is one of many components in a student's educational experience. It would be misguided as well as implausible to attribute a significant, qualitative change in an important educational domain, with associated measurable changes in behaviour, to any single intervention. Similarly, to connect a service-learning experience to significant changes in patient or health system outcomes is also an implausible leap of logic. What, then, can educational researchers be held accountable to demonstrate in the way of evidence?

Complex outcomes, such as critical thinking, civic engagement, altruism and cultural humility are difficult to measure and are likely influenced by multiple factors.[48] Simpson and Courtney[49] point out in their thoughtful review of critical thinking assessment that there is no agreed-upon best tool. Self-report is particularly problematic for representing change in attitudes, value systems and commitments where change in knowledge, and even expressed change in attitudes, do not reliably predict behaviour change. In addition to the strategies for strengthening design and findings noted here, use of mixed methods can verify and solidify the evidence yielded from an individual study, and it can provide the richness that these complex constructs demand. Self-reported data can be strengthened if it is collected in a standardised manner, such as critical incident reports and learner portfolios, and analysed by trained personnel using structured and standardised rubrics and assessment tools. Observational assessments can supplement self-report and other data.

Recommended strategies include peer assessments, focused objective structured clinical examinations, and other direct observations by faculty, community members and other trained observers.[50] Evaluation of educational interventions to address complex learning objectives will never be 'neat' and linear. No single method is perfect, but carefully and appropriately selected and combined approaches are feasible in service-learning pedagogy, will provide stronger evidence in these important educational domains, and test the contribution that service-learning can make to the health professionals' education.

There are several important questions that are not well-addressed in the studies that were found, including dose and durability.

Dose

Is there an exposure threshold in service-learning that is critical? Does a brief exposure, such as in the study by Nokes *et al.*,[13] raise awareness and lead to more informed and lower self-ratings in critical thinking and cultural competence? Would a longer intervention lead to higher self-ratings? The study by Brush *et al.*[11] is the only one that attempted to correlate level of service-learning involvement with educational outcomes, with some indication that higher exposure had greater positive effect in certain domains.

Durability

How durable are the outcomes achieved? Few studies mention durability. Several asked students (short-term) if the service-learning experience affected their interest in serving underserved populations. Results were mixed – for example, positive[8,12,38,41] as well as variable or neutral[45] – and the study by Brush *et al.*[11] found no effect on residency choice. While many factors undoubtedly determine career choices, it is plausible that opportunities and exposures through service-learning courses would validate and reinforce students' nascent interest in career areas that are marginalised, invisible and not valued in the standard curriculum. Leung *et al.*[10] measured durability of improved attitudes towards the elderly after 1 month, and results showed a decrease in both groups, although less erosion in the intervention group. Durability of other outcomes and the relationship between dose and durability of effect were largely unaddressed.

Assessing community and/or service objectives

Finally, in discussing service-learning, it would be remiss to ignore community and service objectives. While this was not the focus of this review, it was notable how few studies mentioned these objectives. It is affirmed that these can be addressed;[51] the more complex questions of the relationship between community and service objectives and students' learning objectives is an important area for further research.

CONCLUSION

Based on this review of service-learning, it is clear that a wide range of health professions educators use service-learning to ensure that their learners are acquiring attributes needed for practice in the twenty-first century. While there is evidence that the use of service-learning helps learners acquire these attributes, the evidence is weak; evaluation needs to begin measuring behavioural changes and possibly even patient outcomes while it also addresses issue of dose and durability.

SUMMARY POINTS

- Service-learning, a structured learning experience that combines community service with student preparation and reflection, is widely used in curricular and extracurricular activities to educate health professions students.
- Service-learning can be an effective strategy to promote and achieve important learning objectives, including clinical skills and discipline relevant knowledge, contextual and conceptual knowledge and skills, thinking skills and approach to learning, professional conduct, and values and commitments.
- Evidence for the effectiveness of service-learning is promising but rests on studies that vary in scope and design. The majority are small, single-course, single-institution studies with short-term follow-up.
- Studies can strengthen the evidence for use of service-learning through:
  - specifying clear hypotheses and measurable educational objectives
  - using mixed methods to bolster findings through triangulation
  - employing validated tools and standard rubrics to measure outcomes
  - enlarging study size and scope by including several programmes within a school or cross-institutional collaboration
  - articulating clear and replicable data analysis methods
  - employing experimental or quasi-experimental design.
- Additional recommendations for strengthening the evidence of service-learning in the health professions and designing programmes that target appropriate learning objectives, with appropriate scope and intensity include defining and measuring:

—achievement of community and service objectives

—students' behaviour change through critical incident reports, learner port-folios, and structured and standardised observations

—appropriate dose – how much, how long and how intensive must a service-learning experience must be in order to achieve its objectives?

—durability – do service-learning experiences have an enduring impact on students?

REVIEW QUESTIONS

- Given the state of the evidence related to service-learning in the health profes-sions, what do you think the most pressing issues are for the next generation of research on this area?
- If you think that service-learning should be a pedagogy required by additional health professions, what evidence would you use to support this assertion?
- As an educator, how does the state of the evidence related to service-learning as pedagogy in the health professions affect your inclination to use this type of pedagogy?

REFLECTIVE QUESTIONS AND EXERCISES

- Select one of the review domains that you think is most important for health professions students to incorporate into their persona and practice. Why do you think this is the most important, and what approach would you use to ensure it is taught and learned?

REFERENCES

1. Liaison Committee on Medical Education. *Standards for Accreditation of Medical Education Programs Leading to the MD Degree.* Available at: www.lcme.org/ (accessed 13 October 2014).
2. Seifer SD. Service-learning: community-campus partnerships for health professions education. *Acad Med.* 1998; **73**(3): 273–7.
3. Kindig D, Stoddart G. What is population health? *Am J Public Health.* 2003; **93**(3): 380–3.
4. Johnson JF. A diabetes camp as the service-learning capstone experience in a diabetes concentra-tion. *Am J Pharm Educ.* 2007; **7**(6): 119.
5. Young S, Bates T, Wolff M, *et al.* Service-learning in healthy aging for medical students and family medicine residents. *Educ Health.* 2002; **15**(3): 353–61.
6. Cox ED, Koscik RL, Olson CA, *et al.* Caring for the underserved: blending service learning and a web-based curriculum. *Am J Prev Med.* 2006; **31**(4): 342–9.
7. Brown JD, Bone L, Gillis L, *et al.* Service learning to impact homelessness: the result of academic and community collaboration. *Public Health Rep.* 2006; **121**(3): 343–8.
8. Roche VF, Jones RM, Hinman CE, *et al.* A service-learning elective in Native American culture, health and professional practice. *Am J Pharm Educ.* 2007; **71**(6): 129.

9. Keselyak NT, Simmer-Beck M, Bray KK, *et al.* Evaluation of an academic service-learning course on special needs patients for dental hygiene students: a qualitative study. *J Dent Educ.* 2007; **71**(3): 378–92.

10. Leung AYM, Chan SSC, Kwan CW, *et al.* Service learning in medical and nursing training: a randomized controlled trial. *Adv Health Sci Educ Theory Pract.* 2012; **17**(4): 529–45.

11. Brush DR, Markert RJ, Lazarus CJ. The relationship between service learning and medical student academic and professional outcomes. *Teach Learn Med.* 2006; **18**(1): 9–13.

12. Brown B, Heaton PC, Wall A. A service-learning elective to promote enhanced understanding of civic, cultural, and social issues and health disparities in pharmacy. *Am J Pharm Educ.* 2007; **71**(1): 9.

13. Nokes KM, Nickitas DM, Keida R, *et al.* Does service-learning increase cultural competency, critical thinking, and civic engagement? *J Nurs Educ.* 2005; **44**(2): 65–70.

14. Elam CL, Sauer MJ, Stratton TD, *et al.* Service-learning in the medical curriculum: developing and evaluating an elective experience. *Teach Learn Med.* 2009; **15**(3): 194–203.

15. Narsavage GL, Lindell D, Chen Y-J, *et al.* A community engagement initiative: service-learning in graduate nursing education. *J Nurs Educ.* 2002; **41**(10): 457–61.

16. Dharamsi S, Richards M, Louie D, *et al.* Enhancing medical students' conceptions of the Can MEDS Health Advocate Role through international service-learning and critical reflection: a phenomenological study. *Acad Med.* 2010; **32**(12): 977–82.

17. Love R. Access to healthy food in a low-income, urban community: a service-learning experience. *Public Health Rep.* 2008; **123**(2): 244–7.

18. Lewis A, Smith D. Defining higher order thinking. *Theor Pract.* 1993; **32**(3): 131–7.

19. Eyler J, Giles D. *Where is the Learning in Service-Learning?* San Francisco, CA: Jossey-Bass; 1999.

20. Paul R, Elder L. *The Miniature Guide to Critical Thinking: concepts and tools.* Santa Rosa, CA: The Foundation for Critical Thinking; 2008.

21. Paul R. *Critical Thinking: what every person needs to know to survive in a rapidly changing world.* Rohnert Park, CA: Center for Critical Thinking and Moral Critique; 1993.

22. Goldberg L, Coufal K. Reflections of service-learning, critical thinking, and cultural competence. *J Coll Teach Learn.* 2009; **6**(6): 39–49.

23. Freire P. *Pedagogy of the Oppressed.* New York, NY: Continuum Books; 2000.

24. *Higher Education: civic mission & civic effects.* Stanford, CA: Carnegie Foundation for the Advancement of Teaching and CIRCLE (the Center for Information and Research on Civic Learning and Engagement); 2006.

25. Kabli N, Liu B, Seifert T, *et al.* Effects of academic service learning in drug misuse and addiction on students' learning preferences and attitudes toward harm reduction. *Am J Pharm Educ.* 2013; **77**(3): 63.

26. Brondani MA, Clark C, Rossoff L, *et al.* An evolving community-based dental course on professionalism and community service. *J Dent Educ.* 2008; **72**(10): 1160–8.

27. Brondani MA. Students' reflective learning within a community service-learning dental module. *J Dent Educ.* 2010; **74**(6): 628–36.

28. Witmer D. Reflective practice: what does it mean for me? *Communique.* 1997; **73**: 47–56.

29. Sullivan WM. Medicine under threat: professionalism and professional identity. *CMAJ.* 2000; **162**(5): 673–5.

30. Coulehan J. Viewpoint: today's professionalism; engaging the mind but not the heart. *Acad Med.* 2005; **80**(10): 892–8.

31. Charon R. Narrative medicine: a model for empathy, reflection, profession and trust. *JAMA.* 2009; **286**(15): 1897–902.

32. Masella RS. Renewing professionalism in dental education: overcoming the market environment. *J Dent Educ.* 2007; **71**(2): 205–16.

33. O'Toole TP, Kathuria N, Mishra M, *et al.* Teaching professionalism within a community context: perspectives from a national demonstration project. *Acad Med.* 2005; **80**(4): 339–43.

34. Buffet SM, Oubre OL, Ariail JC, *et al.* Junior Doctors of Health©: an interprofessional service-learning project addressing childhood obesity and encouraging health care career choices. *J Allied Health.* 2011; **40**(3): e39–44.

35. Falter RA, Pignotti-Dumas K, Popish SJ, *et al.* A service learning program in providing nutrition education to children. *Am J Pharm Educ.* 2011; **75**(5): 85.

36. Davidson RA, Waddell R. A historical overview of interdisciplinary family health: a community-based interprofessional health professions course. *Acad Med.* 2005; **80**(4): 334–8.

37. Fries KS, Bowers DM, Gross M, *et al.* Service learning in Guatemala: using qualitative content analysis to explore an interdisciplinary learning experience among students in health care professional programs. *J Multidiscip Healthc.* 2013; **6**: 45–52.

38. Batra P, Chertok JS, Fisher CE, *et al.* The Columbia-Harlem homeless medical partnership: a new model for learning in the service of those in medical need. *J Urban Health.* 2009; **86**(5): 781–90.

39. Dharamsi S, Ho A, Spadafora SM, *et al.* The physician as health advocate: translating the quest for social responsibility into medical education and practice. *Acad Med.* 2011; **86**(9): 1108–13.

40. DeLuca E, Andrews L, Hale P. You learn how to act: the impact of service with elders on student learning. *J High Educ Outreach Engage.* 2004; **9**(2): 91–105.

41. Gadbury-Amyot CC, Simmer-Beck M, McCunniff M, *et al.* Using a multi-faceted approach including community-based service-learning to enrich formal ethics instruction in a dental school setting. *J Dent Educ.* 2006; **70**(6): 652–61.

42. Redman RW, Clark L. Service-learning as a model for integrating social justice in the nursing curriculum. *J Nurs Educ.* 2002; **41**(10): 446–9.

43. Rubin RW. Developing cultural competence and social responsibility in preclinical dental students. *J Dent Educ.* 2004; **68**(4): 460–7.

44. Jimenez M, Tan-Billet J, Babineau J, *et al.* The promise clinic: a service learning approach to increasing access to health care. *J Health Care Poor Underserved.* 2008; **19**(3): 935–43.

45. Aston-Brown RE, Branson B, Gadbury-Amyot CC, *et al.* Utilizing public health clinics for service-learning rotations in dental hygiene: a four-year retrospective study. *J Dent Educ.* 2009; **73**(7): 358–74.

46. Gelmon S, Holland B, Driscoll A, *et al. Assessing Service-Learning and Civic Engagement: principles and techniques.* Providence, RI: Campus Compact; 2001.

47. Stacy R, Spencer J. Assessing the evidence in qualitative medical education research. *Med Educ.* 2000; **34**(7): 498–500.

48. Kearney KR. Impact of a service-learning course on first-year pharmacy students' learning outcomes. *Am J Pharm Educ.* 2013; **77**(2): 34.

49. Simpson E, Courtney M. Critical thinking in nursing education: literature review. *Int J Nurs Pract.* 2002; **8**(2): 89–98.

50. Cohen JJ. Professionalism in medical education, an American perspective: from evidence to accountability. *Med Educ.* 2006; **40**(7): 607–17.

51. Lattanzi JB, Campbell SL, Dole RL, *et al.* Students mentoring students in a service-learning clinical supervision experience: an educational case report. *Phys Ther.* 2011; **91**(10): 1513–24.

PART IV

Applying evidence-based education in the health professions

CHAPTER 27

Evidence-based education in occupational therapy

....

Anita Witt Mitchell

OVERVIEW

This chapter describes the published evidence related to occupational therapy education, detailing four different aspects: (1) the Scholarship of Discovery, (2) the Scholarship of Integration, (3) the Scholarship of Application, and (4) the Scholarship of Learning and Teaching. Particular emphasis is given to evidence related to clinical reasoning, experiential learning and problem-based learning. Recommendations for future research to advance the practice of evidence-based education in occupational therapy are provided.

CHAPTER OBJECTIVES

Upon completion of this chapter, the reader will be able to:
- describe the four types of scholarship needed to advance occupational therapy education
- describe the status of evidence-based education in occupational therapy in relation to each type of scholarship
- generate ideas for contributing to occupational therapy evidence-based education.

KEY TERMS: occupational therapy education, learning and teaching, Scholarship of Learning and Teaching

Occupational therapy has embraced and is committed to evidence-based practice in the clinic as well as the classroom. Recognising the profession's need to establish the efficacy of both therapeutic and educational practices, the American Occupational Therapy Association described the types of scholarship that contribute to this effort, including the Scholarship of Discovery (SoD), the Scholarship of Integration (SoI), the Scholarship of Application (SoA) and the Scholarship of Learning and Teaching (SoLT). SoD refers to activities which produce and advance new knowledge. In occupational therapy education, this involves conducting research to help explain and inform the understanding of occupational therapy students and the processes involved in their transformation into practitioners. Over time, scholars may develop a body of knowledge specific to occupational therapy education and generate new theoretical perspectives. Assimilating knowledge from occupational therapy and other disciplines through SoI may lay the groundwork for development of conceptual frameworks tailored to the needs of students seeking to grasp the art and science of occupational therapy practice. These frameworks can then be used to develop instructional approaches and methods for SoA and to test these strategies utilising SoLT.[1]

As occupational therapy educators rigorously and systematically study techniques and approaches associated with identified conceptual frameworks and disseminate this information via SoLT, they advance the practice of evidence-based education (EBE). This chapter will examine the state of EBE in occupational therapy from each of these perspectives of scholarship, focusing on prominent topics in the occupational therapy education literature. The information presented is based on literature searches of databases such as CINAHL (Cumulative Index to Nursing and Allied Health Literature), PsycINFO and Scopus, as well as individual searches of occupational therapy journals such as the *American Journal of Occupational Therapy*, the *British Journal of Occupational Therapy*, *Occupational Therapy International* and *Occupational Therapy in Health Care*. References from relevant articles were also utilised. Search terms included 'occupational therapy education', 'occupational therapy students', 'learning' and 'teaching'.

THE SCHOLARSHIP OF DISCOVERY

In the early phase of development of a science, SoD is prevalent as phenomena are described and concepts are developed. In their international systematic mapping review of research related to occupational therapy education, Hooper *et al.*[2] found that most of the papers were descriptive studies that began because of a need to understand a local problem or situation. Many were examples of SoD. Often the studies were related to the complex skills and abilities required of occupational therapy practitioners (e.g. clinical reasoning).

The groundbreaking SoD related to clinical reasoning was initiated in 1986 with a 2-year study sponsored by the American Occupational Therapy Association and the American Occupational Therapy Foundation.[3] These organisations recognised that in order to develop approaches and methods for promoting students' understanding of the intricacies of occupational therapy practice, it was first necessary to engage in

SoD – specifically, to describe the nature of the reasoning process that is essential to competent practice. Often SoD and SoI occur in tandem, and this is the case with the literature related to clinical reasoning. Along with SoD, SoI occurred as investigators incorporated critical thinking research from various disciplines and assimilated those discoveries with the specifics of reasoning used in occupational therapy practice.[3–5]

Although specific theoretical frameworks have not been developed in relation to teaching and learning clinical reasoning in occupational therapy, SoD examining the clinical reasoning of novices and how it differs from the clinical reasoning of expert practitioners[3–5] paved the way for the application of these findings by occupational therapy educators. Educators have utilised various methods and approaches to advance students' clinical reasoning, and researchers have conducted a number of studies to test these methods and approaches.

As is common with SoD studies in occupational therapy education,[2] research contributing to SoD in relation to clinical reasoning has been almost exclusively qualitative, utilising interviews, observations and analyses of videotaped treatment sessions. Since clinical reasoning is a mental process and the aim of these studies was descriptive, this is not surprising. A quantitative measure of students' self-perceptions of their clinical reasoning, the Self-Assessment of Clinical Reflection and Reasoning, has been developed;[6] however, its use in published studies has been limited. Use of this measurement tool and development of a psychometrically sound objective measure of occupational therapy-specific clinical reasoning could allow more rigorous study and advance EBE (both SoD and SoLT) related to clinical reasoning. A theoretical framework specific to the processes involved in teaching and learning occupational therapy clinical reasoning would provide the underpinnings for innovative approaches that could be utilised in SoA and tested through SoLT.

Overall, there is still much to be learned about many aspects of the process of learning and teaching occupational therapy. Further discoveries about the characteristics of students and how they learn occupational therapy could enable development of the theoretical foundations for effective andragogy. Theoretical and conceptual frameworks for educating occupational therapy students would facilitate the systematic development of a body of knowledge to help describe, explain and predict important teaching and learning processes related specifically to occupational therapy. This could direct the focus, support reflection, inform practice and guide interpretation and application of educational research. As researchers investigate issues and problems related to education, educators can apply the findings, using SoA to modify courses, curricula, approaches and methods. Utilising SoLT to test innovations and disseminate the results can further contribute to the advancement of EBE in occupational therapy.[2]

THE SCHOLARSHIP OF INTEGRATION

Occupational therapy educators and scholars have utilised findings from other disciplines to further EBE in occupational therapy. However, educational psychologists have demonstrated how constructs such as motivation, self-efficacy, self-regulated learning, and epistemic and ontological cognition can influence learning and teaching, and yet occupational therapy educators have practised little SoD and SoI in these areas. Until SoD and SoI are further established in occupational therapy education, the relationship of core educational concepts to teaching and learning in occupational therapy will be difficult to elucidate, hindering the development of theoretical and conceptual models. Indeed, to date, occupational therapy education studies have rarely described a conceptual framework for the research.[2]

One educational theory that has been utilised in many occupational therapy programmes is adult learning theory.[7] This theory is the cornerstone for active learning and student-centred approaches such as problem-based learning (PBL).[8] Adult learners are expected to take initiative and contribute to the learning process. There is a shift from a view of the instructor as the authority figure who imparts knowledge to a view in which learning occurs as a result of a collaborative process. The instructor acts as a guide and facilitator, and the learner participates in the construction of knowledge.[9-12]

Few attempts have been made to advance a theory or conceptual framework specifically for occupational therapy education. Fisher[9] developed the Pyramid of Occupational Therapy Learning to facilitate curriculum planning and development. Based on her previous research involving three occupational therapy programmes, she advocated the use of active and experiential approaches to facilitate occupational therapy student learning in four hierarchically arranged areas: (1) student–teacher commitment, trust and communication; (2) medical and scientific knowledge; (3) holistic occupational therapy theories of human performance; and (4) application of occupational therapy theory to patient cases. While Fisher's[9] Pyramid of Occupational Therapy Learning provides practical guidance for curriculum design and development, it offers little theoretical explanation of how occupational therapy students learn the art and science of the profession. Hooper[10,11] offered a more theoretical description of occupational therapy education. She argued for a subject-centred approach, in which students are assisted in connecting each subject in the occupational therapy programme with the core tenets of occupation and its contributions to health and engagement in life. Through this process, students come to understand the assumptions, claims, theories, logic and conceptual structure, or *practice epistemology*, of the profession.[12]

Similar to Fisher,[9] Hooper identified trust and a personal commitment to acting as a co-contributor to the knowledge base as essential components of occupational therapy education. Along with a subject-centred focus, she maintained that this approach would facilitate student 'self-authorship'.[11(p102)] Self-authorship involves the process of developing and maintaining a unique identity as an occupational therapist, something that has been the focus of much of the SoD in occupational therapy education. According to Hooper,[11] a critical part of both subject-centred education and self-authorship is the understanding of the uncertain, complex and temporary nature of knowledge, or sophisticated epistemic and ontological cognition. Similarly, Mitchell[12] described the potential effects of epistemic and ontological cognition on clinical reasoning and evidence-based practice in occupational therapy. She maintained that students with a certain and simple view of knowledge may have difficulty considering contextual variables and tailoring treatment approaches to the needs of the individual client. Both Hooper[11] and Mitchell[12] provide examples of how educators can utilise SoA to facilitate development of students' epistemic and onto-logical cognition. Consistent with adult learning theory, both authors advocate for active and collaborative learning approaches.

While SoI can facilitate the development of a conceptual framework for occupational therapy education, scholars warn against over-reliance on theory from other disciplines. Hooper et al.[2] argue that educational methods and approaches must be influenced by, integrated with and tailored to the profession's practice epistemology. Currently, it appears that more work is required in SoD and SoI to build on and expand the ideas of Fisher,[9] Hooper[10,11] and Mitchell,[12] with the goal of developing a cohesive theoretical and conceptual framework for occupational therapy education. Just as theory is important to clinical practice, it is essential that occupational therapy educators base teaching methods and approaches on well-grounded theoretical and conceptual frameworks.

THE SCHOLARSHIP OF APPLICATION

The lack of theoretical and conceptual groundwork for occupational therapy education has not deterred educators from applying instructional approaches and teaching methods to actual problems encountered in the classroom. Occupational therapy educators have built on the existing SoD and SoI to advocate a variety of approaches and methods from education and other health professions. As Mosey[13] noted, SoA can have value, even without theoretical underpinnings.

Hooper et al.[2] drew a distinction between educational approaches and teaching methods. They used the term *educational approaches* to denote 'broad theoretical and philosophical stances that encompass ideals about the nature of knowledge and content, educator-learner roles, why students learn and through what mechanisms.'[2(p10)] Non-research articles describing and advocating the application of approaches such as active learning, cooperative learning and learner-centred approaches began to appear in the occupational therapy literature in the mid 1990s and have since become prominent.[2,8,10] In fact, active or experiential learning has been widely adopted by occupational therapy educators,[10] and Hooper et al.[2] found that experiential learning was the most frequently addressed educational approach in their mapping review. Besides its general acceptance in the field of education, active learning is consistent with the values, norms and epistemology of the profession.[8,11] Based on constructivist theories of education and consistent with occupational therapy philosophy, experiential approaches provide opportunities for students to practise the application of theory, knowledge and skills in real-life contexts and construct their own understanding. Direct, constructive feedback and student reflection on the activity are also essential components of experiential learning. Proponents of experiential learning contend that it can facilitate the development of clinical reasoning, evidence-based practice, clinical skills and confidence.[14] In comparison, the more recently proposed subject-centred approach has the advantage of avoiding both the idea that knowledge consists of objective facts and the idea that all knowledge is relative and individual-specific. The subject-centred approach creates personal connections between the learner and the subject (i.e. occupation) while facilitating student co-construction of knowledge.[10,11]

Hooper et al.[2] described teaching methods as specific techniques for planning and organising instruction and assessment. Examples include PBL, service-learning, and case-based methods. They noted that teaching methods are not specific to a particular educational approach.[2] For example, case-based methods could be utilised in both learner-centred and cooperative learning approaches. In terms of clinical reasoning in occupational therapy, there is ample SoA in the published literature.[2] Examples of teaching methods endorsed for promoting clinical reasoning include practice with simulated patients or persons with disabilities in the classroom, reading and analysing novels about the experience of having a disability, writing autobiographical papers, conducting interviews, PBL and fieldwork.[4,13,15]

In their review, Hooper et al.[2] found that the most prominent teaching method was PBL. Both experiential learning and PBL have been advocated because of their potential to facilitate advanced problem-solving skills, clinical reasoning, self-directed learning and knowledge co-construction.[2,8] Hooper[10] cautioned that instructional methods in and of themselves do not guarantee that students act as co-constructors of knowledge related to occupation. She advocated explicit, intentional strategies to assist students in connecting topics to occupation and engaging personally with the subject of occupation. SoA addressing these and other educational approaches and methods has spawned a number of conceptual papers describing and promoting their use. SoLT, described in the next section of this chapter, has provided evidence to begin to clarify the effectiveness of these approaches and methods and to enable EBE in occupational therapy.

THE SCHOLARSHIP OF LEARNING AND TEACHING

SoD, SoI and SoA have all contributed to EBE in occupational therapy. SoLT can further that understanding in two ways: (1) by testing hypotheses generated from theories and conceptual frameworks developed via SoD and SoI, and (2) by examining the effectiveness of recommended approaches and methods utilised in SoA. Thus, SoLT can help refine theories and models developed for occupational therapy education as well as inform and enhance the effectiveness of day-to-day practices in the classroom.[15] Since no conceptual or theoretical models have been developed for occupational therapy education, the focus here will be on studies that have investigated the effectiveness of various approaches and teaching methods.

Clinical reasoning

When taking an EBE approach, questions of effectiveness must be asked in relation to the desired outcomes. Utilising SoLT, a number of studies have been conducted to examine the effectiveness of techniques endorsed for facilitating clinical reasoning.

Results of these studies have been mixed. There is evidence that case-based methods,[16,17] PBL across the curriculum or in a course,[18,19] a classroom-as-clinic technique in which students practise with individuals with disabilities in the classroom,[20] and service-learning[21] are all effective methods for promoting occupational therapy clinical reasoning. However, other studies have found that some of these same methods were not effective, e.g. the classroom-as-clinic technique using videotapes rather than 'live' clients,[22] an eight-week PBL course,[23] and a specific PBL technique in which students learn to ask questions facilitating analysis, evaluation, and application.[24] Further inspection of the evidence reveals an interesting trend. That is, qualitative studies involving student reports or perceptions, single case studies, and studies using researcher-designed outcome measures with little or no psychometric data tended to find more positive effects.[16,20,21,25] On the other hand, studies with more rigorous designs or using measures with acceptable psychometric properties tended to find little change in clinical reasoning following the intervention.[20–22,26] The only teaching method which has been consistently associated with improvement in clinical reasoning, regardless of the research design used, is Level II Fieldwork,[27–29] a required part of occupational therapy education in the United States in which students provide services under the supervision of a credentialed occupational therapy for a minimum of 24 weeks.

Additional limitations of these studies are apparent. Most of the study designs were qualitative and one-group 'pre- then post-tests', often with small convenience samples from one occupational therapy programme. No randomised controlled trials have been conducted. In terms of internal validity, studies that involved pre- and post-testing at the beginning and end of a course or curriculum must consider factors other than educational experiences which may have contributed to the changes noted, e.g. maturation, historical factors, motivation, and the particular faculty or courses in the curriculum. The use of study-designed surveys with unknown psychometric characteristics may also have affected the results. Further, there is a need for the development of ecologically valid instruments to measure occupational therapy-specific clinical reasoning. Outcome measures that have been utilised in the extant literature may not be sensitive to the types of clinical reasoning used in occupational therapy. Utilisation of small convenience samples from one programme and lack of information about the characteristics of the sample also limit the external validity of many of the studies. To summarise, at present, the evidence for approaches and methods to promote clinical reasoning is inconclusive. While the best available evidence suggests that longer-term, authentic experiences in fieldwork settings may be effective for facilitating improved clinical reasoning, more research is needed, particularly in relation to didactic methods for enhancing students' reasoning skills and abilities.

Experiential learning

The most prominent educational approach in the occupational therapy education literature is experiential.[2] Qualitative, quantitative and mixed methods studies have been conducted and report positive effects as a result of active learning techniques. A variety of strategies have been studied, including pairing students to practise assessment and intervention in a clinical setting,[15] providing opportunities for students to work with individuals with disabilities in the classroom,[18] and student fabrication of adapted clothing for individuals with disabilities.[19] Outcomes investigated include cognitive dimensions such as clinical reasoning[9,11,12,15,19] and understanding of course material;[9,19] behavioural dimensions such as client-centred care and application of course material;[14] and affective dimensions such as attitudes towards course material and confidence.[15]

Fieldwork is perhaps the ultimate active learning experience.[32] Studies of fieldwork have considered its effects on outcomes such as clinical reasoning,[13,16,17] attitudes towards individuals with mental illness,[31] and occupational therapy knowledge and skills,[32] to name just a few. Only one study measured client outcomes.[31] While some of these studies incorporated specific methods such as tutorials,[31] structured asynchronous online discussions,[27] and specific clinical reasoning activities such as journal writing, reviewing videotaped treatment sessions, reviewing case studies and answering probing questions[28] during fieldwork, others investigated the effect of standard fieldwork experiences.[26,30,33]

While the preponderance of evidence suggests that these experiential learning approaches are effective, caution is in order when considering the results of these studies. Many of the studies, both qualitative and quantitative, relied on student perceptions as the outcome measure. Of the quantitative studies, most involved one-group pre- and post-tests using study-designed questionnaires, and small convenience samples from one programme. Threats to both internal and external validity are apparent. Further studies with increased rigour are needed to provide robust evidence of the effectiveness of experiential learning. Studies comparing the effectiveness of experiential and alternative approaches could prove particularly informative.

Problem-based learning

One of the more commonly investigated teaching methods in the occupational therapy education literature is PBL. PBL is based on constructivism, as learners engage in the construction of knowledge in response to case triggers, or problems. Working in small groups with facilitation by tutors, students determine how to address problems presented in the case. Learners independently research information related to the case problems and the group collaborates to develop strategies to tackle them.[8,34–38]

Proponents of PBL claim that it is effective for improving clinical reasoning; critical reflection; motivation and enjoyment of learning; teamwork; the search, evaluation and utilisation of resources; and synthesis, retention and transfer of knowledge. On the other hand, it has been acknowledged that students who experienced PBL may have poorer knowledge of facts and basic science information, may experience frustration and dissatisfaction during the PBL process, and may focus on the medical model and procedural reasoning rather than occupation-centred practice.[8,34–38] Occupational therapy researchers have studied the effects of PBL across the curriculum,[18] PBL utilised in a single course and a single PBL case.[35] Outcomes measured have included acquisition of intended knowledge and skills,[34,35,37,38] development of teamwork[37] and clinical reasoning.[18,23,24] Most of these studies report positive effects.

However, similar to other areas of occupational therapy education research, studies with more rigorous designs and more objective outcome measures tended to yield non-significant results,[23,24,34] as opposed to less rigorous quantitative or qualitative studies of student perceptions. Concerns related to small convenience samples, study-designed instruments that lack psychometric evidence, and potential response bias also limit the internal and external validity of many of these studies. Thus, despite the fact that a number of studies have been conducted, the educational efficacy of PBL in occupational therapy has not been well established.

CONCLUSION

Based on their review, Hooper *et al.*[2] concluded that EBE in occupational therapy is in the early stages of development. Indeed, there is a need for all types of scholarship. SoD can generate systematic descriptions to further our understanding of occupational therapy students and their education. Incorporating SoI, researchers can build on research from other disciplines and elucidate the complex factors that influence how occupational therapy students learn. Organisation and synthesis of this information will facilitate creation of conceptual frameworks to support profession-specific education. Based on cohesive theories and frameworks derived from SoD and SoI, hypotheses can be generated and tested to revise, enhance and refine the constructs and relationships described by the framework. SoA and SoLT can be utilised to answer specific practical questions that arise and facilitate EBE in occupational therapy.

RECOMMENDATIONS

Advancing EBE in occupational therapy will require all types of scholarship and rigorous research into the numerous factors that influence the effectiveness of various strategies and approaches. Learner attributes such as demographic characteristics, personal experience, epistemic and ontological cognition, preferred learning approaches and educational background – among others – will likely influence the effectiveness of a particular technique. Another important variable is the learning context.[39,40] What 'works' in a large face-to-face programme may not automatically transfer to a small programme that uses interactive videoconferencing, for example. Multi-site studies with large samples could allow characteristics of the context and the learners to be included as variables in the research design, and the effects of an educational method could be considered in light of those variables. In studies with smaller samples in one location, thorough descriptions of the study participants and the learning context could assist readers in interpreting the relevance of the results for the students in their classrooms.

A particularly important aspect of the learning context is the instructor. Instructor experience, skill, beliefs, values and assumptions likely play a role in the successful utilisation of an instructional technique or approach, especially when one considers that few occupational therapy faculty members have formal training as educators.[39] Perhaps, as Tanner[39] asserted, the development of 'reflective instructors who are analytical about their practice and who make iterative instructional decisions based on evidence from the students sitting right in front of them'[39(p329)] is even more important than the approach or technique utilised. Studies of occupational therapy faculty at different stages in their careers could shed light on the characteristics of effective instructors and their practices.

Some argue that there is probably no one way to approach instruction; rather, educators should utilise a variety of – and perhaps all – methods in order to accommodate the needs of diverse student populations.[39] This does not, however, imply that instructional methods should be chosen arbitrarily. On the contrary, it has been argued that teaching and assessment methods should be matched to the desired learning outcome.[39,40] To date, many studies have measured student attitudes and perceptions rather than student knowledge, behaviour, performance in the practice setting, or skill in serving clients.[2] While learners may prefer a particular method or approach, it may not be effective for improving performance in the practice arena. Thus, conclusions about the effectiveness of various methods may depend on the outcome measured.[39] Hooper *et al.*[2] encourage researchers to design studies with compatibility between the approach, the desired level and outcomes of learning, and assessment measures. Currently, more evidence is needed to determine which approaches and methods are most effective for facilitating profession-specific outcomes (e.g. occupation- and client-centred clinical reasoning). Further, valid and reliable instruments to measure these outcomes need to be developed. Studies utilising psychometrically sound measures and comparing the effectiveness of different instructional methods for facilitating particular learning outcomes could provide useful evidence to inform our teaching practices.

When designing studies comparing the effectiveness of instructional approaches and methods, fidelity of implementation must also be considered.[39] Variations in teaching practices that are inconsistent with the intended model could lead to different outcomes in studies purporting to investigate the same teaching strategies. Manualisation could help ensure adherence to the principles of the teaching approach and facilitate replication of effectiveness studies.

Vroman and MacRae[36] stress the importance of EBE, arguing that just as clinically based therapists must be accountable for outcomes, so must educators. Over time, drawing on a variety of types of research designs and all types of scholarship, occupational therapy educators and researchers can gain new insights to enrich our understanding of occupational therapy education. While teaching and learning processes are complex and influenced by many variables, educators have a responsibility to continue working towards a deeper understanding of occupational therapy students and effective methods for facilitating their transformation into effective therapists.

SUMMARY POINTS

- EBE in occupational therapy is in the early stages of development, and there is a need for all types of scholarship to advance our knowledge and understanding.
- Occupational therapy educators have creatively incorporated a wide variety of teaching methods and approaches in the pursuit of effective learning experiences for students, even without a conceptual model.
- The lack of a well-established theoretical and conceptual foundation for occupational therapy education limits our understanding of the underlying reasons for equivocal research findings.
- Methodological flaws and lack of rigour also present challenges when interpreting and building on the available outcome studies.
- Rigorous research with improved methodological quality is needed, including studies measuring behavioural changes in students, transfer of learning to the clinical environment, and the impact on patient treatment.

REVIEW QUESTIONS

- Explain how the SoD, the SoI and the SoA contribute to evidence-based education in occupational therapy?
- How does the SoLT contribute to evidence-based education in occupational therapy?
- What is the evidence around the development of clinical reasoning skills in occupational therapy students through educational activities?
- What is the evidence base for using PBL in occupational therapy as an education method?
- What is the evidence for using experiential learning as an education method with occupational therapy students?

REFLECTIVE QUESTIONS AND EXERCISES

- Consider a technique or approach you are currently using in one of your courses. What evidence do you have of its effectiveness? What does the education literature tell you? Is there evidence from the occupational therapy education literature to support the technique or approach? How can you take a systematic approach to gathering evidence about its effectiveness? How can you disseminate your findings?

- Reflect on the intended and expected outcomes of a course you plan to teach. What types of knowledge, skills, values and attitudes need to be fostered in the course? What does the literature say about effective methods for designing a classroom atmosphere and teaching techniques to facilitate these outcomes? What are the most appropriate ways to assess the outcomes, and how can your assessment provide systematic data-gathering that could contribute to EBE?

- Think about a topic or concept that students in your course have struggled with in the past. Brainstorm and consider a variety of explanations for the students' struggles and consider alternatives for addressing them. Consult the literature for ideas and guidance about how the issues might be addressed effectively. Articulate (to others or in writing) your rationale for a new evidence-based approach to the issue.

- Start a discipline-specific or an interdisciplinary journal club to review education literature. Include both occupational therapy-related and general education literature. Analyse how educational theories and approaches might apply or be adapted for occupational therapy. Utilise the information to design an assignment in a course you are teaching. Systematically gather information about its effectiveness for dissemination at a conference or in a publication.

REFERENCES

1. American Occupational Therapy Association. Scholarship in occupational therapy. *Am J Occup Ther.* 2009; **63**(6): 790–6.

2. Hooper B, King R, Wood W, *et al*. An international systematic mapping review of educational approaches and teaching methods in occupational therapy. *Br J Occup Ther.* 2013; **76**(1): 9–22.

3. Mattingly C, Fleming MH. *Clinical Reasoning: forms of inquiry in a therapeutic practice.* Philadelphia, PA: FA Davis; 1994.

4. Liu KPY, Chan CCH, Hui-Chan CWY. Clinical reasoning and the occupational therapy curriculum. *Occup Ther Int.* 2000; **7**(3): 173–83.

5. Unsworth CA. The clinical reasoning of novice and expert occupational therapists. *Scand J Occup Ther.* 2001; **8**(4): 163–73.

6. Royeen CB, Mu K, Barrett K, *et al*. Pilot investigation: evaluation of clinical reflection and reasoning before and after workshop intervention. In: Crist P, editor. *Innovations in Occupational Therapy Education.* Bethesda, MD: American Occupational Therapy Association; 2000. pp. 107–14.

7. Knowles M. *Self-Directed Learning: a guide for learners and teachers.* Chicago, IL: Follett; 1975.

8. Salvatori P. Meaningful occupation for occupational therapy students: a student-centred curriculum. *Occup Ther Int.* 1999; **6**(3): 207–23.
9. Fisher GS. Successful educational strategies and the Pyramid of Occupational Therapy Learning. *Occup Ther Health Care.* 1999; **12**(1): 33–45.
10. Hooper B. Beyond active learning: a case study of teaching practices in an occupation-centered curriculum. *Am J Occup Ther.* 2006; **60**: 551–62.
11. Hooper B. On arriving at the destination of the centennial vision: navigational landmarks to guide occupational therapy education. *Occup Ther Health Care.* 2010; **24**(1): 97–106.
12. Mitchell AW. Teaching ill-structured problem solving using occupational therapy practice epistemology. *Occup Ther Health Care.* 2013; **27**(1): 20–34.
13. Mosey AC. Partition of occupational science and occupational therapy: sorting out some issues. *Am J Occup Ther.* 1993; **47**(8): 751–4.
14. Knecht-Sabres LJ. The use of experiential learning in an occupational therapy program: can it foster skills for clinical practice? *Occup Ther Health Care.* 2010; **24**(4): 320–34.
15. Neistadt ME. Teaching strategies for the development of clinical reasoning. *Am J Occup Ther.* 1996; **50**(8): 676–84.
16. Lysaght R, Bent M. A comparative analysis of case presentation modalities used in clinical reasoning coursework in occupational therapy. *Am J Occup Ther.* 2005; **59**(3): 314–24.
17. Neistadt ME. Teaching clinical reasoning as a thinking frame. *Am J Occup Ther.* 1998; **52**(3): 221–9.
18. Hammel J, Royeen CB, Bagatell N, *et al.* Student perspectives on problem-based learning in an occupational therapy curriculum: a multiyear qualitative evaluation. *Am J Occup Ther.* 1999; **53**(2): 199–206.
19. Stern P. Student perceptions of a problem-based learning course. *Am J Occup Ther.* 1997; **51**(7): 589–96.
20. Neistadt ME. The classroom as clinic: applications for a method of teaching clinical reasoning. *Am J Occup Ther.* 1992; **46**(9): 814–19.
21. Ciaravino EA. Student reflections as evidence of interactive clinical reasoning skills. *Occup Ther Health Care.* 2006; **20**(2): 75–88.
22. Neistadt ME, Smith RE. Teaching diagnostic reasoning: using a classroom-as-clinic methodology with videotapes. *Am J Occup Ther.* 1997; **51**(5): 360–8.
23. McCarron KA, D'Amico F. The impact of problem-based learning on clinical reasoning in occupational therapy education. *Occup Ther Health Care.* 2002; **16**(1): 1–13.
24. Velde BP, Wittman PP, Vos P. Development of critical thinking in occupational therapy students. *Occup Ther Int.* 2006; **13**(1): 49–60.
25. Benson JD, Provident I, Szucs K. An experiential learning lab embedded in a didactic course: outcomes from a pediatric intervention course. *Occup Ther Health Care.* 2013; **27**(1): 46–57.
26. Lederer JM. Disposition toward critical thinking among occupational therapy students. *Am J Occup Ther.* 2007; **61**(5): 519–26.
27. Coates GLF, Crist PA. Brief or new: professional development of fieldwork students; occupational adaptation, clinical reasoning, and client-centeredness. *Occup Ther Health Care.* 2004; **18**(1–2): 39–47.
28. Scanlan JN, Hancock N. Online discussions develop students' clinical reasoning skills during fieldwork. *Aust Occup Ther J.* 2010; **57**(6): 401–8.
29. Sladyk K, Sheckley B. Clinical reasoning and reflective practice: implications of fieldwork activities. *Occup Ther Health Care.* 2000; **13**(1): 11–22.
30. Kratz G. Evaluation of an occupational therapy training module: adapting clothes for persons with disabilities. *Occup Ther Int.* 1996; **3**(1): 32–48.

31. Beltran RO, Scanlan JN, Hancock N, *et al*. The effect of first year mental health fieldwork on attitudes of occupational therapy students towards people with mental illness. *Aust Occup Ther J.* 2007; **54**(1): 42–8.

32. Packer TL, Paterson M, Krupa T, *et al*. Client outcomes after student community fieldwork in Russia. *Occup Ther Int.* 2000; **7**(3): 191–7.

33. Crabtree JL, Justiss M, Swinehart S. Occupational therapy master-level students' evidence-based practice knowledge and skills before and after fieldwork. *Occup Ther Health Care.* 2012; **26**(2–3): 138–49.

34. Liotta-Kleinfeld L, McPhee S. Comparison of final exam test scores of neuroscience students who experienced traditional methodologies versus problem-based learning methodologies. *Occup Ther Health Care.* 2001; **14**(3–4): 35–53.

35. McCannon R, Robertson D, Caldwell J, *et al*. Students' perceptions of their acquired knowledge during a problem-based learning case study. *Occup Ther Health Care.* 2004; **18**(4): 13–28.

36. Vroman KG, MacRae N. How should the effectiveness of problem-based learning in occupational therapy education be examined? *Am J Occup Ther.* 1999; **53**(5): 533–6.

37. Reeves S, Mann SL, Caunce M, *et al*. Understanding the effects of problem-based learning on practice: findings from a survey of newly qualified occupational therapists. *Br J Occup Ther.* 2004; **67**(7): 323–7.

38. Spalding NJ, Killett A. An evaluation of a problem-based learning experience in an occupational therapy curriculum in the UK. *Occup Ther Int.* 2010; **17**(2): 64–73.

39. Tanner KD. Reconsidering 'what works'. *CBE Life Sci Educ.* 2011; **10**(4): 329–33.

40. Chapman J, Watson J, Adams J. Exploring changes in occupational therapy students' approaches to learning during pre-registration education. *Br J Occup Ther.* 2006; **69**(10): 457–63.

CHAPTER 28

Evidence-based education in physiotherapy

....

Vanina Dal Bello-Haas, Sarah Wojkowski
and Julie Richardson

OVERVIEW

In the past 100 years, the physiotherapy profession has evolved and as a result, entry-level education has undergone parallel extreme changes. This chapter explores five exemplar instructional strategies in physiotherapy education: (1) electronic learning (e-Learning) and technology; (2) problem-based learning (PBL); (3) interprofessional education (IPE); (4) portfolio and electronic portfolio (e-Portfolio); and (5) service-learning and globalisation. A search was conducted for research papers for each exemplar. The majority of papers were excluded after screening by title and abstract, remaining included papers underwent full text narrative review, and the results are presented.

Technology has been used with great diversity in physiotherapy education, such as teaching acquisition of knowledge, technical skills and a broad range of curricular content, and for evaluation and feedback purposes. Some reported student benefits of PBL include greater interest in the subject matter being studied, implementation of positive learning behaviours, transfer of PBL skills to the clinical setting, and being more likely to develop and use research skills. The integration of IPE into physiotherapy academic education has occurred through three main methods: (1) PBL, (2) technology-facilitated learning and (3) integrated practical experiences. Reported benefits are understanding and respecting other healthcare professionals' roles; increased confidence and self-esteem about themselves as healthcare professionals; and improved communication skills with other healthcare providers. In terms of portfolios and e-Portfolios, they are well received by students overall and they positively support learning. Physiotherapy educators have been advocating for a greater inclusion of global health content and curricula, and conceptual frameworks have been proposed to guide the development of global health service-learning for physiotherapy education programmes.

The available research evidence reviewed is largely limited to one particular programme at one particular institution. Future research needs to focus on integrating theoretical frameworks into educational research. In addition, use of valid and reliable outcomes measures, more standardised and rigorous methodology, and comparative research are needed to move evidence-based physiotherapy education forward.

CHAPTER OBJECTIVES

Upon completion of this chapter, the reader will be able to:
- discuss the changes in entry-level physiotherapy education programmes and the factors that have been the impetus for these changes
- outline the knowledge and skills graduates of entry-level physiotherapy education programmes need to possess in order to meet the needs of healthcare and society of the future
- define the terms blended learning; computer-assisted or computer-aided instruction; e-Learning; health informatics; learning technology; optimal international service-learning
- compare and contrast the five phases of international service-learning programme development
- explain the use of the following teaching strategies in physiotherapy education programmes – e-Learning and technology, PBL, IPE, portfolio and e-Portfolio, and service-learning and globalisation
- summarise the current state of the physiotherapy education-related evidence for the following teaching strategies – e-Learning and technology, PBL, IPE, portfolio and e-Portfolio, and service-learning and globalisation
- discuss one benefit and one drawback (based on the current evidence) of each of following teaching strategies in physiotherapy education programmes – e-Learning and technology, PBL, IPE, portfolio and e-Portfolio, and service-learning and globalisation
- describe one recommendation for future research related to physiotherapy education programmes for each of the following teaching strategies – e-Learning and technology, PBL, IPE, portfolio and e-Portfolio, and service-learning and globalisation.

KEY TERMS: physiotherapy, education, e-Learning/technology, problem-based learning, interprofessional education, portfolios, e-Portfolios, service-learning, globalisation

INTRODUCTION

Physiotherapy entry-level education has undergone extreme changes over the past century. Entry-level physiotherapy education has evolved from a 6-month to 1-year training course coinciding with World War I to a diploma programme. Although diversity in physiotherapy education still exists, since the 1980s physiotherapy education programmes have progressed from a diploma programme (still in existence in some African, Asian and eastern European countries) to a 3- or 4-year baccalaureate degree (e.g. European Union countries, the United Kingdom, Australia, New Zealand), a master's degree (e.g. Canada, the United Kingdom, Australia) and a clinical doctorate degree (e.g. the United States, Australia).[1] Numerous factors drive changes in entry-level education, physiotherapy curriculum, delivery methods (including ever-changing healthcare environments and systems), and continuous advances in healthcare and information technology. Currently, theory is considered foundational and is wholly integrated with practice within curricula; physiotherapy entry-level education is scientifically based, with less focus on 'recipe approaches' and observation and opinion-based decision-making; and evidence-based practice is now considered an essential element of physiotherapy programmes worldwide.[1,2]

These education changes are well aligned with evolutionary shifts in the physiotherapy profession. Physiotherapy is an area of study that involves an expansive body of knowledge, and as a profession it has developed a distinct domain. Current physiotherapy speciality areas are numerous and varied, and physiotherapists work with a multitude of client populations. In addition to practising in diverse practice settings, from more traditional settings to schools, hospices and industry, physiotherapists also practise in non-patient care areas including the medico-legal field, health policy and health administration. Direct access to physiotherapy services in many jurisdictions worldwide has resulted in professional autonomy, making physiotherapists responsible for their professional judgements and actions.[3] The outcome of this independent and self-determined authority and accountability for decision-making is an ever-increasing complexity of physiotherapy care and clinical practice environments.

It is well established that today's knowledge will be considered obsolete tomorrow. During the last century there has been an exponential growth of healthcare information, and research evidence and dissemination.[4] Globalisation now affects every aspect of health, healthcare and technology,[5] and as a result it affects entry-level physiotherapy education. An ageing population and an increase in chronic and lifestyle-related diseases have transformed the scope of physiotherapy practice to include prevention, health promotion, wellness and chronic disease management. Client-centred care and interdisciplinary approaches to client assessment and management are considered essential elements of practice. Practice environments now include community-based care and primary care, in addition to hospital-based and rehabilitation settings, providing physiotherapists with emerging role opportunities. The explosion of health, information and communication technology, the necessity to monitor treatment outcomes for effectiveness and reimbursement purposes, and the need for valid outcomes and evidence-based interventions have further broadened the scope of physiotherapy practice to include capitalising on technological advances and research, quality improvement, and programme and business management.

Graduates of today and those of tomorrow need to be independent, self-reliant, and capable of adapting to and meeting the changing healthcare needs of the communities they serve. In addition to being self-directed, lifelong learners, physiotherapy graduates need to be able to think broadly and critically, and need to be able to assess, apply, integrate, and synthesise information from multiple sources. Entry-level education must not only provide students with the requisite attitudes, knowledge, and skills to practice physiotherapy, but must also prepare students for work and life as physiotherapy professionals in ever changing global, social and political contexts, and to meet the needs of healthcare and society of the future.

How can physiotherapy educators best prepare students to practise in a world that is changing and unpredictable? What does the evidence indicate regarding best practice in physiotherapy education? In this chapter, we describe the search methods used to examine a select number of instructional strategy exemplars in physiotherapy education. For each exemplar, a narrative review of the search findings is presented. We discuss the 'state of evidence' for each of the exemplars and make recommendations for future research and considerations.

METHODS

A literature review (full text English-language articles) of select instructional strategy exemplars was conducted using a PICO (*Population, Intervention, Comparison, and Outcome*) approach. Population was defined as physiotherapy and physical therapy students. The following interventions were searched as exemplars: electronic learning (e-Learning) and technology, problem-based learning (PBL), interprofessional education (IPE), portfolio and electronic portfolio (e-Portfolio), and service-learning and globalisation. Because of the dearth of literature expected, no set comparisons or specified publication time periods were defined. Outcome was predetermined to be any educational outcome. Comprehensive searches were conducted using the following databases: MEDLINE (1946–2013), ERIC (Education Resources Information Center; 1966–2013), Embase (1980–2013), CINAHL (Cumulative Index to Nursing and Allied Health Literature; 1982–2013) and the Cochrane Library (1996–2013). One reviewer reviewed all titles and abstracts and full text of papers for a particular exemplar. Papers were included if they described a research study (randomised controlled trial, case-control trial, case study, descriptive study, case report, qualitative study, mixed methods study) of the exemplar in physiotherapy education. Once papers were systematically identified and included, the remaining included papers underwent full text narrative review, and theories or theoretical concepts used, study elements, outcomes and study results were extracted.

RESULTS

After removing duplicates, the search yielded 40 papers for PBL, 21 papers for e-Learning and technology, 15 papers for IPE, 21 papers for portfolios and e-Portfolios, and 34 papers for service-learning and globalisation. Of these papers, the majority were excluded by screening the title and abstract.

ELECTRONIC LEARNING AND TECHNOLOGY

The use of technology to educate physiotherapy students has evolved over the last 10 years. *See* Table 28.1 for common definitions and descriptions of technology-related terms. The literature has many examples of hybrid instructional approaches – enhancing traditional didactic instruction with technology.[6–10] However, in general, the quality of evidence is poor.[11] A 2002 survey of 186 accredited physiotherapy education programmes examined the number of programmes which used or were planning to use computer-assisted instruction (CAI), web-based or web-enhanced courses, or student web-based bulletin boards.[11] The majority of programmes favoured the use of web-based instruction in entry-level physiotherapy programmes and 41.5% of programmes included courses taught at least partially online.[11] Common uses of CAI that have been reported by physiotherapy programmes include providing tutorials, testing students, replacing class meetings, distance learning during clinical education, remediation and extra credit.[12]

TABLE 28.1 Definition and description of key terms related to technology used in education

Key term	Definition and description
Blended learning[13]	Brings together or integrates face-to-face classroom instruction with online activities
Computer-assisted or computer-aided instruction[11]	Computer technology that supplements the delivery of course material that would otherwise be delivered through traditional lecture-based means
e-Learning[14]	The use of electronic media and devices as tools for improving access to training, communication and interaction
	Facilitates the adoption of new ways of understanding and developing learning
Health informatics[15]	Evaluates how health information and knowledge can be effectively used for clinical decision-making
Learning technology[12]	Application of technology for the enhancement of teaching, learning and assessment
	Includes multimedia materials, and networks and communication systems to support learning

Technology has been integrated into physiotherapy education across a spectrum of curricular content – for example, neurological,[8] cardiopulmonary,[6] orthopedic,[16] ethics[13] and clinical decision-making.[10] Three main themes were identified regarding the use of technology in physiotherapy education.

1. Acquisition of knowledge:
   a. technical (e.g. palpation, evaluation)
   b. academic (e.g. clinical reasoning, content specific)
2. Research and/or information gathering (e.g. a student discussion board)
3. Evaluation or feedback.

ACQUISITION OF KNOWLEDGE

Technical

Technology has been used to facilitate physiotherapy students' technical skills.[16] Arroyo-Morales *et al.*[16] completed a randomised controlled trial to examine e-Learning resources for palpation and ultrasound imaging of the knee. One group of students was provided with access to a website (http://ecofisio.com), and a second group was not. The website, which supplemented in-class instruction, included videos of palpation procedures, images illustrating correct placement of ultrasound probes, diagrams of the ultrasound scan, anatomical sections and self-assessments (e.g. multiple-choice questions, short answer questions, jumbled sentence tests). Students without access to the website independently consulted textbooks for supplemental information after in-class sessions. The website was found to be more effective than textbooks for skill acquisition (palpation and ultrasound techniques), but not for knowledge acquisition.[16]

Use of online communities is another example of how technology can be used for the acquisition of skill and knowledge. Wong and Abbruzzese[15] described the use of online communities to analyse gait.[15] Students, in groups, created a multimedia video essay that was viewed and analysed by student peers. Students collaborated online and in face-to-face meetings to provide feedback, clarify rationales, or revise opinions until each group member felt comfortable presenting the video made by every other group member. The majority of students agreed that the assignment enhanced their learning and clinical decision-making abilities.

Academic

Many examples exist related to the use of technology to deliver academic content or supplemental tutorials to physiotherapy students.[6,8-13] The effectiveness of blended learning compared with traditional classroom-based learning on ethics knowledge and knowledge application confidence in physiotherapy students was examined by Dal Bello-Haas *et al.*[13] Four existing units were converted to online modules involving videotaped vignettes, opportunities for topic exploration via asynchronous online discussions, reflections on future practice and critical thinking, and clinical application exercises. One group of students completed the course entirely face-to-face, and the other group completed four online modules and the remainder of the course face-to-face (blended learning). Students in both groups demonstrated statistically significant changes in their confidence related to ethical, legal, professional and healthcare issues after the course. However, level of satisfaction with the blended learning course was related to confidence in computer skills.[13]

RESEARCH AND INFORMATION GATHERING

Maloney *et al.*[17] examined the usage and user experiences of Physeek, an online, keyword-searchable repository of learning resources (lecture slides, practical videos, self-directed learning modules, pre-readings), of students enrolled in the Monash University undergraduate physiotherapy programme (Melbourne, Australia). The database allowed remote access to learning resources, which were developed or identified by faculty, and was intended to support and advance practice competency. Student focus groups and an audit of Physeek utilisation were used to evaluate the value of the resources. Students perceived Physeek to be an efficient and preferred source for learning resources, and were most likely to use this resource close to examinations or to gather information needed during clinical placements. Interestingly, the availability of the Physeek repository did not have a negative impact on attendance at scheduled learning sessions.[17]

EVALUATION AND FEEDBACK

Corrigan and Hardham[7] described the use of technology to provide audio and visual feedback to develop physiotherapy students' self-awareness of performance of clinical skills in simulated tasks; and, evaluate the use of audio and visual feedback as learning and teaching tools. Students in a third-year undergraduate course worked in groups and preselected a case scenario that required the development of a treatment plan to retrain motor skills (walking, standing up). One student role-played the patient described in the scenario, one student was the 'treating' therapist, and a third student videotaped the simulation (all students assumed all roles), and the generated DVD was provided to the lecturer for feedback. The simulated task was found to be useful for student reflection and self-evaluation of their performance, and was well received by the students.[7]

The research indicates that the integration of technology into the education of physiotherapy students has supplemented but not replaced traditional teaching techniques in the areas of acquisition of knowledge, research and information gathering, and evaluation and feedback. However, the quality of evidence is poor.[6] Additionally, issues with integrating technology in physiotherapy education include the time required for familiarisation with the technology (faculty and students) and the cost associated with developing computer-based modules or courses. As technology continues to advance and becomes more widely accessible, there will be a need for additional research to better understand how, or if, the integration of technology can not only support, but perhaps replace the traditional teaching techniques in order to prepare physiotherapy students for technology supported clinical practice after graduation.

PROBLEM-BASED LEARNING

PBL, first described in 1980,[18] is an approach used in physiotherapy curriculum that focuses on problems encountered in clinical practice as the stimulus for learning. Students, working in small groups, use these problems to develop and refine their learning objectives, search for best evidence to address their learning objectives, and use this evidence to discuss and problem solve through the learning objectives. PBL can be a completely integrated curricular approach, can be incorporated in a single course or can be utilised as a transitional approach where students are initially engaged in more traditional curriculum and then transition to PBL.

Although PBL continues to be a foundation for many physiotherapy curricula, there is a paucity of rigorous comparative research. A recent study conducted in Spain used a quasi-experimental design to compare learning preferences and strategies of physiotherapy students engaged in PBL curriculum and those in a conventional lecture-based curriculum.[19] Students within the PBL curriculum reported improvement in understanding the relationship of ideas, greater interest in the subject matter being studied, a decrease in lack of purpose and more integration of the ideas being learned.[19] A further study, which included third- and fourth-year students in a PBL curriculum in Japan, found that students implemented positive learning behaviours, including self-reflection, self-evaluation and self-directedness, into clinical placement experiences.[20]

Van Langenberghe[21] used the Approaches to Studying Inventory to examine the learning approaches of 187 first- and second-year students in a PBL programme. Both cohorts of students demonstrated superior approaches to learning compared with normative data of students undertaking professional education.[21] Titchen and Coles[22] compared the results of the study by Van Langenberghe[21] with students in a traditional physiotherapy programme (N = 48) using the Approaches to Studying Inventory. Students in the PBL programme had higher scores on complex learning in the first year than those in the subject-based programme, but the results were reversed by the end of the second year.[22]

It has been suggested that PBL prepares students both in the preclinical stage of their professional education and for clinical experiences.[23] Semi-structured interviews with clinical supervisors were used to explore how students use skills gained through PBL in practice.[24] Supervisors reported that PBL resulted in positive outcomes for both student education and clinical practice. PBL skills that students transferred to clinical practice settings included effective team skills, an enhanced problem-solving approach, especially in unfamiliar situations, and a holistic approach to patient management.[24]

Another UK study examined physiotherapy students' evaluations of their initial PBL experience during an interprofessional module using the PBL Attitudes Questionnaire and a qualitative evaluation that focused on communication skills and patient-focused approaches to care.[25] Students expressed positive attitudes about their personal learning and team-working skills gained from PBL. Female students expressed a greater confidence in the quality of information provided by other students, and a greater enjoyment of the responsibility of PBL and in working with others.[25]

Some studies report physiotherapy students being more positively engaged with a PBL curriculum than a more traditional curriculum,[26] and research has also focused on whether physiotherapy students are more likely to develop research skills as a result of PBL. Physiotherapy students in Sweden who were engaged in a PBL learning curriculum reported a greater intention of engaging in future research than students in a traditional curriculum, a more positive attitude towards research, and a stronger intention to initiate research and use research evidence to improve practice.[27] The authors concluded that PBL programmes may have a greater impact on shaping students as research consumers and being involved in research compared to traditional education methods.[27]

More recent evidence examining the effect of PBL approaches on student learning and professional competency does not provide high-quality evidence to support the adoption of PBL within the physiotherapy curriculum. Current evidence from quasi-experimental designs and qualitative studies suggests that physiotherapy students trained within a PBL curriculum may transfer skills from the academic setting to a clinical setting and feel prepared to engage in limited research activities. There have been many changes external to professional curriculum such as students using laptops in physiotherapy PBL tutorials, the use of social media to share resources, and many different forms of synthesised evidence that have influenced the process of PBL within current physiotherapy curriculum. A new generation of rigorous studies is required to reflect the current approaches to the implementation of PBL in curricula today.

INTERPROFESSIONAL EDUCATION

IPE occurs when 'students from two or more professions learn about, from and with each other to enable effective collaboration and improve health outcomes'.[28(p1)] The integration of IPE into physiotherapy academic education has occurred through three main methods: (1) PBL, (2) technology-facilitated learning and (3) integrated practical experiences (e.g. not associated with a clinical placement). Regardless of the methodology used to integrate IPE into the academic physiotherapy curriculum, the literature has noted benefits, including understanding and respecting other healthcare professionals' roles; students having increased confidence and self-esteem about themselves as healthcare professionals; and improved communication skills with other healthcare providers.

PROBLEM-BASED LEARNING

Interprofessional PBL (IPPBL) has been successfully implemented with different health professional students, including physiotherapy students, at various points in their education.[29,30] To evaluate students' perceptions of participating in IPPBL, faculty members from medicine, pharmacy, nursing, physiotherapy and occupational therapy collaboratively developed a module focused on a new mother with lower back pain and post-partum depression.[29] Twenty-four health professional students, at various points in their studies, volunteered in the IPPBL, completed a 'pre- then post-test' to evaluate their attitude and knowledge towards interprofessional collaboration, and participated in a post-study focus group. All students reported they agreed or strongly agreed that the module enhanced their understanding of interprofessional teamwork; noted a better understanding of how their own scope of practice 'fit' with other health professionals; and had increased confidence in collaborating with other practitioners.[29]

Hayward et al.[30] integrated three nursing and three physiotherapy students with six high school seniors, from a variety of cultural backgrounds, into groups that were tasked with creating a patient case study. The high school students identified a health condition that affected them or a family member, or that was of interest, and the nursing and physiotherapy students guided the high school students through collection of background information about the disease, and wrote the case study. The integrated learning experience not only introduced the high school students to two health professionals, but it also encouraged the nursing and physiotherapy students to work as mentors and learn from each other. Specifically, the nursing and physiotherapy students noted they refined their listening skills and learned about different cultural values related to healthcare from the high school students.[30]

TECHNOLOGY-FACILITATED LEARNING

The literature includes some innovative approaches to IPE for physiotherapy students through the use of technology. Davies et al.[31] describes the use of WebCT Online learning platform to involve students from multiple professions in interprofessional activities over the final 2 years of their programmes. A trained facilitator guided the online learning experiences either through posing questions or providing support and guidance. While barriers such as technological challenges and lack of participation by some students/student groups were identified, the module was effective in improving student physiotherapists' awareness of roles and issues, and their ability to develop collaborative working relationships. In addition, students reported increased confidence in personal knowledge and skills, and improved interdisciplinary values.[31]

INTEGRATED PRACTICAL EXPERIENCES

Other IPE strategies reported in the literature for physiotherapy learners include practical experiences during academic training[32] or immersion experience in an interprofessional setting.[33] Wamsley et al.[32] created an interprofessional standardised patient exercise with chronic illness as the focus. Physiotherapy students participated with medical, dentistry, nurse practitioner and pharmacy students to complete a 4-hour exercise in a clinical skills facility. Outcome themes focused on professional roles, skills and confidence, with some students expressing greater appreciation of other professionals and learning skills (interview techniques, patient education skills) by observing others. There was a significant increase in team value for all professional students post-interprofessional standardised patient exercise.[32] Ateah et al.[33] instructed students in a classroom setting, prior to integrating a practical IPE experience. The didactic component was also interprofessional, allowing students to participate in interprofessional group discussions. Students then travelled to a clinical site in a remote community for an interprofessional immersion placement. After the IPE experience ended, students reported improved perceptions about other healthcare professionals and increased understanding of other professionals' roles and scope of practice. Interestingly, perceptions of other health professions changed significantly only after the education session and did not increase again following the immersion placement.[33]

IPE in physiotherapy education programmes has not been standardised. However, regardless of strategies used, outcomes of IPE experiences for physiotherapy students include increased understanding and respect for the roles of other professionals in the healthcare system; students having increased confidence and self-esteem about themselves as healthcare professionals; and improved communication with other healthcare providers that extends into clinical settings. Additionally, there is a dearth of evidence related to whether any gains attributed to IPE can be sustained longer term. Although IPE may enhance students' attitudes towards interprofessional collaboration and clinical decision-making ability,[20] currently there is little effectiveness evidence related to collaborative competencies development. Additional and more rigorous research is required to provide evidence about the most effective way to deliver IPE experiences to physiotherapy students.

PORTFOLIOS AND E-PORTFOLIOS

Portfolios, a collection, record or set of materials or evidence that provide a representation of educational or developmental experiences,[34] have been used for many years as methods of student assessment in fine arts, teacher training and nursing education. A portfolio functions as both product and process. As a product, the portfolio is a documentation of learning, while the process of learning occurs through the portfolio development, reflection on learning, and analysis of 'learning moments'.[35]

Although portfolios have traditionally been paper based, the electronic portfolio (often called an e-Portfolio) is viewed as an emerging educational technology and is garnering attention. An e-Portfolio is similar to a traditional portfolio in that the information can be stored in a single location.[36] However, the e-Portfolio is considered to be more interactive, with supplementary benefits. The e-Portfolio can be easily accessed from any computer with an Internet connection.[36,37] Artefacts or evidence of student work can take many forms such including Word documents, video, digital pictures, audio files, hypertext links to uniform resource locators and presentations.[36] In addition, students develop or broaden their computer skills while creating or editing their e-Portfolios.[36] While an e-Portfolio can remain private for the learner, the content can be shared with faculty for assessment purposes, and other audiences such as employers, and accrediting and regulatory agencies.[36,37]

Reflection is now recognised as a critical element of any portfolio or e-Portfolio. In fact, a professional portfolio with reflective activities is an instructional strategy often employed to enhance students' critical thinking and reflective abilities in academic and clinical learning settings.[34,36] Description, results and outcomes of the portfolio papers reviewed are summarised in Table 28.2. All papers describe student benefits – the portfolio and e-Portfolio was overall well received by the students and positively supported learning.[34,36,38,39]

TABLE 28.2 Summary of the portfolio and e-Portfolio literature in physiotherapy education

Author/s, and general description of paper	Outcomes	Limitations
Hayward *et al.*[36] Descriptive paper Culmination of 3 years of work developing an e-Portfolio in a 6½ year DPT programme; physiotherapy programme at Northeastern University, Boston, Massachusetts Development involved four stages: 1. designing a paper-based portfolio model to organise and create linkages among liberal studies, and the professional and experiential components of the DPT programme 2. transforming the model into an electronic format 3. creating a demonstration e-Portfolio and tutorial 4. pilot testing to evaluate the e-Portfolio model (technology, usability)	Student benefits: • e-Portfolio assisted students in organising and archiving relevant products • e-Portfolio provided a visual representation of how student learning evolved over time • e-Portfolio allowed students to appreciate what professional development entails • e-Portfolio encouraged students to integrate, assess and reflect upon their learning • students found the reflective components of the e-Portfolio rewarding and meaningful Design team learning: • diversity of team was enlightening and enhanced learning • cross-pollination of ideas • including students as members of the design team was critical	Limited generalisability Limited pilot testing sample size, with limited student representation across years of the DPT programme
Heijne *et al.*[38] Descriptive paper Implementation of a portfolio in the physiotherapy 3 course (a second-semester course); physiotherapy programme, Karolinska Institutet, Sweden	Student perceptions of the portfolio: • majority of students were satisfied with the portfolio as an assessment tool • portfolio was found to increase student workload • instructions for the portfolio need to be more clearly articulated	Limited theoretical rationale for implementation of a 'showcase portfolio' Specific 'showcase portfolio' modifications not described nor linked with theoretical basis Evaluation of portfolio conducted using author-developed questionnaire only

Author/s, and general description of paper	Outcomes	Limitations
Heijne et al.[38] (cont.) Modified 'showcase portfolio' (only best pieces of student's work included, summative); portfolio made up of three assignments: personal exercise programme; exercise programme for a healthy client; reflection – physical exercise, experience with physical exercise, why physiotherapists need to have integrated knowledge of physical exercise, evidence of physical activity as preventive intervention	Student perceptions of the portfolio peer review: • majority of students were satisfied with the peer review of their portfolio • some students found it difficult to review a student colleague's portfolio	Questionnaire not included in paper; no reported pilot testing or psychometrics properties of questionnaire Limited generalisability
Jensen and Saylor[34] Report of project results; project piloted the use of portfolios as a vehicle for professional development in MPT students (N = 32) at Samuel Merritt College, Oakland, California, and bachelor's (N = 12) and master's (N = 5) nursing students at San Jose State University, San Jose, California Product (portfolios) and evaluation (student and instructor assessments) data were examined for the following purposes: (a) to examine the usefulness of portfolios to facilitate reflection and to assess professional development in students; (b) to identify portfolio components most useful to students and instructors	Student feedback: • benefits included: the opportunity to be reflective and the opportunity to be creative; the portfolio provided structure for organising thoughts and for looking at a progress over time • barriers included: lack of time for reflection; uncertainty due to lack of clear guidelines for format Instructors' perspectives: • journal entry component of portfolio was not useful, as often an emotionless list of tasks and devoid of thinking; portfolios should only include reflective components • portfolios described what and how much students learned within the course	Retrospective analysis Limited description of key qualitative methodology and analysis elements, e.g researcher knowledge, backgrounds, institutional locations, life histories, role of researcher and perspective he or she brings to the study, data saturation, triangulation of data, and so on Limited description of student and instructor assessments Limited generalisability
Senger and Kanthan[39] Descriptive paper	Student perceptions and feedback: • perceptions about the portfolio improved from midterm to final	Limited generalisability Limited theoretical rationale for portfolio components included in paper

(*continued*)

Author/s, and general description of paper	Outcomes	Limitations
Senger and Kanthan[39] (*cont.*) Implementation and evaluation of a learning portfolio introduced in a pathology course (module 2), physiotherapy programme (N = 41 physiotherapy students), University of Saskatchewan, Saskatoon, Canada; examination of drivers and barriers of learning portfolios via self-, peer and instructor assessment The portfolio incorporated assessment of affective and course-specific objectives and the Association for Medical Education in Europe suggestions for portfolio assessment standardisation; the portfolio included weekly mandatory entries – individual class quiz, the class group quiz, the group activity and a one-page self-reflection document – and suggested, voluntary entries, e.g. completion of specially designed online digital games or inclusion of relevant and interesting news articles, list of recommended websites or literary sources; students selected voluntary entries that best displayed their growth and learning over the semester for inclusion in their portfolio	Student perceptions and feedback: (*cont.*) • students, overall, found the development of the portfolio to be a worthwhile experience • some students found the portfolio assisted in identifying effective learning strategies and integrating and organising materials • the portfolio assisted students in developing time management skills and key learning points • the most difficult aspect of the portfolio process was deemed to be maintaining motivation to complete the portfolio elements and finding the time to add documents to, reflect on and personalise the portfolio	Evaluation conducted using author-developed questionnaire; no reported pilot testing or psychometrics properties of questionnaire Descriptive approach to 'open-ended qualitative questions' – saturation and triangulation not reported

Abbreviations: DPT = Doctor of Physical Therapy; MPT = Master of Physical Therapy

SERVICE-LEARNING

The Global Independent Commission on the Education of Health Professionals for the Twenty-First Century concluded that

> all health professionals in all countries should be educated to mobilise knowledge and to engage in critical reasoning and ethical conduct so that

they are competent to participate in patient and population-centred health systems as members of locally responsive and globally connected teams.[5]

The commission argues that global dimensions of health, including leadership, management, policy analysis and communication skills, have been neglected in curricula and are necessary for students to engage in global health initiatives.

Global health is a new paradigm that emphasises collaboration, partnership and the willingness to share knowledge and resources,[40] and physiotherapy educators have advocated for a greater inclusion of global health content and curricula.[41,42] A survey in 2006 found 28% of American programmes (N = 24) and 50% of Canadian programmes (N = 4) had been involved with international service-learning (ISL) experiences in the previous decade.[40] Experiences that students can undertake from a global perspective can be categorised as (a) ISL with equal emphasis on community service and student learning, defined as structured learning experience that combines explicit learning experiences, preparation and reflection with community service,[43] or (b) international clinical education experiences that focus on students acquiring clinical skills and earning clinical education credits.[40]

The evidence to support global health learning experiences within physiotherapy education is limited; however, conceptual frameworks have been proposed to guide the development of global health service-learning within programmes. Pechak and Thompson[44] initially identified and analysed common structures and processes used to establish 'optimal' ISL within physiotherapy education programmes. They used data from interviews with 14 physiotherapy faculty members who had been involved in ISL or some type of international learning experience, and five phases in the development of an ISL programme were identified[44] (*see* Table 28.3). A definition of optimal ISL* based on the conceptual model was developed,[44] and the model has undergone some further modifications.[40]

Black Lattanzi and Pechak[41] proposed an additional framework to be used as a practical tool to develop ISL courses, while considering ethical issues. They describe six principles and three essential stages to guide ISL course planning (*see* Table 28.3). Cultural competency training has been identified as an important component of ISL curriculum, and it has been suggested that prior to the ISL experience students should explore the history, politics, economics, geography and resources of the country.[41] It is also important that students understand how the community conceptualises health and illness and the preferences for health interventions.[41]

Increasingly, physiotherapy academic leaders are exploring how population and public health can be integrated into the curriculum. The formulation of learning goals around personal and social responsibility – civic knowledge and engagement, local and global, intercultural knowledge and competence, ethical reasoning in action

---

* 'Optimal ISL in physical therapist education is defined as a structured program of service and learning experiences as an international site that includes preparation, reflection, and explicit service and learning objectives. This service is performed in partnership with an established community partner that understands the role of physical therapy to address community identified needs, with the goal of creating sustainable change in the community. Program evaluation with service learning components is integrated into the design of the program and enhances ongoing program improvement to the benefit of the students and community.'[44(p2)]

TABLE 28.3 Five phases in the development of an international service-learning programme

Phase	Phase description
1 The *developmental phase*	Involves establishing connections between the committed faculty member and a community partner
	It is important for both partners to clearly communicate what the community needs and what the faculty can offer
2 The *design phase*	Involves operational decisions in five areas:
	1. positioning the ISL content within the overall curriculum
	2. outlining the international service and learning components
	3. selecting students
	4. instrumentalising the plan for ISL
	5. funding the programme
3 The *implementation* phase	Includes increased student involvement in preparation activities such as collecting equipment, and educating and training family members and nonprofessional caregivers
	Students involved in reflection in groups or use journaling in this phase
	Risk management is an important component of this phase
4 The *evaluation*	Assessment of outcomes related to student, department, university and community
5 The final phase, *enhancement*	The faculty member collaborates and communicates with the community partner around how to improve and expand the programme

Note: from Pechak and Thompson;[44] *abbreviation:* ISL = international service-learning

and foundation in skills for lifelong learning – as described for undergraduate public health education, could inform physiotherapy curriculum.[45] It is suggested that skills be developed within diverse communities, so that students gain a global perspective of real-world challenges.[45]

Ethical issues are also important considerations in the development of ISL experiences, as the disparity in resources that exist between the host community and the academic programme has the potential to create a power imbalance. Therefore, ethical issues such as ensuring that the ISL is mutually beneficial, that the experience is not just an opportunity for medical tourism, and that the project has goals that relate to sustainability beyond the life of the ISL experience need to be addressed. It is also suggested that students have a minimum proficiency with the local language.[41] Physiotherapy students and healthcare students in general who participate in global health initiatives as part of their education or training come to understand the social determinants of global healthcare, increase their cultural competency and gain a greater understanding of public health issues.[46]

TABLE 28.4 Six principles and three essential stages to guide international service-learning (ISL) course planning

Principle		Essential stage	
1	Beneficence and non-maleficence guides the project	1	The *pre-experience or planning* stage: • students are trained and equipped
2	Cross-cultural differences that can negatively affect relationships with community partners and project outcomes need to be considered	2	The *field immersion experience* stage: • involves the structured scheduling of activities and assessments
3	Evaluation should include clients, the host community, programme effectiveness and student learning	3	The *post-experience* stage: • occurs back at the educational institution • experience debriefing
4	Students need to be involved in all aspects of the project, including development and assessment, and need to be accountable within the relationship with the host community			
5	The ISL course plan should outline the students' responsibility across all stages of the project			
6	The plan should create a foundation for ethical practice among all the stakeholders			

Note: from Black Lattanzi and Pechak;[41] *abbreviation:* ISL = international service-learning

RECOMMENDATIONS FOR FUTURE RESEARCH

The rationale for evidence-based physiotherapy education parallel those in clinical practice – *to apply the best available evidence to make decisions* so that educators provide students with the most optimal and highest quality educational experiences. Often educational research is viewed as much too complex to investigate, as there are too many extraneous and confounding variables to consider and control. Educational theory and research paradigms and methodologies are viewed as too diverse and difficult to limit, and determining optimum outcomes to measure or evaluate often challenges physiotherapy educational researchers.[47]

Some of the issues with integrating technology in physiotherapy education include the amount of time required for faculty and students to become familiar and comfortable with technology; and, the costs associated with developing a new computer-based module or course. Additionally, although physiotherapy students report using the Internet for learning, this use is mainly for content consumption.[48] As well, many physiotherapy students have a poor understanding of how technologies (e.g. blogs, wikis, podcasts) that can develop collaborative and reflective skills work.[48] The decision to incorporate technology into physiotherapy education requires not only faculty, staff, financial and other resources and support, but also student engagement in the use of the specific technology.

As technology continues to evolve, the assimilation of technology into clinical practice will expand. More and more, physiotherapy students will be employed in practice environments that incorporate technology into client care. Incorporating technology into physiotherapy student entry-level preparation will not only enhance learning during student training, but may also better prepare physiotherapy graduates to embrace technology as part of their clinical practices. Future research needs to determine the most effective way to integrate technology into physiotherapy student education and how to best engage students in the use of technology to maximise learning and knowledge translation.

The review of more recent educational studies examining the effect of PBL approaches on student learning and professional competency does not provide high quality evidence to support the adoption of PBL within physiotherapy curriculum. Current evidence from quasi-experimental designs and descriptive studies suggests that physiotherapy students trained within a PBL curriculum feel prepared to engage in limited research activities and may transfer skills from the academic setting to a clinical setting. Nowadays, physiotherapy students are tech savvy, using laptops in PBT tutorials, social media to share resources, the Internet to search literature, and many different forms of synthesised evidence, all of which are influencing the PBL process. A new generation of high-quality research which examines Generation X and Millennial students within a problem-based curriculum is necessary to understand how the PBL approach and technology use are influencing students' learning, learning processes, and outcomes of importance. If educators are to continue to endorse and engage in PBL approaches, more evidence is required about how PBL contributes to the students' learning considering individual learning styles, curriculum requirements and outcomes compared with other educational approaches.

Although IPE is not new, IPE in physiotherapy education programmes has not been standardised. The National Interprofessional Competency Framework, which includes six interconnecting interprofessional competency domains, will provide a guide for physiotherapy educators; however, little evidence 'exists in regards to whether the gains attributed to IPE can be sustained over time'.[49(p3)] Although IPE may enhance students' attitudes towards IP collaboration and clinical decision-making ability,[15] effectiveness evidence 'in developing collaborative competencies in learners is just starting to emerge'.[50(p3)]

Regardless of strategies used, outcomes of IPE experiences for physiotherapy students include increased understanding and respect for other professionals' roles in the healthcare system; students having increased confidence and self-esteem about themselves as healthcare professionals; and improved communication with other healthcare providers that extends into clinical settings. As Solomon[50] has noted, a common element across the IPE literature is the willingness of instructors to experiment and innovate. However, additional and more rigorous research is required to provide evidence about the most effective way to deliver IPE experiences to physiotherapy students.

Although widely adopted in other health, service, and professional preparation education programmes, the reported use of portfolios and e-Portfolios in physiotherapy education is unknown, and the current literature related to portfolios and e-Portfolios is descriptive. There are many issues to consider when integrating portfolios and e-Portfolios, all of which could be considered as a focus of research, including pedagogical framework and portfolio style, which in turn affects implementation, design and development issues, operational issues, usability issues, assessment issues (e.g. to assess or not to assess; reliability and validity of assessment methods), and accessibility issues in the case of e-Portfolios. Successful portfolio and e-Portfolio integration is, in part, dependent on the purpose for use, which needs to be clearly articulated. Any educational research related to portfolio/ and e-Portfolio use needs to include outcomes that are well aligned with the stated purpose. Research needs to examine best practices and what effective portfolio and e-Portfolio implementation looks like, as well as advantages and disadvantages of use from multiple perspectives.

Globalisation has resulted in increased opportunities for physiotherapy students to undertake clinical placements in middle- and lower-income countries. Students and faculty need to be well prepared for ISL experiences and the frameworks described can be used to develop curriculum. Future research needs to provide evidence of the value of these experiences for all stakeholders in the context of global health and how the relationship between the academic programmes and communities that offer these experiences can be enhanced.

CONCLUSION

Although scholarship related to teaching and learning in physiotherapy has over a 40-year history, the research base for PBL, IPE, e-Learning and technology, portfolio and e-Portfolio, and service-learning and globalisation in physiotherapy education is largely in the developmental stages. The available research evidence is descriptive, limited to one particular programme at one particular institution, and in some cases is not methodologically rigorous enough or of limited quality.

SUMMARY POINTS

- Entry-level physiotherapy education has undergone parallel extreme changes in the past century as a result of evolutionary shifts in the physiotherapy profession.
- Technology in physiotherapy education has been used for teaching acquisition of knowledge and technical skills, for teaching a broad range of curricular content, and for evaluation and feedback purposes.
- The integration of IPE into physiotherapy academic education has occurred through PBL, technology-facilitated learning, and integrated practical experiences. Benefits include understanding and respecting healthcare professionals' roles; increased confidence and self-esteem of students as healthcare professionals; and improved communication skills with other healthcare providers.
- Portfolios and e-Portfolios are well received by physiotherapy students overall and they positively support learning.

- Physiotherapy educators have been advocating for a greater inclusion of global health content and curricula, and conceptual frameworks are available to guide the development of global health service-learning for physiotherapy education programmes.
- In order to move evidence-based physiotherapy education forward, future research needs to incorporate theoretical frameworks, use of valid and reliable outcomes measures, more standardised and rigorous methodology, and comparative research methodology.

REVIEW QUESTIONS

- List three changes in entry-level physiotherapy education programmes and the factors that have been the impetus for these changes.
- Describe three knowledge areas or skills graduates of entry-level physiotherapy education programmes need to possess in order to meet the needs of healthcare and society of the future.
- Define the following terms: blended learning; computer-assisted or computer-aided instruction; e-Learning; health informatics; learning technology; optimal international service-learning.
- Describe the following phases of international service-learning programme development according to Pechak and Thompson:[44] developmental, design, implementation, evaluation and enhancement.
- Explain one use of the following teaching strategies in physiotherapy education programmes: e-Learning and technology, PBL, IPE, portfolio and e-Portfolio, and service-learning and globalisation.
- Summarise one area of current research of the physiotherapy education-related evidence for the following teaching strategies: e-Learning and technology, PBL, IPE, portfolio and e-Portfolio, and service-learning and globalisation.

REFLECTIVE QUESTIONS AND EXERCISES

- Describe one benefit and one drawback (based on the current evidence) of each of following teaching strategies in physiotherapy education programmes: e-Learning and technology, PBL, IPE, portfolio and e-Portfolio, and service-learning and globalisation.
- Explain one recommendation for future research related to physiotherapy education programmes for each of the following teaching strategies: e-Learning and technology, PBL, IPE, portfolio and e-Portfolio, and service-learning and globalisation.

REFERENCES

1. World Confederation for Physical Therapy (WCPT). *WCPT Guideline for Physical Therapist Professional Entry Level Education.* London: WCPT; 2011. Available at: www.wcpt.org/sites/wcpt.org/files/files/Guideline_PTEducation_complete.pdf (accessed 15 January 2014).

2. World Confederation for Physical Therapy. *Policy Statement: evidence based practice.* London: WCPT; 2011. Available at: www.wcpt.org/sites/wcpt.org/files/files/PS_EBP_Sept2011.pdf (accessed 15 January 2014).

3. American Physical Therapy Association (APTA). *Autonomous Physical Therapist Practice: definitions and privileges.* BOD P03-03-12-28 [Position]. Alexandria, VA: APTA; 2009. Available at: www.apta.org/AM/Template.cfm?Section=Home&TEMPLATE=/CM/ContentDisplay.cfm&CONTENTID=6742 (accessed 15 January 2014).

4. Larsen PO, von Ins M. The rate of growth in scientific publication and the decline in coverage provided by Science Citation Index. *Scientometrics.* 2010; **84**(3): 575–603.

5. Frenk J, Chen L, Bhutta ZA, *et al.* Health professionals for a new century: transforming education to strengthen health systems in an interdependent world. *Lancet.* 2010; **376**(9756): 1923–58.

6. Bayliss A, Warden SJ. A hybrid model of student-centered instruction improves physical therapist student performance in cardiopulmonary practice patterns by enhancing performance in higher cognitive domains. *J Phys Ther Educ.* 2011; **25**(3): 14–20.

7. Corrigan R, Hardham G. Use of technology to enhance student self evaluation and the value of feedback on teaching. *Int J Ther Rehabil.* 2011; **18**(10): 579–90.

8. McKeough DM, Mattern-Baxter K, Barakatt E. Effectiveness of a computer-aided neuroanatomy program for entry level physical therapy students: anatomy and clinical examination of the dorsal column-medial lemniscal system. *J Allied Health.* 2010; **39**(3): 156–64.

9. Willett GM, Sharp JG, Smith LM. A comparative evaluation of teaching methods in an introductory neuroscience course for physical therapy students. *J Allied Health.* 2008; **37**(3): e178–97.

10. Bonder BR, Hulisz D, Marsh S, *et al.* An interactive electronic instructional unit on substance abuse. *J Allied Health.* 2006; **35**(3): e215–26.

11. Simpson BP. Web-based and computer assisted instruction in physical therapist education. *J Phys Ther Educ.* 2002; **17**(2): 45–9.

12. Erickson ML. Examining the presence of computer-assisted instruction in physical therapy education. *J Allied Health.* 2004; **33**(4): 255–66.

13. Dal Bello-Haas V, Proctor P, Scudds R. Comparison of knowledge and knowledge application confidence in physical therapist students completing a traditional versus blended learning professional issues course. *J Phys Ther Educ.* 2013; **27**(1): 10–19.

14. Sangra A, Vlachopoulos D, Cabrera N. Building an inclusive definition of e-Learning: an approach to the conceptual framework. *Int Rev Res Open Dist Learn.* 2012; **3**(2): 145–59. Available at: www.irrodl.org/index.php/irrodl/article/view/1161/2146 (accessed 2 August 2013).

15. Wong CK, Abbruzzese L. Collaborative learning strategies using online communities. *J Phys Ther Educ.* 2011; **25**(3): 81–7.

16. Arroyo-Morales M, Cantarero-Villanueva I, Fernandez-Lao C, *et al.* A blended approach to palpation and ultrasound imaging skills through supplementation of traditional classroom teaching with an e-Learning package. *Man Ther.* 2012; **17**(5): 474–8.

17. Maloney S, Chamberlain M, Morrison S, *et al.* Health professional learner attitudes and use of digital learning resources. *J Med Internet Res.* 2013; **15**(1): e7. Available at: www.jmir.org/2013/1/e7/ (accessed 15 January 2014).

18. Barrows H, Tamblyn R. *Problem-Based Learning: an approach to medical education.* New York, NY: Springer; 1980.

19. Castro-Sánchez A, Aguilar-Ferrándiz ME, Matarán-Peñarrocha GA, *et al.* Problem based learning approaches to the technology education of physical therapy students. *Med Teach.* 2012; **34**(1): e29–45.

20. Suzuki S, Maruyama H. Influence of a problem-based learning tutorial on practical training of PT students. *J Phys Ther Sci.* 2010; **22**(1): 81–6.

21. Van Langenberghe H. Evaluation of students' approaches to studying in a problem-based physical therapy curriculum. *Phys Ther.* 1988; **68**(4): 522–9.

22. Titchen AC, Coles CR. Comparative study of physiotherapy students' approaches to their study in subject-centered and problem based-curricula. *Physiother Theory Pract.* 1991; **7**(2): 127–33.

23. Morris J. How strong is the case for the adoption of problem based learning in physiotherapy education in the United Kingdom? *Med Teach.* 2003; **25**(1): 24–31.

24. Gunn H, Hunter H, Haas B. Problem based learning in physiotherapy education: a practice perspective. *Physiotherapy.* 2012; **98**(4): 330–5.

25. Reynolds F. Initial experiences of interprofessional problem-based learning: a comparison of male and female students' views. *J Interprof Care.* 2003; **17**(1): 35–44.

26. Solomon P, Finch E. A qualitative study identifying stressors associated with adapting to problem based learning. *Teach Learn Med.* 1998; **10**(2): 58–64.

27. Kamwendo K, Tornquist K. Do occupational therapy and physiotherapy students care about research? A survey of perceptions and attitudes to research. *Scand J Caring Sci.* 2001; **15**(4): 295–302.

28. Health Professions Network Nursing and Midwifery Office, Department of Human Resources for Health. *Framework for Action on Interprofessional Education and Collaborative Practice.* Geneva: World Health Organization; 2010. Available at: http://whqlibdoc.who.int/hq/2010/WHO_HRH_HPN_10.3_eng.pdf (accessed 22 September 2013).

29. Eccott L, Grieg A, Hall W, *et al.* Evaluating students' perceptions of an interprofessional problem based pilot learning project. *J Allied Health.* 2012; **41**(4): 185–9.

30. Hayward LM, Canali A, Hill A. Interdisciplinary peer mentoring: a model for developing culturally competent health care professionals. *J Phys Ther Educ.* 2005; **19**(1): 28–40.

31. Davies K, Harrison K, Clouder DL, *et al.* Making the transition from physiotherapy student to interprofessional team member. *Physiotherapy.* 2011; **97**(2): 139–44.

32. Wamsley M, Staves J, Kroon L, *et al.* The impact of an interprofessional standardized patient exercise on attitudes toward working in interprofessional teams. *J Interprof Care.* 2012; **26**(1): 28–35.

33. Ateah CA, Snow W, Wener P, *et al.* Stereotyping as a barrier to collaboration: does interprofessional education make a difference. *Nurse Educ Today.* 2011; **31**(2): 208–13.

34. Jensen G, Saylor C. Portfolios and professional development in the health professions. *Eval Health Prof.* 1994; **17**(3): 344–7.

35. Pitts J, Coles C, Thomas P. Enhancing reliability in portfolio assessment: 'shaping' the portfolio. *Med Teach.* 2001; **23**(4): 351–6.

36. Hayward LM, Blackmer B, Canali A, *et al.* Reflective electronic portfolios: a design process for integrating liberal and professional studies and experiential education. *J Allied Health.* 2008; **37**(3): e140–59.

37. Cambridge BL. Digitized student portfolios. In: Cambridge BL, editor. *Electronic Portfolios: emerging practices in student, faculty, and institutional learning.* Washington, DC: American Association for Higher Education; 2001. pp. 53–9.

38. Heijne A, Nordgren B, Hagströmer M, *et al.* Assessment by portfolio in a physiotherapy programme. *Adv Physiother.* 2012; **14**(1): 38–46.

39. Senger JL, Kanthan R. Student evaluations: synchronous tripod of learning portfolio assessment: self-assessment, peer assessment, instructor assessment. *Creat Educ.* 2012; **3**(1): 155–63.

40. Pechak C, Black J. Exploring international clinical education in US-based programs: identifying common practices and modifying an existing conceptual model of international service-learning. *Physiother Theory Pract.* 2014; **30**(2): 94–104.

41. Black Lattanzi J, Pechak C. A conceptual framework for international service-learning course planning: promoting a foundation for ethical practice in the physical therapy and occupational therapy professions. *J Allied Health.* 2011; **40**(2): 103–9.

42. Hayward L, Charrette AL. Integrating cultural competence and core values: an international service-learning model. *J Phys Ther Educ.* 2012; **26**(1): 78–89.

43. Seifer S. Service learning community-campus partnerships for health professions education. *Acad Med.* 1998; **73**(3): 273–7.

44. Pechak C, Thompson J. A conceptual model of optimal international service-learning and its application to global health initiatives in rehabilitation. *Phys Ther.* 2009; **89**(11): 1192–204.

45. Albertine S. Undergraduate public health. *Am J Prev Med.* 2008; **35**(3): 253–7.

46. Stoltenberg M, Rumas N, Parsi K. Global health and service learning: lessons learned at US medical schools. *Med Educ Online.* Epub 2012 Jul 19.

47. Dal Bello-Haas V. Extreme makeover: entry-level physical therapist education edition. *J Phys Ther Educ.* 2013; **27**(1): 3–5.

48. Rowe M, Frantz J, Bozalek V. Physiotherapy students' use of online technology as part of their learning practices: a case study. *S Afr J Physiother.* 2012; **68**(1): 29–34.

49. Lapkin S, Levett-Jones T, Gilligan C. A systematic review of the effectiveness of interprofessional education in health professional programs. *Nurse Educ Today.* 2013; **33**(2): 90–102.

50. Solomon P. Interprofessional education: has its time come? *J Phys Ther Educ.* 2010; **24**(1): 3.

CHAPTER 29

Evidence-based education in speech-language pathology and audiology

*Sarah M Ginsberg, Colleen F Visconti
and Jennifer Friberg*

OVERVIEW

This chapter discusses evidence-based education in communication sciences and disorders (CSD), which includes speech-language pathology and audiology, as a critical consideration to ensure that teaching practices that lead to increased student learning are applied when designing courses and other learning opportunities for CSD students in a manner consistent with our signature pedagogy. The use of evidence-based practice (EBE) and the scholarship of learning and teaching in making pedagogical decisions in the CSD classroom are relatively new for the field. The inclusion of EBE in the decision process has the potential to change both deep and surface structures of the signature pedagogy of CSD. This chapter discusses EBE and signature pedagogy in CSD. In addition, information related to the importance of using active learning strategies is discussed. Specifically, the active learning strategies examined include evidence for the use of academic service-learning and problem-based learning within CSD and other related fields. The chapter concludes by discussing the use of various technologies – such as wikis, blogs, clickers, podcasts, YouTube and other social media – to support learning and actively engage students, while preparing future speech-language pathologists and audiologists. The information presented in the chapter will provide the reader with an overview of the current state of EBE within CSD and the limitations and challenges that we are facing as a discipline.

CHAPTER OBJECTIVES

Upon completion of this chapter, the reader will be able to:

- understand the concept of EBE in relation to CSD
- consider the signature pedagogy of his or her profession and the unique deep and surface demands faced by practitioners therein
- distinguish between passive and active learning strategies
- consider the uses of technology to augment and support teaching and learning in the traditional university classroom.

KEY TERMS: evidence-based education, scholarship of learning and teaching, communication sciences and disorders, active learning, academic service-learning, problem-based learning, technology to support learning, signature pedagogy

---

INTRODUCTION

Speech-language pathology and audiology are related but unique disciplines, often collectively referred to as 'communication sciences and disorders' (CSD). Speech-language pathologists work in a wide variety of settings, including public education, hospitals, rehabilitation facilities and private clinics, where they evaluate the speech, language and swallowing skills of children and adults. When disorders of speech, language, or swallowing are identified – the result of developmental issues, injury or disease processes – speech-language pathologists also develop treatment plans and provide therapeutic services to improve the ability of the individual to communicate or swallow functionally. Working with both children and adults, audiologists prevent, assess and treat hearing and balance disorders. They also dispense amplification systems, such as hearing aids. Audiologists may be employed in schools, hospitals, private clinics and within otorhinolaryngology practices. Audiologists and speech-language pathologists are typically educated in the same programmes at the undergraduate level, with graduate programmes dividing into separate, but related fields. Graduate education focuses on discipline specific knowledge and the development of the clinical skills needed for the specific discipline. For both fields, there is a strong emphasis in clinical and practical experiences.

In considering how CSD curricula are typically structured, it may prove useful to consider the predominant signature pedagogy of our disciplines. Shulman[1] described signature pedagogy as types of teaching that organise the fundamental ways in which future practitioners are educated for their new professions. He suggested that disciplines have a distinctive method of how they educate students that is often relatively consistent across institutions, school types or locations. One aspect of signature pedagogy, the surface structure, can be thought of as the tangible and viewable structures of teaching and learning. By answering questions such as 'How is the information being presented?' and 'What do the students do while learning?' the surface structure of a discipline's signature pedagogy can be uncovered. While there are always exceptions to the broad-brush description of a discipline's signature pedagogy, it is not uncommon for whole generations of professionals within a field to have had very similar educational experiences. In CSD courses, particularly at the undergraduate level, instructors have traditionally provided lectures to the class and conducted assessments through tests and research or term papers.[2]

Another aspect of signature pedagogy, deep structure, reflects why we teach the way we do, and the sequence of learning that is typical for a discipline. In CSD, it is common for students to learn about communication theory first, then normal communication development, followed by disordered communication, and then concluding with clinical and practical experiences, which are often community-based. This structure may reflect the belief that many faculty hold that fundamental theoretical knowledge serves as a prerequisite to learning about normal or disordered communication.[2] As a result of this deep structure, it is not until relatively late in the student's education that he or she begins actual hands-on clinical work in many pro-grammes. Again, not all programmes in all countries will follow this format; however, it is common practice in many universities.

MOVING FORWARD: EVIDENCE-BASED EDUCATION IN CSD

From the big-picture perspective, some of the most significant changes in teaching and learning in CSD reflect a potential shift in the signature pedagogy of our fields. The best evidence from teaching and learning studies reflects the trend seen in many other disciplines' research that suggests that increasing active learning and incorporating technology as appropriate are more effective and satisfying to the learner than traditional 'sit and get' or 'chalk and talk' lectures. As many faculty are consuming the teaching and learning literature from across a wide variety of clinical disciplines, the deep structure thinking of the CSD pedagogy is beginning to shift as faculty understand more about the need to integrate academic and clinical thinking. The surface structure changes to reflect this new way of thinking and faculty are beginning to move away from relying exclusively on the traditional lectures.

The emerging body of evidence within our discipline supports this paradigm shift. CSD faculty have become increasingly interested in the Scholarship of Learning and Teaching (SoLT) work, both as consumers and as researchers. In disciplines such as CSD where evidence-based clinical practice is a priority, there is a need to prioritise evidence-based education (EBE) when considering the most effective ways to educate future clinicians.[3] In order to build an EBE base for what CSD academics do as educators, it is essential that the SoLT work of educational researchers be made more public and accessible, through presentations and publications for peer review and interpretation. Because of a paucity of peer-reviewed publication outlets for CSD-specific SoLT work, CSD faculty have historically shared their work in a variety of contexts: general SoLT journals (e.g. *College Teaching*), textbooks related to SoLT in CSD,[3] book chapters in teaching and learning texts (such as this text), and through presentations at professional conferences. Heightened interest in SoLT has led to increases in visibility of SoLT work within CSD-specific research journals (e.g. *International Journal of*

Speech-Language Pathology and *Contemporary Issues in Communication Sciences and Disorders*) and the publication of a test issue of *Evidence-Based Education (EBE) Briefs*, a CSD-specific, peer-reviewed journal for SoLT work in CSD by Pearson Publishing.[4,5]

In reviewing the above literature and presentations, there are two trends that become clear foci of this work in our disciplines: the use of active learning strategies that focus on the integration of academic and clinical learning and the use of technology in preparing speech-language pathologists and audiologists. These trends will be used to organise and summarise the findings in the current EBE literature in CSD.

ACTIVE LEARNING IN CSD

Active learning occurs when students are able to increase their understanding of a particular concept or idea by actively engaging with someone or something in the instructional environment.[6] At the most basic level, active learning is considered to be the 'intersection of thinking and doing'[3] and is realised when transformative learning is evidenced in non-lecture-based educational experiences. Despite the importance of active learning, there is a lack of empirical research to support its use with students in speech-language pathology and audiology. Thus, we look to the work of other clinically based professions to better understand the appropriate use and application of active learning strategies within CSD.

Understanding that active learning must be designed purposefully, Wrenn and Wrenn[7] described specific dispositions for teachers in establishing active learning classrooms. Specifically, they described that teachers should focus on student learning outcomes, establish opportunities for students to actively engage with course materials, encourage the use of higher level critical thinking skills, and challenge students to develop their own value system to make judgements and determine the value of what is learned.

In CSD, active learning is particularly important as clinical practice is the eventual outcome for most graduates of our training programmes: as clinical practice is active, learning should be as well. As professionals we interact dynamically with our clients, their families and our co-workers. While rote memorisation and studying lecture notes may be necessary for understanding aspects of professional practice such as terminology and processes, they are not the best way for students to learn to be clinicians. Rather, collaborative, hands-on techniques that drive active learning have proven benefits to develop clinical thinking and problem-solving.[8] Further, research would indicate that hands-on, community-based learning is something that the current generation of students craves to aid in their learning, as these characteristics are inherent within students born in the last 25 years.[9] Thus, to foster high-quality learning experiences, active learning is realised in many different ways within CSD programmes. Two of the most popular types of active learning approaches in CSD are academic service-learning (ASL) and problem-based learning (PBL).

ACADEMIC SERVICE-LEARNING

Goldberg *et al.*[10] define academic service-learning ASL as 'experiential and reflective problem-based learning in which students enrolled in an academic course provide needed services to a community partner.'[(p131)] With ASL, course instructors find a community entity (e.g. school, shelter), with an identified need for services and provides those services as part of a course's design. For instance, in a speech sound disorders course, conducting speech screenings for incoming kindergarten students in a particular school or district would be considered ASL. Both parties would benefit from the completion of the project. The school would have help with mass screenings and students would gain experience with administering and interpreting a diagnostic screening test. Student learning could potentially increase because of the experience, not only in their knowledge of speech and language but also in their knowledge of young children. Peters[11] stated that, 'given that the field of CSD is inherently service driven, ASL can be a meaningful addition to both the undergraduate and graduate curricula.'[(pS181)]

Benefits of ASL have been discussed widely and include tangible outcomes, such as increased performance in class, increased understanding of how community partners function and operate, improved leadership skills; and intangible outcomes, such as improved personal and interpersonal development, greater appreciation for learning, and better satisfaction with the learning experience.[10,12] Recently, the *American Journal of Audiology* has published a research supplement within its journal describing how ASL could potentially support learning in undergraduate and graduate training programmes. Beyond the benefits already espoused here, researchers have identified benefits of ASL specific to CSD students. Specifically, active learning can assist in shaping the development of a clinical persona in future speech-language pathologists and audiologists. Across various types of ASL experiences, researchers determined that clinical experiences in 'real life' situations had the benefits of increasing students' interest in committing to a clinical career, improving attitudes towards individuals with disabilities, and furthering students' understanding of different cultures and languages.[13-15] Hoepner *et al.*[4] described assigning students to an 'immersion learning' experience to develop clinical abilities to work with patients with aphasia. By engaging in hands-on, mentored clinical experiences, students were able to increase their knowledge of aphasia, understand how to apply that knowledge, and commit to service excellence as developing clinicians. This level of active engagement with the content increases the likelihood that students will not only recall the information more effectively, but will also be able to integrate, synthesise, and analyse it for more effective application in clinic contexts. If we want our new clinicians to be effective clinical problem solvers and thinkers, giving them experiences in the classroom that help them make these connections is useful.

PROBLEM-BASED LEARNING

PBL is another active learning pedagogical method and is based on the thought that students learn more effectively when actively engaged in solving problems and realising solutions. Taylor and Mifflin[16] describe the progression of PBL in a typical classroom environment: (1) a problem is posed first, with no specific student preparation necessarily preceding the presentation of the problem; (2) students activate/articulate existing knowledge as the starting point of discussion in the problem-solving process; and (3) students engage in systematic reasoning about the problem, including applying new learning.

Research on the use of PBL has found that students engaged in PBL have better retention of content and course information,[17] increased clinical knowledge and performance,[18-20] and improved critical thinking.[21] Additionally, Visconti[17] found that the use of PBL was associated with increased student engagement and more time spent interacting with course content and materials. Furthermore, Greenwald[22] found that utilising PBL within a research methods course enabled the instructor to 'build directly on the student's current level of knowledge in clinical diagnosis and treatment and to help students extend clinical questions into research questions.'(p173)

Even though there are many benefits to using PBL, there are also several challenges associated with its use. The main challenge is using PBLs to design high-quality practical, authentic, real-life problems that are open ended in nature. One way to meet this challenge is to assess the quality of the problems. This can be accomplished by utilising a quality rating scale that assesses the problems based on five characteristics: 'the extent to which the problem (1) leads to learning objectives, (2) is familiar, (3) interests students, (4) stimulates critical reasoning, and (5) promotes collaborative learning.'[23](p43) Another solution is to have students both design and solve the problems. Lee[24] found that student involvement in the creation of the tasks and problem situations lead to an increase in learning authenticity or learning that resembles daily activities of professionals within the field, and enhance task performance and satisfaction. Furthermore, similar to developing clinical skills in the real world some students needed three to five attempts to reach mastery on PBL tasks, but this is dependent on the difficulty of the problem and the sequencing of the problems.[25]

PBL is a pedagogical approach that can be incorporated into a single course[17,22] or across the curriculum of a campus, such as that at University College Dublin.[26] Further, PBL allows for the use of technology,[27] can be used in as an approach for interprofessional education,[26] and is a pedagogical approach that actively engages the learner with the course material. Similar to ASL, PBL creates an opportunity for students to interact with the material at a higher level beyond recall.[28] This interaction allows students to use course content in a way that is meaningful and creates templates for clinical thinking required for successful postgraduate practice. The key to these pedagogical approaches is that the students no longer sit passively and receive the information, but are required to apply it in meaningful ways to real-life situations. This lays the groundwork for the clinical type of thinking and problem-solving that they will engage in whether they work in educational or healthcare-based settings.

TECHNOLOGY AND TEACHING IN CSD

As technology has advanced so too has its use within education and its impact on student learning. As Manning and Johnson[29] point out, 'the term *technology* often refers to the tools that are used to assist in the delivery of a curriculum.'[(p1)] The technology used must fit the learner, the content and the knowledge or skill that you are trying to teach.[30] However, one must remember that the use of technology does not guarantee student learning.[27] Technology needs to be intentionally integrated into the educational approach being used, and has the potential to change not only the way that we teach, but also what students learn.[27] Manning and Johnson[29] provide an in-depth examination of the variety of ways that technology can be used within the classroom, including the use of technology as a way to stay organised through the use of calendars, scheduling tools, and virtual storage and file management systems; to communicate and collaborate through discussion boards, blogs and wikis; to present course content by using tools such as podcasts, YouTube, and screencasting or screen captures; to assess learning by using rubrics, online quizzes, tests or surveys, and e-Portfolios; and to transform your identity by using avatars, virtual worlds or social networking.

Within CSD courses, technology can be used to create learning units to teach basic to more advanced concepts by incorporating PowerPoint presentations, videos, voice threads, among other technology either within or outside of the classroom setting. Utilising these types of technology outside of the classroom setting enables the instructor to flip the classroom. The instructor determines what information would be appropriate for students to learn outside of the classroom setting, which then leaves classroom time for more active learning tasks. Sams and Bergmann[31] pointed out that flipping the classroom is one way to utilise technology in order to create a student-centred classroom. In addition, they concluded that 'videos were valuable in shifting the lower levels of Bloom's taxonomy out of the class'[31(p16)] and allowed class time to be spent on upper levels of the taxonomy. Wikis and discussion boards can also be utilised to actively engage students in learning. Wikis 'allows a group of users to update and edit text collaboratively',[29(p1)] while at the same time maintaining the history of the document. Finan[32] discussed the use of various forms of technology in a speech science course including wikis, and points out the strengths of the wikis being open discussions, freedom of class members to edit the information, use of a variety of resources by students to compliment the discussion, and the responsibility that students then have for searching for and analysing information obtained. Using wikis to support faculty development, Folkins *et al.*[33] developed a wiki for CSD faculty teaching or planning to teach an Introduction to Communication Sciences and Disorders course. This wiki was established to share classroom activities, resources that participants have found useful, assignments, assessment information, textbook recommendations, and general information regarding any topic.

Discussion boards are similar to wikis in that they promote communication among students; however, they are different because students are not creating a collaborative text, but rather reading previous posts and responding to them. The goal of the discussion board is to encourage student communication.[29] Research conducted with

20 oral health and dentistry students found that the use of online reflective group discussions enabled the third-year students to develop a mentoring role and professional leadership attributes, while the first-year students were provided with guidance and support in the development of foundational knowledge of the field.[34] The use of discussion boards was examined in a graduate level Augmentative and Alternative Communication course.[35] Discussion boards were found to be an efficient use of class time by allowing class time to be spent providing additional demonstrations and presentations, since the discussions were taking place outside of the classroom. In addition, the discussion boards were an effective way to generate discussion and student reflections; however, it did require the professor to play a fundamental role in generating prompts and monitoring the discussion.[35] Thus, wikis and discussion boards can be utilised to further develop content knowledge, professional skills, communication and collaboration between students.

Technology in the form of audio and video files has also been utilised within CSD courses. Audio files frequently take the form of podcasts, which are 'audio files saved to a website using RSS technologies that allow users to subscribe to a syndication feed and be automatically notified when new content is available.'[29(p1)] Tools such as Audacity, GarageBand or Propaganda can be utilised to create the audio files. The American Speech-Language-Hearing Association website has podcasts posted on topics including hearing and hearing loss, advocacy, healthcare, literacy, traumatic brain injury, aphasia, early intervention, research, language delay, autism and many others (http://podcast.asha.org/). Podcasts have also been used within undergraduate and graduate courses in CSD. Friberg[36] found that podcasts used within a Professional Issues in Speech Pathology and Audiology course helped students understand course content and procedures, learn about specific professional issues, and retain course content better. The students felt that the use of podcasts within the course enhanced their course experience.

Blood and Blood[37] utilised not only podcasts, but also Google, YouTube, wikis, discussion boards and other technology within their CSD 101 Preventing Hearing Loss online course that 2745 students completed from 2003 to 2011. The students were positive about the learning experience and the online course lead to students being successful in learning 'new knowledge and skills about hearing, hearing loss, and the negative impact of noise across the lifespan.'[37(p4)]

Within the classroom setting audience response systems or clicker technology has been found to be useful in actively engaging students with course content. Clickers are an interactive device that allows the instructor to pose questions and the students to anonymously participate in real time using an audience response device. From a faculty perspective the use of clicker technology was found to increase student participation and engagement by expanding the class discussion through the elimination of group bias, and provides a quick assessment of student learning which therefore enables faculty members to identify areas of confusion.[38] The benefits to students were that they perceived that they increased their understanding of the course content, were better able to identify material that they needed to study further, and the technology made the course fun.[39] In addition, evidence supports the students' perceptions of improved learning in that students using clicker technology scored higher on measures of academic performance than students not using the technology.[39]

The use of technology can be valuable as another tool to increase student engagement with the content to be learned. However, as noted earlier, it is critical for instructors to identify technology that fits the learners and the content that is being taught. Technology used for the sake of entertainment is less likely to increase the effectiveness of teaching and student learning. As the studies cited here show, when the technology increases the students' opportunities to interact with the content being taught, it improves learning outcomes in much the same ways as non-technological-based active learning strategies do. In short, it is seen that any time when students are provided with the opportunity to apply their newfound knowledge in the classroom setting, they are more likely to be effective with that information in clinics.[2]

The disciplines of audiology and speech-language pathology are relatively new to SoLT. The movement of understanding what is happening in CSD learning environments has only begun gaining a foothold in the last 10 years. The research by authors cited in this chapter has done wonders for developing a foundation for EBE in CSD; however, it is only the beginning. While much of the focus of SoLT in CSD referenced here has been on new, more active ways of engaging learners than what were used 20–30 years ago, there is much that is still not known. For instance, various accrediting bodies across the globe mandate specific standards of education and clinical preparation (e.g. standards or mandatory hours of clinical practicum), yet it is unclear whether these mandates reflect best practices in educating future speech-language pathologists and audiologists. Future research will need to focus on informing clinical and educational standards so that CSD pedagogical methods and requirements are based on solid evidence. Additionally, interprofessional education is a topic generating both attention and study from academicians as ways to educate students in complementary fields (e.g. CSD, nursing, nutrition and dietetics, physiotherapy, occupational therapy, social work) to improve job performance and patient outcomes following graduation and licensure. The effectiveness of this model will need to be closely followed to determine its effectiveness as a curricular innovation for students in CSD.

SUMMARY POINTS

- Most disciplines have a signature pedagogy[1] that constitutes the ways in which students are prepared to practise in various professions. This signature pedagogy includes deep (why we teach the way we do) and surface (observable aspects of learning) structures, and interactions between these define contemporary practice in teaching and learning. The signature pedagogy for CSD is emerging as increased attention is being paid to the need to apply evidence-based educational techniques in CSD classrooms and clinics.
- Focus on EBE and the SoLT is relatively new to CSD. At this time, discipline specific outlets are limited. As a result, there is a paucity of work specifically within the professions and there is a dependence on related fields.

- Active learning occurs when students are able to increase their understanding of a particular concept or idea by actively engaging with someone or something in the instructional environment.[6] Two approaches to such learning, ASL and PBL, actively engage students in thinking, applying and synthesising information as part of the learning process with the intention of encouraging deeper, lasting learning by students.
- Technology, the use of tools that can assist in the delivery of a curriculum, have been demonstrated to be effective in teaching and learning in CSD. Technology that has been proven to be valuable includes videos, wikis and discussion boards. Materials found on social media sites, such as YouTube, and podcasts are also useful to faculty in CSD to improve learning, particularly by increasing student engagement.

REVIEW QUESTIONS

- What are the surface and deep structures which support the signature pedagogy of your discipline?
- How does the signature pedagogy of your discipline differ from CSD?
- What are the benefits of using active learning in higher education?
- Identify two active learning strategies that are used in teaching speech-language pathology and audiology students and which could be applied in your own classroom.
- What technologies may be useful to increase the active learning of students in clinical fields?
- What are the benefits of using clicker audience response systems in teaching?

REFLECTIVE QUESTIONS AND EXERCISES

- Think about teaching and learning strategies that have been used in the CSD professions and then consider what strategies could also be applied in your field.
- PBL is used in a number of different health professions to educate students. What are the similarities and differences between how PBL has been used to education CSD students and students from other health professions?
- How might an interprofessional education session that includes CSD, physiotherapy, occupational therapy, and nutrition and dietetics students be structured to promote optimal learning outcomes?

REFERENCES

1. Shulman LS. Signature pedagogies in the professions. *Daedalus*. 2005; **134**(3): 52–9.
2. Brackenbury T, Folkins JW, Ginsberg SM. The signature pedagogy of communication sciences and disorders. *Contemp Iss Commun Sci Disord*. 2014: in press.
3. Ginsberg SM, Friberg JC, Visconti CF. *The Scholarship of Teaching and Learning in Speech-Language Pathology and Audiology: evidence-based education*. San Diego, CA: Plural Publishing; 2012.
4. Hoepner JK, Clark MB, Sather T, *et al*. Immersion Learning at Aphasia Camp. *EBE Briefs: Evidence-Based Education*. Pearson Education; 2012. Available at: www.speechandlanguage.com/wp-content/uploads/2012/11/EBE_briefs_ImmersionLearning.pdf (accessed 14 January 2014).
5. Dudding CC. *Fostering Communication in Online CSD Offerings. EBE Briefs: Evidence-Based Education*. Pearson Education; 2012. Available at: www.speechandlanguage.com/wp-content/uploads/2012/11/EBE_briefs_FosteringComm.pdf (accessed 14 January 2014).
6. Prince M. Does active learning work? A review of the research. *J Eng Educ*. 2004; **93**(3): 223–31.
7. Wrenn J, Wrenn B. Enhancing learning by integrating theory and practice. *Int J Teach Learn High Educ*. 2009; **21**(2): 258–68.
8. Fink LD. *Creating Significant Learning Experiences: an integrated approach to designing college courses*. San Francisco, CA: Jossey-Bass; 2003.
9. Svinicki M. New directions in learning and motivation. In: Svinicki MD, editor. *Teaching and Learning on the Edge of the Millennium: building on what we have learned*. San Francisco, CA: Jossey-Bass; 1999. pp. 5–28.
10. Goldberg L, McCormick Richburg C, Wood L. Active learning through service learning. *Commun Disord Q*. 2006; **27**(3): 131–45.
11. Peters KA. Including service learning in the undergraduate CSD curriculum: benefits, challenges and strategies for success. *Am J Audiol*. 2011; **20**: S181–96.
12. Simons L, Cleary B. The influence of service learning on students' personal and social development. *Coll Teach*. 2006; **54**(4): 307–19.
13. Kaf WA, Strong EC. The promise of service learning in a paediatric audiology course on clinical training with the paediatric population. *Am J Audiol*. 2011; **20**: S220–32.
14. Kaf WA, Barboa LS, Fisher BJ, *et al*. Effect of interdisciplinary service learning experiences for audiologists and speech-language pathology students working with adults with dementia. *Am J Audiol*. 2011; **20**: S241–9.
15. Reading S, Padgett R. Communication connections: service learning and American sign language. *Am J Audiol*. 2011; **20**: S197–202.
16. Taylor D, Mifflin B. Problem-based learning: where are we now? *Med Teach*. 2009; **30**(8): 742–63.
17. Visconti CF. Problem-based learning: teaching skills for evidence-based practice. *Perspect Iss High Educ*. 2010; **13**(1): 27–31.
18. Baker CM, McDaniel AM, Pesut DJ, *et al*. Learning skills of masters students in nursing administration: Assessing the impact of problem-based learning. *Nurs Educ Perspect*. 2007; **28**(4): 190–5.
19. Leahy MM, Dodd BJ, Walsh IP, *et al*. Education for practice in the UK and Ireland: implementing problem-based learning. *Folia Phoniatr Logop*; 2006: **58**(1): 48–54.
20. Weismer M. Problem-based learning: benefits and risks. *Teach Prof*. 2007; **21**(2): 5.
21. Schmidt H, van der Molen H, te Winkel WWR. Constructivist, problem-based learning does work: a meta-analysis of curricular comparisons involving a single medical school. *Educ Psychol*. 2009; **44**(4): 227–49.
22. Greenwald ML. Teaching research methods in communication disorders: a problem-based learning approach. *Commun Disord Q*. 2006; **27**(3): 173–9.
23. Sockalingam N, Rotgans J, Schmidt H. Assessing the quality of problems in problem-based learning. *Int J Teach Learn High Educ*. 2012; **24**(1): 43–51.

24. Lee HW. User-design approach in problem development and its effect on authenticity, performance, and satisfaction in problem-based learning. *Asian-Pacific Educ Res*. 2012; **21**(3): 526–34.

25. Kuruganti U, Needham T, Zundel P. Patterns and rates of learning in two problem-based learning courses using outcome based assessment and elaboration theory. *Can J Scholarsh Teach Learn*. 2012; **3**(1): 1–13.

26. Barrett T, Cashman D, editors. *A Practitioners' Guide to Enquiry and Problem-Based Learning*. Dublin: UCD Teaching and Learning; 2010.

27. Donnelly R. Using technology to support project and problem-based learning. In: Barrett T, Mac Labhrainn I, Fallon H, editors. *Handbook of Enquiry and Problem Based Learning*. Galway: CELT; 2005. pp. 157–77. Available at: www.nuigalway.ie/celt/pblbook/chapter16.pdf (accessed 14 January 2014).

28. Bloom BS. *Taxonomy of Educational Objectives: the classification of educational goals. Handbook I: cognitive domain*. New York, NY: Longmans, Green; 1956.

29. Manning S, Johnson KE. *The Technology Toolbelt for Teaching*. San Francisco, CA: Jossey-Bass; 2011.

30. Morrison GR, Ross SM, Kemp JE. *Designing Effective Instruction*. 5th ed. Hoboken, NJ: John Wiley & Sons; 2007.

31. Sams A, Bergmann J. Flip your students' learning. *Educ Leader*. 2013; **70**(6): 16–20.

32. Finan DS. Speech science education: roll over Beethoven. *Perspect Speech Sci Orofac Disord*. 2008; **18**(1): 22–30.

33. Folkins JW, Behrman A, Self TL, *et al*. A wiki to support teaching the course: introduction to Communication Sciences and Disorders. *Perspect Iss High Educ*. 2012; **15**(1): 3–10.

34. Tsang AKL. Online reflective group discussion: connecting first year undergraduate students with their third year peers. *J Scholarsh Teach Learn*. 2011; **11**(3): 58–74.

35. McCarthy J, Schock M, Zojwala R. Electronic discussion boards to enhance graduate student learning in AAC [Poster]. *The American Speech-Language-Hearing Association convention*; Miami, FL; 2006.

36. Friberg JC. The use of supplementary podcasting as an instructional tool in an online classroom setting. *Perspect Iss High Educ*. 2008; **11**(2): 61–6.

37. Blood IM, Blood GW. Podcasts, Google, and YouTube – Oh My! An innovative online course for university students on preventing hearing loss. *Perspect Pub Health Iss Rel Hear Bal*. 2011; **12**(1): 4–12.

38. Visconti CF. Audience response systems: a mode for enhancing student learning [Poster]. *The American Speech-Language-Hearing Association convention*. Miami, FL; 2006.

39. Powell S, Straub C, Rodrigues J, *et al*. Using clickers in large college psychology classes: academic achievement and perceptions. *J Scholarsh Teach Learn*. 2011; **11**(4): 1–11.

CHAPTER 30

Evidence-based education in nursing and midwifery

....

Lisa McKenna

OVERVIEW

Evidence-based practice has been a focus of nursing and midwifery education for many years. Students are encouraged to apply their clinical decisions on best available evidence for practice. In the delivery of education, nursing and midwifery academics have reported on a vast amount of related research resulting in an extensive body of knowledge. However, much of the research reports on small-scale, localised studies that make broader application difficult. This chapter presents an overview of evidence-based education in the disciplines of nursing and midwifery. While recognising the existing value and scope of evidence available, it is argued that there is a need for larger scale studies involving teaching and learning strategies and learning outcomes, and interpretations of smaller studies through systematic reviews and meta-analyses to facilitate greater applicability into other contexts, not only in nursing and midwifery, but into other health professions.

CHAPTER OBJECTIVES

Upon completion of this chapter, the reader will be able to:

- outline strengths and weaknesses in the evidence base for education in nursing and midwifery
- identify differences in evidence-based education between nursing and midwifery
- identify areas for priority development of evidence to inform education across the two disciplines.

KEY TERMS: evidence-based education, midwifery, nursing

INTRODUCTION

Evidence-based practice has been widely advocated and taught in the disciplines of nursing and midwifery for many years. Nurses and midwives have engaged in diverse research aimed at improving patient care and prevention of illness, as well as educationally focused research around teaching and learning in the two disciplines. Yet, evidence to support teaching and learning varies in quality and scope.[1] This chapter argues that internationally educators have engaged in extensive research around education in nursing and midwifery. Despite this, there is still a need for rigorous research that seeks to evaluate the effectiveness of teaching and learning interventions and further informs evidence-based education, in particular with relation to curricula and teaching and learning methodologies.

EVIDENCE-BASED EDUCATION

The practice of nursing and midwifery education entails a range of activities including teaching, coordinating and evaluating learning in classroom and clinical environments, as well as designing and implementing curricula. However, as Emerson and Records[2] assert, these activities are 'not sufficient to build the scientific knowledge base required for that education to take place.'[(p359)]

There is no doubt that nurses and midwives have readily engaged in educationally focused research activities. In an analysis of journal publications by Australian nurses between 2004 and 2008, Wilkes and Jackson[3] found nursing education to be the second most highly researched topic, constituting 24.3% of publications in Australian journals, and the sixth-highest topic internationally. Yet, despite the high engagement in education research, Oermann[4] argued that

> Nurse educators often make their decisions about what and how to teach based on tradition, how they were taught, or expert opinion without thinking about whether evidence might be available to guide their educational practices.[(p250)]

Thus, despite having evidence available, and professional competencies for educators articulating the requirement for application of evidence-based teaching practice, educators may still not be teaching from an evidence-based position.[5] This raises two main possibilities: either the available research is unsuitable to use to inform teaching practice, or there is reluctance in applying evidence to teaching practice. It can be surmised, therefore, that a divide exists between the educational research being conducted, its influence on teaching and learning practices and its overall utilisation.

THE CURRENT STATE OF PLAY IN NURSING AND MIDWIFERY

Research in nursing education has a long history in comparison with other health professions. There are increasing numbers of journals dedicated to this specific aspect of nursing and indications that nursing education research continues to grow (*see* Table 30.1). Yet, a large gap seemingly exists between the research being conducted and its application into practice. While educators regularly teach students about evidence-based clinical practice, it is unclear whether they also use evidence to inform their own teaching practice.[1] One reason postulated for nursing academics' difficulty in translating existing research to their teaching is the often localised, and small scale of, studies undertaken, and use of tools individually developed by the particular researcher.[4] Furthermore, like other areas of nursing and midwifery

TABLE 30.1 Journals specific to nursing, midwifery and health professional education

Education category	Journal title
Nursing and midwifery education specific	*Clinical Simulation in Nursing*
	International Journal of Nursing Education Scholarship
	Journal for Nurses in Staff Development
	Journal of Continuing Education in Nursing
	Journal of Nursing Education
	Nurse Educator
	Nurse Education in Practice
	Nurse Education Today
	Nursing Education Perspectives
	Teaching and Learning in Nursing
Health professional education	*Advances in Health Sciences Education*
	Education for Health
	Focus on Health Professional Education
	International Journal of Clinical Skills
	Simulation in Healthcare
	The Clinical Teacher
	Work-based Learning in Primary Care

research, there has been considerable emphasis on qualitative research, which while adding important knowledge to the existing evidence base around education, may not be generalisable to other populations or settings, or may be difficult to translate into practice. Further impacting on the ability of researchers to conduct large-scale education research is the difficulty in securing funding for non-scientific research. Particularly noteworthy in the context of increasingly complex and evolving disciplines is that limited nursing and midwifery education research examines such important aspects as curriculum development, ideal curriculum structure or testing of pedagogical approaches.

EVIDENCE GENERATION IN NURSING EDUCATION

The literature highlights particular areas where research in nursing education is more common. Broadly speaking, such research often falls into one of four main categories: (1) clinical education, (2) teaching approaches, (3) student-focused and (4) curriculum-related research. Table 30.2 provides a summary of commonly emerging research topics in nursing education journals. Most often, there are reports of practical aspects of nursing education, while notably there is an overall lack of research into effective pedagogical foundations for teaching and learning interventions. Moreover, often, student-focused education is undertaken with undergraduate students, with some beginning to emerge on graduate entry programmes. Less student-focused research examines the experiences of postgraduate students, either in clinical or theoretically based programmes, or at doctoral level, highlighting a need for more evidence in these areas.

Over many years, there has been an abundance of research exploring multiple facets of clinical education in nursing, hence the evidence base in that area is strong. Such research has explored a broad array of topics such as evaluating the effectiveness of different local partnerships/collaborations between academia and practice, such as dedicated education units (DEUs), or other models for the delivery of education. In DEUs, students work more closely alongside clinical staff who provide their coaching and mentoring. Academic staff engage in a less hands-on role through guiding clinical staff on aspects of education and encouraging research within the unit. Mulready-Shick et al.[6] recently undertook a randomised controlled trial to evaluate the effectiveness of DEUs on student learning. They found that these delivered more significant learning outcomes and higher-quality education than traditional clinical teaching models where groups of students are taught in the clinical setting by an academic staff member.[6] Much research has also considered the teaching of clinical practice with extensive available literature around clinical teaching, facilitation, mentor and preceptor roles,[7-9] and students' perspectives on their clinical learning experiences.[10-12] For example, McIntosh et al.[13] conducted focus groups with 120 final-year midwifery students in the United Kingdom, exploring their perceptions of learning to be midwives. Little research, however, has examined pedagogical issues associated with the structure of clinical placements or clinical learning and their impact on student learning outcomes.

TABLE 30.2 Contemporary research areas in nursing education

Broad category	Common foci
Clinical education	Clinical education models (e.g. dedicated education units)
	Clinical skills
	Clinical teaching and facilitation
	Competency
	Preceptorship and mentorship
Teaching approaches	Case-based learning
	Critical thinking
	e-Learning and use of multimedia
	Peer-assisted learning
	Portfolios
	Problem-based learning
	Simulation
	Small educational interventions
Student-related	Attitudes and perceptions
	Attributes (e.g. empathy, communication skills)
	Professional identity and socialisation
	Recruitment, retention and attrition
	Student experience
	Transition to professional practice
Curriculum-related	Accelerated or second degree programmes
	Cultural safety and competency
	Informatics
	Interprofessional education
	Patient safety
	Primary care
	Quality

Varying amounts of research have explored pedagogical approaches to nursing education, however, there remain significant gaps. Of particular note in this area, over recent years there has been a strong trend towards research into simulation in nursing. In one example, Buykx et al.[14] developed a simulation-based educational model using a patient actor to assist nursing students to develop their emergency management and clinical skills in patient deterioration. These researchers applied the model to undergraduate nursing students, undergraduate and postgraduate midwifery students, and registered nurses, concluding that the model was both effective and adaptable to different learner groups.[14] Yet, evidence suggests that educators may still not readily understand its value to their teaching. It continues to be argued that there remains a clear need for further research demonstrating 'efficacy of simulation in nurse education and to build a supporting evidence base.'[15(p245)] Clearly, while research is being readily undertaken into simulation in nursing contexts, it may not be providing substantive evidence to support implementation into teaching practice. Besides simulation, only pockets of research have examined effectiveness of teaching and learning approaches and new, potentially valuable, innovations.

While some research exists, there is still much scope to examine aspects related to the nursing curriculum more broadly. Some recent studies have focused on new approaches to nursing curricula such as accelerated and graduate entry programmes, usually for individuals with qualifications in other disciplines to become entry-level nurses.[16] However, more work needs to be undertaken on traditional nursing curricula and their suitability in a rapidly changing world. Research around how nursing education is delivered, what content should be covered in contemporary nursing courses, and teaching of particular topic areas is particularly lacking.

There has been a steady stream of research exploring development of nursing students throughout their journeys as students and into the transition of being professional practitioners.[17–20] Some studies have explored development of professional attributes, such as empathy,[21,22] caring and communication skills.[23] However, little is available to inform those trying to develop such attributes about the most effective means for achieving such ends, that is, the teaching and learning strategies that can be employed to most effectively facilitate the development of such attributes.

While nurses have been active researchers in the education space for a long period, the scope of resulting research has been variable. Some areas, such as clinical education and simulation, have been well researched, while others, such as curriculum development approaches and pedagogical research, are more limited. There is clearly a need for a focused approach to the generation of evidence to support nursing education. In the United States, Valiga and Ironside[24] advocate the need for creating a national agenda for nursing education research to ensure the education that is delivered is scientifically informed. However, it could be argued that this is not an issue limited to one country, but rather an issue for educators within the nursing profession internationally to strive to address.

EVIDENCE GENERATION IN MIDWIFERY EDUCATION

In many countries, midwifery has been subsumed until recent years under the umbrella of nursing. In Australia, direct entry, undergraduate midwifery education was first introduced in 2002. Prior to this time, a nursing qualification was required for entry into postgraduate midwifery programmes.[25] As a result, the specific evidence base for teaching and learning in midwifery has been previously dependent upon what was conducted in nursing, despite the two disciplines having very different philosophies of care and scope of clinical practice.[26] Given this, midwifery education's own evidence base is much more limited in breadth and relatively recent.

The discipline is yet to have its own professional journal dedicated to its education and currently that appears to be the case well into the future. Midwifery researchers are much fewer in number and across the discipline generally there is much to be done. Areas of education research are evolving but have focused to date largely on clinical education and students' course experiences (*see* Table 30.3). There is a clear need for more research that informs pedagogical approaches to midwifery education, not merely an assumption that what works in nursing will work for midwifery. In addition, there is a particular gap in research that supports the philosophical tenets of wellness and woman-centredness in midwifery curricula within clinical learning contexts that are medicalised and interventionist,[27] as well as in other areas such as the provision of childbirth education by midwives.[28]

TABLE 30.3 Contemporary research areas in midwifery education

Broad category	Common foci
Clinical education	Clinical assessment
	Clinical education models
	Continuity of care and follow-through journeys
	Competence
	Clinical teaching
	Preceptorship and mentoring
Teaching approaches	Simulation
	Storytelling
Student-related	Attitudes and perceptions
	Attributes (e.g. empathy, communication skills)
	Professional identity and socialisation
	Recruitment, retention and attrition
	Student experience
	Transition to professional practice
Curriculum	Interprofessional education
	Quality

KEY ISSUES FOR NURSING AND MIDWIFERY EDUCATION EVIDENCE GENERATION

The previous analysis of nursing and midwifery education research highlights the existence of a number of key issues that warrant closer attention. First, much of the existing research conducted is based on perceptions or experiences of students or educators. Often, this is undertaken using qualitative methods with findings difficult to transfer to other populations. Second, there is a dearth of research into the effectiveness of actual teaching methods used by educators. Third, much of the existing research is based on small populations, again making generalisability difficult.

PERCEPTIONS-BASED RESEARCH

An extensive number of studies in nursing and midwifery education research have examined perceptions of students and/or staff with regard to a range of aspects relating to education. Abundantly occurring is research relating to student or staff perceptions of clinical learning or placements. While perceptions-based research is important, such approaches provide little direction for guiding evidence-based education practice. These are generally small-scale studies, they notably employ a variety of methodologies and they often employ qualitative approaches.[9,10,17] Hence, while such research is of interest to educators, findings may be applicable only to local contexts in which they have been conducted and have limited ability to inform best practice education more broadly.

RESEARCHING TEACHING AND LEARNING APPROACHES

One of the limitations in research in nursing and midwifery education is a lack of research into teaching methods commonly employed by educators, and their effectiveness that can directly inform curricula. Such studies have the ability to inform best practice in education for optimal student learning outcomes. In a study at one Australian university, McKenna et al.[29] used scenarios with simulated patients to examine final-year nursing students' history taking skills. Video recordings were reviewed and analysed, resulting in identification of deficits in students' skills in interpersonal interactions, questioning techniques and missed cues requiring further questioning. Focus groups with students further affirmed the existence of deficits in history taking skills. Findings directly informed curriculum change to ensure students more effectively developed their history taking skills.[29]

The teaching of clinical skills is fundamental in nursing and midwifery. However, the evidence to inform effective teaching of these is limited in many areas.[30] As a result, many skills are taught using traditional approaches, despite the potential for more effective methods. Comparing different approaches for teaching a particular skill can lead to identifying best practice. In a large American study, Kardong-Edgren et al.[31] compared two approaches to teaching cardiopulmonary resuscitation to nursing students: an instructor-led approach with traditional manikins and a computer-based course. They measured compression rates, depth and hand placement, as well as volume of ventilation. Students who had the computer-based approach performed better on compression depth, ventilation volume and correct hand placement. Hence, their findings supported use of the computer-based approach.[31] In a subsequent study, Oermann et al.[32] examined the impact of monthly cardiopulmonary resuscitation practice at 3, 6, 9 and 12 months on nursing students' skill performance. In this study, the researchers used a control group who did not receive the monthly practice. They found that the study group retained their ability to ventilate and continued to improve, while the control group demonstrated a significant loss in their compression ability over a 12-month period. The researchers concluded that regular practice was fundamental to retaining effective performance levels.[32]

RESEARCHING THE CURRICULUM

Interestingly, despite the extensive variation in nursing curricula internationally, there is little research evidence base to inform curriculum development and content. In a systematic review of curriculum evaluation, Roxburgh et al.[33] in the United Kingdom concluded that there was insufficient evidence to support curriculum decision-making with their review identifying some localised studies with limited rigour. The researchers advocated the need for rigorous research around nursing curricula that includes content through to outcomes.[33] In one of the few available studies that could be used to inform curriculum development, Kumm and Fletcher[34] reported on one American nursing school's process of curriculum reform that employed a systematic three phase approach with a combination of theory, research findings, and faculty participation to inform development. Such approaches to research and scholarship are vital to inform future directions and best practice for nursing education and ensure that graduates produced meet workplace and professional expectations.

Nursing and midwifery education is continually evolving. Research around new and innovative curricula is important to understanding the impact of such education programmes and needs of students entering. For example, in some countries, such as the United States and Australia, accelerated pre-registration programmes for graduates from other disciplines are gaining in popularity.[16,35] Students can vary greatly from those entering traditional education programmes, hence may have different educational needs. Extensive research is needed to examine these programmes to ensure they meet student and industry needs. McKenna and Vanderheide[16] reported on characteristics of students entering one such programme in Australia, finding higher proportions of male students than traditional courses, as well as extensive cultural and professional diversity, aspects that need to be considered in the way such programmes are delivered. More research is needed in this area to assess the subsequent impact of such learners on the profession.

POTENTIAL IN SYSTEMATIC REVIEWS

The use of systematic reviews has recently begun to gain momentum in nursing education and offers much in informing teaching and learning. This approach offers possibilities to collate abundant small-scale studies into meaningful outcomes that can inform education and further research. In one study, Cant et al.[36] employed systematic review to examine best approaches to objective assessment of nursing students' clinical skills. The study accessed research conducted between January 2000 and May 2011. Initial search yielded 92 publications, which after consideration of inclusion criteria, resulted in 16 being included. Variety was found in the types of skills assessments employed. Analysis resulted in the conclusion that objective assessments of clinical skills, such as objective structured clinical examination, were necessary in nursing education. However, there was a need for further research to ensure valid and reliable assessment tools. The authors recommended a large study with consideration being giving to development of nationally consistent assessment tools for clinical skills assessments.[36]

In another example, Eick et al.[37] conducted a systematic review of clinical placement-related student attrition in nursing education. Their review included both quantitative and qualitative studies from 1995 to July 2011. A total of 18 studies met their inclusion criteria. Findings suggested that personal factors influenced an individual student's decision to leave his or her course, and this was often based around the student's belief in his or her own abilities and peer support. The researchers concluded that approaches to reducing student attrition needed to be multifaceted. Furthermore, they identified methodological issues relating to the definition of placement-related attrition within existing research.[37]

RECOMMENDATIONS

Healthcare systems are changing continually. There is a resulting need for nursing and midwifery curricula to respond to changes, both theoretically and clinically, including how material is delivered to learners.[38] It is unsatisfactory to deliver education based on traditional, out-dated approaches just because this is how it has always been done. The need for research around nursing and midwifery curricula is imperative to guide innovative and responsive curricula. In particular, there is a need for 'sound data about graduates' performance and the effects on client care, both of which may be linked to the educational and philosophical approaches that underlie nursing education programs.'[39(n.p.)]

There is a clear need for more rigorous studies, including, where possible, randomised controlled trials of particular education innovations. Yet, it is acknowledged that the realities of conducting larger-scale investigations, such as lack of funding and access to large populations, may limit these. With a dearth of larger, but a wealth of smaller and potentially valuable, studies available to guide nursing and midwifery educators, it is also recommended that systematic reviews and meta-syntheses would allow for critique and collation of findings and make them more accessible to inform teaching and learning. Generally speaking, there appears to be a need for more pedagogical evidence for the interventions being employed by nursing and midwifery educators.

CONCLUSION

While nursing and midwifery academics are experienced at teaching evidence-based practice, they are less inclined to use evidence themselves to inform their teaching and learning. There is need 'to facilitate the paradigm shift, preparing nurse educators to question how they assess, teach and evaluate students.'[40(p245)] Investment in developing teaching staff in nursing and midwifery towards using, and developing, evidence to support and inform their teaching and learning practices, as well as to continue building the body of evidence on which to base education practice is important. This is especially necessary within the current climate of education change and curriculum renewal.

SUMMARY POINTS

- The need for evidence-based practice has been a focus of nursing and midwifery education for many years. Students are instructed how to apply their clinical decisions on best available evidence for practice.
- Nursing and midwifery academics and researchers have generated a vast array of evidence on education over recent decades. Applying this evidence into education practice has been difficult because of the size and scale of many studies undertaken.
- This chapter has explored evidence-based education across the disciplines of nursing and midwifery. In light that much valuable evidence exists, there is a need for larger-scale studies to inform education practice.
- Interpretations of groups of smaller studies through systematic reviews and meta-analyses will assist with applicability into other education settings, not only in nursing and midwifery but also in other health professions, and enhancing usability of existing evidence.
- Furthermore, there is a need for more research focusing on the effectiveness of teaching and learning strategies and their learning outcomes.

REVIEW QUESTIONS

- What are the biggest challenges facing nursing and midwifery evidence-based education? What strategies could be employed to assist tackling these?
- What areas should nursing and midwifery education researchers and academics focus most heavily on developing?
- Nursing and midwifery were traditionally task-focused occupations without strong evidence bases to support practice change. How can nursing and midwifery educators be encouraged to embrace evidence-based education over their traditional practices?

REFLECTIVE QUESTIONS AND EXERCISES

- Identify an area related to your own teaching practice. Conduct a review of existing evidence on that topic. Is there evidence to inform your teaching? What could you do differently?
- Develop a short list of potential research projects you could develop for evidence that could support your own teaching in either nursing or midwifery.

REFERENCES

1. Ferguson L, Day DA. Evidence-based nursing education? Myth or reality? *J Nurs Educ*. 2005; **44**(3): 107–15.
2. Emerson RJ, Records K. Today's challenge, tomorrow's excellence: the practice of evidence-based education. *J Nurs Educ*. 2008; **47**(8): 359–70.
3. Wilkes L, Jackson D. Trends in publication of research papers by Australian-based nurse authors. *Collegian*. 2011; **18**(3): 125–30.
4. Oermann MH. Approaches to gathering evidence for educational practices in nursing. *J Contin Educ Nurs*. 2007; **38**(6): 250–5.
5. Australian Nurse Teachers' Society (ANTS). *Australian Nurse Teacher Competencies 2010*. Sydney, NSW: ANTS; 2010.
6. Mulready-Shick J, Flanagan KM, Banister GE, *et al*. Evaluating dedicated education units for clinical education quality. *J Nurs Educ*. 2013; **52**(11): 606–14.
7. Walker S, Dwyer T, Moxham L, *et al*. Facilitator versus preceptor: which offers the best support to undergraduate nursing students? *Nurse Educ Today*. 2013; **33**(5): 530–5.
8. Hallin K, Danielson E. Being a personal preceptor for nursing students: registered nurses' experiences before and after introduction of a preceptor model. *J Adv Nurs*. 2009; **65**(1): 161–74.
9. Richards J, Bowles C. The meaning of being a primary nurse preceptor for newly graduated nurses. *J Nurses Staff Dev*. 2012; **28**(5): 208–15.
10. Baglin MR, Rugg S. Student nurses' experiences of community-based practice placement learning: a qualitative exploration. *Nurse Educ Pract*. 2010; **10**(3): 144–52.
11. James A, Chapman Y. Preceptors and patients – the power of two: nursing student experiences on their first acute clinical placement. *Contemp Nurse*. 2009; **34**(1): 34–47.
12. Houghton CE, Casey D, Shaw D, *et al*. Students' experiences of implementing clinical skills in the real world of practice. *J Clin Nurs*. 2013; **22**(13–14): 1961–9.
13. McIntosh T, Fraser DM, Stephen N, *et al*. Final year students' perceptions of learning to be a midwife in six British universities. *Nurse Educ Today*. 2013; **33**(1): 1179–83.
14. Buykx P, Cooper S, Kinsman L, *et al*. Patient deterioration simulation experiences: impact on teaching and learning. *Collegian*. 2012; **19**(3): 125–9.
15. Miller A, Bull RM. Do you want to play? Factors influencing nurse academics' adoption of simulation in their teaching practices. *Nurse Educ Today*. 2013; **33**(3): 241–6.
16. McKenna L, Vanderheide R. Graduate entry to practice in nursing: exploring demographic characteristics of commencing students. *Aust J Adv Nurs*. 2012; **29**(3): 49–55.
17. Newton J, McKenna L. The transitional journey through the graduate year: a focus group study. *Int J Nurs Stud*. 2007; **44**(7): 1231–7.
18. Ostini F, Bonner A. Australian new graduate experiences during their transition program in a rural/regional acute care setting. *Contemp Nurse*. 2012; **41**(2): 242–52.
19. Theisen JL, Sandau KE. Competency of new graduate nurses: a review of their weakness and strategies for success. *J Contin Educ Nurs*. 2013; **44**(9): 406–14.
20. Thomas CM, Bertram E, Allen RL. The transition from student to new registered nurse in professional practice. *J Nurses Staff Dev*. 2012; **28**(5): 243–9.
21. McKenna L, Boyle M, Brown T, *et al*. Levels of empathy in undergraduate nursing students. *Int J Nurs Pract*. 2012; **18**(3): 246–51.
22. Ward J, Cody J, Schaal M, *et al*. The empathy enigma: an empirical study of decline in empathy among undergraduate nursing students. *J Prof Nurs*. 2012; **28**(1): 34–40.
23. Zavertnik JE, Huff TA, Munro CL. Innovative approach to teaching communication skills to nursing students. *J Nurs Educ*. 2010; **49**(2): 65–71.
24. Valiga TM, Ironside PM. Crafting a national agenda for nursing education research. *J Nurs Educ*. 2012; **51**(1): 3–4.

25. McKenna L, Rolls C. Bachelor of Midwifery: reflections on the first 5 years from two Victorian universities. *Women Birth.* 2007; **20**(2): 81–4.

26. Fahy K. An Australian history of the subordination of midwifery. *Women Birth.* 2007; **20**(1): 25–9.

27. Thomas BG. An evidence-based strategy for midwifery education. *Evid Based Midwifery.* 2007; **5**(2): 47–53.

28. Hotelling BA. Toward more evidence-based practice. *J Perinat Educ.* 2005; **14**(1): 46–9.

29. McKenna L, Innes K, French J, *et al.* Is history taking a dying skill? An exploration using a simulated learning environment. *Nurse Educ Pract.* 2011; **11**(4): 234–8.

30. Oermann MH. Toward evidence-based nursing education: deliberate practice and motor skill learning. *J Nurs Educ.* 2011; **50**(2): 63–4.

31. Kardong-Edgren SE, Oermann MH, Odom-Maryon T, *et al.* Comparison of two instructional modalities for nursing student CPR skill acquisition. *Resuscitation.* 2010; **81**(8): 1019–24.

32. Oermann MH, Kardong-Edgren SE, Odom-Maryon T. Effects of monthly practice on nursing students' CPR psychomotor skill performance. *Resuscitation.* 2011; **82**(4): 447–53.

33. Roxburgh M, Watson R, Holland K, *et al.* A review of curriculum evaluation in United Kingdom nursing education. *Nurse Educ Today.* 2008; **28**(7): 881–9.

34. Kumm S, Fletcher KA. From daunting task to new beginnings: Bachelor of Science in Nursing curriculum revision using the new essentials. *J Prof Nurs.* 2012; **28**(2): 82–9.

35. Ziehm SR, Uibel IC, Fontaine DK, *et al.* Success indicators for an accelerated masters entry nursing program: staff RN performance. *J Nurs Educ.* 2011; **50**(7): 395–403.

36. Cant R, McKenna L, Cooper S. Assessing preregistration nursing students' clinical competence: a systematic review of objective measures. *Int J Nurs Pract.* 2013; **19**(2): 163–76.

37. Eick SA, Williamson GR, Heath V. A systematic review of placement-related attrition in nursing education. *Int J Nurs Stud.* 2012; **49**(10): 1299–309.

38. Kenner CA, Pressler JL. Trends in nursing education. *Nurse Educ.* 2011; **36**(5): 179–80.

39. Iwasiw CL, Goldenberg D, Andrusyszyn M-A. Extending the evidence base for nursing education. *Int J Nurs Educ Scholarsh.* 2005; **2**: Editorial.

40. Patterson BJ, McAleer Klein J. Evidence for teaching: what are faculty using? *Nurs Educ Perspect.* 2012; **33**(4): 240–5.

CHAPTER 31

Evidence-based education in paramedics

Brett Williams and Dale Edwards

OVERVIEW

While the paramedic clinical workforce is guided and measured against evidence-based practice principles, the same is certainly not true when it comes to evidence-based education in the Australian paramedic discipline. This chapter brings together the latest educational evidence, underpinned by the pedagogical and policy issues currently facing the discipline. A brief historical overview of the transition from vocational to tertiary-level education is also provided. The remaining sections of the chapter outline the key areas currently under examination and provide the paramedic discipline with an overview and blueprint of contemporary evidence-based education.

CHAPTER OBJECTIVES

At the conclusion of this chapter the reader should be able to:

- summarise the transition to paramedic education and the impact this transition has had on current evidence-based education in Australia
- distinguish between pre- and post-employment models of education
- compare and contrast clinical placement learning and exposure to learning opportunities
- relate the different aspects of simulation and its effects on clinical learning in paramedicine
- identify the impact on student experiences and engagement during clinical placement learning.

KEY TERMS: clinical learning, clinical placements, paramedicine, simulation, tertiary education, vocational education and training

INTRODUCTION

Paramedic education has been undergoing substantial change over the past 2 decades within Australia, with the emergence of tertiary models of education replacing the more traditional vocational education programmes. Paramedic education prior to the mid 1990s was the providence of industry, with or without partnerships with formal vocational education and training (VET) providers. Since the mid 1990s, universities have welcomed the paramedic education sector, bringing with them a changing educational and pedagogical landscape.

The first bachelor's programmes in paramedicine in Australia were offered as conversion programmes for existing paramedics to undertake further study and upgrade to a degree. The earliest of these programmes was conducted at Charles Sturt University in 1994, with Victoria University of Technology (now Victoria University) following suit in 1995.[1] Since this first foray into the tertiary sector there has been a progression of universities implementing paramedic programmes; currently there are 17 universities offering programmes in paramedicine,[2] 10 of which have been operating for less than 5 years.

Early drivers for paramedic education to enter the tertiary sector in paramedicine were primarily around raising the professional status of the discipline, developing an esoteric body of knowledge, and making claims of profession rates of pay.[1,3] This early push came more from the grass-roots level of the discipline rather than from healthcare, organisational or government sector imperatives. This soon changed, however, as the growth and expansion in the paramedic role brought with it a demand for paramedics with a more broad level of knowledge of not only their own scope of practice but also the wider health system. Throughout this somewhat rapid change process there has been little exploration of the evidence underlying the models of education for paramedics. The focus of this chapter is to explore the evidence-based education in the paramedic discipline. Particular attention on how this evidence has influenced or changed practice will be discussed on two broad topics: clinical placements and clinical exposure.

PARAMEDIC EDUCATIONAL CHANGE

Paramedic education within Australia is currently delivered by both the tertiary and the VET sectors.[4] The VET sector model involves an apprenticeship-style post-employment approach, where students must first gain employment with an ambulance service and then progress through a VET qualification, usually a Diploma of Paramedical Sciences or similar. The tertiary education sector predominantly offers a pre-employment model of education, in which a student enters a degree programme and seeks employment on successful completion of that programme. There are additional pre-employment paramedic programmes offered through Australia within the VET sector; however, these programmes are often not recognised as suitable for employment within the statutory ambulance services.[2]

The model of education delivery within the tertiary sector is subject to variation depending on the university; however, there are common themes employed. Figure 31.1 outlines the two predominant models of paramedic education currently

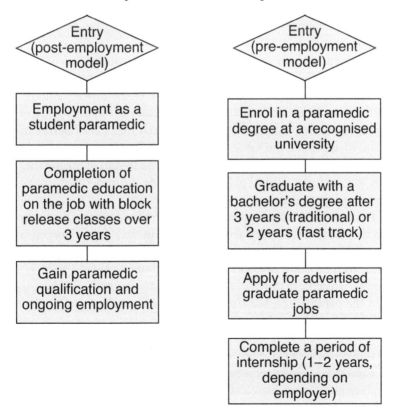

FIGURE 31.1 Models of paramedic education[4]

available in Australia. While Figure 31.1 reflects the more common bachelor's degree, there are variations to the tertiary approach that include double degrees, as well as master's degree programmes for students transitioning into paramedicine from other health disciplines. Regardless of the specific degree undertaken, the stages outlined in Figure 31.1 are common to all.

CLINICAL PLACEMENT AND CLINICAL EXPOSURE IN PARAMEDIC EDUCATION

In discussing the value of the clinical placement, or the professional experience placement, it is necessary to first explore its origins in paramedic education. As previously highlighted, less than 20 years ago paramedic education was centred on vocational training programmes – the aforementioned post-employment model. Throughout these programmes, students would undertake block-release periods from the operational paramedic roster to participate in theory classes, between which, the student would work as a second person on an operational emergency ambulance. While there were defined learning goals for some of the periods in which students worked on an ambulance (periods of clinical practicum), there were also many times when there were no defined learning experiences to complete. Paramedic students in the post-employment model therefore were exposed to learning experiences (as opposed to defining learning outcomes), and preceptors for the majority of their time working on an ambulance.[4]

The learning experience in the post-employment model was opportunistic in nature; the human resources priorities of the organisations dictated the model rather than any planned learning paradigm. This is, however, fortunately aligned to experiential learning theory,[5] and the more recent socio-cultural theories of learning, in that students were immersed in experiences from which they could derive meaning on a daily basis. To approach the same level of learning and achievement, the modern tertiary model of paramedic education has followed a hybrid of the nursing and medical models, as it includes clinical placements during the undergraduate years and an internship following graduation.

One of the stated outcome requirements of accredited paramedic programmes in Australia is that the graduate paramedic, at the end of their degree programme 'should have the core foundation elements to practice under supervision.'[6(p1)] Furthermore, at the end of an internship period a paramedic graduate should be able to practise independently.[6] To achieve this goal there is a need to ensure there is adequate clinical exposure in the paramedic education programme to position the graduate to meet these standards of work-readiness.

The nature and level of clinical exposure across paramedic programmes is diverse, with some universities offering more clinical exposure than some others. For example, Hou *et al.*[7] conducted a review of paramedic education literature and identified a range of clinical placement hours, from 280 hours at one university through to 640 hours at another. However, the range of sources identified to provide these data are from 2003 through to 2009, with no recent evidence base reported in the literature. Furthermore, while there is a clear expectation of clinical experience in tertiary paramedic pro-grammes, there is no quantification beyond an expectation that there be 'adequate clinical experience.'[6(p1)]

THE RELATIONSHIP BETWEEN CLINICAL PLACEMENT AND STUDENT ACHIEVEMENT

The clinical placement experience can have a positive, as well as negative, impact on the student learning experience,[8] and it can influence the likelihood of students' suc-cess in their education programme.[9] While there is a lack of literature on the impact of clinical placements on overall student success, one study from the United States identified a relationship between the quality of clinical exposure during clinical internships and overall success of the student.[9] Furthermore, this study could identify no relationship between length of placement and overall student success. This finding is in some ways supported by an Australian study that found there was inadequate opportunity for skills performance while on paramedic clinical placement.[10]

The lack of evidence surrounding the relationship between length of clinical experience in paramedic programmes and paramedic student success brings into focus the need to explore what is meant by *adequate clinical experience* and how this can be achieved. The standard applied in the accreditation of entry-level paramedic programmes includes 'sufficient patients, simulated patients and clinical training facilities'[6(p1)] to achieve this requirement.

SIMULATION IN PARAMEDIC CLINICAL EDUCATION

Paramedic education and ongoing training has primarily made use of simula-tions (role plays, DVDs, manikins) and hands-on authentic exposure on clinical placements.[11] Simulation training allows paramedic students to practise and con-solidate their clinical problem-solving skills, practical and assessment skills, and 'non-technical skills' such as empathy and communication in a controlled and safe environment.[12] Simulation training allows this practice to occur in a risk-free and controlled environment.[13,14] As such, simulation training can conceivably contribute to a reduction in healthcare errors made by paramedics plus a reduction in the cost of clinical education.[13] It has also been suggested that simulation training can act as a supplement to clinical placements when such opportunities are limited.[13,15] While simulation training is anecdotally viewed as primarily the use of manikins in an assessed scenario, there are studies emerging that demonstrate the broader uses and perhaps more accurate definitions of simulation.[16]

Williams and Brown[17] investigated the effectiveness of DVD simulations in the education of healthcare students, including paramedic students. They also inves-tigated the potential for DVD simulations to supplement clinical placements for paramedic students. Four academic departments at Monash University (nursing, paramedics, occupational therapy and physiotherapy) developed 11 clinical DVD simulations regarding cases such as asthma, fractured neck of femur, drug overdose, traumatic brain injury and acute myocardial infarction. The DVD simulations used actors to play the patients and practising healthcare professionals to play the health-care professional roles. Undergraduate students from the four departments viewed the DVD simulations. The students' perceptions of clinical relevance of the simula-tions were assessed using questionnaires and focus groups. The authors found that, overall, the students responded positively to the DVD simulations in terms of the learning potential and clinical relevance to their practice. Some of the advantages of DVD simulations that were addressed in the focus groups included the usefulness for preparation for clinical placements, as a tool for reinforcing learning, and as a supple-ment for the wasted learning opportunities students reported experiencing while on clinical placements. Students also highlighted some shortcomings of the DVD simula-tions; for example, all student groups believed that, while the DVD simulations were an effective learning tool, the simulations were not as effective as clinical placements and therefore should not replace hands-on clinical placements. The students also suggested the realism of the cases in the DVD simulations was questionable. It was indicated that the simulations would have a greater impact on the students' learning if they were real-life cases.

Another type of simulation training includes the use of virtual simulation. Power[14] conducted a virtual simulation workshop at a university in the United Kingdom for paramedic students to practise skills and assessment. The simulated scene involved a road traffic collision with three casualties. Paramedic students who utilised the virtual simulations worked in pairs on computer terminals with their own avatar and were able to communicate face-to-face with one another and with the other professionals involved. The objective of the virtual simulations was to have the paramedic students work in teams to manage the scene, assess and treat the casualties. The developers of the simulations were hoping that certain factors of paramedic practice would be addressed in the scenarios, including communication, teamwork, scene management and patient care, critical thinking and clinical decision-making. Power[14] found that the students were able to utilise the virtual simulation programme well with only a few minutes of training and that the students had few issues with the usability of the programme. Power[14] felt that virtual simulations were advantageous in paramedic education, as they allow the creation of scenarios and environments that would be otherwise difficult to create in real-life. They also provide a safe and controlled simulation environment for students to practise in. Despite these advantages, Power[15] recognised some shortcomings, including the possible issues for some students with technological usability and the expensive and labour-intensive nature of developing and implementing such a programme in paramedic education.

Literature regarding the effectiveness of simulation training in paramedic educa-tion is sparse; however, Wyatt et al.[18] demonstrated in their study that it could improve clinical performance for paramedic students. In their study, Wyatt et al.[18] investigated whether clinical simulations using a human patient simulator in the education of paramedics in trauma management could reduce subsequent error rates in clinical performance. The participants involved student paramedics and qualified intensive care paramedics. Wyatt et al.[18] noticed the most significant improvement in clinical performance following the simulation-based learning was in the student paramedics. Those students who participated in the simulation-based learning performed better than those who participated in case-based learning.

While studies have shown the use of simulations in assisting student paramedics in learning and mastering clinical skills and assessment, studies have also investigated the use of simulation in the continuing professional development of qualified pre-hospital healthcare providers. Lammers *et al.*[19] conducted a study with the objective of identifying problem areas in paramedic knowledge and skills in regard to paedi-atric emergencies, using simulated paediatric emergency scenarios. The study was conducted with paramedics from five paramedic agencies in Michigan. The research-ers designed and validated three clinical assessment modules using three different paediatric simulator manikins of varying technological complexity. Each simulation required participating paramedics to carry out an assessment of the 'patient', identify the problem (e.g. cardiac arrest, asthma, sepsis) and decide on and deliver the appro-priate treatment according to the Michigan State Model Pediatric Protocols. Each module used a different type of simulation manikin. Module 1 used a low-fidelity training manikin, which can generate cardiac arrhythmias and create pulses for palpa-tion. It does not have lung or heart sounds or spontaneous breathing, so therefore it requires an instructor to provide clinical information for the scenario. Module 2 used an intermediate-fidelity manikin, which can also generate heart and lung sounds. Module 3 used a high-fidelity simulator. This manikin was computer-controlled and could produce cardiac arrhythmias, pulses, lung and heart sounds, spontaneous and variable breathing patterns, and seizure-like activity. The participants' performance was scored according to checklists of steps to be performed throughout the scen-arios and whether these steps were performed in a timely fashion and in the correct sequence. The participants performed the scenarios with a partner who played the role of an intermediate emergency medical technician with limited experience. Through the use of the simulations, Lammers *et al.*[19] were able to determine certain deficiencies in paramedic skills in regard to paediatric emergencies.

THE STUDENT EXPERIENCE IN CLINICAL PLACEMENT

Clinical placements are an integral aspect of paramedic education and provide a practical, real-life linkage for students' theoretical knowledge.[8] Although there is an acknowledged limited capacity to achieve clinical placements throughout the health sector,[6] this capacity has been reduced over time, with some programmes finding it necessary to reduce clinical placement hours.[7,10] This theory–practice linkage is a critical step in the development of paramedic students' education.[8,17] The literature regarding clinical placements for paramedic students is limited. While clinical place-ments are important to the learning development of paramedic students, there are often only restricted numbers of placements available.[17] There are also a number of factors that call into question the effectiveness of clinical placement and the reliance on these placements as the sole, practical, hands-on learning experience for the paramedic students.

An important factor relating to the effectiveness of clinical placements for para-medic education is the students' perceptions and feelings of the placements. Boyle *et al.*[8] investigated paramedic students' views on their clinical placements. The authors addressed factors such as the students' reception by qualified paramedics and their overall impression of the placements in terms of learning opportunities. Boyle *et al.*[8] found that, while the wide majority of the participants reported that their clinical placement was a positive experience, approximately half also reported they were not made to feel welcome at the ambulance branch by paramedic staff. Similarly, a study by Wray and McCall[20] reported that many students felt unwelcome on clinical place-ment and unwanted by the on-road paramedic educators. Waxman and Williams[21] also found evidence of the same theme in their study, regarding student concerns about gaining employment in ambulance services in Australia. These negative feelings towards, and perceptions of, clinical placement can be detrimental to the student's learning and professional identity development.[21] In order for an effective learning experience to occur for the student, there needs to be a willingness to educate from the supervising paramedic and a relatively positive relationship between educator and student.[21]

Clinical placement is an important aspect of student education in which students are generally able to employ the assessment and practical skills they have learned in a real-life, supervised setting.[8] Examples of such hands-on practice include vital signs assessments, assessing patient injuries, teamwork, building rapport, utilising equipment and professionalism. Students are also able to employ communication skills with real-life patients, paramedics and other healthcare professionals. This hands-on experience is very important in forming the theory–practice link for stu-dents.[8] Michau *et al.*[10] found that 70% of third-year paramedic students participating in their study reported they were regularly afforded the opportunity to attend and manage cases during their clinical placements. A further 30% reported being able to regularly assist the attending paramedic in their management.[22] In their study, Boyle *et al.*[8] found that 88% of students reported they were afforded some form of hands-on experience while on placement.[8] However, one-third of student respondents were excluded from hands-on experience while on placement.[9] Michau *et al.*[10] also found that for the third-year students, less than 50% of learned skills were practised during the clinical placements. This raises concern that the students are not receiving adequate hands-on practice during these clinical placements; some of which is less than 6 months before they enter the paramedic workforce. Some of the potential bar-riers to students' participation and inclusion in hands-on experience during clinical placements includes the student's skill level, motivation and confidence, and whether the case was life-threatening.[9] This concern leads to assumptions that perhaps fur-ther supplemental learning procedures need to be put in place to rectify this, such as increased targeted simulation training.

Some commentators on the issue of clinical placement have stated that simply sending students on clinical placements does not necessarily guarantee learning will occur.[8] This led to some paramedic researchers coining the term 'learning lottery'.[22] It can be seen from the discussion earlier in this chapter that the students' feelings about, and perceptions of, clinical placements can effect whether they perceive the experience as positive or negative. Also, there are a variety of factors that affect the degree to which the student is allowed the opportunity to engage in hands-on experience while on clinical placement. An additional factor that affects the learning outcomes of clinical placement is 'downtime'. 'Downtime' is a reality of the paramedic discipline, and as such it is a reality for students on clinical placement. Michau *et al.*[10] found that the average amount of downtime experienced by students while on clinical placement was 4 hours for rural placements and 1 hour for metropolitan placements. The majority of students included in the study by Michau *et al.*[10] reported that the opportunity for structured learning activities during these prolonged periods of downtime would be beneficial.[8]

Supervision of students in the health professions is a significant factor in the success of the clinical placement, with several authors citing the importance of the clinical supervisor.[22-25] In both the pre-employment and the post-employment models of paramedic education, the role of the preceptor is of significant importance. Post-employment students have access to paramedics who act in the role of preceptor during most, if not all, of their time in the workplace (excluding intensive teaching blocks), whereas students coming through the pre-employment tertiary model achieve this exposure during clinical placements and during their internship following employment with an ambulance service.[4]

Most of what we know about preceptors in paramedicine comes from research into the clinical placement experience of the student.[11] There has been little research into the preparedness of paramedics to undertake the preceptor role, or into their experiences of that role. What can be found in the literature appears contradictory and presents a demand for further research.

CONCLUSIONS

While the paramedic discipline has seen recent and somewhat rapid transformations in its education and training moving from the VET sector to the tertiary sector, it is nonetheless well placed to integrate principles of evidence-based education into its curricula nationally and into accreditation and benchmarking processes. This chapter has explored the evidence relating specifically to clinical placement education, providing examples of where evidence-based education has, and is, playing an important role in providing direction and policy change based on empirical work.

SUMMARY POINTS

- Tertiary-level education has provided paramedicine with opportunities to closely examine its approach to evidence-based education.
- While clinical placement education is critical for the education and training of paramedic students, a number of issues continue to exist in that domain.
- Simulation takes many forms; its benefits are many and varied. Further theoretical and empirical work is required on its true benefits for paramedicine.
- While national education standards exist in paramedicine, many aspects of curricula design, assessment and clinical placement learning are disjointed and based on a limited number of evidence-based education approaches.

REVIEW QUESTIONS

- What are the key pedagogical differences between vocational and tertiary-level education?
- Are pre-employment models more appropriate in professionally oriented disciplines such as paramedicine?
- Can you really *measure* and *guarantee* quality learning during paramedic clinical placements?
- What level of simulation fidelity is required to ensure professional competency?

REFLECTIVE QUESTIONS AND EXERCISES

- How many hours or specific learning activities are required to reach competency or accreditation for a programme? How can this be achieved in a completely unpredictable working environment where no two jobs are ever the same?
- Why can't simulation replace elements of clinical placement hours?
- Are there alternative pedagogical approaches in minimising the theory–practice gap?
- What is meant by work-readiness and job-readiness and where does the current state of play leave paramedicine?

REFERENCES

1. Lord B. The development of a degree qualification for paramedics at Charles Sturt University. *Australas J Paramed.* 2003; **1**(1–2): 13.
2. Council of Ambulance Authorities. *Accredited Courses.* www.caa.net.au/education/accredited-courses (accessed 21 July 2013).
3. DeWit A. Against the odds: tertiary education for ambulance paramedics in Victoria, Australia. *Australas J Emerg Care.* 1997; **4**(3): 19–22.

4. Edwards D. Paramedic preceptor: work readiness in graduate paramedics. *Clin Teach.* 2011; **8**(2): 79–82.
5. Yardley S, Teunissen P, Dornan T. Experiential learning: AMEE Guide No. 63. *Med Teach.* 2012; **34**(2): e102–15.
6. Council of Ambulance Authorities (CAA). *Guidelines for the Assessment and Accreditation of Entry-Level Paramedic Education Programs.* Melbourne, VIC: CAA; 2010. Available at: www.caa.net.au/attachments/article/91/PEPAP_Guidelines_Reviewed_MAY_2010.pdf (accessed 21 July 2013).
7. Hou X-Y, Rego J, Service M. Review article: paramedic education opportunities and challenges in Australia. *Emerg Med Australas.* 2013; **25**(2): 114–19.
8. Boyle MJ, Williams B, Cooper J, *et al.* Ambulance clinical placements – a pilot study of students' experience. *BMC Med Educ.* 2008; **8**: 19.
9. Salzman J, Dillingham J, Kobersteen J, *et al.* Effect of paramedic student internship on performance on the national registry written exam. *Prehosp Emerg Care.* 2008; **12**(2): 212–16.
10. Michau R, Roberts S, Williams B, *et al.* An investigation of theory-practice gap in undergraduate paramedic education. *BMC Med Educ.* 2009; **9**: 23.
11. Alinier G. Skills benefits of advanced simulation training. *J Paramed Pract.* 2007; **1**(9): 369.
12. Boyle M, Williams B, Burgess S. Contemporary simulation education for undergraduate paramedic students. *Emerg Med J.* 2007; **24**(12): 854–7.
13. Peate I. Using simulation to enhance safety, quality and education. *J Paramed Pract.* 2011; **3**(8): 429.
14. Power P. Enhancing the student learning experience through interactive virtual reality simulation. *J Paramed Pract.* 2011; **3**(8): 447–9.
15. Williams B, Brown T, Scholes R, *et al.* Can interdisciplinary clinical DVD simulations transform clinical fieldwork education for paramedic, occupational therapy, physiotherapy, and nursing students? *J Allied Health.* 2010; **39**(1): 3–10.
16. Jones C, Jones P, Waller C. Simulation in prehospital care: teaching, testing and fidelity. *J Paramed Pract.* 2011; **3**(8): 430–4.
17. Williams B, Brown T. Clinical teaching and learning in paramedic education: is there a link between classrooms and clinical placements? *Australian College of Ambulance Professionals.* Conference paper. Auckland, New Zealand. 2009: 15–17 October.
18. Wyatt A, Fallows B, Archer F. Do clinical simulations using a human patient simulator in the education of paramedics in trauma care reduce error rates in preclinical performance? *Prehosp Emerg Care.* 2004; **8**(4): 435–6.
19. Lammers RL, Byrwa MJ, Fales WD, *et al.* Simulation-based assessment of paramedic pediatric resuscitation skills. *Prehosp Emerg Care.* 2009; **13**(3): 345–56.
20. Wray N, McCall L. 'They don't know much about us': educational reform impacts on students' learning in the clinical environment. *Adv Health Sci Educ.* 2009; **14**(5): 665–76.
21. Waxman A, Williams B. Paramedic pre-employment education and the concerns of our future: what are our expectations? *Australas J Paramed.* 2012; **4**(4): 4.
22. Williams BMB. Should undergraduate paramedic clinical placements be a 'learning lottery? *Primary Health Care Research Evaluation and Development.* Conference paper. Shepparton, VIC; 2007.
23. Billay D, Myrick F. Preceptorship: an integrative review of the literature. *Nurse Educ Pract.* 2008; **8**(4): 258–66.
24. Bury G, Janes D, Bourke M, *et al.* The advanced paramedic internship: an important clinical learning opportunity. *Resuscitation.* 2007; **73**(3): 425–9.
25. Jelinek G, Weiland T, Mackinlay C. Supervision and feedback for junior medical staff in Australian emergency departments: findings from the emergency medicine capacity assessment study. *BMC Med Educ.* 2010; **10**(1): 74.

CHAPTER 32

Evidence-based education in radiography

. . . .

Curtise KC Ng

OVERVIEW

The notion of evidence-based education is not a new idea in academic settings. However, it seems the culture of using education research evidence to inform teaching is still developing in academic institutions. The purpose of this chapter is to review the recent radiography education research literature, with the outcomes informing radiography educators on some better (evidence-based) strategies applicable to their daily teaching. A comprehensive literature search was conducted using the ScienceDirect and Informit databases, and by using the keywords 'learning and teaching' and 'radiography' to identify English peer-reviewed original research articles focusing on pre-registration radiography educational strategies and published in the last 10 years.

Thirty-two articles met the inclusion criteria and were included in the literature review. These articles reported positive findings relating to the use of 10 student-centred learning strategies: (1) constructive alignment, (2) fully online learning, (3) blended learning, (4) reflective learning, (5) clinical education, (6) simulated learning, (7) interprofessional education, (8) enquiry-based learning, (9) multidimensional assessment and (10) portfolio. The evidence provided in the articles suggests these strategies are able to enhance different aspects of radiography education.

Radiography educators should consider applying these strategies to their daily teaching, so as to achieve evidence-based education. Evidence suggests the breadth and depth of evidence for evidence-based education in radiography needs to be strengthened. It is recommended that further research should be conducted; for example, to evaluate the use of these strategies in a programme scale involving larger sample size and multiple sources of evidence including student learning performance, so as to strengthen the existing evidence base. In this way, a higher level of evidence-based education practice could be attained.

CHAPTER OBJECTIVES

Upon completion of this chapter, the reader will be able to:
- outline the different education approaches that have been used in radiography
- summarise the current body of educational research evidence related to radiography that has been published to date
- make recommendations for future educational research activities in the education of radiography students.

KEY TERMS: evidence-based education, radiography education, student-centred learning, adult learning

---

INTRODUCTION

The notion of evidence-based education is not a new idea in academic settings. However, it seems the culture of using education research evidence to inform teaching is still developing in academic institutions. Quality of education research and difficulty in locating the evidence are considered to be the factors hindering the development of evidence-based education.[1] The purpose of this chapter is to review the recent radiography education research literature, with the outcomes informing radiography educators on some better (evidence-based) strategies applicable to their daily teaching. Further research directions are also provided for them to engage in the higher level of evidence-based education practice, i.e. evidence establishment when such evidence is unavailable.[1]

SEARCH STRATEGY USED

A comprehensive literature search was conducted using the ScienceDirect and Informit databases, and by using the keywords 'learning and teaching' and 'radiography' to identify articles focusing on radiography educational strategies. The article inclusion criteria were as follows:
- pre-registration radiography education focused
- published between 2004 and 2013
- with primary research findings
- peer-reviewed
- written in English.

Articles belonging to any of the following categories were excluded:
- post-registration radiography education

- literature review
- without findings
- commentary
- conference abstract.

CURRENT STATUS OF RADIOGRAPHY EDUCATION RESEARCH

Thirty-two articles were identified in the literature search and these covered a range of education research areas including constructive alignment (n = 2), fully online learning (n = 2), blended learning (n = 4), reflective learning (n = 1), clinical education (n = 7), simulated learning (n = 4), interprofessional education (IPE) (n = 1), enquiry-based learning (EBL) (n = 5), multidimensional assessment (n = 3) and portfolio (n = 3). All strategies involved in these studies are student-centred and based on Knowles[22] adult learning theory. They are discussed in the following sections.

CONSTRUCTIVE ALIGNMENT

Constructive alignment is an educational theory proposed by Biggs,[3] which merges a number of theories for curriculum planning, such as constructivism and instructional design, to maximise students' learning. Constructivism emphasises students' learning as constructed by themselves through learning and teaching activities (LTAs), while instructional design focuses on the alignment of learning objectives or intended outcomes with assessment. Constructive alignment refers to the establishment of learning objectives or intended outcomes with appropriate cognitive demands for students relevant to the context, the planning of LTAs that facilitate students' construction of learning towards meeting the objectives, and appropriate assessment strategies that can measure that expected level of cognitive development of the objectives.

In the study conducted by Castle,[4] a questionnaire was used to assess critical thinking skills of 48 second-year and 51 third-year radiography students. The questionnaire findings indicated the majority of students perceived their radiography programme able to promote critical thinking skills development. However, their written assignment results showed their skills were limited. Castle[5] applied the constructive alignment theory to review the curriculum. Learning outcomes and assessment items specific to critical thinking skills development were added to each year of study. Although the curriculum review resulted in an increase of students' critical thinking skills level from poor to average, further improvement would be possible if the LTAs were better aligned with the new learning outcomes and assessments. This is also a requirement of the constructive alignment theory.[3]

FULLY ONLINE LEARNING

The fully online learning offers a flexible learning environment and students can have a high level of control over their study pace[6] (e.g. self-directed noted in the adult learning theory).[5,7] This approach allows the students to revisit learning materials, conveniently leading to active engagement, which is a pathway for deep learning.[6,8] The knowledge acquired through deep learning would be retained longer than via the traditional (didactic) instruction. The students would also become more independent and motivated to learn.[8,9]

In Shanahan's study,[8] the Blackboard platform was used to provide a fully online information literacy module to 41 students. Questionnaires were used to collect students' self-reported performances on information literacy skills, such as use of a journal database, Boolean operators, and search narrowing and expansion before and after the intervention. The study findings showed the students' information literacy skills were improved dramatically and the effect had been retained for 7 months after the intervention. However, it was acknowledged that the purposefully (carefully) designed learning activities for the online platform were the key to success.

Similar positive findings and comments on fully online learning were also noted in the study by Messer and Griffiths[6] on the use of a commercial online course (Ciris; Ciris Healthcare Ltd, Cambridge, United Kingdom) to teach 35 third-year radiography students about the issue of clinical governance. The student participation was voluntary. The questionnaire results revealed learning taken place among students, and usefulness of the learning materials and online platform was recognised. The current evidence suggests a carefully planned online learning package would be able to facilitate deep learning, and increase independence and motivation of students for lifelong learning.[6,8]

BLENDED LEARNING

Blended learning involves the use of both online and face-to-face channels for instruction delivery.[10–12] It provides similar benefits to the fully online learning, such as being flexible and self-directed leading to active engagement.[7,13–15] However, this approach is considered as more robust than the fully online learning[10] because it could potentially address different learning needs of students.[7,13] Some students would prefer face-to-face learning while others may incline to more flexible learning means.[14] Also, the classroom interactivity could help the students to develop essential interpersonal skills for the radiography profession.[13,15]

The four blended learning studies identified in the literature search showed positive findings on this approach.[7,13–15] In the study conducted by Lorimer and Hilliard[13] and involving 102 students, podcasts (audio downloads) with PowerPoint slides were used to replace 2-hour traditional lectures, and face-to-face tutorials were substituted for another 2-hour lecture. Students' engagement and classroom interactivity were increased when compared with the traditional setting, as the students spent around double the amount of time to study the materials online and through the use of tutorials. Although White and Cheung[14] reported blended learning (through the use of the WebCT platform and one 2-hour lecture) did not change the academic performance of their 73 students, they appreciated the flexible learning environment in this approach. Chapman and Oultram[7] indicated in their study with nine students that the reduction of face-to-face contact time in blended learning would allow staff members to focus on more important tasks such as learning facilitation. However, it appears the appropriate balance between online and face-to-face components was not addressed in these studies.[7,15]

REFLECTIVE LEARNING

Reflective practice is crucial in the radiography profession. Through critically reviewing past experiences, new insights would be obtained to inform better clinical practice, and integration of theory and practice would be achieved. It is common to incorporate reflective learning elements into a radiography programme, so as to prepare students to become reflective practitioners upon graduation.[16]

Abrahams[16] implemented a 1-year reflective tutorial programme for five radiography students to explicitly promote the use of reflection for improving their practice. There were five sessions within the programme and these covered topics of learning styles and reflection, reflection-on-action, reflection-in-action and reflection-on-reflection. The students were required to complete reflective writings on these topics after the sessions. The evaluation questionnaire findings revealed all students perceived the tutorial programme was useful. However, two out of five respondents indicated they would not engage in reflective practice in the future. Further study is required to investigate this unexpected finding.

CLINICAL EDUCATION

Clinical education is indispensable to any radiography programme because of the practice-based nature of the profession.[17-19] The major focus of the identified studies is related to determining ways for enhancing clinical education programmes by using surveys, except one that was based on students' performance data.[17-23] Currie and Wheat[17] compared 40 first-year students' assessment results before and after placement. They found the first-year placement would strengthen students' understanding and suggested the placement should be introduced earlier in any radiography programme. A similar finding was also noted in Bolderston et al.'s[20] study on students' experiences in clinical placement. However, Currie and Wheat[17] and Ogbu[18] indicated not every clinical centre would be able to meet the stage of progress of individual students. Bridge et al.[21] conducted a survey of practices and facilities of clinical departments. The outcomes were used to match individual students' needs with the nature of clinical centres.

Clinical skills workshop, orientation, documentation and learning contract were identified as useful ways to ensure that students were clear about learning objectives and goals prior to the placement.[22,23] Well-trained clinical and university supervisors were found to be crucial during the placement.[19,20,23] Well-trained supervisors would be able to provide appropriate tutorials and feedback to help students to progress.[20,23] Most important, these supervisors could potentially address the common problem of clinical assessment: the lack of reliability.[19]

SIMULATED LEARNING

Simulated learning is common in radiography education. Resources such as anatomical models, live actors and virtual reality systems can be used to mirror clinical situations for students to develop clinical skills.[24] Every student can experience a range of clinical settings, which sometimes are not available during the placement, enriching the students' clinical exposure.[9,24–26] It is also considered as complementary to the clinical placement for improving quality of clinical education and hence reducing students' attrition rate which is crucial to maintain adequate radiography workforce.[9,24,26]

Thoirs *et al.*[24] used online questionnaires and interviews to survey 205 Australian academic, clinical and accrediting stakeholders for obtaining their perception of simulated learning. The participants believed the simulated learning was complementary to the clinical placement, especially for early stages of clinical skills development, but that it could not be a replacement because of the complexity of real situations. However, the respondents also suggested there would be a potential of 10%–20% of clinical placement hour reduction if a simulated learning programme was well designed, such as the Virtual Environment Radiotherapy Training (VERT) system (Vertual Ltd, East Yorkshire, United Kingdom).

James and Dumbleton's[26] survey study on the VERT revealed that students' positive learning outcomes would rely on departmental factors such as provision of adequate training, time and resources to staff for proper implementation of programmes. The staff members in Green and Appleyard's[25] study provided both group demonstration and individual guided practicals for students to use the VERT. The students indicated their clinical skills and confidence were improved by the programme. Nisbet and Matthews[9] applied a range of pedagogies including constructive alignment, EBL, reflective learning and peer tutoring to develop a student workbook on the VERT. Their students valued the session contents and reported learning gained from following the workbook to use the VERT.

INTERPROFESSIONAL EDUCATION

Interprofessional collaboration has been identified as one of the best strategies to address the complex challenges in healthcare, such as the ageing population. IPE can be used to prepare healthcare students for this collaboration upon graduation. According to the World Health Organization, 'IPE occurs when two or more professions learn about, from and with each other to enable effective collaboration and improve health outcomes.'[27(p1)] However, the development of IPE appears to be still in the early stage. Currently, the theory in its practice is developing, but Knowles'[2] adult learning theory seems to be commonly associated with IPE.[28] There was only one article related to IPE identified in the literature search. Turner *et al.*[29] reported the use of IPE in the research project module of their undergraduate radiography programme. Their students were asked to determine expertise and knowledge required for completing projects and approach relevant staff members from other disciplines. Effective collaboration between radiography students and staff from other professions such as medical physics, information technology and oncology was found. For example, the findings of one student project contributed to improvement of clinical protocols for their centre, which was an outcome of effective collaboration leading to healthcare improvement.

ENQUIRY-BASED LEARNING

In the EBL or enquiry-based learning approach, a trigger is given to students to initiate their learning facilitated by staff.[30] When the trigger is in the form of a problem, the learning is known as problem-based learning.[31,32] Generic skills development of students is considered as its major benefit.[30-33] Deep learning would apparently happen when the students actively engage in tasks required by the trigger or problem, leading to better study results.[31]

Higgins et al.[33] used the grounded theory method to study the process of EBL of eight first-year students. The benefits perceived by the participants included development of generic skills and attributes such as team working, communication and confidence, and applied understanding on subject matters for better clinical practice. Similar benefits were noted in other survey studies. However, these studies also found additional skills development such as time management, leadership, conflict resolution, problem-solving and critical thinking through the EBL process.[30 32]

Elsie et al.[32] investigated academic performances of 24 students who experienced the EBL over 6 years and found improvement in their results. A similar finding was revealed in Foster's[34] study on seven students enrolled in one module with the EBL. Elsie et al.[32] acknowledged the improvement was due to the increasing ability of staff to deliver the EBL over time. However, reliability and validity of assessment for the EBL were still issues within this pedagogy.[30-32,34] Elsie et al.[31,32] suggested the use of portfolios to address these concerns, and this was also the assessment used in their studies.

MULTIDIMENSIONAL ASSESSMENT

The reliability and validity of assessment is a common issue in radiography education. This issue is related not only to the assessment tool itself but also to the abilities of assessors. Reliability represents reproducibility or consistency of assessment result, while validity refers to the result reflecting the intended items assessed or not.[35] Hall and Durward[36] conducted a study on retention of anatomy knowledge of 51 students. The findings showed both second- and third-year students were able to retain more than 99% of anatomy knowledge after 10 and 22 months, respectively, when multiple-choice questions (MCQs) was used as the assessment tool. However, only a 67%–77% retention rate was noted in the short answer questions section. The authors suggested retrieval cues of MCQs contributed to its high retention rate, but they could only assess factual recall and were unable to gauge higher-level skills such as analysis, interpretation, synthesis and application. MCQs should not be used as a single assessment for students' knowledge. Multidimensional strategy would be useful to increase the reliability and validity of student assessment and also to encourage deep learning.

Kench et al.[37] conducted a survey study on perceptions of 100 students on group project peer assessment. The students indicated peer assessment should be used to determine individuals' marks based on group results, which was a more fair process to avoid 'social loafing' and 'free-riding'. Tan et al.[35] pointed out in their online survey study on staff perception of assessment that the fairness and equity of assessment could not be simply based on the multidimensional assessment strategy. Training of assessors also contributed to this issue to a great extent.

PORTFOLIO

Portfolio pedagogy requires students to collect evidence (artefacts) from their learning experiences, select the representing evidence from the collection and reflect on the selected evidence to illustrate their learning achievement.[38] The portfolio model would be able to integrate all assessment tools within a multidimensional assessment strategy for gauging complex intellectual capabilities and hence maximise the outcomes from the multidimensional assessment.[39]

Mubuuke et al.[40] used the portfolio as the assessment for their EBL curriculum. Thirty-five students were required to experience two different settings of portfolio assessment. The first setting did not have any restriction in number of artefacts included in the portfolio and staff members assessed all contents. The second setting required the students to orally present two artefacts selected from the portfolio, and assessment was only conducted on the selected artefacts. Both the students and staff indicated in their evaluation questionnaire and focus group surveys that evidence selection was important in the portfolio process. This arrangement could reduce the workload of both students and staff, making it more practical and sustainable. The sustainability could also be ensured when the portfolio was a compulsory requirement.

Ng et al.[39] developed a portfolio framework based on questionnaire survey and literature review for assessing students' competence development throughout a radiography programme. They identified that critical reflection of learning experiences during the portfolio building process was able to facilitate the students to perceive the linkage between individual, separate outcomes from the multidimensional assessment. The portfolio was the place for the students to put the linked pieces of evidence together to provide a simple, clear and manageable display of their competence attainments. In order to improve efficiency of portfolio building process, Ng et al.[38] conducted another study to develop a web database portfolio system based on their previous portfolio framework. The students were only required to provide essential ingredients of portfolio (e.g. selected evidence and written account or justification of evidence provided). The electronic system managed the rest for the students. The evaluation results of the system revealed its functionalities were well aligned with the portfolio pedagogy of 'collect', 'select' and 'reflect', and quality portfolio processes were also found.

RECOMMENDATIONS FOR FUTURE RESEARCH

There do not seem to have been many radiography education research articles published in the past 10 years (*see* Table 32.1). Only 32 original research articles were found. Although the evidence to support the use of the identified strategies was provided in these articles, some evidence might not be strong because it was based on a subject or module, a small number of samples and a limited variety of data. This phenomenon is also noted in other disciplines.[1] When radiography educators adopt any strategy discussed, they should consider implementing it as a research study on a programme scale involving a larger sample size and multiple sources of evidence, including learning performance, so as to strengthen the existing evidence base. Two pedagogy-specific future research directions were also identified in the previous discussion. They are the determination of appropriate balance between online and face-to-face components in blended learning and factors affecting the transfer of reflection skills from university learning to clinical practice after graduation.

TABLE 32.1 Summary of radiography education research articles identified

Author/s	Country of origin	Study design	Cross-sectional or longitudinal	Study participants	Sample size	Data collection method/s	Specific outcome measure/s	Key finding/s	Study limitation/s
Constructive alignment									
Castle (2006)[4]	United Kingdom	Quantitative	Cross-sectional	2nd and 3rd year students	2nd year: 48 3rd year: 51	Questionnaire and assessment performance review	Self-perceived and actual critical thinking skills	75% of 2nd and 90% of 3rd year students perceived the course able to promote critical thinking skills; however, the mean assessment score was lower than 60%	Unable to show the effect of constructive alignment directly
Castle (2009)[5]	United Kingdom	Quantitative	Cross-sectional	1st, 2nd and 3rd year students	1st year: 132 2nd year: 115 3rd year: 96	Assessment performance review	Actual critical thinking skills	Mean assessment score: 5.22–6.36 (scale: poor, 0–3; average, 4–6; good, 7–9)	Unable to confirm the long-term effect of constructive alignment
Fully online learning									
Messer and Griffiths (2007)[6]	United Kingdom	Quantitative and qualitative	Cross-sectional	Final-year students	35	Questionnaire	Perception of learning experience, technical issues and learning materials	100% (17/17) of students indicated learning taken place 68.6% (24/35) of respondents thought the online platform was beneficial to study	Small sample size No learning performance data collected Only studied one learning module

(continued)

Author/s	Country of origin	Study design	Cross-sectional or longitudinal	Study participants	Sample size	Data collection method/s	Specific outcome measure/s	Key finding/s	Study limitation/s
Shanahan (2007)[8]	Australia	Quantitative and qualitative	Longitudinal	2nd year students	41	Pre- and post-intervention questionnaires and follow-up interviews	Self-reported information literacy skills	Pre-intervention: 38% (14/37) of students used journal database. Post-intervention: 100% (35/35). 7 months after intervention: 100% (17/17)	Small sample size. Only studied one subject
Blended learning									
Chapman and Outram[7] (2008)	Australia	Quantitative	Cross-sectional	Professional development year students	Conventional cohort: 4 eLearning: 5	Record of face-to-face and telephone support	Hours of face-to-face support and no. of phone calls	Face-to-face hours: 9.7–42 (conventional); 3–6.5 (eLearning). No. of phone calls: 2–18 (conventional); 0–6 (eLearning)	Very small sample size. No learning performance data collected
Lorimer and Hilliard[13] (2009)	United Kingdom	Quantitative	Longitudinal	Students of a radiography module and staff	102	Interim and end-of-module questionnaires	Perception of learning experience and no. of hours studying online materials	Interim: 77.5% of students preferred blended learning. End of module: average no. of hours studying online materials = 3.5–4	No learning performance data collected. Only studied one learning module
White and Cheung (2006)[14]	Hong Kong	Quantitative and qualitative	Longitudinal	Students of a radiography subject	73	Questionnaire and assessment performance record	Perception of learning experience and subject result	Questionnaire: about 70% of students indicated online materials facilitated preparation ahead of face-to-face classes. Pre- (2000–02) and post- (2003–04) intervention subject results were similar	Only studied one subject

Author/s	Country of origin	Study design	Cross-sectional or longitudinal	Study participants	Sample size	Data collection method/s	Specific outcome measure/s	Key finding/s	Study limitation/s
Bleiker et al. (2011)[15]	United Kingdom	Quantitative and qualitative	Cross-sectional	1st and 2nd year students	1st year: 60 2nd year: 50	Questionnaire	Perception of usefulness of virtual learning environment in blended learning	Mean values of questions: 3.9–4.6 (1st year); 3.7–4.3 (2nd year)	No learning performance data collected Only studied one learning module Unable to evaluate the whole blended learning programme
Reflective learning									
Abrahams (2012)[16]	Australia	Quantitative and qualitative	Cross-sectional	Professional development year students	5	Questionnaire	Perception of the reflective learning programme	100% (5/5) of students suggested the reflective learning programme was useful 40% (2/5) of respondents indicated they would not engage in reflective practice in the future	Very small sample size No learning performance data collected
Clinical education									
Currie and Wheat (2005)[17]	Australia	Quantitative	Longitudinal	1st year students in 2003 and 2004	40	Written test and retest	Students' academic performance before and after clinical placement	There was a 9.1% of mean score improvement after clinical placement	Small sample size Only studied one learning module

(continued)

Author/s	Country of origin	Study design	Cross-sectional or longitudinal	Study participants	Sample size	Data collection method/s	Specific outcome measure/s	Key finding/s	Study limitation/s
Ogbu (2008)[18]	Nigeria	Quantitative and qualitative	Cross-sectional	3rd, 4th and 5th year students	3rd year: 62 4th year: 60 5th year: 56	Questionnaire	Self-perceived clinical placement experience	Students indicated they had positive placement experience overall; however, they disagreed that clinical centres offered adequate resources for learning enhancement (mean: 3.59)	No learning performance data collected
Adams et al. (2004)[19]	Australia	Quantitative and qualitative	Cross-sectional	Final-year students	21	Questionnaire	Self-perceived clinical placement experience	62% (13/21) of students agreed their clinical performances were assessed by clinical and university supervisors in a way matching their expectation.	Small sample size No learning performance data collected
Bolderston et al. (2008)[20]	Canada	Qualitative	Cross-sectional	Final-year students, recent graduates and staff	Final-year students and recent graduates: 6 Staff: 5	Interview	Clinical placement experiences of students with English as second language	Key themes identified: communication, differences and dealing with it; one sub-theme example: clinical learning environment more preferable than classroom	Small sample size No learning performance data collected
Bridge et al. (2013)[21]	Australia	Quantitative	Cross-sectional	Staff	12	Questionnaire	Clinical practice of placement centres	No. of case types: 59 Technology with high usage: IMRT (12.0%, 122/1014) and PET fusion (11.2%, 114/1014)	No finding of the effectiveness of mapping exercise provided

Author/s	Country of origin	Study design	Cross-sectional or longitudinal	Study participants	Sample size	Data collection method/s	Specific outcome measure/s	Key finding/s	Study limitation/s
Halkett et al. (2011)[22]	Australia	Quantitative	Longitudinal	3rd year students	27	Pre-, interim and post-questionnaires	Improvement of students' confidence after attending communication workshops	Students' self-perceived confidence level increases were statistically significant (p < 0.002–0.038)	Students' communication skills not accessed
Chapman and Oultram (2007)[23]	Australia	Quantitative and qualitative	Cross-sectional	Students attending a clinical placement centre	23	Questionnaire and interview	Perception of usefulness of clinical orientation programme	96% (22/23) of students indicated the orientation programme was useful	Small sample size; No learning performance data collected
Simulated learning									
Nisbet and Matthews (2011)[9]	United Kingdom	Quantitative and qualitative	Cross-sectional	1st, 2nd and 3rd year students	Not provided	Questionnaire	Experience of using the VERT with workbook	81% of students indicated learning gained from using the VERT with workbook; 73% of respondents valued the content of the session	Sample size not provided; No learning performance data collected
Thoirs et al. (2011)[24]	Australia	Quantitative and qualitative	Cross-sectional	Educators, clinicians, representatives from professional body	205	Questionnaire and interview	Perception of simulated learning	62.9% (100/159) of respondents used simulated learning techniques in teaching; 48.2% (27/56) and 26.8% (15/56) of participants thought simulated learning could not replace clinical placement and were unsure, respectively	No learning performance data collected

(continued)

Author/s	Country of origin	Study design	Cross-sectional or longitudinal	Study participants	Sample size	Data collection method/s	Specific outcome measure/s	Key finding/s	Study limitation/s
Green and Appleyard (2011)[25]	United Kingdom	Quantitative and qualitative	Cross-sectional	1st and 2nd year students	1st year: 23 2nd year: 21	Randomised controlled trial, questionnaire and interview	Effect of virtual environment on skill development	89% (39/44) and 80% (35/44) of respondents suggested the use of VERT could improve their confidence and skills, respectively	Small sample size Only studied one learning module
James and Dumbleton (2013)[26]	United Kingdom	Quantitative and qualitative	Cross-sectional	Clinical centre managers	53	Questionnaire and interview	VERT utilisation in clinical placement centres	79% (26/33) of respondents indicated VERT was useful for students' clinical skill development but provision of adequate training, time and resources to staff were the top 3 (out of 12) factors affecting the outcome	No learning performance data collected

Interprofessional education

Author/s	Country of origin	Study design	Cross-sectional or longitudinal	Study participants	Sample size	Data collection method/s	Specific outcome measure/s	Key finding/s	Study limitation/s
Turner et al. (2012)[29]	Canada	Qualitative	Cross-sectional	Staff and final-year students	Not provided	Informal feedback	Perception of interprofessional education	Effective collaboration between students and staff of different disciplines was identified as a benefit of interprofessional education	Sample size not provided Only studied one learning module Study design not rigorous

Enquiry-based learning

Author/s	Country of origin	Study design	Cross-sectional or longitudinal	Study participants	Sample size	Data collection method/s	Specific outcome measure/s	Key finding/s	Study limitation/s
Naylor (2011)[30]	United Kingdom	Quantitative and qualitative	Cross-sectional	Staff and 1st year students	1st year: 35 Staff: not provided	Questionnaire interview and informal feedback	Perception of enquiry-based learning in an imaging technology module	91% (32/35), 86% (30/35) and 71% (25/35) of students suggested the benefits of enquiry-based learning were team working skills, presentation skills and confidence developments, respectively	Small sample size Only studied one learning module No learning performance data collected

Author/s	Country of origin	Study design	Cross-sectional or longitudinal	Study participants	Sample size	Data collection method/s	Specific outcome measure/s	Key finding/s	Study limitation/s
Elsie *et al.* (2009)[31]	Uganda	Quantitative and qualitative	Cross-sectional	Staff and 1st, 2nd and 3rd year students	1st year: 12 2nd year: 12 3rd year: 11 Staff: 10	Questionnaire and interview	Attitudes and perceptions of students and staff on problem-based learning	100% (35/35) of students indicated they developed generic skills through problem-based learning 100% (10/10) of staff expressed concern about assessing students' performance	Small sample size No learning performance data collected
Elsie *et al.* (2010)[32]	Uganda	Quantitative and qualitative	Cross-sectional	Staff and 2nd and 3rd year students	2nd year: 13 3rd year: 11 Staff: 7	Questionnaire, interview and assessment performance review	Students' academic performance and perception of problem-based learning	An increasing trend of student assessment mean score was noted 100% (24/24) of students and 100% (7/7) of staff suggested students' lifelong learning skill was developed through problem-based learning 100% (7/7) of staff expressed concern about assessing students' performance	Small sample size
Higgins *et al.* (2013)[33]	United Kingdom	Qualitative	Cross-sectional	1st year students	8	Interview	Experience of inquiry-based learning	Students experienced development of generic skills and attributes such as team working, communication and confidence, and applied understanding on subject matters	Only studied one learning module No learning performance data collected

(*continued*)

Author/s	Country of origin	Study design	Cross-sectional or longitudinal	Study participants	Sample size	Data collection method/s	Specific outcome measure/s	Key finding/s	Study limitation/s
Foster (2008)[34]	United Kingdom	Quantitative	Longitudinal	Students with and without dyslexia	With dyslexia: 3 Without dyslexia: 4	Assessment performance review	Dyslexic students' assessment performance in a problem-based learning module	Problem-based learning had a positive effect on assessment of performance	Small sample size Only studied one learning module
Multidimensional assessment									
Tan et al. (2013)[35]	Canada	Quantitative and qualitative	Cross-sectional	Clinical educators	75	Questionnaire	Perception of clinical educators on competence assessment	58% (43/74) of clinical educators believed formal training in education would make them more comfortable to assess students	No learning performance data collected
Hall and Durward (2009)[36]	United Kingdom	Quantitative	Longitudinal	2nd and 3rd year students	2nd year: 23 3rd year: 28	Written test and retest	Anatomy knowledge retention	2nd and 3rd year students were able to retain more than 99% of knowledge after 10 and 22 months, respectively, when MCQs were used as the assessment tool; however, only 67%–77% of retention rate was noted in the short answer questions section	Small sample size Only studied one learning module
Kench et al. (2009)[37]	Australia	Quantitative and qualitative	Cross-sectional	Final-year students	100	Questionnaire	Perception of peer assessment	Students thought they should assess other members when working in a group situation (mean: 3.82)	Only studied one learning module
Portfolio									
Ng et al. (2009)[38]	Hong Kong	Quantitative and qualitative	Cross-sectional	Students and staff	Students: 62 Staff: 3	Questionnaire	Perception of electronic portfolio practice	Mean values of questions regarding system functionality alignment with the portfolio pedagogy were 3.33–4.67	No learning performance data collected

Author/s	Country of origin	Study design	Cross-sectional or longitudinal	Study participants	Sample size	Data collection method/s	Specific outcome measure/s	Key finding/s	Study limitation/s
Ng et al. (2008)[39]	Hong Kong	Quantitative and qualitative	Cross-sectional	3rd year students, and local and overseas staff	3rd year: 28 Local: 28 Overseas: 10	Questionnaire	Perception of competence development and assessment strategies in a radiography programme	A 1-year interval should be adequate for students to advance their competence from a lower to a higher level in a radiography programme 44.4% (4/9) of staff used portfolio as the clinical placement assessment	No learning performance data collected
Mubuuke et al. (2010)[40]	Uganda	Quantitative and qualitative	Cross-sectional	Staff and 1st, 2nd and 3rd year students	1st year: 12 2nd year: 12 3rd year: 11 Staff: 15	Questionnaire and interview	Perception of portfolio assessment	100% (50/50 and 15/15) of students indicated portfolios should be assessed and indicated satisfaction with the arrangement of evidence selection for the portfolio, respectively 87% (13/15) of staff could complete portfolio marking in 2 weeks	No learning performance data collected

Abbreviations: IMRT = intensity-modulated radiation therapy; MCQs = multiple-choice questions; no. = number; PET = positron emission tomography; VERT = Virtual Environment Radiotherapy Training system

CONCLUSION

Ten evidence-based strategies were identified in the literature review on 32 radiography education research articles: (1) constructive alignment, (2) fully online learning, (3) blended learning, (4) reflective learning, (5) clinical education, (6) simulated learning, (7) IPE, (8) EBL, (9) multidimensional assessment and (10) portfolio. The benefits of these strategies discussed in the chapter were based on the evidence provided in the identified articles. Educators should consider applying these strategies to enhance their radiography programmes, so as to achieve evidence-based education. Evidence suggests the breadth and depth of evidence for evidence-based education in radiography need to be strengthened. It is recommended that further research should be conducted. Some future research directions were suggested for the educators to engage in the higher level of evidence-based education practice.

SUMMARY POINTS

- The education approaches in radiography are varied and include online learning, blended learning, reflective learning, clinical education, simulated learning, IPE, EBL, multidimensional assessment and portfolio.
- The body of educational research in radiography is small and continues to evolve.
- The future education of radiography students will involve more technology as advances occur.

REVIEW QUESTIONS

- What are some of the educational strategies that have been used with radiography students?
- How has problem-based learning been utilised with radiography students?
- How has IPE been applied with radiography students?
- What types of educational technology have been used with radiography students?

REFLECTIVE QUESTIONS AND EXERCISES

- Think about what educational strategies could be used to promote psychomotor development in radiography students.
- What types of learning goals could be achieved with radiography students in the same classroom as physiotherapy, occupational therapy, nutrition and dietetics, nursing, midwifery and paramedic students?
- How could different types of social media (e.g. Twitter, YouTube, Facebook) be used as an educational tool with radiography students?

REFERENCES

1. Davies P. What is evidence-based education? *Br J Educ Stud.* 1999; **47**(2): 108–21.
2. Knowles M. *The Adult Learner: a neglected species.* 4th ed. Houston, TX: Gulf Publishing Company; 1990. pp. 194–5.
3. Biggs J. Enhancing teaching through constructive alignment. *High Educ.* 1996; **32**(3): 347–64.
4. Castle A. Assessment of the critical thinking skills of student radiographers. *Radiography.* 2006; **12**(2): 88–95.
5. Castle A. Defining and assessing critical thinking skills for student radiographers. *Radiography.* 2009; **15**(1): 70–6.
6. Messer S, Griffiths M. An online clinical governance learning package for student radiographers. *Radiography.* 2007; **13**(2): 95–102.
7. Chapman N, Oultram S. Piloting e-Learning in a radiation oncology department. *J Med Imaging Radiat Sci.* 2008; **39**(2): 81–5.
8. Shanahan MC. Information literacy skills of undergraduate medical radiation students. *Radiography.* 2007; **13**(3): 187–96.
9. Nisbet H, Matthews S. The educational theory underpinning a clinical workbook for VERT. *Radiography.* 2011; **17**(1): 72–5.
10. Rovai AP, Jordan HM. Blended learning and sense of community: a comparative analysis with traditional and fully online graduate courses. *Int Rev Res Open Dist Learn.* 2004; **5**(2): 1–13.
11. Ginns P, Ellis R. Quality in blended learning: exploring the relationships between on-line and face-to-face teaching and learning. *Internet High Educ.* 2007; **10**(1): 53–64.
12. Garrison DR, Kanuka H. Blended learning: uncovering its transformative potential in higher education. *Internet High Educ.* 2004; **7**(2): 95–105.
13. Lorimer J, Hilliard A. Incorporating learning technologies into undergraduate radiography education. *Radiography.* 2009; **15**(3): 214–19.
14. White P, Cheung AKY. e-Learning in an undergraduate radiography programme: example of an interactive website. *Radiography.* 2006; **12**(3): 244–52.
15. Bleiker J, Knapp KM, Frampton I. Teaching patient care to students: a blended learning approach in radiography education. *Radiography.* 2011; **17**(3): 235–40.
16. Abrahams K. Evaluation of a reflective learning programme for radiation therapy graduates. *Radiographer.* 2012; **59**(2): 40–5.
17. Currie GM, Wheat JM. The first year clinical placement for undergraduate medical radiation science students: tool or toil? *Radiographer.* 2005; **52**(2): 18–22.
18. Ogbu SOI. Radiography students' perceptions of clinical placements: a Nigerian perspective. *Radiography.* 2008; **14**(2): 154–61.
19. Adams EJ, Adamson BJ, Poulos A. An insight into the students' perspective of a nuclear medicine clinical education program. *Radiographer.* 2004; **51**(3): 111–15.
20. Bolderston A, Palmer C, Flanagan W, *et al.* The experiences of English as second language radiation therapy students in the undergraduate clinical program: perceptions of staff and students. *Radiography.* 2008; **14**(3): 216–25.
21. Bridge P, Carmichael M, Brady C, *et al.* A snapshot of radiation therapy techniques and technology in Queensland: an aid to mapping undergraduate curriculum. *J Med Radiat Sci.* 2013; **60**(1): 25–34.
22. Halkett GKB, McKay J, Shaw T. Improving students' confidence levels in communicating with patients and introducing students to the importance of history taking. *Radiography.* 2011; **17**(1): 55–60.
23. Chapman NA, Oultram SC. Enhancing the RT student clinical experience: Newcastle Mater Hospital Radiation Oncology Department. *Radiography.* 2007; **13**(2): 159–63.
24. Thoirs K, Giles E, Barber W. The use and perceptions of simulation in medical radiation science education. *Radiographer.* 2011; **58**(3): 5–11.

25. Green D, Appleyard R. The influence of VERT™ characteristics on the development of skills in skin apposition techniques. *Radiography*. 2011; **17**(3): 178–82.

26. James S, Dumbleton C. An evaluation of the utilisation of the Virtual Environment for Radiotherapy Training (VERT) in clinical radiotherapy centres across the UK. *Radiography*. 2013; **19**(2): 142–50.

27. World Health Organization (WHO). *Framework for Action on Interprofessional Education & Collaborative Practice*. Geneva: WHO; 2010.

28. Hean S, Craddock D, Hammick M, *et al*. Theoretical insights into interprofessional education: AMEE Guide No. 62. *Med Teach*. 2012; **34**(2): e78–101.

29. Turner A, Zhou R, Tran C, *et al*. Translating theory to practice: the use of interprofessional student research teams to model interprofessional collaborative practice: what we learnt. *J Med Imaging Radiat Sci*. Epub 2012 Jan 27.

30. Naylor S. An evaluation of an enquiry based learning strategy for the science of imaging technology. *Radiography*. 2011; **17**(4): 319–22.

31. Elsie K, Francis B, Gonzaga MA. Attitudes and perceptions of students and teachers about problem based learning in the radiography curriculum at Makerere University, Uganda. *Eur J Radiol*. 2009; **1**(4): 156–62.

32. Elsie K, Gonzaga MA, Francis B, *et al*. Evaluation of ultrasound training in the problem based learning radiography curriculum at Makerere University, Uganda. *Radiography*. 2010; **16**(4): 314–20.

33. Higgins R, Hogg P, Robinson L. Towards a research informed teaching experience within a diagnostic radiography curriculum: the level 4 (year 1) student holistic experience. *Radiography*. 2013; **19**(1): 62–7.

34. Foster I. Enhancing the learning experience of student radiographers with dyslexia. *Radiography*. 2008; **14**(1): 32–8.

35. Tan K, Dawdy K, Di Prospero L. Understanding radiation therapists' perceptions and approach to clinical competence assessment of medical radiation sciences students. *J Med Imaging Radiat Sci*. 2013; **44**(2): 100–5.

36. Hall AS, Durward BR. Retention of anatomy knowledge by student radiographers. *Radiography*. 2009; **15**(3): e22–8.

37. Kench PL, Field N, Agudera M, *et al*. Peer assessment of individual contributions to a group project: student perceptions. *Radiography*. 2009; **15**(2): 158–65.

38. Ng CKC, White P, McKay JC. Development of a web database portfolio system with PACS connectivity for undergraduate health education and continuing professional development. *Comput Methods Programs Biomed*. 2009; **94**(1): 26–38.

39. Ng CKC, White P, McKay JC. Establishing a method to support academic and professional competence throughout an undergraduate radiography programme. *Radiography*. 2008; **14**(3): 255–64.

40. Mubuuke AG, Kiguli-Malwadde E, Kiguli S, *et al*. A student portfolio: the golden key to reflective, experiential, and evidence-based learning. *J Med Imaging Radiat Sci*. 2010; **41**(2): 72–8.

CHAPTER 33

Evidence-based education in pharmacy

Judith T Barr and Lynne M Sylvia

OVERVIEW

The objectives of this chapter are to determine the current status of best evidence pharmacy education (BEPE), defined as implementation by pharmacy teachers in their practice of methods and approaches to pharmacy education based on the best evidence available, and to compare the quality and quantity of evidence of active learning strategies in pharmacy education as reported in volumes 72 (published in 2008) and 76 (published in 2012) of the *American Journal of Pharmaceutical Education* (*AJPE*). A comprehensive literature search was conducted for the first objective, while hand searches of volumes 72 and 76 of the *AJPE* were used for the second. The second objective was prompted by the Accreditation Council for Pharmacy Education's 2007 accreditation standards recommending 'active learning strategies', a recommendation that the council then strengthened in its 2011 revision of the standards. While studies employing BEPE were not identified, a task force of the American Association of Colleges of Pharmacy assessed the current status of BEPE and provided recommended steps for conducting and applying best evidence to the process of pharmacy teaching. Manuscript criteria for the *AJPE* were strengthened for a category of article, Instructional Design and Assessment, to provide an article template consisting of five sections: Introduction, Design, Evaluation, Assessment and Summary. The search of the two *AJPE* volumes yielded seven active learning articles in 2008 and 21 in 2012. Only four of the seven articles from 2008 included both a comparison group and assessment of knowledge outcomes; 8 of the 21 articles from 2012 had both, including two reports on randomised controlled trials. As faculty strive to improve their classes and laboratories, they would benefit from a repository of high-quality studies, organised by subject content and educational strategies. These can be aggregated to yield meaningful systematic reviews and meta-analyses. Faculty will then have the resources to practise BEPE.

CHAPTER OBJECTIVES

Upon completion of this chapter, the reader will be able to:
- describe the teaching methods typically utilised in pharmacy education
- outline the BEPE principles
- articulate how active learning is used as an education strategy with pharmacy students
- outline the current evidence available related to pharmacy education.

KEY TERMS: best evidence pharmacy education (BEPE), best practice, pharmacy education, active learning

---

INTRODUCTION

Clinical pharmacy, as defined by the American College of Clinical Pharmacy, is a scientifically rooted discipline in which pharmacists apply evidence and evolving science to the care of individual patients.[1] Clinical decision-making based on conscientious and judicious use of current evidence is the foundation of contemporary pharmacy practice.

To prepare pharmacy graduates for contemporary practice, the evidence-based approach to clinical decision-making is reinforced throughout the professional programme in pharmacy leading to the Doctor of Pharmacy (PharmD) degree. Early in the professional years of the PharmD programme, courses such as research methods, drug information and drug literature evaluation establish the framework for an evidence-based practice. In the later years of the professional degree programme, students are taught to apply an evidence-based approach to clinical problem-solving in courses such as pharmacotherapeutics and disease state management. This approach is then refined during the experiential components of the programme, in which students learn to modify population-based evidence by incorporating patient-specific information to create medication therapy management plans for individual patients. The current accreditation standards and guidelines for the programme, as established by the Accreditation Council for Pharmacy Education (ACPE), state:

> the college or school must ensure that graduates are competent, at a minimum, to … *provide population-based care*, through the ability to develop and implement population-specific, evidence-based disease management programs and protocols based upon analysis of epidemiologic and pharmacoeconomic data, medication-use criteria, medication use review, and risk-reduction strategies.[2(p23)]

In addition to the content of the PharmD curriculum, the current accreditation standards and guidelines for American schools and colleges of pharmacy are specific to pedagogy: '[colleges and schools should be committed] to a culture that, in general, respects and … promotes use of teaching methods shown to enhance student learning.'[2(p3)] The accreditation standards and guidelines also refer to the use of 'proven teaching and learning methodologies' and the use of 'teaching and learning techniques that promote: knowledge base development; integration, application, and assessment of principles; critical thinking and problem solving; and professionalism.'[2(p29)] Colleges and schools of pharmacy are encouraged to be innovative in their methodologies and to integrate active learning strategies throughout the curriculum.

Based on a review of the current accreditation standards and guidelines for pharmacy education, it is clear that the content of the PharmD curriculum should be evidence based. What remains less clear are the teaching and learning methods that produce graduates who are competent practitioners. What evidence is available to support the use of 'proven teaching and learning methodologies' in pharmacy? What are these methodologies and how were they validated? In keeping with the evidence-based approach to decision-making initially described by Sackett et al.,[3] this chapter has been designed to answer these questions. In particular, our first research question for this chapter is: '*What is the current status of best evidence pharmacy education (BEPE)?*' BEPE is defined as 'implementation by pharmacy teachers in their practice of methods and approaches to pharmacy education based on the best evidence available.'[4(p1)] Our second research question is: '*What is the evidence, albeit not "best evidence", of the effectiveness of active learning strategies in pharmacy education, the strategies singled out as teaching and learning methods by the ACPE in its accreditation standards?*'[2]

SEARCH STRATEGY

To answer our first research question, a search of the academic literature, restricted to English-language articles, was performed using the following bibliographic systems: MEDLINE (1996 to June 2013), CINAHL (Cumulative Index to Nursing and Allied Health Literature; 1981 to the present), Web of Knowledge (1985–2013) and ERIC (Education Resources Information Center; 1966 to the present). The search terms were 'best evidence', 'pharmacy education', 'pharmacy', 'evidence-based education' and 'Best Evidence Pharmacy Education (BEPE)'. In MEDLINE, the search term 'pharmacy education' was also linked with the terms 'meta-analysis' or 'systematic review'. The following journals were manually searched using the same key words: the *American Journal of Pharmaceutical Education* (*AJPE*; 2001–13), the *Journal of Pharmacy Teaching* (1990 and 2007), *Currents in Pharmacy Teaching and Learning* (2009–13) and the *International Journal of Pharmacy Teaching and Practices* (2010–13). The reference lists and bibliographies of the retrieved papers were also reviewed for pertinent articles.

In order to answer our second research question, given the guidelines of this chapter, a more restrictive search was conducted. 'Active learning' is a collective term encompassing many teaching strategies that may or may not be used as keywords by a bibliographic indexer. Therefore, given concerns about the comprehensiveness of results from a database search for 'active learning in pharmacy', an in-depth but time-limited hand search was performed of the 'Research' and the 'Instructional Design and Assessment' sections of volumes 72 (six issues, published in 2008) and 76 (10 issues, published in 2012) of the *AJPE*. Inclusion criteria for articles were as follows: evidence-based, comparison group studies; interventions involving one of seven active learning pedagogies (audience response systems, discussion-based learning including deliberative discussion, patient simulation, problem-based learning including case-based learning, inquiry-based learning, process-oriented inquiry learning, team-based learning); modification to teaching strategies in a didactic classroom or associated laboratory; and inclusion of an outcome measure evaluating cognitive knowledge acquisition. Exclusion criteria were as follows: descriptive studies, pre-post only studies, studies evaluating introductory or advanced pharmacy practice experiences and only perception or student attitude outcome measures.

APPRAISAL OF THE EVIDENCE: BEST EVIDENCE PHARMACY EDUCATION

Our literature search yielded four papers specific to BEPE. Three were commentaries published in 2002,[5] 2003[6] and 2007,[7] encouraging pharmacy educators to approach curricular decision-making and teaching using evidence-based thinking. Beck[5] stated that 'if we approach decisions about our curricula and teaching strategies like we do in our laboratories or patient care environments, we will achieve our desired educational outcomes.'[(p87)] In 2002, Beck, as Chair of the Council of Faculties of the American Association of Colleges of Pharmacy (AACP), charged a task force on BEPE. The task force was specifically charged to review the evidence-based approach to medical education, or Best Evidence Medical Education (BEME), and assess its applicability to pharmacy education. Beck[5] noted:

> some may argue that pharmacy education lacks sufficient research literature within the discipline to make evidence-based decisions; however, evidence-based thinking includes consideration of established educational principles and the research of other health professional educators has applicability.[(p87)]

In 2004, the task force on BEPE published a White Paper on BEPE; this report by the task force was the fourth paper captured in our literature search.[4]

To date, this White Paper provides the most comprehensive assessment of the current status of BEPE. The task force explored the *notion* (rather than the *practice*) of BEPE by examining four areas: (1) evidence-based decision-making and its teaching, (2) using evidence in the content of teaching, (3) using evidence in the process of teaching and (4) the relationship between BEPE and the scholarship of teaching.[4] The task force endorsed a definition of BEPE modelled after that of BEME. The practice of

BEPE should be systematic, involve the gathering and critical assessment of relevant information before an action is taken, and apply to both the content and the process of teaching. Consistent with evidence-based medicine, evidence-based pharmacy education should involve the integration of the educator's experience with the 'best available external evidence obtained through a systematic search in order to implement effective instruction.'[4(p1)]

There are a number of recommended steps for applying best evidence to the process of pharmacy teaching (*see* Figure 33.1). Note that BEPE should begin with the identification of the desired educational outcome(s) to teaching, consistent with the practice of evidence-based medicine as described by Sackett *et al.*[8] After this first step of identifying measurable educational outcomes, the second step is a systematic search of the academic literature, recommended to identify best evidence. Both electronic and manual searches of the literature are recommended. Sources of evidence may include both experimental and experiential data (e.g. outcome assessment data obtained from one's own institution, personal experience with a teaching technique, a

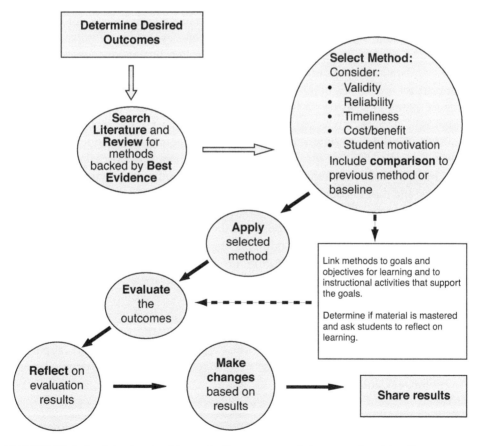

FIGURE 33.1 Applying best evidence to the process of pharmacy teaching (from Hammer *et al.*[4])

professional colleague's experience with a technique). The third step is to evaluate the evidence before taking action (e.g. choosing the study method or process of teaching). Assessment of the evidence should be performed using a structured approach with consideration given to the quality, utility, extent, strength, target group and setting of the evidence (e.g. the QUESTS method[9]). The fourth step would be the application of the teaching method to the course, curriculum or experiential setting. Step five involves evaluation of the outcome, evaluation of the process and reflection. Sharing of the experience with the larger teaching and learning community constitutes the final step in the process of BEPE. As noted by the task force, these proposed steps to BEPE are closely related to the six standards of the scholarship of teaching. By gathering, evaluating and applying the education-based evidence, the practice of BEPE supports a more scholarly approach to teaching and learning.

In 2004, BEPE was described as more of a notion than a practice; however, since this time, strides have been made within academic pharmacy to develop an infrastructure for BEPE. One significant move in the direction towards BEPE was the adoption in 2004 of revised criteria for manuscripts submitted to the *AJPE* in the category of Instructional Design and Assessment. The revised criteria, coined the IDEAS format, require authors not only to describe their experience with instructional innovation but also to provide evidence of assessment and evaluation of outcomes.[10] The term IDEAS is an acronym for Introduction, Design, Evaluation, Assessment and Summary, the structural format for articles in this section. The IDEAS format provides a template for the sharing of the scholarship of teaching in pharmacy, and it promotes evidence-based practices. In 2009, IDEAS was revised to offer further direction and guidance to authors of educational research in pharmacy.[11] Currently, manuscripts on instructional design submitted to the *AJPE* are required to include an evidence-based approach to support the improvements in the learner's knowledge, attitudes or performance. The revised criteria offer guidance on the types of data to use to assess outcomes, and they encourage assessment of additional aspects of the teaching process including time efficiency and institutional costs.[11] Adherence with the IDEAS format or comparable criteria throughout the pharmacy education literature may serve as one step forward on the continuum to BEPE.

To answer our first research question, no 'best evidence in pharmacy education' empirical articles were identified from the current literature search. Moreover, the database searches failed to identify any meta-analyses or systematic reviews of topics in pharmacy education to guide educators in the application of BEPE principles to pharmacy education. However, the hand search of *AJPE* issues revealed several review articles; only one, summarising the evidence on the use of virtual patients in pharmacy education, met the criteria of a systematic search (e.g. detailed search description, evidence tables).[12]

APPRAISAL OF THE EVIDENCE: ACTIVE LEARNING IN PHARMACY

In 2007, the ACPE's accreditation standards and guidelines included the mention of a specific type of pedagogy: active learning. 'Instructors should employ active learning strategies and encourage students to ask questions wherever possible.'[12(p1)] In a foot-note, 'active learning' was defined as:

> a style of teaching that requires the learner to formulate answers to questions based on acquired knowledge while continuing to search for new knowledge that may provide better, more complete answers. Active learning enhances a student's ability to think in an independent and critical manner.[12(p1)]

Active learning has been used since at least 300 BC, when Socrates encouraged students to learn through questioning. But what *evidence* was available to the ACPE to support the guideline that 'active learning strategies' should be used in pharmacy education (*see* Table 33.1)? While 'best evidence' of active learning did not exist in pharmacy education, evidence did exist in the scientific community. In 1991, Bonwell and Eison's[13] evidence-based report to the Association for the Study of Higher Education advocated the use of active learning to create excitement in the classroom. In 1999 the National Research Council synthesised the research findings from the developing field of 'the science of learning'; its report, *How People Learn: Brain, Mind, Experiences, and School*,[14] linked scientific findings to recommendations for changes in classroom activities and student learning strategies. Quoting from that report:

> The new science of learning is beginning to provide knowledge to improve significantly people's abilities to become *active learners* who seek to understand complex subject matter and are better prepared to transfer what they have learned to new problems and settings.[14(p1)]

Evidence supporting active learning strategies has developed in scientific fields such as physics, engineering and others.[16-18] The National Science Foundation has established CELEST (the Center of Excellence for Learning in Education, Science and Technology) to further the science of learning and development of evidence-based education.

Are active learning strategies being used in US schools and colleges of pharmacy? In spring 2010, Stewart *et al.*[18] surveyed the faculty members (N = 2013) of the AACP to determine if and what active learning strategies they were using. While only 59% (n = 1179) of the AACP faculty members responded, collectively they came from 95% of US pharmacy schools. Of the responding faculty, 87% used at least one active-learning strategy in their classroom. However, there are serious problems in drawing conclusions from these survey results: (a) not all pharmacy faculty are AACP members, creating potential for a biased sample; (b) only 59% of AACP members responded, further creating potential for sample and response bias; and (c) faculty were asked to indicate if they used any of the strategies, but no information was collected on frequency of use (e.g. how often within a course or within how many courses). Therefore, an accurate estimate of the frequency and intensity of use of active learning strategies in courses and classes in US pharmacy programmes is unknown.

TABLE 33.1 Active learning strategies included in a survey of US colleges and schools of pharmacy regarding curriculum content[18]

Strategy	Brief description
Audience response systems and clickers	Use of remote control devices by students to anonymously respond to multiple-choice questions posed by the instructor; can be integrated into traditional lectures; often termed 'active learning'
Discussion-based learning, including deliberate discussions	Use of communication among learners (both synchronous and asynchronous) as a teaching modality; can be used with strategies such as case studies
Interactive spaced education	Use of repetition of content at spaced intervals combined with testing of that content; developed and used heavily within the context of medical education
Interactive web-based learning	Use of web-based modules to deliver content and assess student understanding in an interactive format
Patient simulations	Use of human patient simulators in a laboratory environment to teach providers to respond to a variety of physiologic emergencies and situations
POGIL and discovery learning	Use of exercises specifically designed to lead teams of students through stages of exploring data, developing concepts based on that data, and applying the concepts
PBL, including case-based learning	Use of cases or problem sets meant to be explored in self-managed teams of students (with facilitators); PBL sessions precede any discussion of content by instructor
Team-based learning	Use of small student groups to facilitate discussion, case study exploration or other aspects of content; preparation required in advance, and content integrated throughout the class by the facilitator (expert)
Traditional laboratory experiences	Use of traditional laboratory and benchtop experiences to provide hands-on learning experiences

Note: adapted from Table 1 in Steward et al.;[18] *abbreviations:* POGIL = practice-oriented global inquiry learning; PBL = problem-based learning

In 2011, the ACPE issued a revised version[2] of its accreditation standards and guidelines from 2007.[12] Among the revisions were the addition of three more references to active learning (italics added): (1) 'curriculum committees would strive for consistency of course syllabi to include … *identification of active learning strategies employed*'[(p1)] (guideline 10.2); (2) 'the development of critical thinking *through active learning strategies and other higher order pedagogical strategies*'[(p1)] (guideline 11.2); and (3) '*Active learning strategies* include …'[(p1)] (guideline 11.2).

Given that no meta-analysis has been published for best practices in pharmacy education, the answer to our second research question is that it is not known what is the best practice related to the use of active learning strategies in pharmacy education.

However, the change in increased specificity for the inclusion of active learning in the updated standards from 2011, compared with the standards from 2007, does suggest a corollary to our second research question: *Does ACPE's increased emphasis on active learning have a parallel in an increased number of active learning studies in pharmacy education and do the latter studies provide increased rigour of evidence-based study design and measurement of knowledge outcomes?* To answer this question we compared active learning articles in the two volumes of the *AJPE* subsequent to the adoption of each version of the ACPE accreditation standards and guidelines. Are the active learning articles published in 2008 (Volume 72), 1 year after adoption of the 2007 accreditation standards and guidelines, different from the active learning articles published in 2012 (Volume 76), 1 year after adoption of the 2011 revision of the standards? As the specificity of the ACPE active learning guidelines increased from 2007 to 2011, was there any change in the strength of the evidence of effectiveness of active learning to improve student knowledge outcomes as published in the journal of the AACP?

TABLE 33.2 Comparison incorporating active learning articles published in the *American Journal of Pharmaceutical Education* in 2008 and 2012

Variable	Number of articles in 2008 (Volume 72)	Number of articles in 2012 (Volume 76)
Issues	6	10
Research articles	37	56
Research articles involving active learning	1	1
Research articles with 'active learning' in the title	0	0
Research articles involving active learning with comparative effectiveness study design	0	0
Research articles involving active learning with knowledge outcomes	1	0
Research articles with both comparative effectiveness design and knowledge outcomes	0	0
IDA articles	27	58
IDA articles involving active learning	7	21
IDA articles with 'active learning' in the title	2	11
IDA articles involving active learning with comparative effectiveness study design	4	8
IDA articles involving active learning with knowledge outcomes	4	15
IDA articles with both comparative effectiveness design and knowledge outcomes	4	8

Abbreviation: IDA = Instructional Design and Assessment

Table 33.2 presents comparative findings between the active learning studies that appeared in the 'Research' or 'Instructional Design and Assessment' sections of the six issues of the 2008 *AJPE* (Volume 72) and the 10 issues of the 2012 *AJPE* (Volume 76). Of the 37 'Research' articles in 2008 and the 56 articles in 2012, only one article in each volume described an active learning intervention. Neither included a comparison population and only the 2008 article assessed a knowledge outcome. Of the 27 'Instructional Design and Assessment' articles in 2008, seven reported active learning studies, and only four had both a comparison group and measured knowledge outcomes. In 2012, there were 58 'Instructional Design and Assessment' articles that included 21 active learning studies, of which eight included both criteria, including two randomised controlled trials. The use of a 'pre- then post-test' design and student perception surveys were the primary reasons for studies to be excluded. Table 33.3 provides further descriptive information of active learning studies that included both comparison groups and knowledge assessment. Nearly all studies documented that active learning led to improved knowledge outcomes over the control group. Overall, the active learning studies increased in quantity and quality from 2008 to 2012.

Based on this analysis, several caveats are worth mentioning. First, in total, there were 30 active learning articles published in the *AJPE* during these 2 years; however, only 13 of these articles included 'active learning' in the article's title, an important fact to consider when designing bibliographic search strategies. This prompts the second caveat: 'active learning' encompasses a range of methods to engage students during the teaching and learning process, and it is not a homogenous activity. Of the 12 articles that did include a comparison group and measured knowledge outcomes, six different active learning strategies were studied across a range of subject content. Therefore, a third caveat relates to the generalisability of the findings. As faculty consider applying the results of these studies to their teaching, they should consider that there may be interaction effects among educational strategies, subject content and placement in the pharmacy curriculum. What is effective with one active learning method with one type of subject content in one group of students may not be generalisable to another method with a different subject content. Further studies using strong research design and meaningful outcomes will increase our confidence in the applicability of the findings.

RECOMMENDATIONS

It is obvious to pharmacy faculty that they need to keep current with the best evidence in the science of their subject content or clinical practice. However, less obvious to faculty is the need to remain current with the best available evidence concerning the pedagogy that best assists students in learning the content. A need exists to create a culture that recognises the equal value of combining what is the best scientific evidence with what is the best evidence to aid the student in learning that science. Therefore, more emphasis should be placed within the pharmacy academy to acculturate faculty to evidence-based educational practices and to provide incentives for the use of available evidence in the design of their classes and learning activities.

TABLE 33.3 Characteristics of articles incorporating comparative effectiveness design and knowledge outcomes published in the *American Journal of Pharmaceutical Education* in 2008 and 2012

Journal page	Citation	School or college of pharmacy	Type of active learning	Subject content	Design	Comparator	Comparative outcomes	Test versus control result
American Journal of Pharmaceutical Education, **2008, Volume 72**								
28	Ernst and Colthorpe[19]	University of Queensland	Interactive web-based, discussion-based learning	Respiratory physiology	Concurrent and nonconcurrent cohorts	2 years prior: traditional 1 year prior: partial implementation of Web	Summative knowledge examination (Also* perceptions)	Improvement in respiratory physiology questions between web-based and traditional in renal physiology questions, but not renal pharmacology questions ($p < 0.001$)
29	Dupuis and Persky[20]	University of North Carolina	CBL	Clinical pharmacokinetics	Concurrent and nonconcurrent cohorts	Self and traditional previous years	Summative examination (Also attitudes)	CBL higher scores in final exam and after first case, but higher in traditional after second case ($p < 0.005$)
31	Alsharif and Galt[21]	Creighton University	CBL	Two-semester medicinal chemistry	Concurrent and nonconcurrent cohorts	On/off campus Traditional previous year	Quizzes and summative exams (Also perceptions)	CBL class, both on- and off-campus, improved over examination and course scores in both semesters of the course ($p < 0.005$)
103	Letassy *et al.*[22]	University of Oklahoma	TBL and CBL	Endocrine module in pharmaceutical care series	Nonconcurrent cohort	Traditional previous years	Unit and final examinations (Also perceptions)	'Students performed similarly or better on unit examinations and achieved higher grades in the courses when developed in TBL format.'

(*continued*)

Journal page	Citation	School or college of pharmacy	Type of active learning	Subject content	Design	Comparator	Comparative outcomes	Test versus control result
American Journal of Pharmaceutical Education, 2012, Volume 76								
14	Albano and Brown[23]	North Dakota State University	Cases, COL	Physical assessment	Nonconcurrent cohort	Traditional previous year	Examination and PCOA (Also perceptions)	On PCOA, COL students scored higher than national mean on pathophysiology and patient assessment than in the previous year. Traditional group 'did not do as well relatively or marginally'
27	Haack and Phillips[24]	Drake University	Discussion-based learning	Cultural competence	Concurrent cohort	Traditional previous year	Cultural competence inventory assessment	Overall inventory scores same; better in subscores for cultural competence and cultural encounters
28	Lupu *et al.*[25]	Duquesne University	Patient simulation: mock patient counselling	Motivational interviewing	Randomised controlled trial	Written dialogue and peer role-play	Test, interviewing skills, confidence, attitudes	All improved; mean change in knowledge scores in mock patient group higher than in written group. Interview skills trending higher in mock patient
31	Persky[26]	University of North Carolina	TBL	Pharmacokinetics	Nonconcurrent cohort	Previous year recitation group format	Examination (Also impact on subsequent class)	Synthesis-level examination questions significantly better in TBL. TBL associated with higher grades in subsequent clinical pharmacokinetics course

Journal page	Citation	School or college of pharmacy	Type of active learning	Subject content	Design	Comparator	Comparative outcomes	Test versus control result
84	Dunham et al.[27]	University of Michigan	Interactive web-based preparation for laboratory	Laboratory portion of drug assay course	Nonconcurrent cohort with/without computer introduction	5 previous years	Online quiz, final exams, perceptions	Final practical examination improved, from 82.7% prior to use of web tools, to 86.2% with partial use of web tools, to 91.2% fully implemented ($p < 0.001$)
86	Ray et al.[28]	University of Tennessee	Patient simulation	Drug-induced diseases	Randomised controlled trial	Written case	Knowledge test: immediately and 25 days later	Test scores improved in both written and simulation case, but no difference in retention
112	Kolluru[29]	Texas A&M University	TBL	Medicinal chemistry	Nonconcurrent cohort	Traditional previous year	Final examination (Also perceptions)	Average examination grade in TBL was higher than traditional ($p = 0.002$)
196	Pierce and Fox[30]	Shenandoah University	POGIL, flipped classroom	Renal pharmacotherapy	Nonconcurrent cohort	Traditional previous year	Final examination (Also perceptions)	Student performance on the 16 final examination questions relating to the renal module significantly improved in the POGIL group

Note: * the 'also' outcome measure obtained in active learning population only; *abbreviations:* CBL = case-based learning; COL = cooperative learning; PCOA = Pharmacy Curriculum Outcomes Assessment; POGIL = process-oriented guided learning; TBL = team-based learning

Web-based educational resources should be developed to diffuse this information to faculty members.

A development of a repository of pharmacy educational studies is a first step in aggregating best available evidence. At a minimum, studies must have strong research designs that include comparison group studies with meaningful knowledge outcomes. The repository should be organised by curricular or subject content, pedagogic approach and study design. For topics with sufficient studies, systematic reviews with meta-analyses should be conducted and published. Topics lacking sufficient evidence should be identified. The importance of these topics should be priorities, a special call for studies on this topic should be issued, and a themed-issue of a pharmacy education journal feature the studies that result from the call.

Pharmacy educators must continue to encourage the scientific rigour of pharmacy education study design. The IDEAS format with documentation of outcomes assessment is a good first step, but weak designs and student perception studies appear in the Instruction Design and Assessment section of the *AJPE*. To more clearly identify the stronger studies, these could be kept in the Instruction Design and Assessment section, while others could be removed to an 'Education Reports' section. This emphasis on stronger study designs will increase the internal validity of the study's conclusion. A method to increase the external validity of studies would be to develop pharmacy education research collaborations among colleges and schools of pharmacy to increase the generalisability of research findings.

The steps will take time to develop. In the interim, when a pharmacy question is of a general health professional (or interprofesssional) nature, faculty can consider existing BEME Collaboration reviews. By the end of 2014, the BEME Collaboration will have published 29 reviews.[31] While the majority pertain to medical education only, several encompass the health professional educational literature and summarise the evidence of the effectiveness of audience response systems[32] and of case-based learning.[33] Pharmacy educators considering the use of these strategies could use the systematic reviews as a generic foundation for the steps in planning a pharmacy-specific education intervention and evaluation.

CONCLUSION

At present, BEPE still remains more of a notion than a practice. While the AACP's White Paper from 2004 developed an agenda to include best evidence into the design of educational pedagogy, the field is awaiting its first BEPE review. The IDEAS format in the *AJPE* has the potential to increase the rigour of *AJPE* articles. This appears to have started already, as evidenced by a comparison of the *AJPE* articles from 2008 and 2012 describing active learning interventions: both the quantity and the quality of the studies have increased. Efforts must continue to emphasise the scholarship of teaching and learning and the publication of well-designed pharmacy educational studies.

SUMMARY POINTS

- BEPE is used to promote high-quality evidence in pharmacy education.
- Active learning principles are frequently used in pharmacy education.
- The search of the *AJPE* volumes from 2008 and 2012 yielded seven active learning articles in 2008 and 21 in 2012.
- The body of pharmacy education research continues to grow.

REVIEW QUESTIONS

- What are the BEPE principles?
- How have active learning principles been applied in pharmacy education contexts?
- What is the current state of evidence-based education in a pharmacy education context?

REFLECTIVE QUESTIONS AND EXERCISES

- What types of education research would be appropriate for pharmacy education?
- Think about how pharmacy students could be included in an interprofessional education class with other health professional students.
- How could a problem-based education approach be implemented in a pharmacy curriculum?

REFERENCES

1. American College of Clinical Pharmacy (ACCP). *Clinical Pharmacy Defined.* Lenexa, KS: ACCP; 2005. Available at: www.accp.com/about/clinicalPharmacyDefined.aspx (accessed 17 July 2013).
2. Accreditation Council for Pharmacy Education (ACPE). *Accreditation Standards and Guidelines for the Professional Program in Pharmacy Leading to the Doctor of Pharmacy Degree.* Version 2.0. Chicago, IL: ACPE; 2011. Available at: www.acpe-accredit.org/pdf/FinalS2007Guidelines2.0.pdf (accessed 17 July 2013).
3. Sackett DL, Rosenberg WM, Gray JM, *et al.* Evidence-based medicine: what it is and what it isn't. *BMJ.* 1996; **312**(7023): 71–2.
4. Hammer DP, Sauer KA, Fielding DW, *et al.* White Paper on best evidence pharmacy education (BEPE). *Am J Pharm Educ.* 2004; **68**(1): 24.
5. Beck DE. Pharmacy educators: can an evidence-based approach make your instruction better tomorrow than today? *Am J Pharm Educ.* 2002; **66**(1): 87–8.
6. Lubaway WC. Evaluating teaching using the best practices model. *Am J Pharm Educ.* 2003; **67**(3): 87.
7. DiPiro JT. Good teaching is good science. *Am J Pharm Educ.* 2007; **71**(1): 10.

8. Sackett DL, Straus SE, Richardson WS, *et al. Evidence-Based Medicine: how to practice and teach EBM.* 2nd ed. London, UK: Churchill Livingstone/Harcourt; 2000.

9. Harden RM, Grant J, Buckley G, *et al.* BEME Guide No. 1. Best Evidence Medical Education. *Med Teach.* 1999; **21**(6): 553–62.

10. Poirier T, Crouch M, Hak E, *et al.* Guidelines for manuscripts describing instructional design or assessment: the IDEAS format. *Am J Pharm Educ.* 2004; **68**(4): 92.

11. Poirier T, Crouch M, MacKinnon G, *et al.* Updated guidelines for manuscripts describing instructional design and assessment: the IDEAS format. *Am J Pharm Educ.* 2009; **73**(3): 55.

12. Accreditation Council for Pharmacy Education (ACPE). *Accreditation Standards and Guidelines for the Professional Program in Pharmacy Leading to the Doctor of Pharmacy Degree.* Version 2.0 (track changes). Chicago, IL: ACPE; 2011. Available at: www.acpe-accredit.org/pdf/S2007Guidelines2.0_ChangesIdentifiedInRed.pdf (accessed 13 August 2013).

13. Bonwell CC, Eison JA. *Active Learning: creating excitement in the classroom.* ASHE-ERIC Higher Education Report No. 1. Washington, DC: George Washington University School of Education and Human Development; 1991.

14. National Research Council. *How People Learn: brain, mind, experience, and school.* Washington, DC: National Academies Press; 2000.

15. Hake RR. Interactive-engagement versus traditional methods: a six-thousand-student survey of mechanics test data for introductory physics courses. *Am J Phys.* 1998; **66**(1): 64–74.

16. Prince M. Does active learning work? A review of the research. *J Eng Educ.* 2004; **93**(3): 223–31.

17. Barr JT. What matters in large classroom teaching? In: Sylvia LM, Barr JT, editors. *Pharmacy Education: what matters in learning and teaching?* Burlington, MA: Jones & Bartlett; 2010. pp. 105–32.

18. Stewart DW, Brown SD, Clavier CW, *et al.* Active-learning processes used in US pharmacy education. *Am J Pharm Educ.* 2011; **75**(4): 68.

19. Ernst H, Colthorpe K. Expanding voluntary active-learning opportunities for pharmacy students in a respiratory physiology module. *Am J Pharm Educ.* 2008; **72**(2): 28.

20. Dupuis RE, Persky AM. Use of case-based learning in a clinical pharmacokinetics course. *Am J Pharm Educ.* 2008; **72**(2): 29.

21. Alsharif NZ, Galt KA. Evaluation of an instructional model to teach clinically relevant medicinal chemistry in a campus and a distance pathway. *Am J Pharm Educ.* 2008; **72**(2): 31.

22. Letassy NA, Fugate SE, Medina MS, *et al.* Using team-based learning in an endocrine module taught across two campuses. *Am J Pharm Educ.* 2008; **72**(5): 103.

23. Albano CB, Brown W. Integration of physical assessment within a pathophysiology course for pharmacy. *Am J Pharm Educ.* 2012; **76**(1): 14.

24. Haack S, Phillips C. Teaching cultural competency through a pharmacy skills and applications course series. *Am J Pharm Educ.* 2012; **76**(2): 27.

25. Lupu AM, Stewart AL, O'Neil C. Comparison of active-learning strategies for motivational interviewing skills, knowledge, and confidence in first-year pharmacy students. *Am J Pharm Educ.* 2012; **76**(2): 28.

26. Persky A. The impact of team-based learning on a foundational pharmacokinetic course. *Am J Pharm Educ.* 2012; **76**(2): 31.

27. Dunham MW, Ghirtis K, Beleh M. The use of virtual laboratories and other web-based tools in a drug assay course. *Am J Pharm Educ.* 2012; **76**(5): 84.

28. Ray SM, Wylie DR, Rowe AS, *et al.* Pharmacy student knowledge retention after completing either a simulated or written patient case. *Am J Pharm Educ.* 2012; **76**(5): 86.

29. Kolluru S. An active-learning assignment requiring pharmacy students to write medicinal chemistry examination questions. *Am J Pharm Educ.* 2012; **76**(6): 112.

30. Pierce R, Fox J. Vodcasts and active-learning exercises in a 'flipped classroom' model of a renal pharmacotherapy module. *Am J Pharm Educ.* 2012; **76**(10): 196.

31. BEME Collaboration. *Published Reviews*. Available at: http://bemecollaboration.org/Published+Reviews/ (accessed 26 August 2013).
32. Nelson C, Hartling L, Campbell S, *et al.* The effects of audience response systems on learning outcomes in health professions education: a BEME systematic review. BEME Guide No. 21. *Med Teach*. 2012; **34**(6): e386–405.
33. Thistlethwaite J, Davies D, Ekeocha S, *et al.* The effectiveness of case-based learning in health professional education: a BEME systematic review. BEME Guide No. 23. *Med Teach*. 2012; **34**(6): e421–44.

CHAPTER 34

Evidence-based education in nutrition and dietetics

······································

Deborah MacLellan

OVERVIEW

A dietitian is a health professional with expertise in foods and nutrition. Dietetic education typically involves two phases: knowledge acquisition (usually in a university setting) and skills development (usually in a practicum setting). The purpose of this chapter is to present the current research evidence related to the education of nutrition and dietetics students. A search of the literature between 1990 and the present identified 36 studies directly related to dietetic education. These studies were limited by small sample sizes, single time points and voluntary participation in most cases; however, they did provide some useful insights into best practices in dietetic education. Evidence is presented in relation to how the curriculum for dietetic education is developed, the strategies or techniques being used to teach dietetic students, and the methods of assessment being used to evaluate knowledge and skill development. It was concluded that dietetic education is heavily reliant on expert opinion and students' preferences and perspectives. Few studies evaluated student outcomes or tried to determine if what was learned translated into practice. Much of what we do in dietetic education is not grounded in evidence. It would appear that this is an understudied area, possibly due to the fact that there is no dedicated journal for dietetic education and therefore little incentive to conduct pedagogical research. There is a significant gap in our knowledge and understanding of what we do in dietetic education which needs to be filled if we are to meet the needs future generations of dietitians.

CHAPTER OBJECTIVES

Upon completion of this chapter, the reader will be able to:

- outline the entry-level competency standards and curriculum development in dietetics education
- describe strategies used in dietetics education
- specify the assessment tools available to evaluate knowledge and skill development in dietetics students.

KEY TERMS: dietitian, competency standards, clinical skills, practicum experience

---

INTRODUCTION

According to the International Confederation of Dietetic Associations (ICDA), an organisation representing dietetic associations throughout the world,

> a dietitian is a person with legally recognised qualifications (in nutrition and dietetics) who applies the science of nutrition to the feeding and education of groups of people and individuals in health and disease.[1(p4)]

How one becomes a dietitian varies among member countries in the ICDA; however, at a minimum, a bachelor's degree and a supervised practicum experience of at least 500 hours is recommended.[2] As with all health professions, it is widely recognised that dietetic practice needs to be grounded in evidence. However, it has been acknowledged that many of the decisions about best practices in dietetic education are based on expert opinion rather than scientific evidence.[3] The purpose of this chapter is to present the current research evidence related to the education of nutrition and dietetics students. A comprehensive literature review was conducted and studies from January 1990 to February 2012 related to evidence-based education were identified using electronic databases (CINAHL [Cumulative Index to Nursing and Allied Health Literature], MEDLINE, Web of Science). Studies were excluded if they were reported in conference abstracts only or were presented as perspectives in practice or were an opinion piece rather than a research study. Reference lists of included studies were also searched for other potentially relevant studies. The review included 36 articles published between 1990 and 2013. The majority of studies were descriptive in nature and would be considered level III evidence (evidence from case, correlation, and comparative studies). Limitations included small sample sizes, single time points and voluntary participation. Regardless of these limitations, the studies provide some useful insights into best practices in dietetic education.

The findings are divided into three sections: how the entry-level competency standards and curriculum for dietetic education are developed, the strategies or techniques being used to teach dietetic students, and the methods of assessment being used to evaluate knowledge and skill development.

ENTRY-LEVEL COMPETENCY STANDARDS AND CURRICULUM DEVELOPMENT

As mentioned earlier, the ICDA recommends that, at a minimum, dietetic education and training should involve a bachelor's degree and a practicum experience of at least 500 hours.[1] This standard was developed by consensus with member association representatives and approved by the Board of Directors of the ICDA in 2004 and was based on data from a study designed to determine the basic level of education required by member countries at that point in time.[2] It is known that not all countries are in compliance with this recommendation and that there is a range of requirements around the world.[1] However, the 23 countries that are in compliance have national standards for their programmes related to the course content, examinations, student assessment and/or supervised practical placement.[1] These standards are typically set by either a government body or the national dietetic association.

In countries with established dietetic education programmes (such as Australia, Canada, the United Kingdom and the United States), dietetic education is based on developing entry-level competencies. These standards include the knowledge, skills and attitudes required to graduate from a dietetic education programme and enter dietetic practice.[4] The standard-setting process generally starts with the identification of these requisite practice skills, attitudes and knowledge, usually through consultations with members of their respective national dietetic associations, expert committees and interviews with key stakeholder groups. Thus, in terms of levels of evidence, for the most part it would appear that dietetic competency standards are based on the lowest level of evidence (level IV).

Australia was the first country to use practice information, gathered in a systematic way, to inform national competency standard development.[5] The first national competency standards for Australian dietitians were published in 1993 and developed through a process which involved consultation with academic dietitians from around the country and validation by new graduates.[5] These standards were reviewed in 1998 by another group of new graduates and other stakeholders, which resulted in only minor changes. In 2007, Ash *et al.*[6] used a mixed methods approach to review the entry-level competencies. They interviewed 19 new graduates to find out what they did in a normal day using a 'Core Activities Interview' guide and analysed that data to identify the knowledge, skills and attitudes required by an entry-level dietitian. These were then compared with the earlier competency review to identify gaps. This process has subsequently been used in Canada to develop a set of integrated competencies for dietetic education.[6]

National competency standards provide a framework for dietetic education and are meant to be flexible to allow individual programmes to create their own curriculum in their own context.[7] However, this flexibility does not always provide enough guidance for entry-level practice. Cant and Aroni[8] conducted a two-phase mixed methods study to identify the necessary core skills and to validate performance criteria for nutrition education and counselling. They included the voices of clients in addition to the perspectives of dietitians to elicit clients' views about dietitians' skills and attributes related to these practice areas. Based on their data, they identified

42 performance criteria that they then used to develop an eight-step nutrition education model. Although it is recognised that there are many possible ways to conduct a
nutrition education and counselling session and to achieve entry-level competencies
in these areas, this type of study is very helpful, in that it identifies more specifically
for new practitioners the steps they need to take to develop the necessary skills and
competencies.

Shafer and Knous[9] have argued for the importance of a learner-centred approach
to curriculum development and the need to understand dietetic students' cognitive
and affective behaviours. They asked dietetic students (N = 18) to complete three surveys (the Cognitive Behavior Survey, the Rosenberg Self-Esteem Scale and the Goal
Analysis Questionnaire), first in a professional practice course and then 2 years later
in an advanced nutrition course. Their findings indicated that students failed to gain
reflective and conceptual thinking skills and their views of the learning experience
were more negative in the upper-level course. Of particular concern was the finding
that competition was the primary learning motivator both at baseline and follow-up.

These authors note that students who are motivated by a desire to outperform
others are more likely to use learning methods such as rote memorisation rather than
the critical and reflective thinking that is necessary for professional dietetic practice.
Further, problem-solving abilities are compromised in a competitive environment.

Another key factor in developing a learner-centred curriculum and learning
activities to ensure that students develop the necessary competencies is to understand
how dietetic students learn. A study by Palermo et al.[10] with 129 Australian dietetic
students from years one to four, demonstrated that students

> were equally balanced in their preferences for active and reflective learn-
> ing, but were more strongly aligned towards intuitive, verbal and global
> learning than towards sensing, visual and sequential learning. The pro-
> portion of students preferring different learning styles remained fairly
> stable over the years, although there was a higher preference for reflective
> learning in the year four cohort.[(p110)]

This is interesting in light of the finding by Shafer and Knous[9] that the competitive
nature of dietetic education does not support the development of reflective thinking.
However, this might be explained by the fact that the students in the study by Palermo
et al.[10] were in an integrated dietetic internship programme; thus the competition
to achieve an internship was not present. These findings suggest that an integrated
approach is more conducive to the development of critical and reflective thinking
skills. However, only one study could be found that explored the question of whether
or not dietetic internship should be integrated with the academic programme or
offered separately after graduation. Lordly and Travers[11] conducted a survey to determine graduate and employer perceptions of an integrated model of dietetic education.
A self-administered questionnaire was used to collect quantitative and qualitative data
from programme graduates (N = 24) and their first employers (N = 19) and results
indicated that participants perceived the integrated programme to be an acceptable

alternative. Further, they noted that the integrated programme allowed them to be exposed to a wide variety of experiences and enabled them to take more responsibility for their own learning.[11]

Two studies were found that discussed current specific curriculum content areas. In 2010, Knoblock-Hahn and Scharff[12] conducted an online survey with 153 dietetic programme directors to assess the extent to which cultural competency is included in dietetics education programmes in the United States. It is widely recognised that dietitians need to be able to work effectively in cross-cultural situations and thus competency standards in the United States include the need for dietetic students to have opportunities to develop cultural competence. Knoblock-Hahn and Scharff[12] found a discrepancy between what programme directors thought should be included in the curriculum related to cultural competency and what they were currently providing. Of particular concern was the fact that content areas related to knowledge were more likely to be included than those related to skills and attitudes and very few programmes had a required course in cultural competency, suggesting that dietetic students have limited opportunities to study this topic in any depth.

Similarly, Vickery and Cotugna[13] conducted a study to determine the extent to which complementary and alternative medicine was being offered in dietetics programmes in the United States. They sent a survey to the directors of all dietetics programmes in the country and received responses from 92 (34% response rate). Almost all programmes included complementary and alternative medicine instruction in some form in their curriculum and most directors indicated that they thought this was an important topic. However, only seven programmes had a course dedicated to this topic and only three programmes required that students take the course. It was concluded that although current curricula is providing some complementary and alternative medicine topics a core of knowledge is lacking, indicating that students are not being adequately prepared in this area. It is unknown if this situation has improved since this study was conducted in 2006.

The practicum experience in dietetic education typically varies in length and can be either integrated with the academic component or completed on a postgraduate basis. The rationale for determining the length of the practicum experience is unclear. For example, a recent study by Thompson[14] found that the practicum experience in Jamaica is 52 weeks, while in Trinidad and Tobago it is only 36 weeks. This difference was attributed to the local system and structure; however, what that means is unclear. Hughes and Desbrow[15] found that the length of the practicum experience was not as important as the types of experiences that a student is exposed to during the practicum. They collected data from three cohorts of student dietitians (N = 59) in Australia to determine the types of cases students were exposed to, what students were allowed to do in those placements, and what activities preceptors were involved in while supervising those students. Their results showed that there was a lot of variability in the types of experiences that students were exposed to and that the minimum number of placement experiences needed to achieve entry-level competence was 47. They concluded that it might be better to suggest a minimum number of placement exposures rather than mandating a specific number of placement weeks.

STRATEGIES USED IN DIETETIC EDUCATION

What are the best practices in teaching strategies in dietetic education? Traditionally, the academic component of dietetic education has been delivered via lectures and labs while the practicum component provided the hands-on experience needed for practice. Dietetic education relies on practising dietitians to supervise the practicum component of dietetic education. Typically, these supervisors are referred to as 'preceptors.' Given the critical role that these individuals play in the education and training of dietitians, it is concerning that there are so few studies of their educational needs. Taylor et al.[16] found that preceptors need training in five key areas: (1) basic teaching skills, (2) time management strategies, (3) methods for coaching students, (4) adult learning styles and (5) methods for providing constructive feedback.

Dietitians are expected to be able to think critically, make decisions about complex issues in practice and be self-directed learners. Most of the research related to the strategies used in dietetic education focuses on the methods used to assist students to develop these skills including: problem-based learning (PBL), concept mapping, double-entry journals, arts-based approaches, service-learning, and computer-assisted instruction (CAI) and online learning. However, in all cases, no objective outcome measures of these skills were included and thus, for the most part, we only have students' or preceptors' perceptions of students' abilities in these areas and the effectiveness of these teaching strategies and approaches.

PBL has been shown to be useful in dietetic education to help students develop clinical reasoning, decision-making, and problem-solving skills by simulating real-life experiences.[17] In 2004, ChanLin and Chan[17,18] published two studies related to PBL in dietetics. These researchers developed a web-based module on drug and nutrient interactions that used a PBL approach. In the first study, they explored students' experiences with PBL and found that most were positive about this instructional approach and thought that it helped them to explore problems and develop skills that could be applied in practice. In the second study, they compared a PBL approach using web-based instructional design with a traditional web-based learning approach to determine if there were any differences in student learning outcomes. Results suggested that PBL students performed significantly better and had more opportunity to develop skills in analysing problems and identifying learning resources. However, whether or not students are able to transfer that learning to other problems and into practice was not assessed.

In 2007, ChanLin and Chan[19] extended their research in PBL by exploring the use of an electronic forum to provide learning support to students. Experts from fields related to the problem were invited to participate in discussion forums with students. Data from these forums, along with student interviews, written reflections and group projects was analysed using content analysis. Results indicated that students were very positive about the support provided by these experts. Furthermore, analysis of their group projects indicated that they had achieved a deeper level of understanding of the course content. These authors concluded that students require two types of support to facilitate their learning: cognitive (related to course content) and affective (related to students' feelings of self-efficacy and confidence).

Concept maps are used in dietetic education to help students understand how key concepts are linked. Studies have shown that they can enhance learning and help dietetic students learn to be more self-directed. Roberts et al.[20] used concept mapping with undergraduate students in a diet therapy course. Their results indicated that students believed that they had developed better critical thinking, problem-solving and collaboration skills. More recently, Molaison et al.[21] used concept mapping to teach nutrition assessment to dietetic interns. They asked interns to draw a concept map based on a case study of a patient with renal disease at the beginning and end of their internship placement. These concept maps were then evaluated by trained internship preceptors using standardised scoring criteria. Results showed that there was a significant difference between the scores on the pre-assessment map versus the post-assessment map. Further, interns' perceptions of the use of concept mapping as a learning tool were very positive. Similar to the findings of Roberts et al.,[20] interns in the study by Molaison et al.[21] thought that they were more self-directed in their learning and that they had a much deeper understanding of medical nutrition therapy as a result of learning how to use concept maps.

Nahikian-Nelms and Nelms[22] used double-entry journals to assist dietetic interns to develop critical thinking skills. They asked nine students to keep a double-entry journal of their experiences on clinical placement. On one side of the page, students were asked to record objective data about their experience; on the other side of the page they were asked to record their subjective responses to the objective data. After 8 weeks, students were asked about the usefulness of the process. Results indicated that the journal writing process enabled students to organise their thoughts and the reflection helped them to develop a deeper understanding of what they were learning. However, although the authors concluded that journal writing can enhance students' critical thinking skills, it must be noted that this conclusion was based on students' perceptions only; there were no objective measures of critical thinking skills in this study. Further, their sample size was very small and it is unknown if the results are generalisable.

Arts-based (narrative, storytelling) approaches in dietetic education have been studied by several researchers over the past 5 years. Dietetic practice is often said to be both a science and an art; however, most emphasis has been on the science aspect. In fact, dietetic educators have been criticised as being too objective and relying too much on scientific evidence and thereby ignoring the relational and emotional aspects of dietetic practice.[23] A qualitative study by Brady and Gingras[23] explored students' perspectives on the use of stories in pedagogy, curriculum and inquiry in an undergraduate nutrition course. Ten students completed a qualitative survey; four of these students agreed to participate in a follow-up focus group. In general, students had very positive comments about the use of storytelling in the classroom and felt that it enriched their understanding and fostered personal growth. More specifically, storytelling helped them to be more creative in their approach and to learn how to listen, a key skill in nutrition counselling. Lordly[24] also found that storytelling can enhance the teaching and learning environment in dietetic education. She used an exploratory, descriptive research methodology to investigate the impact of storytelling during a one-semester course on nutrition through the life cyle. During each class period, either the students or the instructor had the opportunity to tell a story related to the course material. During the final class period, students were invited to complete a 28-item survey that included both closed and open-ended questions. Fifteen students completed the survey. Results indicated that the students valued the storytelling aspect of the course and believed that the stories helped them make connections between the course material and 'real life'. The stories helped them to talk about the emotional aspects of dietetic practice and enhanced their reflective abilities.

Service-learning is a learning strategy that gives students the opportunity to combine meaningful community service with reflection to assist then in developing team and interpersonal skills. Horacek et al.[25] published an article describing the development of an interprofessional learning community that involved students from nursing, dietetics, social work, and child and family studies. The learning community was designed as a 3-credit-hour course and included an interdisciplinary service-learning component and the opportunity for reflective journaling. Students (N = 41) were asked to evaluate the course using an anonymous self-assessment survey which was primarily designed to assess students' understanding of their cultural and communication competence as a result of taking the course. It was concluded that the service-learning experiences helped students to assess their cultural competence more accurately and to recognise that they were not as open-minded as they initially thought they were. In addition, students thought that the experience contributed towards their professional development and helped them to develop the ability to understand and solve problems using a 'wider, multidisciplinary lens'.[25(p14)]

CAI and online learning technologies appear to have been used in dietetics education since the mid 1990s. In 1995, Raidl et al.[26] conducted a study to determine whether or not CAI was useful in helping dietetic students develop clinical reasoning skills. They developed three computer-assisted tutorial programmes for use in their diet therapy course: (1) a tutorial programme designed to teach critical reasoning skills using a cardiovascular disease case study; (2) a drill and practice programme that consisted of questions about the cardiovascular system from a textbook; and (3) a simulation test programme that was designed to evaluate students' use of the clinical reasoning skills they learned in the tutorial programme. Students were first given a lecture on cardiovascular disease and then randomly assigned to one of three groups: group one used the drill and practice programme followed by the simulation test programme; group two used the tutorial programme followed by the simulation test programme; group three was given only the simulation test programme (no CAI). Results showed that the students who did the tutorial programme had much higher scores on the simulation test than the other students. Thus it was concluded that the use of a CAI programme enhanced clinical reasoning skills, possibly due to the opportunity for students to actively apply their learning.

In 2002, Litchfield et al.[27] used a key features exam to evaluate the development of clinical competency in an online instruction programme (e.g. critical thinking, ability to work cooperatively and communicate effectively). A key features exam is made up of clinical case scenarios. Students are then asked questions that focus only on those elements that are considered crucial to resolving the case. Three classes of dietetic students (N = 75) were divided into two groups (those with and those without online instruction) and then asked to complete 'pre- then post-test' key features exams. Their results indicated that those students who had completed the online instruction module had significantly greater improvement on the key features exams in nutrition support and pediatric nutrition but not on the renal key features exam. These researchers concluded that the online technology resulted in a gain of critical thinking skills and clinical competency but acknowledged that competency is very complex and difficult to assess.

More recently, Herriot et al.[28] developed a CD-ROM to help students develop the skills needed to conduct a nutritional assessment and develop a nutrition care plan in a simulated environment. They then conducted a mixed methods study (questionnaires and focus groups) to evaluate its effectiveness as a teaching tool. All second-year dietetic students (N = 34) and seven final-year students participated in the study as part of their undergraduate degree programme. Students rated the programme design and content very highly and most believed that it helped to prepare them for practice, but only 24% of them preferred using the programme to traditional lectures.

Their preference was to use the CD-ROM in combination with traditional lectures rather than as a standalone learning tool. Advantages identified included flexibility, variety and interactivity, and content (opportunity to observe a dietetic interview and comprehensive insight into the interview process). Disadvantages included technical problems, access, content (final-year students were concerned that second-year students may assume the dietetic interview shown was the 'set way' of performing a dietetic consultation, and instruction method – lack of tutor support). Again, there were limitations with this study. There was no control group, the questionnaire was not tested for construct validity and it was not possible to determine if students were able to transfer the skills learned into practice.[28]

ASSESSMENT OF KNOWLEDGE AND SKILL DEVELOPMENT

Once competency standards have been set, curricula developed and teaching and learning strategies have been identified, it is important to develop assessment tools to evaluate the learning outcomes. How are these assessment tools developed and what evidence do we have that they are effective in assessing knowledge and skill development in dietetics?

Pender and de Looy[29] conducted a study to define the key clinical skills necessary for a competent dietetic student practitioner and to devise a reliable assessment tool to measure and track performance in these key skill areas throughout the period of clinical placement. A group of dietetic educators in Scotland, in collaboration with academic colleagues, agreed on the key skill areas deemed by the group to be fundamental to the student practitioner and then developed criteria (tools) against which the student performing skills during clinical placement could be measured or assessed. They identified four core skills: (1) writing, (2) interviewing, (3) skills associated with dietary assessment technique and (4) oral and presentation skills.

Each of these four key skills was further divided into constituent skill performance components; each of these elements could then be measured independently. The tools were pretested in 10 student observations conducted by experienced dietitians prior to the study. The pretested tools were then used by 27 experienced practitioners to record observation of skill performance of 43 student dietitians undertaking the period of 31 weeks' clinical placement during the study period in eight participating centres. Assessment of performance of skills was measured using a visual analogue scale, consisting of a horizontal line of known length (100 mm) with a brief text description at the 0 and 100 mm anchor points. The 50 mm point was taken to represent adequate skill performance; the 100 mm point was taken to represent optimal skill acquisition and performance. Observers were asked to mark the scale at the point which best described skill performance. The visual analogue scale score data for each of the individual component skills were correlated with length of training. In other words, as the training progressed, students' performance improved. Most students achieved a high level of attainment at just over halfway through the training. The assessment tool was considered easy to use, to be valid and appears to be independent of observer bias or error (it is not clear how they assessed validity).[29]In the United Kingdom, all dietetic students are required to develop a portfolio as a means of collecting evidence demonstrating competency achievement. However, the tools used for assessment can differ between placement sites and thus concerns have been raised about the reliability of this method of assessment. Brennan and Lennie[30] conducted an online survey with dietetic students (N = 114) to determine their perceptions and experiences of the use of the portfolio in assessment of practice placements. Most students believed that the portfolio helped them monitor their strengths and weaknesses and agreed that the portfolio was a valuable learning experience. However, they were concerned about the amount of paperwork involved and felt that there were inconsistencies in the assessment of the portfolios by different supervisors. Volders *et al.*[31] also found that dietetic students believe that portfolios are useful in tracking skill development and facilitating regular feedback opportunities. They conducted a study designed to describe the use and evaluation of a clinical teaching and learning portfolio in a nutrition and dietetics programme in Australia and concluded that the portfolio is a valuable assessment tool for clinical placements. However, it must be noted that this study only evaluated the use of portfolios in one placement. Thus, the inconsistencies in assessments between placements were not an issue for them.

In 2010, Lennie and Juwah[32] conducted an online survey with 111 dietitian preceptors and follow-up interviews with 14 dietetic departments to determine the assessment methods being used in dietetic practice placements in the United Kingdom. They found that the median number of assessment tools being used by these departments was eight. Assessment activities included observation, reflection, presentations, projects and case studies. These authors concluded that it is important to standardise assessment processes and tools and to provide adequate training for preceptors to ensure consistency between placements as well as ensure a benchmark of competence throughout the country.

Objective structured clinical examinations (OSCEs) have been used by many health professions to test the development of skills. In 2004, Pender and de Looy[33] conducted a study to identify the key clinical skills needed by student dietitians and then developed an OSCE to assess students' performance of those skills. A project team consisting of six experienced dietitians from the fields of education and practice met to agree upon the key skills needed by students about to enter clinical placements and to discuss and agree how these identified skills would be tested. Four skills were identified as being required for good clinical practice: (1) discriminatory, (2) communication, (3) interpretation and (4) food knowledge. Each skill was examined at a testing station that involved an activity designed to test the skill. A pilot study on the OSCE, including the organisation of stations, the sensitivity and use of test materials, and the impact on student behaviour was completed prior to the main study with eight senior students. The OSCE was then delivered to 37 preclinical students. Four of the test candidates failed in at least one of the skills areas. These students also performed poorly during their clinical placements. Just over half (57%) of students returned the post-OSCE questionnaires. Of these students, 95% reported a positive experience and that initial anxiety diminished as the test progressed.[33]

Lambert *et al.*[34] investigated dietetic skills to determine which ones can be assessed by different activities in a dietetic OSCE and identified which tasks students perform better. The study also explored whether the design of activities, in particular the time allowed for each activity, was influential in students' performance. An OSCE made up of six activities or stations was designed to test students' key clinical dietetic skills at the end of their second year of academic studies. Two activities were 'active' using standardised patients to test communication skills, as well as either 'discriminatory skills' or 'interpretation and food knowledge skills'. The other four activities made up the 'passive stations', which tested students' knowledge and practical skills. Resource requirements to examine 35 students in 1 day were substantial (four academic examiners, four clinical examiners, four actors, two invigilators, one OSCE coordinator, one independent assessor and an individual responsible for timing the whole process). The proposed activities for each station were piloted and reviewed by a group of four qualified dietitians and changes were made to the approach, actors scripts, instructions, and structured marking tools as necessary. To ensure objectivity and inter-assessor reliability at the active stations, a clinical examiner marked the activity on a structured marking tool and an academic examiner validated the marks awarded. An independent objective observer also ensured that, where duplicate stations were run, there was equality of student experience. Immediately after the OSCE, students voluntarily completed a questionnaire to assess their opinions regarding the adequacy of preparation, design, timing, environment, facilities, resources and the instructions for both active and passive stations of the OSCE.

The best performing OSCE stations for students were the active stations with actors, which demonstrated an appropriate level of communication and consultation skills for this stage of training. The station at which students performed least well involved knowledge of portion sizes and carbohydrate content of specific foods. Students responded positively to the OSCE; negative comments related to the length of time allotted to stations. The researchers concluded that OSCEs are an effective form of assessment for key clinical and practical skills but the design of the activities is time consuming and requires careful development to ensure reliability and validity.[34] Objectivity is critical to this form of assessment and can be both a strength (e.g. by ensuring reliability) and a weakness (e.g. by not recognising the way the activity was performed).

Hawker *et al.*[35] described the use of a preclinical OSCE for the assessment of clinical skills in undergraduate dietetic students. Students (N = 193) completed the OSCE at the end of their third year of a 4-year programme, just prior to doing their first clinical placement. Results indicated that there was a strong relationship between the OSCE scores and students' scores at the end of their clinical placements. These authors recommended the use of an OSCE as a method of formative assessment to identify students who are likely to do less well in the first clinical placement so that supports can be put into place earlier.

Communication skills are critical for dietitians and underpin all areas of practice. However, there is limited research into students' attitudes towards learning such skills or how best to teach these skills. Power and Lennie[36] conducted a cross-sectional study to identify dietetic students' attitudes towards learning communication skills. An online questionnaire was sent to all undergraduate and postgraduate dietetic education programmes in the United Kingdom. Three hundred students responded (33% response rate). Their findings indicated that students had positive attitudes towards learning communication skills; however, enthusiasm diminished as they progressed in their studies. First-year students were significantly more positive than fourth-year students. Given the importance of good communication skills in dietetic practice, this finding is of concern. It may reflect a lack of emphasis on communication in the curriculum or possibly students felt that they had already learned how to communicate by fourth year and therefore did not see the importance of lifelong learning and practice.

Finally, Vickery *et al.*[37] conducted a study to evaluate the effectiveness of a nutrition counselling course by comparing the counselling skills of students who took the course (which included mock counselling sessions) with students who had practice opportunities but no formal education. They found that while students in both groups demonstrated respect for their clients, those who had taken the course used more effective counselling strategies and performed significantly better than those students who had not taken the course. Students with 'practice only' experience modelled their counselling behaviours after their preceptors who may or may not have had adequate training themselves. Thus, it was concluded that a mix of counselling theory and practice is necessary for skill development. This study also raises a concern about the type of experience students receive during their practicum. If preceptors are not adequately trained themselves, then students are at risk of learning how to do something that is 'wrong'.

CONCLUSION

Dietetics has come a long way since the early days of the profession but it is clear from this overview of the evidence underpinning dietetic education that we still have a long way to go. We have been relying too heavily on expert opinion and data from other health professions and have not encouraged research in dietetic pedagogy. This is interesting given the recent emphasis on evidence-based practice in dietetics. This has to change if we are to meet future needs. In a recent article in the *Journal of the American Dietetic Association*, Boyce[38] challenged dietitians to look beyond traditional classroom-based education and consider different routes to registration and credentialing with the goal of preparing dietitians for several different careers during their lifetimes. This has to change if we are to meet future needs. What are the best practices in dietetic education that would allow the profession to achieve this goal? The answer to that question is largely unknown at the present time. Hopefully, this review will prompt dietetic educators to take action in this area, to build on the evidence presented and raise the status of the scholarship of teaching and learning in dietetics.

KEY AREAS FOR FUTURE RESEARCH

It is obvious from this review that there are many gaps in the area of evidence-based education in dietetics and nutrition. Key areas for future research should include:

- more systematic exploration of the competencies required by dietitians
- alternatives to traditional classroom-based education
- different pathways to registration and credentialing
- more learning outcome-based research
- an exploration of the use of arts-based activities in dietetic education to enhance critical thinking skills
- an exploration of the need for specialised training and how that should be accomplished
- the definition of entry-level competency and how it should be achieved (There are several questions that could be explored in this area: Who decides what type of bachelor's degree is required to become a dietitian? How is the practicum experience developed? How long does the practicum experience have to be in order to ensure students achieve entry-level competency? What types of experiences do students have to be exposed to during those practicum experiences? Should the practicum experience be integrated with the academic experience or is it better to separate the two?)

SUMMARY POINTS

- Dietetic education typically involves two phases: knowledge acquisition and skills development.
- The current research evidence related to dietetic education is limited by small sample sizes, single time points and, in most cases, voluntary participation; however, it does provide some useful insights into best practices in dietetic education.
- There is a variety of strategies used to teach dietetic students, and there is a variety of assessment methods being used to evaluate knowledge and skill development.
- Dietetic education is heavily reliant on expert opinion, and students' preferences and perspectives of what is done in dietetic education is not grounded in evidence.

REVIEW QUESTIONS

- What will the education needs of dietitians in the future be?
- How do we decide what is included in dietetic education?
- What evidence do we have that dietetic education and training is effective in preparing students for practice?
- What is the best way to educate students to prepare them for the complex realities of dietetic practice?
- Are we preparing students for a profession or training them for a career?

REFLECTIVE QUESTIONS AND EXERCISES

- Dietitians have traditionally been trained in a positivist tradition to consider food as a source of nutrients and to seek the 'right' way to eat. Thus, we are often referred to as the 'food police'. Our clients expect to be told what they can and cannot eat when they come to see us. What needs to happen in the education and training of dietetic students to dispel this notion?
- The social context of nutritional health is often ignored by dietitians, who are trained to focus on the science of nutrition. How can we engage dietetic students in ways that help them to understand the social and cultural contexts of the work that they will be doing?

REFERENCES

1. International Confederation of Dietetic Associations (ICDA). *Dietitians Around the World: their education and their work*. Toronto, ON: ICDA; 2008.
2. Soerensen MA; International Confederation of Dietetic Associations (ICDA). *The Education and Work of Dietitians (2004)*. Toronto, ON: ICDA; 2004.
3. Gingras J. The educational (im)possibility for dietetics: a poststructural discourse analysis. *Learn Inq*. 2009; **3**(3): 177–91.
4. Ash S, Phillips S. What is dietetic competence? Competency standards, competence and competency explained. *Aust J Nutr Diet*. 2000; **57**(3): 147–51.
5. Litchfield RE, Oakland MJ, Anderson J. Promoting and evaluating competence in on-line dietetics education. *J Am Diet Assoc*. 2002; **102**(10): 1455–8.
6. Ash S, Dowding K, Phillips S. Mixed methods research approach to the development and review of competency standards for dietitians. *Nutr Diet*. 2011; **68**(4): 305–15.
7. Phillips S, Ash S, Tapsell L. Relevance of the competency standards to entry level dietetic practice. *Aust J Nutr Diet*. 2000; **57**(4): 198–207.
8. Cant R, Aroni RA. Validation of performance criteria for Australian dietitians' competence in education of individual clients. *Nutr Diet*. 2009; **66**(1): 47–53.
9. Shafer KJ, Knous BL. A longitudinal study of cognitive and affective behaviour in a didactic program in dietetics: implications for dietetic education. *J Am Diet Assoc*. 2001; **101**(9): 1051–4.
10. Palermo C, Walker KZ, Brown T, *et al*. How dietetics students like to learn: implications for curriculum planners. *Nutr Diet*. 2009; **66**(2): 108–12.
11. Lordly DJ, Travers KD. Dietetic internship: evaluation of an integrated model. *Can J Diet Pract Res*. 1998; **59**(4): 199–207.
12. Knoblock-Hahn AL, Scharff DP, Michael E. Cultural competence in dietecs education: Where are we now and where do we need to go? *Topics in Clinical Nutrition*. 2010; **25**: 323–34.
13. Vickery CE, Cotugna N. Complementary and alternative medicine education in dietetics programs: eExistent but not consistent. *J Am Diet Assoc*. 2006; **106**(6): 860–6.
14. Thompson PY. Trends in training for nutritionists and dietitians in the Caribbean. *Nutr Diet*. 2012; **69**(3): 226–30.
15. Hughes R, Desbrow B. An evaluation of clinical dietetic student placement case-mix exposure, service delivery and supervisory burden. *Nutr Diet*. 2010; **67**(4): 287–93.
16. Taylor EL, Hasseberg CM, Anderson MA, *et al*. Dietetic preceptor educational needs from the preceptor, student, and faculty perspectives. *J Allied Health*. 2010; **39**(4): 287–92.
17. ChanLin L-J, Chan K-C. PBL approach in web-based instruction. *J Instr Psychol*. 2004; **31**(2): 98–105.
18. ChanLin L-J, Chan K-C. Assessment of PBL design approach in a dietetic web-based instruction. *J Educ Comput Res*. 2004; **31**(4): 437–52.
19. ChanLin L-J, Chan K-C. Integrating inter-disciplinary experts for supporting problem-based learning. *Innov Educ Teach Int*. 2007; **44**(2): 211–24.
20. Roberts CM, Sucher K, Perrin DG, *et al*. Concept mapping: an effective instructional method for diet therapy. *J Am Diet Assoc*. 1995; **95**(8): 908–11.
21. Molaison EF, Taylor KA, Erickson D, *et al*. The use and perceptions of concept mapping as a learning tool by dietetic internship students and preceptors. *J Allied Health*. 2009; **38**(3): e97–103.
22. Nahikian-Nelms ML, Nelms RG. Use of double-entry journals in a required dietetic course: encouraging critical thinking skills. *J Nutr Educ*. 1994; **26**(2): 93–6.
23. Brady JL, Gingras JR. Dietetics students' experiences and perspectives of storytelling to enhance food and nutrition practice. *Transformative Dialogues: Teach Learn J*. 2012; **6**(1): 1–12.
24. Lordly D. Once upon a time …. Storytelling to enhance teaching and learning. *Can J Diet Pract Res*. 2007; **68**(1): 30–5.

25. Horacek T, Brann L, Erdman M, *et al*. Interprofessional learning community: educating dietetic and other health profession students through an interdisciplinary, service-learning experience. *Topics Clin Nutr*. 2009; **24**(1): 6–15.

26. Raidl MA, Wood OB, Lehman JD, *et al*. Computer-assisted instruction improves clinical reasoning skills of dietetics students. *J Am Diet Assoc*. 1995; **95**(8): 868–73.

27. Litchfield RE, Oakland MJ, Anderson JA. Relationships between intern characteristics, computer attitudes, and use of online instruction in a dietetic training program. *Am J Dist Educ*. 2002; **16**(1): 22–36.

28. Herriot AM, Bishop JA, Truby H. The development and evaluation of Student Training, Education and Practice for Dietetics CD-ROM: a computer-assisted instruction programme for dietetic students. *J Hum Nutr Diet*. 2004; **17**(1): 35–41.

29. Pender FT, de Looy AE. Monitoring the development of clinical skills during training in a clinical placement. *J Hum Nutr Diet*. 2004; **17**(1): 25–34.

30. Brennan KM, Lennie SC. Students' experiences and perceptions of the use of portfolios in UK preregistration dietetic placements: a questionnaire-based study. *J Hum Nutr Diet*. 2010; **23**(2): 133–43.

31. Volders E, Tweedie J, Anderson A. Advancements in nutrition and dietetics teaching and learning: Evaluating the student portfolio. *Nutr Diet*. 2010; **67**(2): 112–16.

32. Lennie SC, Juwah C. Exploring assessment for learning during dietetic practice placements. *J Hum Nutr Diet*. 2010; **23**(3): 217–23.

33. Pender FT, de Looy AE. The testing of clinical skills in dietetic students prior to entering clinical placement. *J Hum Nutr Diet*. 2004; **17**(1): 17–24.

34. Lambert L, Pattison DJ, de Looy AE. Dietetic students' performance of activities in an objective structured clinical examination. *J Hum Nutr Diet*. 2010; **23**(3): 224–9.

35. Hawker JA, Walker KZ, Barrington V, *et al*. Measuring the success of an objective structured clinical examination for dietetic students. *J Hum Nutr Diet*. 2010; **23**(3): 212–16.

36. Power BT, Lennie SC. Pre-registration dietetic students' attitudes to learning communication skills. *J Hum Nutr Diet*. 2012; **25**(2): 189–97.

37. Vickery CE, Cotugna N, Hodges PAM. Comparing counseling skills of dietetics students: a model for skill enhancement. *J Am Diet Assoc*. 1995; **95**(8): 912–14.

38. Boyce B. Future connections summit on dietetics practice, credentialing, and education: summary of presentations on shaping the future of the dietetics profession. *J Am Diet Assoc*. 2011; **111**(10): 1591–9.

CHAPTER 35

Summary, recommendations for future activities and conclusion

....

Ted Brown and Brett Williams

Evidence-based medicine (EBM) introduced a new paradigm within healthcare practice. Several derivations of EBM have emerged since Sackett *et al.*[1] initially coined the term, including evidence-based nursing, evidence-based healthcare and evidence-based practice (EBP). EBP is currently the most commonly used term within the allied healthcare professions when referring to clinical practice based on valid, rigorous empirical evidence. Since the vast majority of healthcare curricula include units of study focused on EBP principles and applications to clinical practice, it leads to the notion that the educational methods being used to promote the learning and teaching of this body of knowledge should also be based on sound empirical evidence. In other words, the approaches and methods being used to educate future healthcare practitioners should be grounded in sound, reliable, empirically based evidence. However, while the EBP and EBM drum is being beaten with increasing fervour, it appears that less attention, less funding and fewer resources are devoted to the evidence-based education (EBE) of future healthcare practitioners. Furthermore, to add to these issues, these challenges are non-discriminate, being faced across different education sectors and educational providers. Despite this, however, there is a growing number of articulate, skilled and productive health professional educational researchers (many of whom are authors within this text) who are actively contributing to the growing body of evidence in this arena.

Sacket *et al.*[1] stated that EBM is based on the integration of clinical expertise, patient values and the best evidence available when making decisions about the care and treatment of patients. If the framework outlined by Sackett *et al.*[1] was generalised to the EBE of health professional students, then it would involve (a) academic and fieldwork educators' knowledge and expertise, (b) health professional students' values and perceptions and (c) the health professional education scholarship of learning and teaching (SoLT) best evidence available.[2,3] This definition fits with the three key components that Ginsberg and colleagues[4] propose make up EBE: (1) SoLT,

(2) pedagogical content knowledge and (3) teacher–learner interaction. This suggests that the way that EBM and EBP ensure the best quality care for patients and families underpinned by best healthcare evidence, also implies that health professional students should be the 'clients' who receive innovative, contemporary, relevant learning and teaching experiences based on best education evidence.

The intent of this edited book was to bring together a range of expertise in EBE related to health professional education; contemporary educational approaches and methods that have at least a starting level of emerging evidence; best practice examples in the SoLT; and health discipline-specific summaries and systematic reviews of educational research. From this emerge a number of recommendations and suggestions to assist moving the health professional EBE agenda forward internationally. This agenda will provide the opportunity for developing a blueprint or road map for the following: individual healthcare practitioners; health practitioner professional associations; health practitioner regulatory bodies; universities and colleges that offer health professional education programmes; health professional educators and researchers; agencies that accredit health professional education programmes; practice education providers; state or provincial and federal governments; research funding agencies; and publishers of scholarly journals.

To promote EBE, individual health practitioners can:

- acknowledge the importance and significance of EBE principles as well as EBP standards in their daily clinical and professional practice
- attend, engage with and support EBE initiatives at local, state, national and international conferences
- ensure that any continuing professional development (CPD) events they attend are based on sound EBE principles and findings
- question organisers and presenters at CPD sessions about what EBE principles they are using
- use instructional methods with students completing fieldwork and practice education placements that are underpinned by EBE
- contribute to or be involved with quality assurance, programme evaluation or research initiatives linked to EBE.

To foster EBE, health practitioner professional associations can:

- generate a position statement about the principles of EBE and its importance, both for entry-level student education and for the education of clients and families that practitioners provide services for
- encourage health professional university and college education programmes to base their curricula, instrumental methods, modes and assessment approaches on valid and reliable EBE principles
- ensure that conferences sponsored by the association have an EBE stream where educationalists, researchers, policymakers and fieldwork providers can present their findings
- provide seed funding for projects related to EBE of entry-level students, practitioners and clients.

To facilitate EBE, health practitioner regulatory bodies can:
- ensure that policies designed to regulate the scope of practice, clinical roles and professional behaviour of health practitioners include a section on basing education-related activities on the SoLT findings
- require that CPD activities that practitioners attend, and which count towards CPD requirements (e.g. points or hours) mandated by regulatory bodies, are based on EBE principles and findings.

To uphold EBE and SoLT programmes, universities and colleges that offer health professional education programmes can:
- include dedicated units or courses that focus on EBP principles and also demonstrate how these principles can be extended to educational activities, particularly those related to patient and family education
- promote health professional students to be critical, independent thinkers and also expect their learning experiences to be based on sound, critical SoLT evidence
- ensure that health education programmes abide by the requirements specified in the professional accreditation guidelines related to implementing their curriculum
- provide teaching and learning awards for academic staff who demonstrate an aptitude for EBE and SoLT initiatives
- embed EBE and SoLT activities in annual performance appraisals of health professional academic, research and education-focused staff
- offer small competitive grants that health professional academic, research and education-focused staff who wish to complete EBE research projects can apply for
- provide more dedicated research funding and resourcing of EBE initiatives
- better coordinate efforts, funding and resources between individual health professions, departments, faculties and institutions towards EBE activities
- provide master's and PhD scholarships available to health professional students who wish to pursue EBE- and SoLT-related topics
- have postdoctoral fellowships available for early-career researchers in the area of health professional EBE.

To encourage EBE activities, individual health professional education departments located in universities and colleges can:
- instil a culture of EBE within the respective health professional departments, schools and faculties
- reward staff who demonstrate SoLT initiatives as part of their role as health professional educators
- create consortiums or collaborations to move their EBE agendas forwards by the pooling of resources, funding and expertise between health professional education programmes in the same discipline from different universities
- provide teaching and learning awards for health professional academic staff who engage in EBE and SoLT projects
- embed EBE activities in annual performance appraisals of health professional academic staff.

To promote EBE schemes, individual health professional educators and researchers can:

- make it known to health professional students that the learning and teaching approaches they are utilising are based on sound SoLT principles
- undertake research about the SoLT activities, thus making a contribution to the health professional EBE body of knowledge
- ensure the teaching and learning methods used are evidence-based
- collaborate with other health professional educations and researchers on education-related research
- write up and submit EBE research findings to peer-reviewed journals, e.g. BEME reviews
- serve on the editorial boards and peer-review submissions for journals that publish EBE research-related manuscripts
- organise a health professional EBE symposium or colloquium at the university or college where they work
- present at national or international professional conferences to raise the awareness of health professional EBE-related research
- attend and/or present at EBE-specific conferences and symposiums
- involve honours, master's and doctoral students in health professional education SoLT research and EBE activities
- have mentoring opportunities between experienced health professional education researchers and early career education researchers.

To facilitate EBE, agencies that accredit health professional education programmes can:

- ensure that health professional education programmes that are being initially accredited or are applying for re-accreditation provide evidence of EBE activities
- specify one of the accreditation points is that units and courses taught to health professional students must be based on best evidence principles and that evidence of this must be provided by the applicants.

To enable EBE for health professional practice education, fieldwork education providers can:

- ensure that methods used to instruct health professional students completing practice education or fieldwork placements are based on sound SoLT evidence
- encourage health professional students to use best SoLT evidence principles when providing education and training sessions for patients and their families
- collaborate with university-based educators and researchers in health professional EBE initiatives.

To assist health professional EBE, state or provincial and federal governments:

- provide funding for universities and colleges for health professional EBE initiatives
- ensure that it is mandated by government policy that health professional students

arc the recipients of teaching and learning strategies that are based on best SoLT evidence

● effective and appropriate dissemination strategies are provided.

To aid EBE activities, research funding agencies can:
● provide education-specific funding for research projects related to the SoLT of health professional students
● have master's and PhD scholarships available to health professional students who wish to pursue EBE-related topics
● have postdoctoral fellowships available for early-career researchers in the area of health professional EBE.

To distribute and promote the update of EBE findings, publishers and editors of scholarly journals can:
● create more peer-reviewed journals dedicated to publishing quality manuscripts based on EBE topics including health professional EBE
● publish special issues of already existing health professional discipline-specific journals dedicated to EBE
● provide opportunities for open access to high-quality health professional SoLT evidence.

In conclusion, the education of future health professional students is an important and essential activity. It ensures that we have adequate numbers of health practitioners to provide care and services to clients and their families in times of need. It is imperative that the teaching and learning methods used to educate the next generation of health-care professionals is based on best evidence. In other words, we need to ensure that adequate resources, time, funding and attention that are applied to EBP enterprises are also available for EBE projects. Both healthcare and higher education funding have limited resources; therefore, we need to ensure the services provided are efficient and effective. EBP and EBE are one way to ensure that all activities, both client or patient care and student education, are based on the best empirical evidence available.

REFERENCES

1. Sackett DL, Straus SE, Richardson WS, *et al. Evidence-Based Medicine: how to practice and teach EBM.* 2nd ed. London: Churchill Livingstone; 2000.
2. Boet S, Sharma S, Goldman J, *et al.* Medical education research: an overview of methods. *Can J Anaesth.* 2012; **59**(2): 159–70.
3. Greenhalgh T, Macfarlane F, Plumb L, *et al.* Transferability of principles of evidence based medicine to improve educational quality: systematic review and case study of an online course in primary health care. *BMJ.* 2003; **326**(7381): 142–5.
4. Ginsberg SM, Friberg J, Visconti C. *Scholarship of Teaching and Learning in Speech-Language Pathology and Audiology: evidence-based education.* San Diego, CA: Plural Publishing; 2012.

Index

Entries in **bold** refer to tables and boxes; entries in *italics* refer to figures.

CPD with Radcliffe

You can now use a selection of our books to achieve CPD (Continuing Professional Development) points through directed reading.

We provide a free online form and downloadable certificate for your appraisal portfolio. Look for the CPD logo and register with us at: www.radcliffehealth.com/cpd

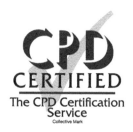

T - #0062 - 090625 - C0 - 246/171/30 - PB - 9781909368712 - Gloss Lamination